Recent Advances in Cardiovascular Medicine

Incorporating Ocular-based Artificial intelligence for systemic diseases and 3D printing technologies

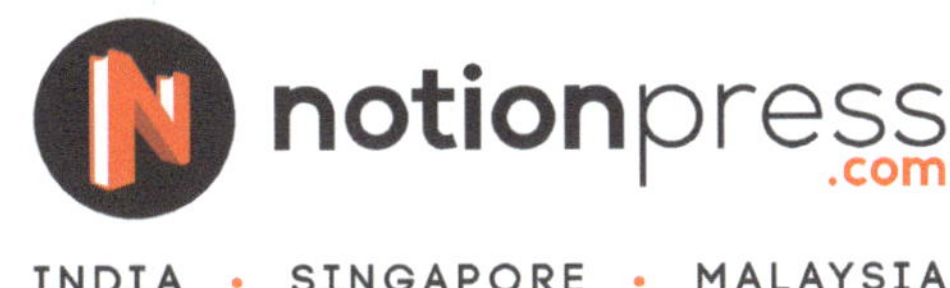

ISBN
Paperback 979-8-89066-980-3
Hardcase 979-8-89066-994-0

Recent Advances in Cardiovascular Medicine

Incorporating Ocular-based Artificial intelligence for systemic diseases and 3D printing technologies

Prof. (Dr.) K. C. VERMA
MBBS, DCH, MD, DM (CARDIOLOGY) FICP (USA),
FRSTM & H (Lond), FCSI (India)
Senior Consulting Heart Specialist and Formerly
Prof. in Cardiovascular and Thoracic Unit
Govt. Medical College, Jammu (J&K)

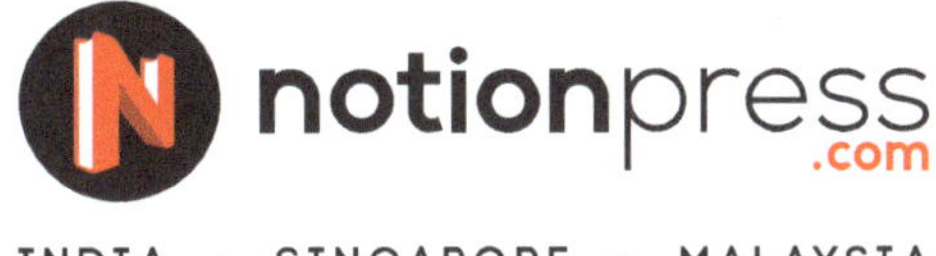

INDIA • SINGAPORE • MALAYSIA

ACKNOWLEDGEMENT

I am indebted to the various scientific workers and research scholars whose names have been mentioned in respective chapter of bibliography and whose basic work became the foundation of each chapter of this book.

I am also very grateful to my wife Dr (Mrs) Urmil Kanta Verma, formerly Prof. in the department of blood transfusion medicine and pathology for providing me a perfect congenial atmosphere and all material and moral support needed for writing such a voluminous book **"Recent Advances In Cardiovascular Medicine"**

To my grand children, Advita, Sidhant Leena, Meera and Deven.

(Author)

FOREWORD

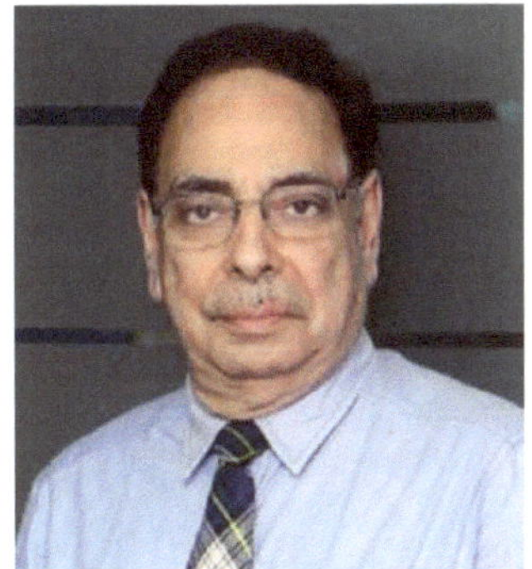

Dr KC Verma an eminent cardiologist practising in Jammu (J&K) has done a commendable job in writing a book ***"Recent advances in cardiovascular medicine*** "The book is an exhaustive work covering all aspects of the current management.. It gives details of entire subject on the various innovations which have taken place over the past a few years ,particularily on impotant topics on ***Artificial Intelligence and 3D printing*** .A brief description regarding newer drug therapies in hypertension, chronic heart failure,Anticoagulants in post coronary intervensions and noval antiplatelet drugs in the prevention of atherosclerosis.have been outlined.

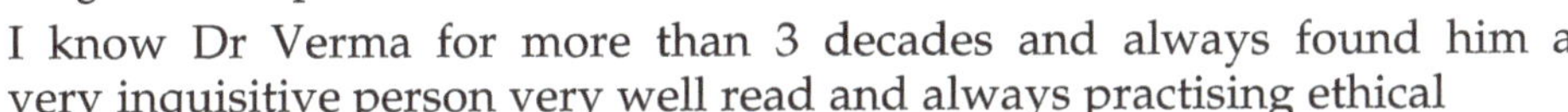

I know Dr Verma for more than 3 decades and always found him a very inquisitive person very well read and always practising ethical medicine. He has been an excellent teacher for his younger colleagues.The book should be of a great help to the practising cardiologists/Reserch scholars /cardiac fellows /cardiology residents and DM cardiology scholars in revising and refreshing their already acquired knowledge . it would ,therefore,have a greater repurcussion in managing their patient with current techniques with mjnjmal cost and least morbidity and mortality.

I recommend this very well written book for all the busy physicians and cardiologists who want evidence based guidance for treating their patients.

Prof. Upendra Kaul

MD DM FCSI FSCAI FAPSIC FACC FAMS

Awarded Padmashiri and Dr BC Roy Award
Chairman Batra Heart Centre,
Dean
Academics and Research, Batra Hospital and Medical Research Centre, New Delhi

Dedication

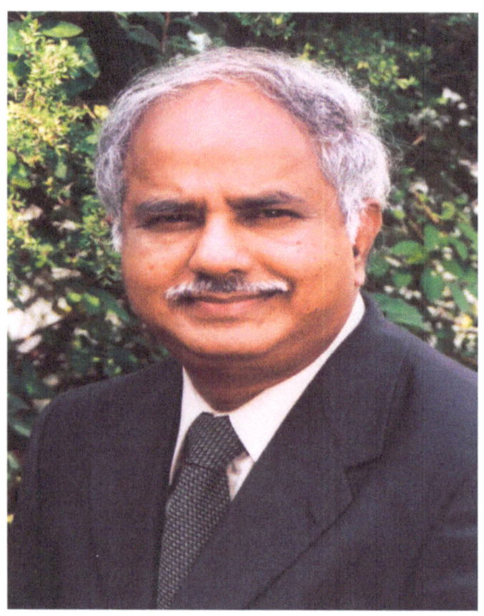

Dr.Dabbala Rajagopal "Raj" Reddy

Dabbala Rajagopal "Raj" Reddy (born 13 June 1937) is an Indian-born American computer scientist and a winner of the Turing Award. He is one of the early pioneers of artificial intelligence and has served on the faculty of Stanford and Carnegie Mellon for over 50 years. He was the founding director of the Robotics Institute at Carnegie Mellon University. He was instrumental in helping to create Rajiv Gandhi University of Knowledge Technologies in India, to cater to the educational needs of the low-income, gifted, rural youth. He is the chairman of International Institute of Information Technology, Hyderabad. He is the first person of Asian origin to receive the Turing Award, in 1994, known as the Nobel Prize of Computer Science, for his work in the field of artificial intelligence.

Reddy is the University Professor of Computer Science and Robotics and Moza Bint Nasser Chair at the School of Computer Science at Carnegie Mellon University. From 1960, he worked for IBM in Australia.He was an Assistant Professor of Computer Science at Stanford University from 1966 to 1969. He joined the Carnegie Mellon faculty as an associate professor of Computer Science in 1969. He became a full professor in 1973 and a university professor, in 1984.

Artificial Intelligence Research

Reddy's early research was conducted at the AI labs at Stanford, first as a graduate student and later as an assistant professor, and at CMU since 1969.His AI research concentrated on perceptual and motor aspect of intelligence such as speech, language, vision and robotics. Over a span of five decades, Reddy and his colleagues created several historic demonstrations of spoken language systems, e.g., voice control of a robot,large vocabulary connected speech recognition, speaker independent speech recognition, and unrestricted vocabulary dictation.Reddy and his colleagues have made seminal contributions to Task Oriented Computer Architectures, Analysis of Natural Scenes,Universal Access to Information, and Autonomous Robotic Systems.Hearsay I was one of the first systems capable of continuous speech recognition. Subsequent systems like Hearsay II, Dragon, Harpy, and Sphinx I/II developed many of the ideas underlying modern commercial speech recognition technology as summarized in his recent historical review of speech recognition with Xuedong Huang and James K. Baker. Some of these ideas—most notably the "blackboard model" for coordinating multiple knowledge sources—have been adopted across the spectrum of applied artificial intelligence

Awards and honors

He is a fellow of the AAAI, ACM, Acoustical Society of America, IEEE[and Computer History Museum.. Reddy is a member of the United States National Academy of Engineering, American Academy of Arts and Sciences, Chinese Academy of Engineering, Indian National Science Academy, and Indian National Academy of Engineering. He has been awarded honorary doctorates (Doctor Honoris Causa) from SV University, Universite Henri-Poincare, University of New South Wales, Jawaharlal Nehru Technological University, University of Massachusetts, University of Warwick, Anna University, IIIT (Allahabad), Andhra University, IIT Kharagpur, Hong Kong University of Science and Technology, Rajiv Gandhi University of Knowledge Technologies, and Carnegie Mellon University.\ In 1994 he and Edward Feigenbaum received the Turing Award, "for pioneering the design and construction of large scale artificial intelligence systems, demonstrating the practical importance and potential commercial impact of artificial intelligence technology."In 1984, Reddy was awarded the French Legion of Honour by French President François Mitterrand. Reddy also received Padma Bhushan, from the President of India in 2001,the Okawa Prize in 2004, the Honda Prize in 2005, and the Vannevar Bush Award in 2006

(Dr K C VERMA MD DM)

Preface

Science and technology are constantly changing fields. New research and experience broaden the scope of information and knowledge. Over the past few years ,numerous innovations have been taken place and it was a herculeous task to choose a few of them (list of chapters in the content section of this book) to make the foundation of this book**"Recent advances in cardiovascular medicine"**

Conventionally,the diagnosis of cardiovascular disease is made by obtaining routine 12-leads ECG, Echocardiography and cardiovascular CT technology.Even among these technologies ,newer innovations have been taken place such as new 80-lead ECG system,which helps to detect silent myocardial Infarct, Heart Sciences MyoVista ECG Device shows promise in detecting abnormal cardiac function, Wavelet ECG In Development may offer new data for cardiac diagnostics and Artificial Intelligence integration into ECG, Similarily newer cardiovascular CT technology for diagnosis of cardiovascular diseases and transformative technology of 3D printing in congenital heart diseases are worth mentioning and certainly likely to help for making better diagnosis.and management.

Recently introduced Artificial intelligence technology which has been shown to revolutionize. the scientific technologies in almost all the scientific fields including cardiovascular sciences such as Artificial Intelligence in cardiovascular imaging for risk stratification in CAD ,current and future applications of Artificial Intelligence in CAD, Machine Learning and Artificial Intelligence to Improve Peripheral artery disease management ,Artificial Intelligence and automation in valvular heart diseases, ,Artificial Intelligence in the diagnosis and management of cardiac arrhythmias and Ocular images-based Artificial Intelligencei in diagnosis of systemic diseases Including Cardiovascular Ailments.

Other topics which have been selected in this book are advances and future directions in Cardiac Pacemakers, Robotic assisted cardiac interventions, Recent advances in the diagnosis and treatment of chronic heart failure, Special procedures in the management of critical heart diseases Cell and Gene therapies for heart disease.,current and future state, Management of heart failure with implantation of newer devices,and Recent advances in drug therapy in cardiovascular diseases

Since it was not possible to accommodate the detailed descriptions of the other newer innovations in the field of Cardiology,hence brief notes and marginal comments have been added at the end this manuscript.

This book in its present format and educative contents of various selective chapters ,is certainly would be very informative ,particularily better understanding of recently introduced Artificial intelligence technology, to research scholars, practicing cardiologists, post-gradutes including DM cardiology ,senior residents of cardiology and medicine.

KCVERMA

Contents

Newer Advances In

Cardiovascular Medicine

(Over view)

ARRHYTHMIAS

New professional guidelines on conduction system pacing (June 2023)

Conduction system pacing is a pacing method that directly stimulates the cardiac conduction system at the His bundle or left bundle branch to resynchronize right and left ventricular contraction and thereby improve left ventricular function. For the first time, the Heart Rhythm Society, Asia Pacific Heart Rhythm Society, and Latin American Heart Rhythm Society published guidelines on the use of conduction system pacing to establish cardiac resynchronization therapy (CRT) . For patients with heart failure (HF), the guidelines suggest that conduction system pacing is reasonable in patients who cannot undergo traditional CRT with a coronary sinus lead but is not typically the first choice for establishing CRT. In patients with HF who have an indication for CRT, CRT pacing with a coronary sinus lead is preferred, but for patients who cannot undergo this method of pacing, CRT with conduction system pacing is an alternative approach.

Dual-chamber leadless pacing (June 2023)

Available single-chamber leadless pacing systems do not support atrial pacing or consistent atrioventricular synchrony. An investigational dual-chamber leadless pacing system was evaluated in a prospective multicenter study of nearly 300 patients with sinus node dysfunction or atrioventricular block Implantation was successful in nearly all patients, and the primary safety end point of freedom from complications (device- or procedure-related) at 90 days was met. The system also met performance goals for atrial pacing and atrioventricular synchrony. These findings suggest that leadless pacing may become an option for a broader range of indications including sinus node dysfunction and atrioventricular block.

Personalized accelerated pacing in patients with heart failure with preserved ejection fraction (April 2023)

Pacing may improve cardiac performance among patients with heart failure with preserved ejection fraction (HFpEF), but trials of pacing in this population have not demonstrated benefit. In a recent trial that included over 100 patients with asymptomatic or mild HFpEF who had a pre-existing pacing system, patients to personalized accelerated programming (ie, a backuppacing rate determined by an algorithm) had improved quality-of-life scores when compared with those programmed to a back-up rate of 60 beats per minute However, the trial's small sample size, incomplete blinding, and subjective outcome limit the broad application of this approach. Optimal therapy for HFpEF includes self-care, pharmacologic therapy, and pacing with standard programming for any underlying rhythm abnormality.

CARDIACI MAGING

Predictive value of 3D-derived right ventricular ejection fraction (June 2023)

Three-dimensional (3D) echocardiography-derived right ventricular ejection fraction (RVEF) provides a more comprehensive assessment of right ventricular function than commonly used two-dimensional or one-dimensional parameters. The predictive value of 3D-derived RVEF was assessed by a meta-analysis of 10 studies of over 1900 patients with a variety of cardiovascular conditions . Reduction in RVEF was more strongly associated with adverse outcomes than alterations in other echocardiographic measures of right ventricular systolic function. This finding suggests that 3D-derived RVEF measurements may enhance risk stratification in patients with cardiovascular disease.

CONGENITAL HEART DISEASE, ADULT

Incidence and predictors of Fontan-associated liver disease (February 2023)

Patients who have undergone a Fontan operation are at risk for liver disease (Fontan-associated liver disease [FALD]), but data on the incidence and risk factors for this complication are limited. In a retrospective study of over 1000 post-Fontan patients, liver cirrhosis developed in 13 percent and hepatocellular carcinoma in 1 percent at 20 years after Fontan operation . High central venous pressure and severe atrioventricular valve regurgitation were risk factors for the development of cirrhosis or hepatocellular carcinoma. These data suggest potential targets for surveillance and prevention of FALD.

Long-term risk of ventricular septal defect (January 2023)

Limited data are available on long-term outcomes in adults with congenital ventricular septal defects (VSDs). In a population-based cohort study comparing 8000 patients with VSDs with over 80,000 matched controls for a median of more than 20 years, the risks of heart failure, arrhythmia, infectious endocarditis, and pulmonary hypertension were elevated in patients with unrepaired or surgically repaired VSDs [6]. Among patients with unrepaired VSDs, the risk of morbidity accelerated after age 40 years, and at a younger age in patients with repaired VSDs. These findings underscore the importance of long-term clinical follow-up in adults with VSDs.

CORONARY HEART DISEASE, STABLE

Increased cardiac events in Black females with ischemia with no obstructive coronary arteries (March 2023)

Black females with ischemia with no obstructive coronary arteries (INOCA) have a higher cardiovascular risk burden, more atypical symptoms, and delayed diagnosis and treatment compared with females of other races and ethnicities. In a study of nearly 600 females with INOCA, of whom 17 percent were Black, Black females had a higher risk of major adverse cardiovascular events and cardiovascular mortality compared with females of other races and ethnicities . Patient and provider education about INOCA symptoms, diagnosis, and treatment may be needed to prevent these disparities.

HEART FAILURE

New professional guidelines on conduction system pacing (June 2023)

Conduction system pacing is a pacing method that directly stimulates the cardiac conduction system at the His bundle or left bundle branch to resynchronize right and left ventricular contraction and thereby improve left ventricular function. For the first time, the Heart Rhythm Society, Asia Pacific Heart Rhythm Society, and Latin American Heart Rhythm Society published guidelines on the use of conduction system pacing to establish cardiac resynchronization therapy (CRT) . For patients with heart failure (HF), the guidelines suggest that conduction system pacing is reasonable in patients who cannot undergo traditional CRT with a coronary sinus lead but is not typically the first choice for establishing CRT. In patients with HF who have an indication for CRT, CRT pacing with a coronary sinus lead is preferred, but for patients who cannot undergo this method of pacing, CRT with conduction system pacing is an alternative approach.

Remote pulmonary artery pressure monitoring in patients with heart failure (June 2023)

In patients with heart failure (HF), remote pulmonary artery (PA) pressure monitoring may lead to changes overload and the need for hospitalization. Ina recent trial that included nearly 350 patients with HF, patients assigned to remote PA pressure monitoring had a lower risk of HF hospitalization and a small increase in quality-of-life scores compared with those receiving standard care [8]. However, similar to other trials of hemodynamic monitoring in patients with HF, methodologic issues (eg, inability to blind patients and clinicians to device placement) limit the generalizability of these findings to practice. In highly selected patients with HF, placement of a PA pressure monitor is an option for chronic disease management

Personalized accelerated pacing in patients with heart failure with preserved ejection fraction (April 2023)

Pacing may improve cardiac performance among patients with heart failure with preserved ejection fraction (HFpEF), but trials of pacing in this population have not demonstrated benefit. In a recent trial that included over 100 patients with asymptomatic or mild HFpEF who had a pre-existing pacing system, patients randomly assigned to personalized accelerated programming (ie, a backup pacing rate determined by an algorithm) had improved quality-of-life scores when compared with those programmed to a back-up rate of 60 beats per minute.However, the trial's small sample size, incomplete blinding, and subjective outcome limit the broad application of this approach. Optimal therapy for HFpEF includes self-care, pharmacologic therapy, and pacing with standard programming for any underlying rhythm abnormality.

Use of an algorithm to determine venue of care in patients with heart failure (April 2023)

In patients with heart failure (HF) who present to the emergency department, the decision to discharge or admit is often determined on a case-by-case basis. In a recent trial that included nearly 5500 patients with HF who were randomly assigned to triage with a decision-support algorithm (ie, triage to home- or hospital-based management based on risk of readmission) or usual care, those in the decision-support group had a lower risk of death or rehospitalization within 30 days [9]. The largest differences in management occurred in high-risk patients who were more likely to be admitted in the decision-support group. In patients with HF who present to the emergency department for evaluation, the decision to discharge or admit may be improved with the use of a decision-support algorithm

Heart failure specialist consultation prior to discharge (March 2023)

In patients with heart failure (HF), medical therapy reduces the risk of morbidity and mortality, but these therapies may be inappropriately discontinued or changed among patients who are hospitalized. In a recent trial that included nearly 100 patients with HF who were hospitalized for any cause, mandatory virtual consultation with a HF specialist prior to discharge increased the use of optimal medical therapy for HF when compared with usual care [10]. In the usual care group, the use of optimal medical therapy actually decreased when compared with admission. In patients with HF admitted to noncardiology services, consultation with a HF specialist prior to discharge may increase the use of optimal medical therapy.

Thiazide diuretics to augment diuresis in heart failure (February 2023)

In patients hospitalized with heart failure (HF), the simultaneous use of a loop diuretic and a thiazide diuretic may augment diuresis, but the safety and efficacy of this approach is unknown. In a trial that included over 300 inpatients with acutely decompensated HF who were receiving treatment with a loop diuretic, patients randomly assigned to receive additional therapy with hydrochlorothiazide (HCTZ) or placebo had similar changes in patient-reported dyspnea scores after 72 hours of therapy [11]. Patients assigned to HCTZ had more weight loss but a greater decrease in kidney function and a higher risk of hypokalemia. We typically attempt combination diuretic therapy with a thiazide or other nonloop diuretic agent in patients with acutely decompensated HF who are refractory to high doses of loop diuretics (eg, furosemide equivalent of 200 mg/day).

Changes to heart failure therapy in patients recently hospitalized for heart failure (February 2023)

Patients with heart failure (HF) benefit from optimal medical therapy, but it is unclear whether patients recently hospitalized with HF can safely undergo rapid changes to their pharmacologic regimen. In a trial in nearly 1100 patients hospitalized with HF who were randomly assigned to high-intensity care (drug adjustment to target within two weeks of discharge and clinical surveillance) or to usual care, patients assigned to or adjusted toward their target doses.

high-intensity care were more likely to achieve target doses of primary therapies for HF with reduced ejection fraction (eg, sacubitril-valsartan, beta blockers) and had a lower risk of hospital readmission by 180 days [12]. Although overall adverse effects were more frequent in the high-intensity care group, rates of serious adverse events were similar between the groups. In highly selected inpatients scheduled for discharge who can reliably undergo frequent observation in the outpatient setting, HF medications can be added

Torsemide or furosemide for diuresis after heart failure hospitalization (January 2023)

Torsemide and furosemide have different pharmacologic properties, but it is unknown whether one agent is superior to the other in patients with heart failure (HF). In a trial in nearly 2900 patients hospitalized with HF who were randomly assigned to treatment with furosemide or torsemide prior to discharge, the rates of all-cause mortality and all-cause hospitalization at 12 months were similar between the groups [13]. However, immediate crossover between treatments and the open-label design may have obscured differences in diuretic efficacy. In patients recovering from acutely decompensated HF without known resistance to a specific diuretic, furosemide and torsemide are reasonable options for outpatient diuresis.

LIPID DISORDERS

Bempedoic acid for patients intolerant to statins (March 2023)

Statins are the preferred therapy for dyslipidemia in most patients, but nearly 10 percent of patients have statin intolerance. In a randomized trial of nearly 14,000 patients at high risk for cardiovascular disease who were unable or unwilling to take statins due to adverse effects, patients assigned to bempedoic acid had a lower risk of major adverse cardiovascular events than placebo (11.7 versus 13.3 percent) [14]. However, gout, cholelithiasis, and increases in serum creatinine, uric acid, and hepatic enzymes were slightly more common with bempedoic acid. Bempedoic acid may be used in statin-intolerant patients who require modest lipid lowering, but side effects must be monitored.

PREVENTIVE CARDIOLOGY

Contribution of inflammation to cardiovascular risk in patients receiving statin therapy (April 2023)

In patients with an indication for statin therapy, lipid lowering therapy has an anti-inflammatory effect but may not completely reduce inflammation, which may contribute to atherosclerotic cardiovascular disease. In an analysis of over 31,000 patients from three clinical trials of statin therapy, baseline levels of high-sensitivity C-reactive protein (CRP), a biomarker of residual inflammatory risk, were associated with incident major adverse cardiovascular events and cardiovascular mortality . By contrast, baseline levels of low-density lipoprotein cholesterol (LDL-C), a biomarker of residual cholesterol risk, were not associated with major adverse cardiovascular events but were associated with cardiovascular mortality. These findings suggest that among patients receiving statin therapy, residual inflammation may be a stronger predictor for cardiovascular risk than LDL-C.

Bempedoic acid for patients intolerant to statins (March2023)

Statins are the preferred therapy for dyslipidemia in most patients, but nearly 10 percent of patients have statin intolerance. In a randomized trial of nearly 14,000 patients at high risk for cardiovascular disease who were unable or unwilling to take statins due to adverse effects, patients assigned to bempedoic acid had a lower risk of major adverse cardiovascular events than placebo (11.7 versus 13.3 percent) . However, gout, cholelithiasis, and increases in serum creatinine, uric acid, and hepatic enzymes were slightly more common with bempedoic acid. Bempedoic acid may be used in statin-intolerant patients who require modest lipid lowering, but side effects must be monitored.

TRANSPLANTATION

Comparison of donor hearts procured after circulatory death or brain death in heart transplantation (June 2023)

The use of donor hearts obtained after declaration of circulatory death (DCD) may increase the number of available donor hearts for transplantation, but may also increase the risk of graft dysfunction compared with donor hearts obtained after declaration of brain death (DBD). In a recent randomized trial in nearly 200 heart recipients, recipients assigned to transplantation with a DCD donor heart had similar six-month survival compared with those assigned to receive a DBD donor heart; postoperative graft dysfunction at 30 days was higher among recipients of a DCD donor heart. While these results suggest comparable short-term survival among recipients of a DCD or DBD donor heart, certain issues in the trial design and analysis (such as crossover from the DCD to the DBD group and important differences in baseline characteristics between the groups) limit the interpretation of the findings. In highly selected recipients and donors, survival after heart transplantation with a DCD donor heart may be similar to that with a DBD donor heart

VALVULAR HEART DISEASE

Tricuspid valve prolapse in patients with mitral valve prolapse (June 2023)

Patients with significant primary mitral regurgitation (MR) commonly have tricuspid regurgitation, but the frequency of tricuspid valve prolapse (TVP) is not well defined. In a study of nearly 500 patients with primary MR, over one-third of patients with mitral valve prolapse (MVP) had TVP on cardiac magnetic resonance imaging; TVP was not identified in patients without MVP . Patients with TVP were more likely to have severe MR and moderate or severe tricuspid regurgitation. These findings identify TVP as an important cause of tricuspid regurgitation in patients with MVP.

Transcatheter edge-to-edge repair for tricuspid regurgitation (April 2023)

Patients with refractory symptomatic severe tricuspid regurgitation (TR) may benefit from tricuspid valve intervention, but tricuspid valve surgery commonly entails high operative risk. In an open-label trial in which 350 symptomatic patients with severe TR were randomly assigned to transcatheter edge-to-edge repair (TEER) or continued medical management, patients in the TEER group experienced an improvement in quality of life and reduction in severity of TR but no change in the risks of mortality or hospitalization . These findings suggest a potential role for TEER as a less invasive alternative to tricuspid valve surgery in symptomatic patients with severe TR. TEER devices for the tricuspid valve are approved for use in Europe but not in the United States.

Five-year outcomes of transcatheter mitral repair for secondary mitral regurgitation (March 2023)

Transcatheter edge-to-edge repair (TEER) reduces secondary mitral regurgitation (MR), but the durability of clinical benefit has not been established. Five-year outcomes were recently reported from a randomized trial that compared TEER with medical therapy alone in over 600 patients with moderate-to-severe or severe (3+ or 4vV+) secondary MR and symptomatic heart failure despite maximal medical therapy At five years, TEER reduced all-cause mortality and hospitalization for heart failure compared with medical therapy alone. For selected patients with moderate-to-severe to severe secondary MR who are symptomatic despite optimum medical therapy, we suggest TEER.

Early surgical valve replacement versus conservative management for asymptomatic severe aortic stenosis (February 2023)

Management options for patients with asymptomatic severe aortic stenosis include surgical aortic valve replacement (SAVR), transcatheter aortic valve mplantation, and conservative management. In a meta-analysis that included two randomized controlled trials and 10 observational studies (over 4000 patients) comparing early SAVR with conservative management, early SAVR was associated with lowerall- cause mortality, cardiovascular mortality, and heart failure hospitalization. The risks of stroke and myocardial infarction were similar with early SAVR and conservative management. These findings support a role for early SAVR in selected patients with asymptomatic severe aortic stenosis.

Prognostic factors for isolated severe tricuspid regurgitation (January 2023)

Patients with severe tricuspid regurgitation (TR) commonly have left-sided valve disease that impacts prognosis, but prognostic data in patients with isolated severe TR and no significant left-sided valve disease are limited. In a study of over 600 patients with isolated severe TR, 23 percent died and 10 percent were hospitalized for heart failure over a median of 26.5 months.Adverse prognostic factors included pulmonary hypertension, elevated blood urea nitrogen levels, decreased albumin levels, and left atrial enlargement. These data may help guide risk-stratified management of isolated severe TR

Five New Technologies Transforming Cardiac Care

Cardiovascular diseases (CVD) are on the rise across the globe due to lifestyle disorders. According to the World Health Organisation (WHO), diseases such as stroke and ischemic heart disease roughly account for 17.7 million deaths only in India. This number includes a large set of younger populations. COVID-19 pandemic is acting as a trigger as the virus alone can be a cause for heart attack. The World Heart Federation (WHF) observes September 29, every year as World Heart Day. This year the objective for World Heart Day 2021 is Globally harnessing the power of digital health to improve awareness, prevention, and management of CVD. Cardiac care has witnessed a significant transformation over the last decade. With Artificial intelligence (AI) and machine learning (ML) playing an important role, cardiologists and cardiac surgeons are bringing unprecedented revolutions in cardiac treatment mechanisms.

These technological advancements are facilitating early detection and treatment of critically ill patients thus, improving outcomes.Let us delve into the work-in-progress technologies that can change the meaning of cardiac care.

Personalized heart models

Have you ever heard of patient-specific 3D models of heart that can aid a doctor in understanding the nature of heart disease? Scientists at University College London have developed such 3D-printed models from MRI scans of children born with heart defects (congenital heart diseases). These models can also boost patients' and their families' understanding of the heart condition. The same team is also working to produce computer simulations, to help a surgeon planning surgery for such children. This personalized approach in cardiac care will help surgeons and patients decide on the best treatment modalities.

Skin patch to counterstroke

A simple skin patch may help in improving the survival chances of stroke victims Unbelievable but true. Researchers at the University of Nottingham are working on a skin patch that can be applied in an ambulance immediately after a patient suffers a suspected stroke attack. This patch, which delivers the drug glyceryl trinitrate, can widen blood vessels and lower blood pressure, thereby reducing the potential damage caused by stroke.Starting treatment within an hour of stroke could revolutionize stroke care. Treating patients inside the ambulances on the way to the hospital will save vital time and aid recovery.Scientists are hoping, if this patch is safe to use, it can be used by paramedics in the ambulance also or in places where conventional treatment facilities are not available.

Implantable heart-rhythm monitors

Most heart failure patients may experience an irregularity in heart rhythm. It can be too slow, too fast, or irregular. Presently we are using ECG recording to trace an irregularity in heart rhythm. ECG can give you a picture of that moment only. What if a doctor wants to track rhythm over a longer period to have a better understanding of the patient's health? Researchers are working on implantable cardiac monitors. These are tiny devices that can be implanted under the skin for recording heart rhythm

Nano Materials For Fighting Cholestrol

We all know fatty deposits in blood vessels are one of the most common causes of various cardiovascular diseases. Though statins can help to lower the levels of low-density lipoprotein (LDL) in the blood, they can affect other tissues like muscles making some people intolerant to statins. Scientists are working on nanomaterials. These nanomaterials can deliver cholesterol-lowering drugs exactly to the sites where they are needed most. Nanomaterials are incredibly small but have very high stability. They biodegrade on their own once the drugs have been delivered to specific sites.

Use of Artificial intelligence (AI) and Machine Learning (ML) to interpret heart condition

Let's start with the basics. Artificial intelligence is the ability of a machine to solve those complex problems that would otherwise require human intervention. Advances in technology have made it possible for machines to accurately and quickly analyze large amounts of data This learning improves decision-making, accurate diagnosis, and treatment planning by detecting specific patterns in patient data. Cardiovascular doctors and scientists are now combining artificial intelligence with clinical practice for better care. Here are two examples of how doctors are using AI forbetteroutcomes For people with stroke – the computer trained to analyze CT data, can examine the scan, diagnose the stroke, and thus saving valuable time.Preventing heart problems – Applying AI to ECGs can be used to detect any abnormality in the heart pump, which if left untreated can lead to heart failure.

Bibliography and Acknowledgement

Brugts JJ, Radhoe SP, Clephas PRD, et al. Remote haemodynamic monitoring of pulmonary artery pressures in patients with chronic heart failure (MONITOR-HF): a randomised clinical trial. Lancet 2023.

Costa GNF, Cardoso JFL, Oliveiros B, et al. Early surgical intervention versus conservative management of asymptomatic severe aortic stenosis: a systematic review and meta-analysis. Heart2023;109:314.

Eckerström F, Nyboe C, Redington A, Hjortdal VE. Lifetime Burden of Morbidity in Patients With Isolated Congenital Ventricular Septal Defect. J Am Heart Assoc 2023; 12:e027477.

Guta AC, El-Tallawi KC, Nguyen DT, et al. Prevalence and Clinical Implications of Tricuspid Valve Prolapse Based on Magnetic Resonance Diagnostic Criteria. J Am Coll Cardiol 2023.

Inuzuka R, Nii M, Inai K, et al. Predictors of liver cirrhosis and hepatocellular carcinoma among perioperative survivors of the Fontanoperation.Heart2023;109:276.

Knops RE, Reddy VY, Ip JE, et al. A Dual-Chamber Leadless Pacemaker.NEnglJMed2023.

Lee DS, Straus SE, Farkouh ME, et al. Trial of an Intervention to Improve Acute Heart Failure Outcomes. N Engl J Med 2023; 388:22.

Luu JM, Malhotra P, Cook-Wiens G, et al. Long-Term Adverse Outcomes in Black Women With Ischemia and No Obstructive Coronary Artery Disease: A Study of the WISE (Women's Ischemia Syndrome Evaluation) Cohort. Circulation 2023; 147:617.

Mebazaa A, Davison B, Chioncel O, et al. Safety, tolerability and efficacy of up-titration of guideline-directed medical therapies for acute heart failure (STRONG-HF): a multinational, open-label, randomised,trial.Lancet2022;400:1938.

Mentz RJ, Anstrom KJ, Eisenstein EL, et al. Effect of Torsemide vs Furosemide After Discharge on All-Cause Mortality in Patients Hospitalized With Heart Failure: The TRANSFORM-HFRandomized Clinical Trial. JAMA 2023; 329:214.

Nishiura N, Kitai T, Okada T, et al. Long-Term Clinical Outcomes in Patients With Severe Tricuspid Regurgitation. J Am Heart Assoc2023;12:e025751.

Nissen SE, Lincoff AM, Brennan D, et al. Bempedoic Acid and Cardiovascular Outcomes in Statin-Intolerant Patients. N Engl J Med 2023; 388:1353.

Reddy YNV, Koepp KE, Carter R, et al. Rate-Adaptive Atrial Pacing for Heart Failure With Preserved Ejection Fraction: The RAPID-HF Randomized Clinical Trial. JAMA 2023; 329:801.

Schroder JN, Patel CB, DeVore AD, et al. Transplantation Outcomes with Donor Hearts after Circulatory Death. N Engl J Med2023;388:2121.

Stone GW, Abraham WT, Lindenfeld J, et al. Five-Year Follow-up after Transcatheter Repair of Secondary Mitral Regurgitation. NEnglJMed2023;388:2037.

Stone GW, Lindenfeld J, Abraham WT, et al. Transcatheter Mitral-Valve Repair in Patients with Heart Failure. N Engl J Med 2018;379:2307.

Trulls JC, Morales-Rull JL, Casado J, et al. Combining loop with thiazide diuretics for decompensated heart failure: the CLOROTIC trial. Eur Heart J 2023; 44:411.

CHAPTER

Newer Innovations In Electrocardiography

The invention of the electrocardiograph by Dutch physiologist Willem Einthoven in 1902 gave physicians a powerful tool to help them diagnose various forms of heart disease, especially arrhythmias and acute myocardial infarction. The discovery of x-rays in 1895 and the invention of the electrocardiograph 7 years later inaugurated a new era in which various machines and technical procedures gradually replaced the physician's unaided senses and the stethoscope as the primary tools of cardiac diagnosis. These sophisticated new approaches provided objective information about the structure and function of the heart in health and disease.

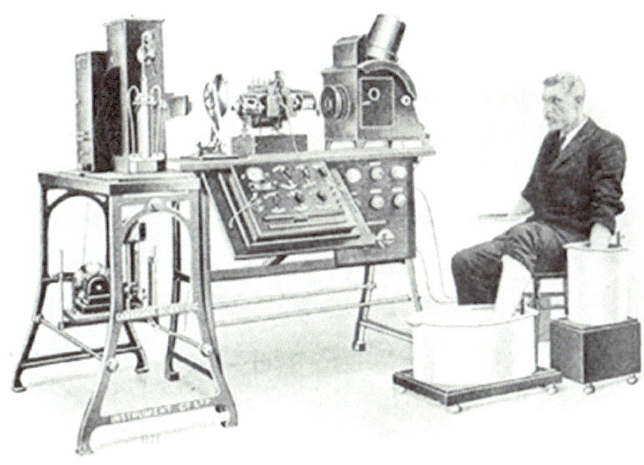

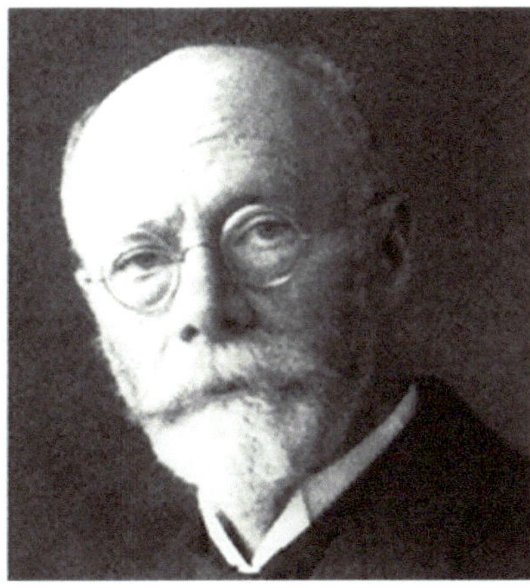

Fig. 1.1 Willem Einthoven and his ECG machine Dutch physician Willem Einthoven is considered as the father of the modern day ECG machine. He invented the string galvanometer in 1901 and this lead to the invention of the first practical clinical ECG machine around the same time. He was also the first to coin the term "electrocardiogram" in 1893. Most of the working principles and methods of reading an electrocardiogram still in use to this day were originally conceived by Willem Einthoven. For his invention, he received the 1924 Nobel Prize in Physiology or Medicine.

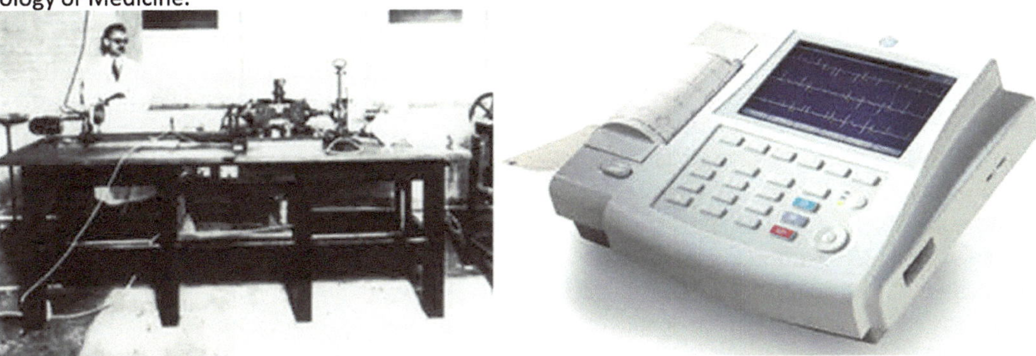

Fig. 1.2 Left: ECG machines in the 1920s. Right: Modern day ECG machine

Electrocardiography is a commonly used, noninvasive procedure for recording electrical changes in the heart. The record, which is called an electrocardiogram (ECG or EKG), shows the series of waves that relate to the electrical impulses that occur during each beat of the heart. The results are printed on paper and/or displayed on a monitor to provide a visual representation of heart function. The waves in a normal record are named P, Q, R, S, and T, and follow in alphabetical order. The number of waves may vary, and other waves may be present.

Basic Principles involved in Electrocardiography

The ECG device detects and amplifies the tiny electrical changes on the skin that are caused when the heart muscle depolarizes during each heart beat. At rest, each heart muscle cell has a negative charge, called the membrane potential, across its cell membrane. Decreasing this negative charge toward zero, via the influx of the positive cations, Na^+ and Ca^{++}, is called depolarization, which activates the mechanisms in the cell that cause it to contract. During each heartbeat, a healthy heart will have an orderly progression of a wave of depolarisation that is triggered by the cells in the sinoatrial node, spreads out through the atrium, passes through the atrioventricular node and then spreads all over the ventricles. This is detected as tiny rises and falls in the voltage between two electrodes placed either side of the heart, which is displayed as a wavy line either on a screen or on paper. This display indicates the overall rhythm of the heart and weaknesses in different parts of the heart muscle. Usually, more than two electrodes are used, and they can be combined into a number of pairs (For example: left arm (LA), right arm (RA), and left leg (LL) electrodes form the three pairs LA+RA, LA+LL, and RA+LL). The output from each pair is known as a lead. Each lead looks at the heart from a different angle. Different types of ECGs can be referred to by the number of leads that are recorded, for example 3-lead, 5-lead, or 12-lead ECGs . A 12-lead ECG is one in which 12 different electrical signals are recorded at approximately the same time and will often be used as a one-off recording of an ECG, traditionally printed out as a paper copy. Three- and 5-lead ECGs tend to be monitored continuously and viewed only on the screen of an appropriate monitoring device, for example during an operation or whilst being transported in an ambulance. There may or may not be any permanent record of a 3- or 5-lead ECG, depending on the equipment used.

Who Performs The Procedure And Where Is It Performed?

The electrocardiograph is conducted by a fully trained technologist and may be done in the cardiologist's office, a testing facility, or at a hospital patient's bedside. The technologist, or perhaps a nurse or nurse practitioner, will take the patient's medical history, educate them about the procedure they are about to undergo, and help them relax. The results of the electrocardiograph will be interpreted by a qualified physician, usually a cardiologist.

Clinical Indications of Electrocardiography

- Enlargement of the heart
- Congenital heart defects involving the conducting (electrical) system
- Abnormal rhythm (arrhythmia) – rapid, slow or irregular heart beats
- Damage to the heart, such as when one of the heart's arteries is blocked (coronary occlusion)
- A heart attack, in emergency situations
- A previous heart attack
- Abnormal position of the heart
- Heart inflammation – pericarditis or myocarditis
- Cardiac arrest during emergency room or intensive care monitoring
- Disturbances of the heart's conducting system
- Imbalances in the blood chemicals (electrolytes) that control heart activity.
- Monitoring the baby's heart during labor
- Telemonitoring the heart rhythm

Medical History Prior to Performing Procedure

There is no need to restrict food or drink prior to the test. You should always let your doctor know what medications you are taking before you have an ECG, and if you have any allergies to adhesive tapes that may be used to attach electrodes.

Technique of Obtaining Electrocardiogram:

Before the procedure:

- Your doctor or the technician will explain the procedure to you and offer you the opportunity to ask any questions that you might have about the procedure.

- Generally, fasting is not required before the test.
- Notify your doctor of all medications (prescribed and over-the-counter) and herbal supplements that you are taking.
- Notify your doctor if you have a pacemaker.
- Based on your medical condition, your doctor may request other specific preparation.

During Procedure

An ECG may be performed on an outpatient basis or as part of your stay in a hospital. Procedures may vary depending on your condition and your doctor's practices.

- You will be asked to remove any jewelry or other objects that may interfere with the procedure.
- You will be asked to remove clothing from the waist up. The technician will ensure your privacy by covering you with a sheet or gown and exposing only the necessary skin.
- You will lie flat on a table or bed for the procedure. It will be important for you to lie still and not talk during the procedure, so as not to interfere with the tracing.
- If your chest, arms, or legs are very hairy, the technician may shave or clip small patches of hair, as needed, so that the electrodes will stick closely to the skin.
- Electrodes will be attached to your chest, arms, and legs.
- The lead wires will be attached to the skin electrodes.
- Once the leads are attached, the technician may key in identifying information about you into the machine's computer.
- The ECG will be started. It will take only a short time for the tracing to be completed.
- Once the tracing is completed, the technician will disconnect the leads and remove the skin electrodes

After The Procedure

- You should be able to resume your normal diet and activities, unless your doctor instructs you differently.
- Generally, there is no special care following an ECG.
- Notify your doctor if you develop any signs or symptoms you had prior to the test (for example, chest pain, shortness of breath, dizziness, or fainting).
- Your doctor may give you additional or alternate instructions after the procedure, depending on your particular situation.

Types of Electrocardiograms: The types of ECG include:

12 lead ECG test – with standard ECG machine: This is the modern adaptation of the original Willem Einthoven ECG machine based on the Einthoven's Triangle principles. It is the standard ECG machine used in clinical settings today. In 1942 Emanuel Goldberger added 3 more leads known as augmented limb leads (aVR, aVL and aVF) to Willem Einthoven's limb leads (I, II & III) and six chest leads (V1, V2, V3, V4, V5 & V6) forming the basis of the 12 lead ECG. The patient lies down. No movement is allowed during this time, as electrical impulses generated by other muscles may interfere with those generated by your heart. This type of ECG usually takes five to 10 minutes.

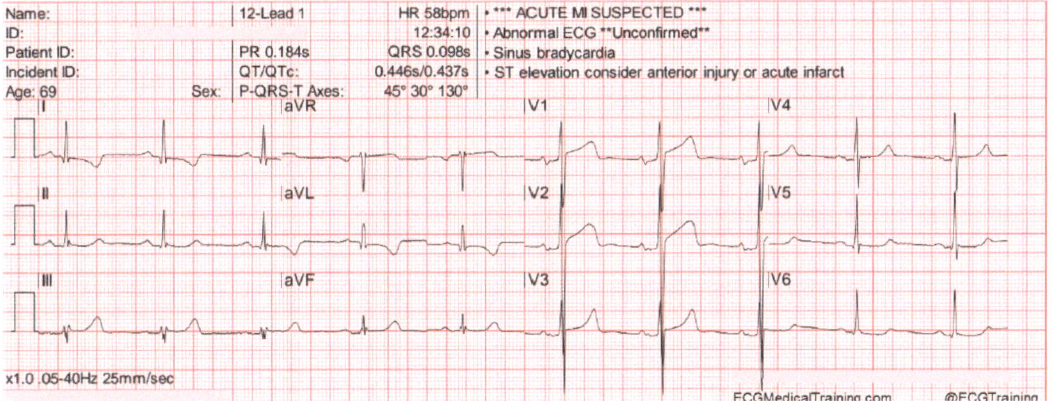

Fig. 1.3 (A) The six-step method for 12-lead ECG interpretation. 1) Rate and rhythm 2) Axis determination 3) QRS duration (intervals) 4) Morphology 5) STEMI mimics 6) STEMI mimics 6) STEMI (Ischemia, injury, infarct) "Step 7" is a rule I started throwing in to remind students that one should always interpret an ECG (or any other diagnostic test) in light of the history and clinical presentation.

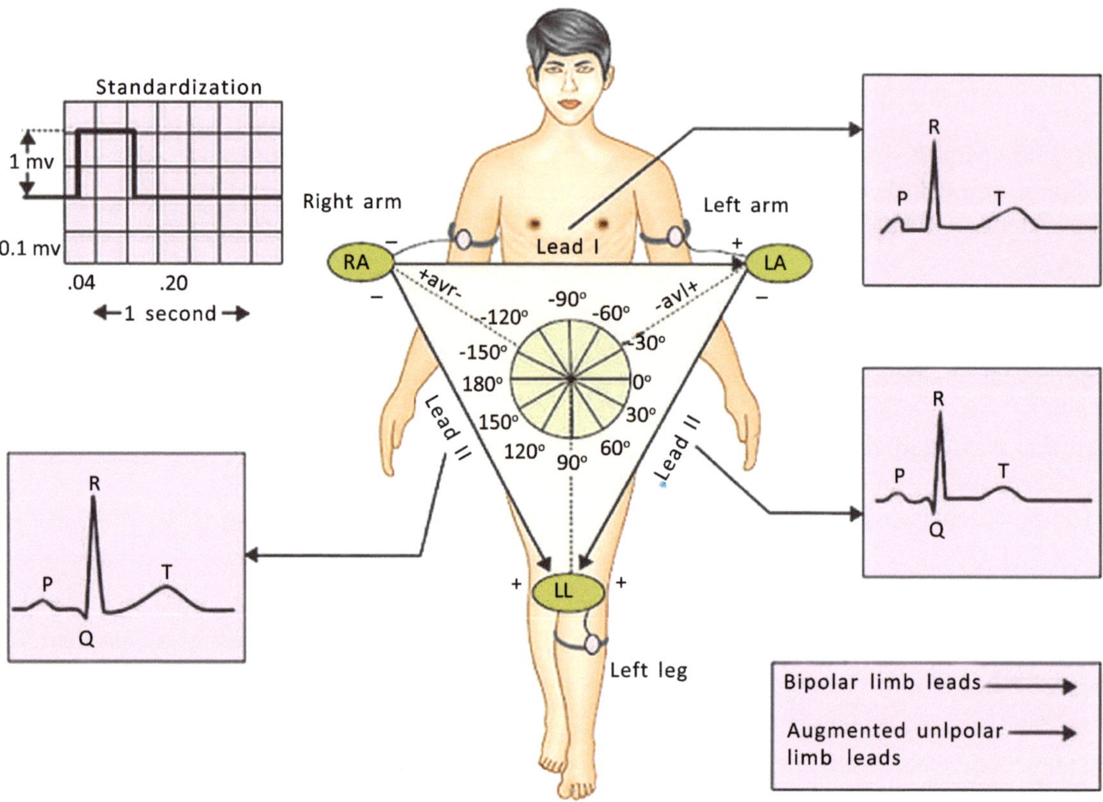

Fig. 1.3 **(B)** Enthoven s triangle. Lead 1 measures the potential difference between the left and right arms. Since the right arm carries the negative electrode the resultant direction of the lead 1 vector is obtained by bisecting the angle between the left arm and a point directly opposite the right arm. The resultant directions of leads 11 and 111 are obtained in a similar way. RA – Right arm, LA – Left arm and F – Foot.

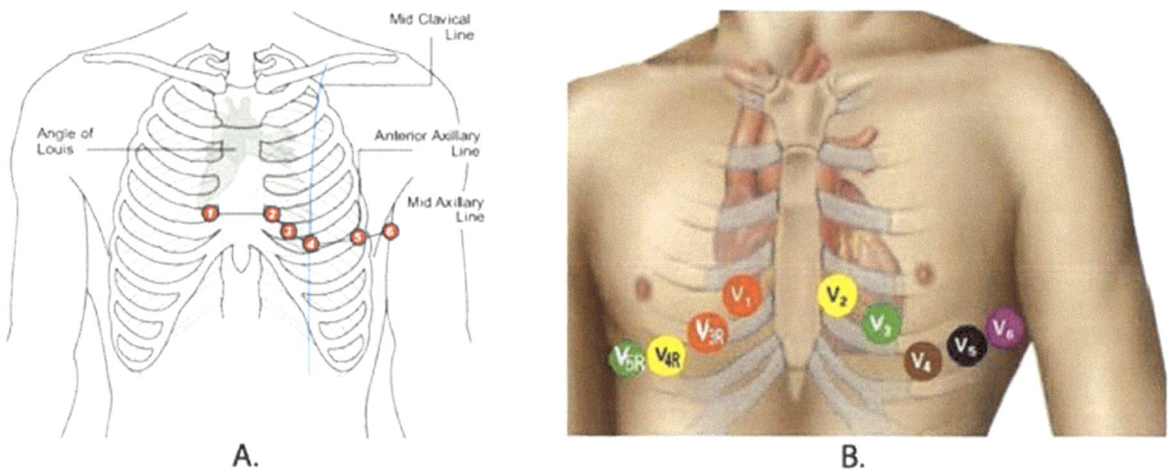

Fig. 1.4 A Precardial six leads placement over the cheast. B. Both left and right sided leads over the chest.

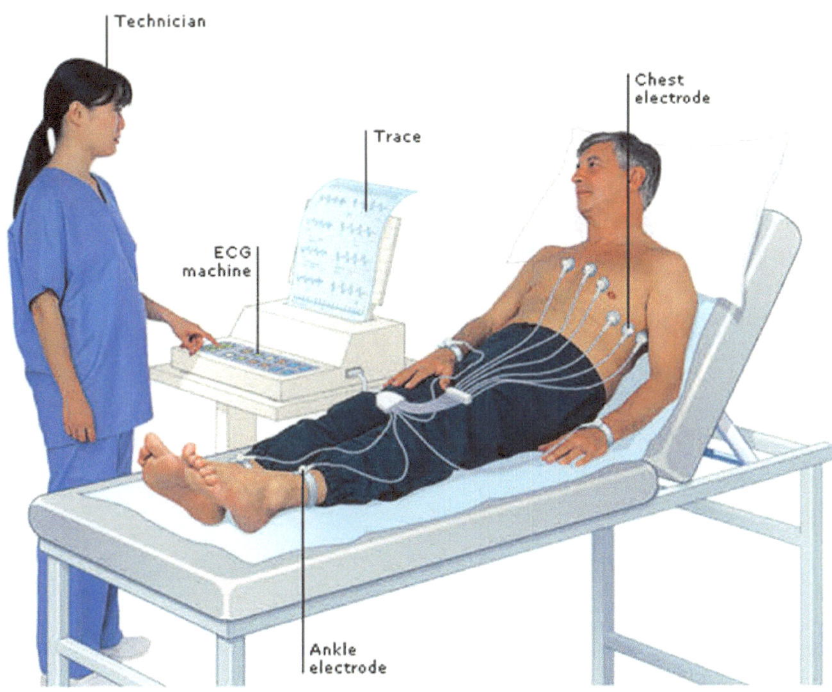

Fig. 1.5 Trained nurse obtaining electrocardiographic trace of patient after application of limb and chest electrodes

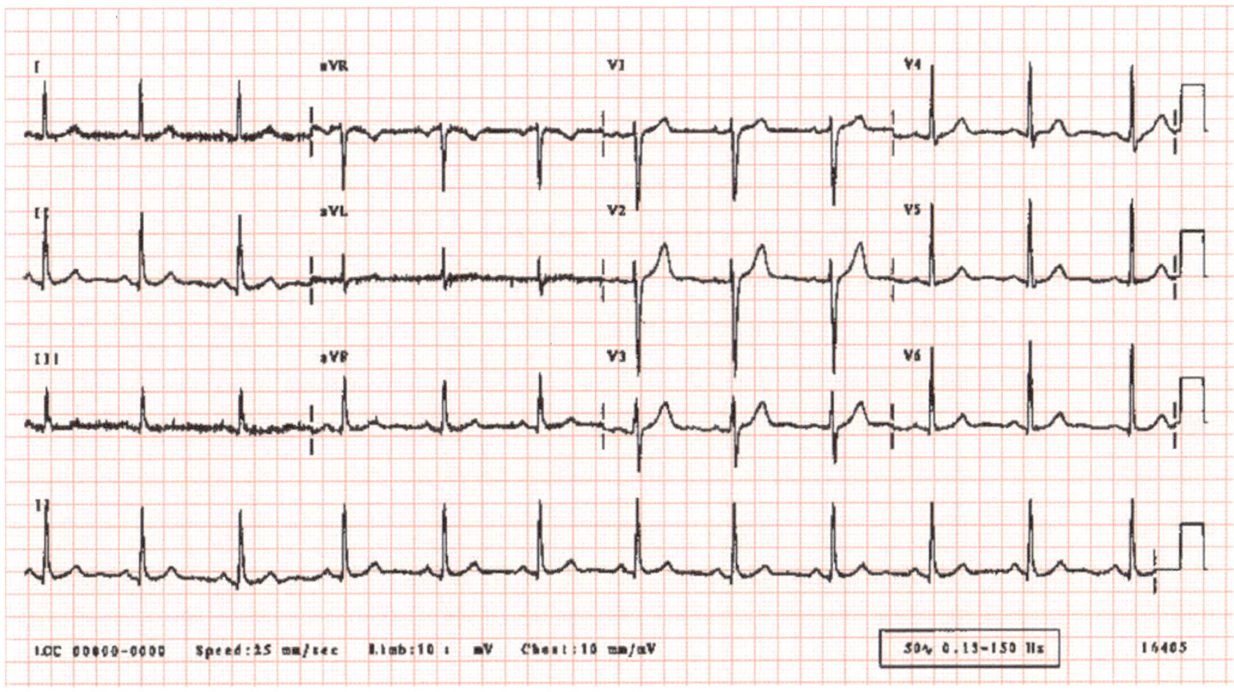

Fig. 1.6 12- Lead ECG trace showing normal morphology of P wave,P-R interval QRS, duration, T wave, ST segment, normal sinus rhythm and dominant R wave in V5 & V6 with rS Pattern in V1&V2 in a normal adult

The 12 leads provide 12 different views of the heart from different angles and this helps the doctor visualize the location of the abnormality in the patient's heart. A 12 lead ECG is critical for doctors to make the right decision when diagnosing or monitoring a patient.

It is important to note that a 12 lead ECG has just 10 physical electrodes placed on the skin surface at various positions. 4 Electrodes are placed on the hands and feet of the patient. 6 Electrodes are placed on the chest of the patient. The 12 views (12 leads) are derived from the combination of electric signals from these 10 electrodes by the ECG machine.

3 Lead ECG monitoring

A 3-lead ECG is used for continuous monitoring of heartbeat, heart rate, and heart rhythm in critical situations, like when the patient is under anesthesia, in surgery or being transported in an ambulance to a health center. 3-lead ECG monitoring requires the use of 4 electrodes that are placed on each of the limbs. It is also used in combination with other medical devices like an echocardiogram (ultrasound scan of heart).

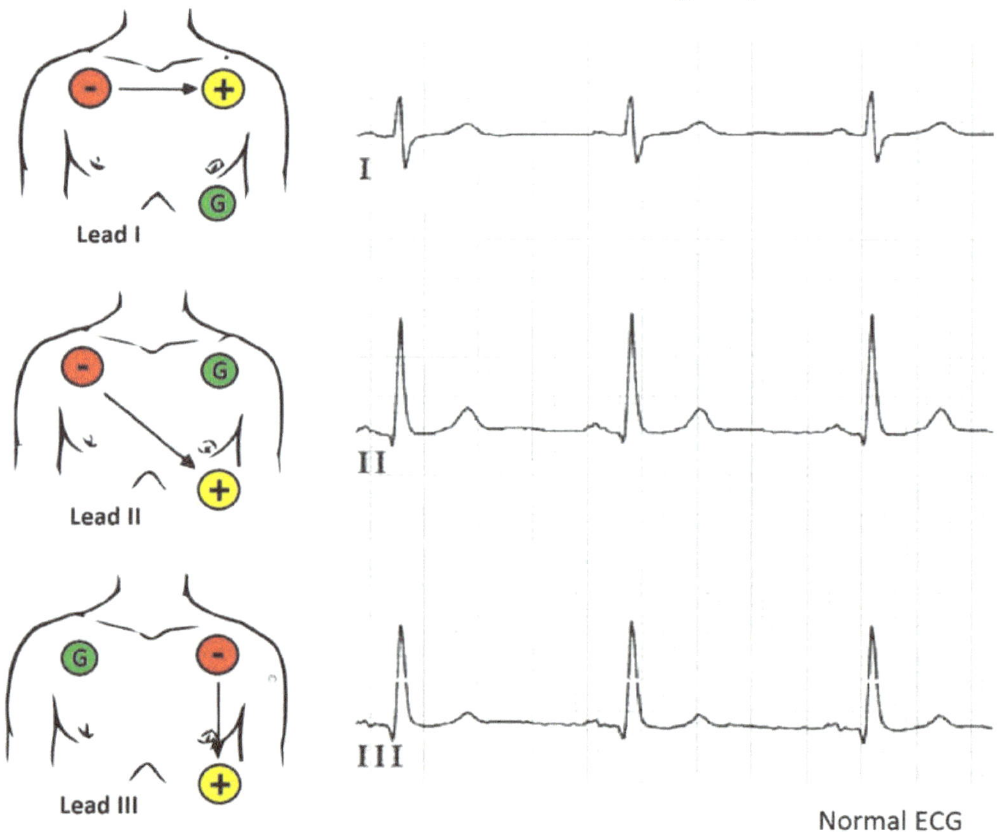

Fig. 1.7 3 Lead ECG monitoring

5 Lead ECG monitoring

Occasionally a 5 lead ECG is also used for monitoring purposes. It uses 4 electrodes like a 3 lead ECG with an additional 5th electrode placed on the chest. Usually these devices do not produce a print out of the electrocardiogram and may not store the information for further review. 3 and 5 lead variations of ECG monitoring does not provide detailed views like a 12 lead ECG, but is most often sufficient for monitoring purposes. A 12 lead ECG is the standard equipment of choice for diagnosing heart disease in a clinical situation.

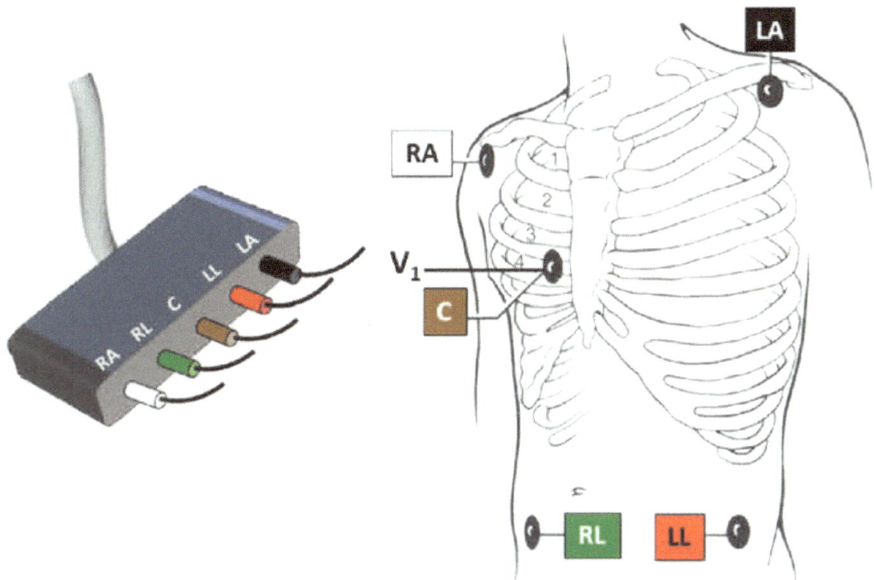

Fig. 1.8 3 Lead ECG monitoring

Single lead monitoring system

The heart of NetGuard is a very small wireless EKG monitor, weighing less than an ounce. The monitor communicates with a standard personal computer (PC) at a nurse's station, which gives an alert and an EKG display when a dangerous rhythm is detected. A nurse typically would confirm the alert and call an emergency "code" in accordance with hospital protocol. One PC has the capacity to cover 50 patients. The system architecture of NetGuard provides for total coverage of a hospital. The NetGuard system is also economical. The cost of the wireless system components, including the reusable portion of the EKG monitor, is a fraction of the cost of conventional monitors. The single-use component of the monitor, including batteries, electrode and adhesive pad are packaged together in a detachable unit that mates neatly with the reusable electronic unit. The batteries in the NetGuard monitor last three days — three times longer than conventional telemeters. Cost of the single-use component has not yet been established but will be affordable based on Datascope's market research.

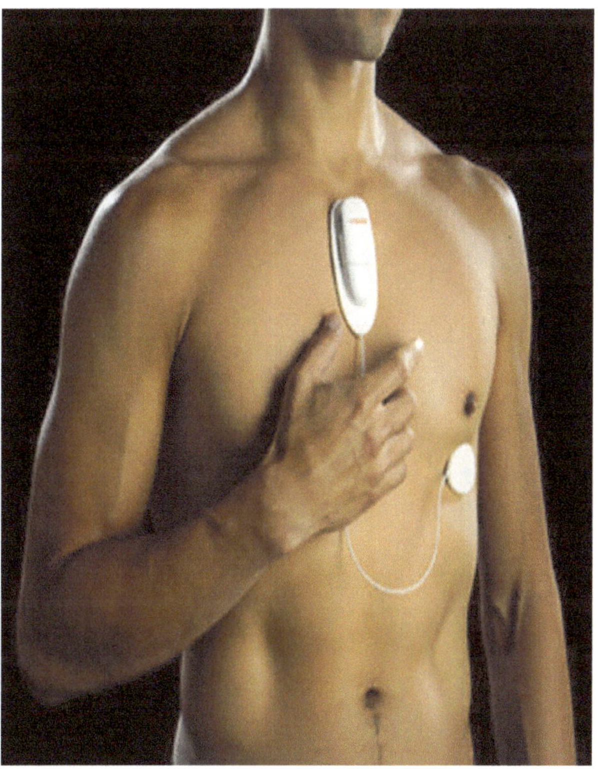

Fig. 1.9 Single lead NetGuard a very small wireless EKG monitor

Ambulatory ECG

Ambulatory or Holter ECG is performed using a portable recording device that is worn for at least 24 hours. The patient is free to move around normally while the monitor is attached. This type of ECG is used for patients whose symptoms are intermittent and may not appear during a resting ECG. People recovering from heart attack may be monitored in this way to ensure proper heart function. The patient usually records symptoms in a diary, noting the time so that their own experience can be compared with the ECG. Holter Monitor is a portable ECG monitor that can be worn by a patient for duration of 24 to 48 hours while the device continuously monitors the heart rhythm. It has fewer leads than a normal clinical ECG machine. The patient is free to move around and go around their usual daily routines. This medical device is useful for detecting abnormalities in heart rhythm that could be easily missed during a clinical ECG test, which last less than a minute. The device is returned to the doctor at the end of the monitoring period and the data from the device is retrieved and analyzed.

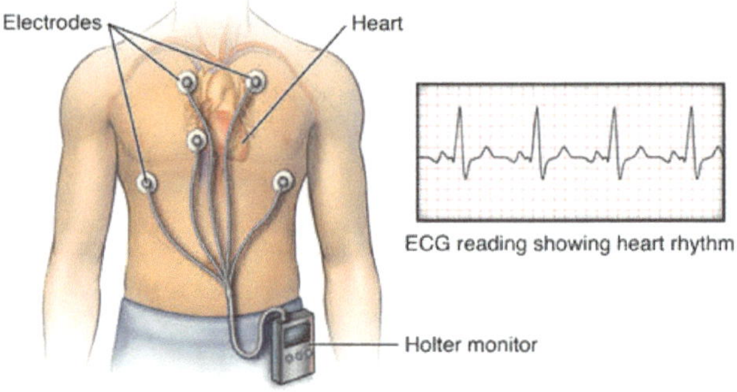

Fig. 1.10 Different leads on the chest along with recorder of Holter monitoring system

Cardiac stress test

This test is used to record a patient's ECG while the patient rides on an exercise bike or walks on a treadmill. This type of ECG takes about 15 to 30 minutes to complete.

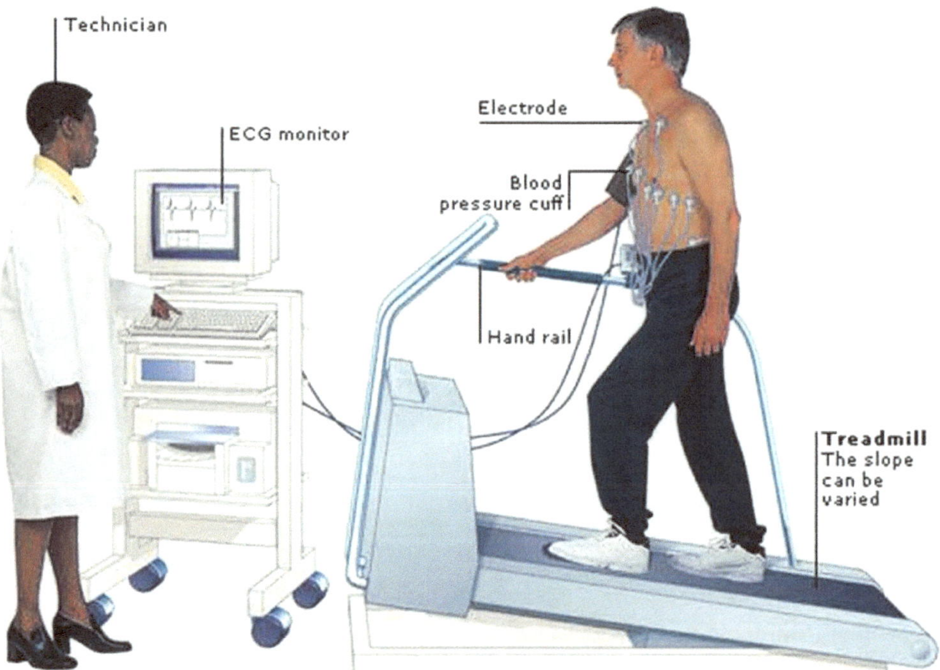

Fig. 1.11 Morphological features of Treadmil machine along with monitor and recording/ printing equipment kept over a specially designed trolley, BP instrument and patient performing a treadmill test

Wireless ECG

This is a modern day innovation of the traditional clinical ECG machine with similar functional capabilities. Electrodes do not have wirers directly attached to the recording or monitoring machine. These electrodes can transmit the signal wirelessly over to the receiver in the ECG machine.Wireless ECG machine can offer more flexibility for the patients. This is especially useful when combined with a treadmill test where the lack of cables can offer more freedom of movement during the test.

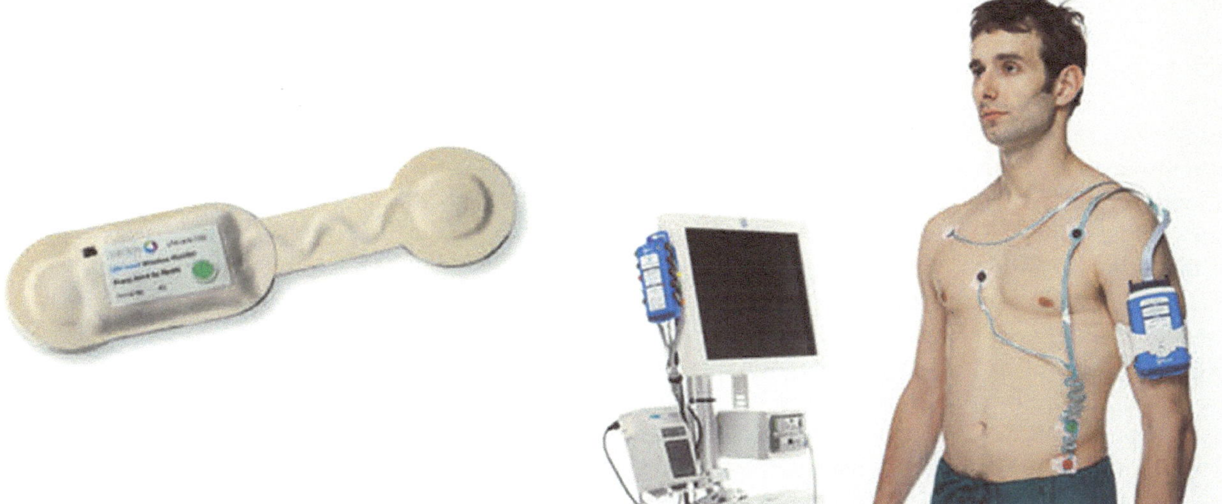

Fig. 1.12 Right: 5 Lead wireless ECG sensor with seprate transmitter and receiver. © LifeSync. Left: Low cost compact wireless ECG sensor. © Isansys Lifecare.

Cardiac Event Recorder

Sometimes the symptoms may not appear during the ECG and a Holter Monitor test. In such cases, the doctor may suggest a cardiac event recorder that can be worn continuously for an extended period of time (2-4 weeks). The device is the size of a deck of cards and cables to the recording device connect the electrodes. Unlike the Holter monitor, an Event recorder does not continuously record the heart rhythm.When the patient is experiencing the symptoms, he or she can activate the recorder, the device will record the incident. Depending on the model of the device, multiple events can be recorded in the internal memory. The data can be transferred to the consulting doctor for detailed analysis and the doctor can make a more accurate diagnosis based on data obtained during the abnormal incident.

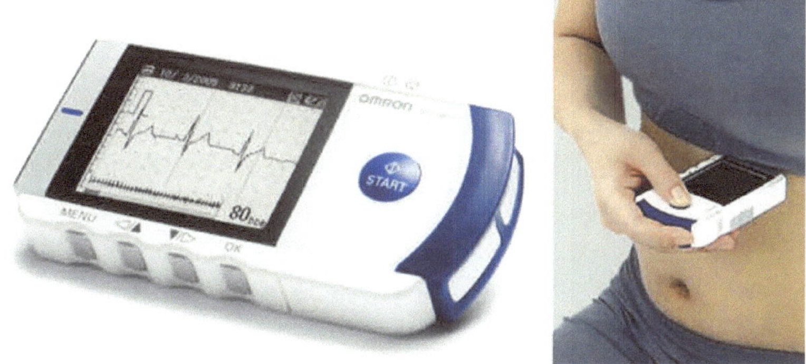

Fig. 1.13 Features of Cardiac Event Recorder

Cardiac Loop Recorder

A loop recorder is a compact USB pen drive sized medical device to monitor the heart function. It can be attached to the surface of the skin around the area of the patient's heart. It continuously records the heart rhythm for a certain duration, depending on the memory capacity of the device and when the device memory is full, it starts overwriting from the beginning of the recording. Hence the name, loop recorder. An event recorder can miss the starting of an abnormal heart activity due to the delay in initiating the record function. A loop recorder has a record button that when pressed can save the immediate few minutes prior to the start of the abnormal heart activity and continue recording for few additional minutes and then stop recording. This way the entire episode is captured and not overwritten. When the patient experiences an abnormality the recorder can be set to automatically record the incident or can manually instruct the device to record the incident. A loop recorder can be worn for many days or weeks (up to 30 days), while the patient goes around the routine day-to-day activities. It can be removed during showering or swimming.

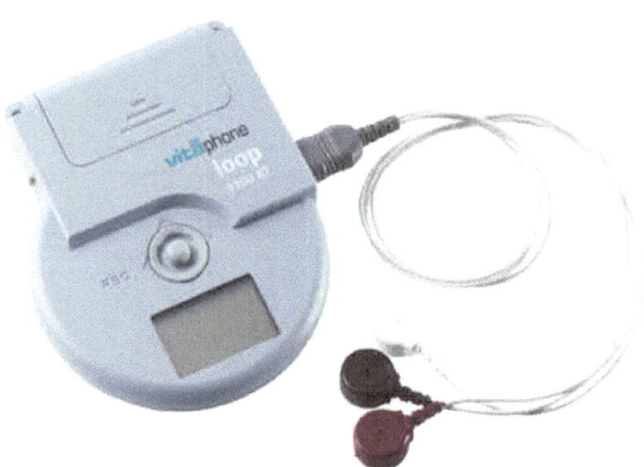

Fig. 1.14 Features of cardiac loop recorder

Implantable Loop Recorder (ILR)

ILR is a miniature loop recorder that can be implanted between the chest skin and the rib cage, above the heart. Like the loop recorder it can be programmed to automatically start recording when an abnormality is detected is detected in the heart rhythm.

It can also be activated by an external trigger device that the patient can carry around in the form of a wrist band or a remote control. This is more suitable for patients who experience symptoms that cannot be monitored easily within the 30 days' period of a normal external loop recorder. The device can have a battery life of up to 3 years and is very suitable for long term continuous monitoring in high-risk patients.

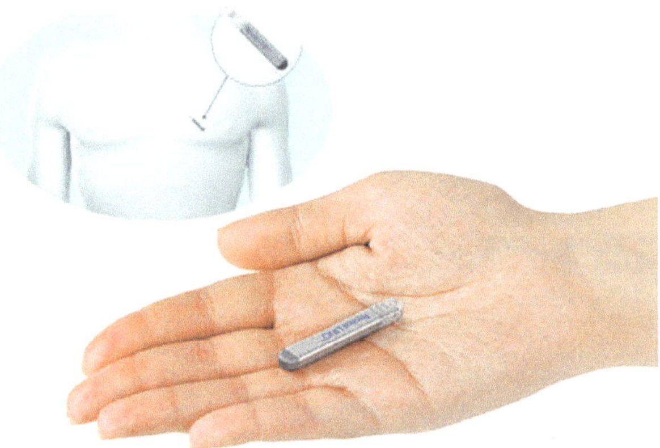

Fig. 1.15 Features of implantable loop recorder (ILR)

Standard 12-lead ECG in a Telecardiology Consultation Service

Telecardiology is one of the oldest applications in telemedicine, and has been largely applied during the last 10-20 years. Telecardiology encompasses a wide variety of applications and is one of the fastest-growing fields in telemedicine. Telecardiology in some fields such as emergency and chronic care undoubtedly improves

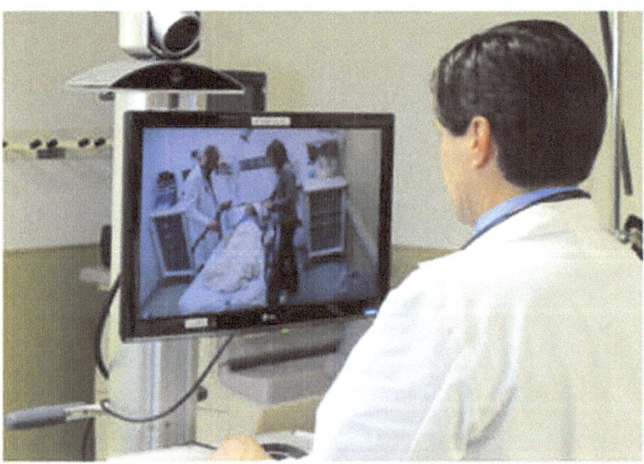

Fig. 1.16 The patient is being monitored in ICCU in a remote center through tele-cardiology system

the quality of health care and helps to contain rising costs. ECG consultations between general practitioners and specialists encompass a wider spectrum of clinical entities, including non-urgent patient care. An internet-based telecardiology centre for ECG consultations have been established globally, including India . The centre provides physicians with comprehensive ECG consultations, including description of the ECG findings, case urgency, need for further examinations, and recommendations for therapeutic strategy, like changes in medication or need for hospital admission.

Fetal Electrocardiography

Monitoring the baby's heart using electrocardiography (ECG) plus cardiotocography (CTG) during labor provides some modest help for mothers and babies when continuous monitoring is needed. Strong uterine contractions during labor reduce the flow of maternal blood to the placenta. The umbilical cord may also be compressed during labor, especially if the membranes are ruptured. Usually the baby has sufficient reserve to withstand this effect but some may become distressed. Electronic heart monitoring may be suggested if the doctors think the baby is not getting enough oxygen during labor. Two different methods may be used. CTG measures the baby's heart rate together with the mother's uterine contractions. An ECG measures the heart's electrical activity and the pattern of the heart beats. This involves an electrode being passed through the woman's cervix and attached to the baby's head. This review of six randomised controlled trials, including a total of 16,295 women, found that monitoring the baby using ECG plus CTG resulted in fewer blood samples needing to be taken from the baby's scalp, and less surgical assistance with the birth, than with CTG alone. There was no difference in the number of caesarean deliveries and little to suggest that babies were in better condition at birth.

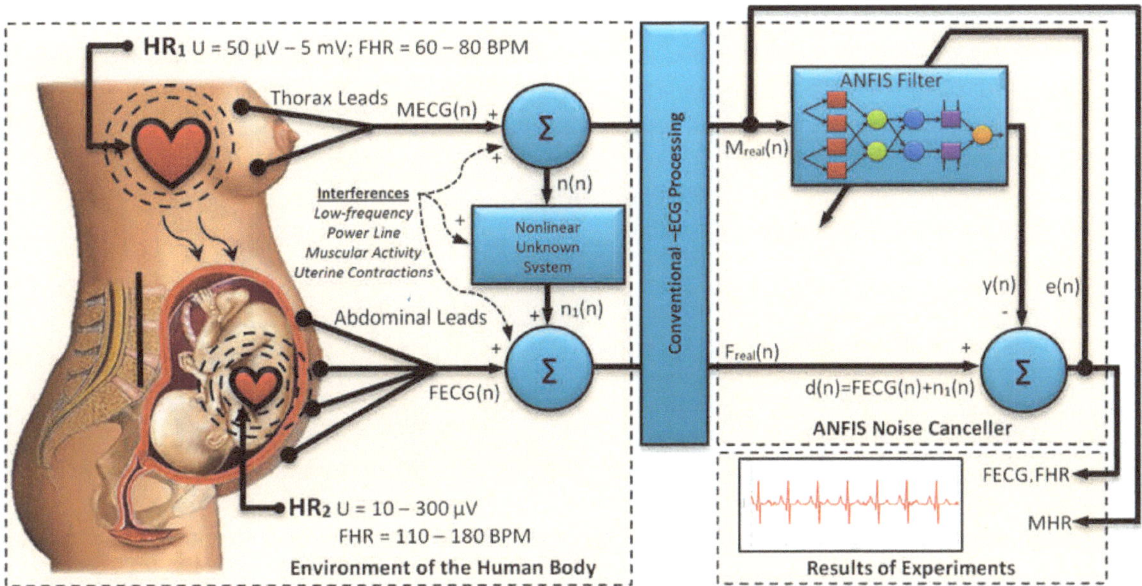

Fig. 1.17 The experimental system designed for ECG monitoring using adaptive neuro-fuzzy inference systems (ANFIS)

Immediately after an ECG procedure

The electrodes are removed. An ECG is completely painless and non-invasive, as the skin is in no way penetrated. The doctor can interpret the results of your ECG straightaway, based on your medical history, symptoms and clinical examination.

Risks in Performing Electrocardiogram

An electrocardiogram is a safe procedure. There may be minor discomfort, similar to removing a bandage, when the electrodes taped to your chest to measure your heart's electrical signals are removed. Rarely, a reaction to the electrodes may cause redness or swelling of the skin.A stress test, in which an ECG is performed while you exercise or after you take medication that mimics effects of exercise, may cause irregular heartbeats or, rarely, a heart attack. These side effects are caused by the exercise or medication, not the ECG itself. There is not any risk of electrocution during an electrocardiogram. The electrodes placed on your body only record the electrical activity of your heart. They don't emit electricity.

New 80-lead ECG System Helps Detect Silent Myocardial Infarct

Saint Francis Hospital in Evanston, Ill. had become the first hospital in Illinois to offer the new PRIME ECG made by Heartscape Technologies, which has a disposable vest containing 80 electrocardiogram leads that detect heart rhythm and blockages in 360-degrees of the heart.

The new vest is expected to help identify heart attacks that might otherwise go undiagnosed. Traditional ECG tests contain only 12-leads that are applied only to the front of a patient's torso and can not monitor electrical impulses in the back or side areas of the heart, which may have undetected blockages and may be the source of chest pain. With the new ECG test, in 10 minutes or less, physicians will know more about the patient and the patient's heart condition than ever before, the hospital said.

PRIME ECG provides physicians with a full 360-degree view of the heart's arteries, without surgical intervention, and can more rapidly and accurately identify closed arteries that might go unnoticed using traditional ECG equipment. Clinical research has shown that the use of large numbers of electrode sites about the front, sides and posterior of the torso provides valuable diagnostic information that can lead to earlier diagnosis for many acute coronary syndrome (ACS) patients. This procedure has traditionally been called body surface mapping (BSM).

"The 80-lead ECG is the next step in advancing emergency cardiac care. Traditional tests do not detect all heart attacks or heart muscle damage or blockages in all patients. This test is an additional safeguard that can be used on patients experiencing chest pain who have tests that are otherwise normal," said Shahriar Dadkhah, M.D., FACC, cardiologist and director of cardiology research at Saint Francis Hospital.

Dr. Dadkhan said the test can catch about 20 out 100 silent heart attacks, which would otherwise go undetected with 12-lead ECG equipment.

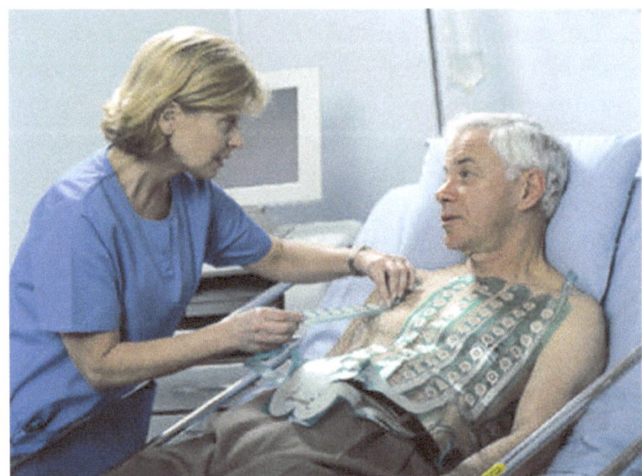

Fig.1.18 The nurse is applying PRIME ECG vest over the chest containing 80 electrocardiogram leads that detect heart rhythm and blockages in 360-degrees of the heart.

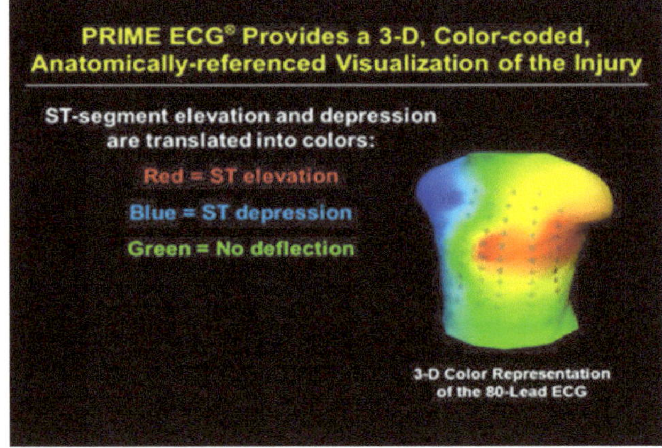

Fig.1.19 The application of PRIME ECG vest over the chest provides a 3-D color-coded, anatomically–referenced visualization of myocardial injury

HeartSciences MyoVista ECG Device Shows Promise in Detecting Abnormal Cardiac Function

Device uses continuous wavelet transform signal processing and artificial intelligence to predict left ventricular diastolic dysfunction

HeartSciences announced the results of a clinical study of its electrocardiography device that applies continuous wavelet transform signal processing and artificial intelligence. The study was serially conducted at The Icahn School of Medicine, Mount Sinai Hospital, New York, N.Y., and the West Virginia University (WVU) Heart and Vascular Institute, Morgantown, W. Va. The results were published online and in the April 17, 2018 issue of *Journal of the American College of Cardiology* (*JACC*).

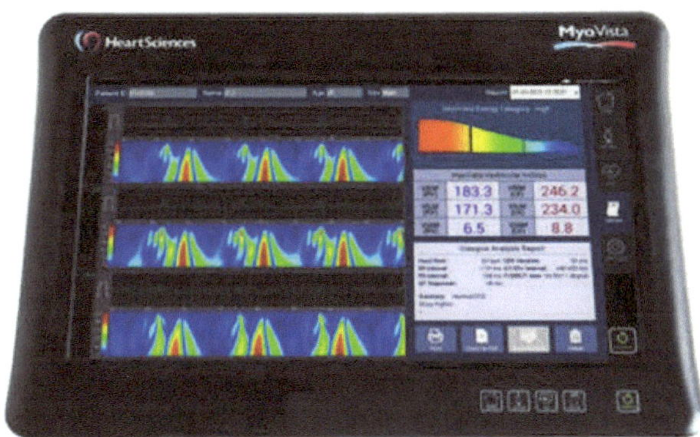

Fig.1.20 Electrocardiography device that applies continuous wavelet transform signal processing and artificial intelligence for the "Prediction of Abnormal Myocardial Relaxation from Signal Processed Surface ECG

The article titled "Prediction of Abnormal Myocardial Relaxation from Signal Processed Surface ECG" presents the results from the investigator-initiated clinical study that focused on evaluating the feasibility of MyoVista Wavelet ECG (wavECG) as a diagnostic tool for predicting myocardial relaxation abnormalities. Abnormal relaxation is an early feature of many types of heart disease and a key characteristic of left ventricular diastolic dysfunction (LVDD).

It is typically detected using echocardiographic imaging. LVDD is a strong predictor of cardiovascular and all-cause mortality.1 Ischemia, hypertension, diabetes, valvular disease and reduced systolic function are all associated with LVDD.

Results from the feasibility study demonstrate MyoVista patented technology can detect myocardial relaxation abnormalities associated with LVDD. The study results demonstrated 80 percent sensitivity and 84 percent specificity, with an area under the curve of 91 percent for the prediction of low (e'), an echocardiographic parameter widely used in determination of LVDD. Prediction of low (e') also correctly identified 23 out of 28 study subjects (82 percent) with significant underlying coronary artery disease. Additionally, MyoVista wavECG prediction of relaxation abnormalities also allowed recognition of subjects with more advanced stages of DD and concurrent CAD with significantly more incremental value compared with clinical variables and conventional ECG information.

What results can be expected from the procedure

Your doctor will look for a consistent, even heart rhythm and a heart rate between 50 and 100 beats a minute. Having a faster, slower or irregular heartbeat provides clues about your heart health, including:

Heart rate. Normally, heart rate can be measured by checking your pulse. But an ECG may be helpful if your pulse is difficult to feel or too fast or too irregular to count accurately.

Heart rhythm. An ECG can help your doctor identify an unusually fast heartbeat (tachycardia), unusually slow heartbeat (bradycardia) or other heart rhythm irregularities (arrhythmias). These conditions may occur when any part of the heart's electrical system malfunctions. In other cases, medications, such as beta blockers, psychotropic drugs or amphetamines, can trigger arrhythmias.

Heart attack. An ECG can often show evidence of a previous heart attack or one that's in progress. The patterns on the ECG may indicate which part of your heart has been damaged, as well as the extent of the damage.

Inadequate blood and oxygen supply to the heart. An ECG done while you're having symptoms can help your doctor determine whether chest pain is caused by reduced blood flow to the heart muscle, such as with the chest pain of unstable angina.

Structural abnormalities. An ECG can provide clues about enlargement of the chambers or walls of the heart, heart defects and other heart problems.

What can you expect at home?

The patient can resume normal activities immediately. The ECG is non-invasive and doesn't involve medications (such as anesthetics) or require recovery time.

Here are a few trends to watch for in electrocardiogram (ECG, or if you prefer the original German EKG) systems. The biggest advancement in ECG systems in recent years has been the movement to greater interoperability and digital formats. But other technologies are beginning to be integrated into ECG systems, such as aids to properly place leads, artificial intelligence and a ways to extract additional information from ECGs to increase diagnostic value.

Here are some trends in these newer ECG systems:

ECG Systems Moving to Full Digital Formats

In the past decade, ECG systems have moved from technology that was largely not compatible with different vendors' cardiology reporting systems or electronic medical record (EMR) systems. The main focus of older generation systems was on a paper printout, but today's systems now require easy IT interface, compatibility and digitally stored waveforms to be compatible with increasingly paperless hospitals that use the EMR to access

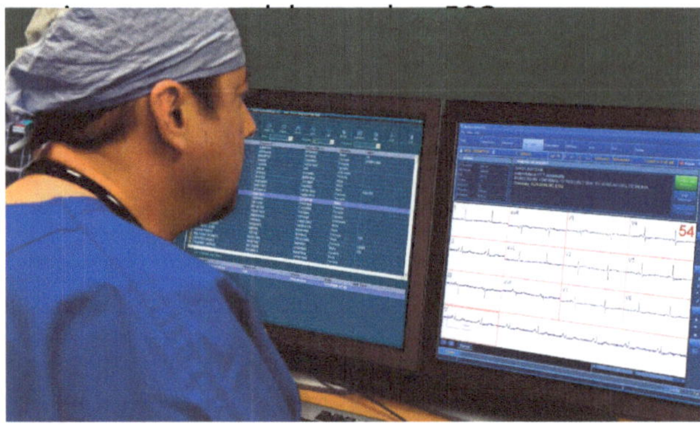

Fig.1.21 ECG Systems Moving to Full Digital Formats

The movement to digital formats has allowed the use of digital calipers and waveform analysis algorithms. It also enables electronic storage and communications of the data with the patient's electronic medical record. Automation to help speed the reading the waveforms and report on them is also offered by some vendors. Digital ECG management and reporting systems also have become standard features on all cardiovascular information systems (CVIS). For this reason, many ECG systems and ECG management systems now offer vendor-agnostic integration with other vendors' ECG system data.

Many of the major vendors in the ECG market sell multiple types of systems that are aimed at different markets, from smaller and less sophisticated versions, to premium systems.

This is to address the different needs of a large, busy, urban hospital which are not the same as those of physician offices or small remote sites.

Technology to Aid ECG Lead Placement Assistance

Improper lead placement in clinics and offices can be an issue leading to poor ECGs. Schiller offers a solution to this issue with its Cardiovit FT-1 ECG system. It has a 3-D rendering of a patient on the device's screen, which shows where each lead needs to be placed. The user can rotate the images on the touch screen to see where the leads go and can easily identify where any issues are when the system automatically alerts them about misplaced leads. The goal is to improve the speed and accuracy of ECGs using a better form of visualization than the traditional black and white 2-D pictures. The system changes the lead placements of the body rendering based on the type of exam being performed using a drop down menu.

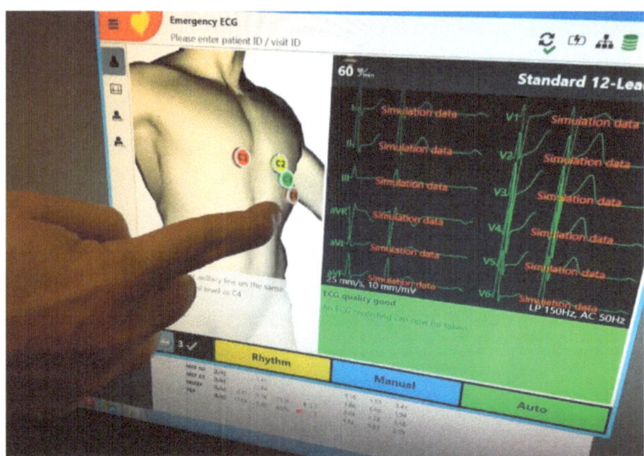

Fig.1.22 ECG System Uses 3-D Interactive Image to Show Proper Lead Placements

Wavelet ECG In Development May Offer New Data for Cardiac Diagnostics

Start-up company HeartSciences has been developing a new type of ECG system that may offer a new way of looking at the heart. Rather than the basic electrical activity waveforms standard ECG has used for a century, the MyoVista Wavelet ECG (wavECG) system uses continuous wavelet transform (CWT) signal processing to provide new frequency and energy information

These colorful waveforms offer more data and can be used to detect cardiac relaxation abnormalities associated with left ventricular diastolic dysfunction (LVDD). The company says its research shows that almost all forms and co-morbidities of heart disease are associated with LVDD, including hypertension, diabetes, valvular disease, ischemia and reduced systolic function.

The MyoVista wavECG uses AI-based algorithms to analyze the data from the transformed ECG signal using continuous wavelet signal processing. The AI categorizes the overall wavECG analysis as either "Normal," "Borderline" or "Abnormal" for risk of abnormal LV relaxation.

The MyoVista is designed to be a low-cost electrocardiographic testing system to provide physicians with new information to improve patient risk-assessment related to heart disease. The MyoVista Device also provides all the information and capabilities of a full-featured conventional resting 12-lead ECG within the same test.

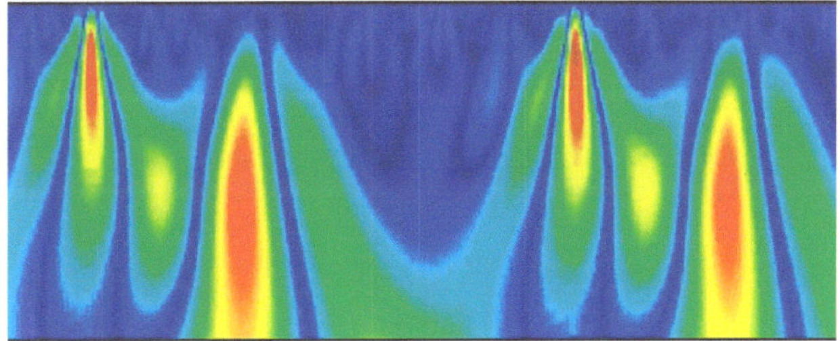

Fig.1.23 MyoVista Wavelet ECG (wavECG) system uses continuous wavelet transform (CWT) signal processing to provide new frequency and energy information

AI Integration Into ECG

Like many facets of healthcare, artificial intelligence is being developed to aid ECG interpretation. Artificial intelligence (AI) can examine ECG waveforms to pinpoint patients at higher risk of developing a potentially dangerous arrhythmia or of dying within the next year. The AI can take a deeper dive to extract more information out of the waveforms that may not be apparent, even for an experienced reader. Several such studies have been presented at the American Heart Association (AHA) meeting over the past two years and published in cardiology journals. These types of algorithms will likely be seen appearing as options on the next generations of ECG systems.

In November 2020, the FDA cleared AliveCor's next generation of interpretive AI-based personal electrocardiogram (ECG) algorithms for its Kardia device to detect atrial fibrillation and a wide range of cardiac conditions.

ECG Market Leading Vendors Move Toward Vendor Neutral Interfaces

One of the big issues for larger hospitals or healthcare systems several years ago was the lack of interoperability between ECG systems and ECG management systems because many operated using proprietary programing. In the last few years, many vendors have moved toward using open platform standards that are easier to interface with other vendors' technology, including use of DICOM format waveforms and HL7 IT interfaces.

The ECG market has many vendors, but it is dominated by six big companies: GE Healthcare, Philips Healthcare, Nihon Kohden Corp., Medtronic, Spacelabs Healthcare and Schiller AG. Combined, these companies had more than 55 percent of the ECG market share in 2018, according to the healthcare market research firm DataM Intelligence.

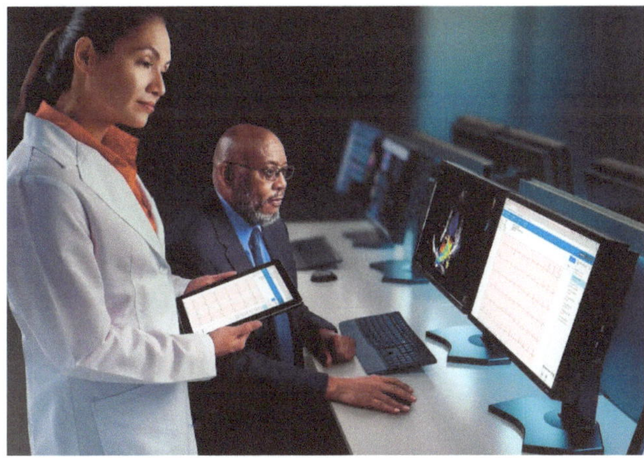

Fig.1.24 ECG System using DICOM format waveforms and HL7 IT interfaces.

GE Healthcare is a good example of a vendor that has undergone change to increase interoperability because of complaints from customers. While GE has held a large portion of the ECG market share, prior to 2016 the vendor required hospitals to use GE ECG systems and the GE Muse ECG management system to guarantee interoperability. To solve this, GE introduced a new version of Muse in 2016 that allowed greater connectivity with other vendors' ECG systems,including newer, adhesive-based wearable Holter and event monitors

Hill-Rom Holdings has built a strong ECG business over the last six years by purchasing two major ECG vendors. It acquired Welch Allyn in 2015 for $2.05 billion, and in 2017 acquired Mortara Instrument for $330 million. Hill-Rom's goal has been to build patient monitoring systems that offer best-in-class ability to integrate with various vendors' EMR systems.

The main diagnostic ECG market is made up of 12-lead resting ECG systems. This is followed by stress ECG systems and then the remote cardiac monitor segment, which included Holter monitors and cardiac event monitors. Today, all of these devices should be able to integrate into a central ECG management system or they will face replacement.

The Need to Record and Interpret Consumer-grade ECGs in the Future

In the past 5 years, there has been an explosion in wearable and handheld ECG enabled devices and smartphone apps that allow anyone to record a 1-6 lead ECG. There also has been a lot of interest by cardiologists in these systems, like the AliveCor Kardia device or the Ekos ECG-enabled stethoscope. These systems are seen as a fast and easy way to better triage patients and get immediate information before sending a patient for more involved exams

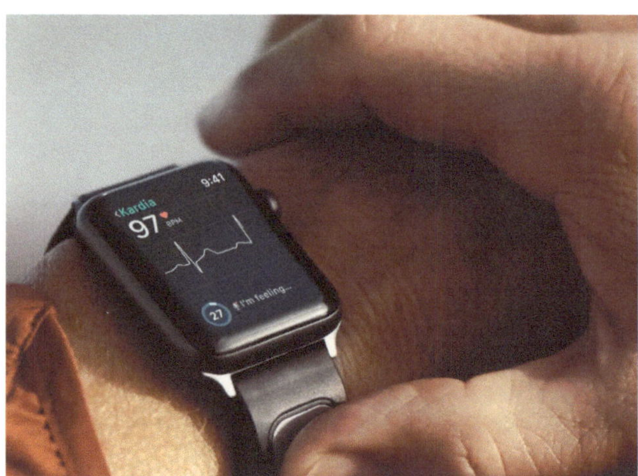

Fig.1.25 The AliveCor Kardia device or the Ekos ECG-enabled stethoscope.

The Kardia device allows iPhones, or directly through the Kardia watch, to record a 30-second ECG strip and AI algorithms, then automatically assess the waveforms for various arrhythmias. These waveforms and interpretation can then be e-mailed to the person's doctor.

The newer generation of implantable cardiac monitors like the Medtronic LINQ, and numerous wearable, clinical-grade, stick-on cardiac monitors now offer interfaces with patients' mobile devices so they can mark events. This data also is transmitted to a physician's office or automated ECG remote monitoring system.

In the coming years, all of these types of ECG data will likely need to be integrated into ECG management systems to allow for a complete picture of the patient's cardiac history. This is part of a larger movement that was included in the Affordable Care Act (ACA) requirements that look to get patients more involved as a participant in their own care. Now that the technology exists and is proliferating, the question is how and where to integrate this data into the patient record.

Artificial Intelligence Examining ECGs Predicts Irregular Heartbeat, Death Risk

Two studies presented at AHA, from the same group of researchers, are among the first to use artificial intelligence to predict future events from an ECG rather than to detect current health problems

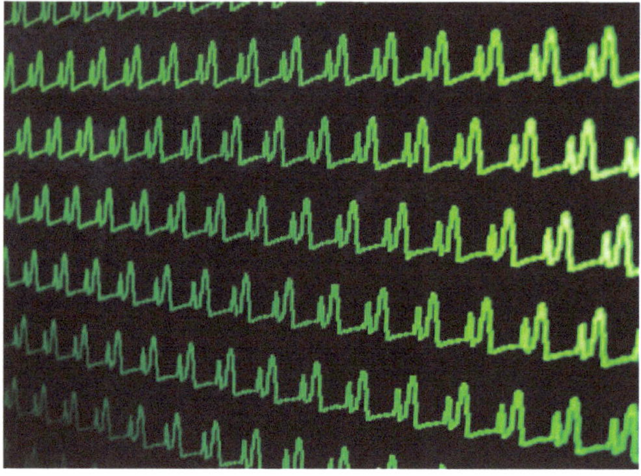

Fig.1.26 showing as how Artificial intelligence can examine electrocardiogram (ECG) test

Artificial intelligence can examine electrocardiogram (ECG) test results, a common medical test, to pinpoint patients at higher risk of developing a potentially dangerous irregular heartbeat (arrhythmia) or of dying within the next year, according to two preliminary studies to presented at the American Heart Association's Scientific Sessions 2019 — November 16-18 in Philadelphia.

BIBLIOGRAPHY AND ACKNOWLEDGEMENT

- Ades P A. Grunvald MH: Cardio-pulmonary exercise testing before and after conditioning in older coronary patients, Am. Heart J. 1990, 120 : 585-589.
- Ades PAt Waldmann ML. Gillespie C. A controlled trial of exercise training in older coronary patients. 1.Genontol A BioI. Sci Med. Sci. 1995, 50 A: M7-MlI.
- Armon Y. Cooper DM, Flores R, Zanconato S. Basstow TJ. Oxygen uptake dynamics during high intensity exercise in children and adults. 1. Apply Physiol., 1991, 70 : 841-848.
- Attia, Z.I., et al., Screening for cardiac contractile dysfunction using an artificial intelligence-enabled electrocardiogram. Nat Med, 2019. 25(1): p. 70-74.
- Becker RC. Alpert JS: Electrocardiographic ST segment depression in coronary heart disease. Am Heart J 1988; 1I5 : 862- 868. Berger RD, Akselrod S, Gordon D, Cohen RJ. An efficient algorithm for spectral analysis of heart rate variability. IEEE TBME 1986;9:900-904.
- British Columbia Guidelines and Protocols; Ambulatory ECG Monitoring (Holter Monitor and Patient-Activated Event Recorder). 2004 (Revised 2007).ACP/ACC/AHA Task Force on Exercise Testing. JACC 1990; 16(5): 1061-1065.
- Gerson MC, McHenry PL. Resting U wave inversion as a marker of stenosis of the left anterior descending coronary artery. Am J Med. 1980 Oct;69(4):545-50. PMID: 7424944
- Girish MP, Gupta MD, Mukhopadhyay S, Yusuf J, Sunil Roy TN, Trehan V. U wave: an important noninvasive electrocardiographic diagnostic marker. Indian Pacing Electrophysiol J. 2005 Jan 1;5(1):63-5.
- Jenkins HML. Thirty years of electronic intrapartum fetal heart rate monitoring: discussion paper. J R Soc Med 1989 Apr; 82(4):210-214.
- Kennedy RG. Electronic fetal heart rate monitoring: retrospective reflections on a twentieth-century technology. J R Soc Med 1998 May; 91(5): 244–250.
- Kowey PR, Kocovic DZ; Cardiology patient pages. Ambulatory electrocardiographic recording. Circulation. 2003 Aug 5;108(5):e31-3.
- Misra, S., et al., Initial validation of a novel ECGI system for localization of premature ventricular contraction sand ventricular tachycardia
- Neilson JP. Fetal electrocardiogram (ECG) for fetal monitoring during labour. Cochrane Database Syst Rev. 2012 Apr 18;4
- Novotny, T., et al., Data analysis of diagnostic accuracies in 12-lead electrocardiogram interpretation by junior medical fellows. JElectrocardiol,2015.48(6):p.988-94.
- Oudijk MA, Kwee A, Visser GH, Blad S, Meijboom EJ, Rosén KG. The effects of intrapartum hypoxia on the fetal QT interval. BJOG2004Jul;111(7)656-660.
- Phibbs, BP. Advanced ECG: Boards and Beyond (2nd edition), SaundersElsevier2006.
- Rajaganeshan, R., et al., Accuracy in ECG lead placement among technicians, nurses, general physicians and cardiologists. International Journal of Clinical Practice, 2008. 62(1): p. 65-70.
- Sameni R, Clifford GD. A review of fetal ECG signal processing; issues and promising directions. Open Pacing ElectrophysiolTherJ.2010Jan;3:4–20.
- Surawicz B, Knilans T. Chou's Electrocardiography in Clinical Practice (6th edition), Saunders 2008.
- Terkelsen CJ, Nørgaard BL, Lassen JF, Gerdes JC, Ankersen JP, Rømer F, et al. Telemedicine used for remote prehospital diagnosing in patients suspected of acute myocardial infarction. JInternMed.2002;252:412-20.
- van Dam, P.M., et al., New Computer Program for detecting 12 Lead ECG Misplacement using a 3D Kinect Camera, in Computing in cardiology, A. Murray, Editor. 2013
- van Dam, P.M., T.F. Oostendorp, and A. van Oosterom, ECGSIM: Interactive Simulation of the ECG for Teaching and Research Purposes. Computing in Cardiology 2010. 37:
- Wagner, GS. Marriott's Practical Electrocardiography (11th edition), Lippincott Williams & Wilkins 2007.
- WillemEinthovenBiography.https://www.tue.nl/en/university/departments/biomedical-engineering

Advances in Echocardiography

CHAPTER 2

More than 60 years have passed since Inge Edler and Hellmuth Hertz began using M-mode echocardiography as a diagnostic tool for cardiovascular disease in 1953 .Over the past 60 years, echocardiography has evolved from a simple M-mode imaging technique to an array of technologies that include two-dimensional (2D) imaging, pulsed and continuous wave Doppler, color flow and tissue Doppler, transesophageal echocardiography, and three-dimensional (3D) echocardiography Although 3D technique has changed rapidly in recent years, and the time needed for 3D image acquisition and analysis has gradually decreased ,it is still difficult to incorporate 3D echocardiography into daily clinical practice. Hence, 2D echocardiography remains the first-choice imaging technique in clinical use. When 2D echocardiography is used to assess left ventricular volume and systolic function, good image quality with clear visualization of endocardial border is required for accurate assessment of left ventricular volume and function .However, suboptimal image quality is estimated to occur in approximately 20% of all patients undergoing echocardiography. Suboptimal image quality may lead to misdiagnosis or the need for additional, often unnecessary, and costly tests. In order to overcome this problem, novel 2D echocardiographic imaging technologies have been introduced in recent years, which have significantly enhanced the image quality of 2D echocardiography. In addition, new on-cart 3D quantification software can greatly reduce the analysis time for 3D volume quantification and facilitate the incorporation of 3D quantitative analysis into daily examination workflow. The following is a general overview of two new echocardiographic technologies.

Echocardiography is a well-established imaging modality that plays a pivotal role in the evaluation of patients with known or suspected heart disease. Over the past 45 years, the technique has evolved from a simple M-mode tracing to a family of technologies that include two-dimensional (2D) imaging, pulsed and continuous wave spectral Doppler, color flow Doppler, tissue Doppler, and transesophageal echocardiography (TEE)).The combined use of these modalities allows a comprehensive anatomic and functional evaluation of cardiac chambers, the pericardium, ascending and descending aorta, and native or prosthetic valves. The conversion more than 10 years ago of analog to digital signal processing revolutionized the field of ultrasound. Instruments became smaller, image resolution progressively improved, and digital image storage allowed for more accurate quantification and comparison with previous studies. It also opened the door for exciting new door for exciting new developments in transducer technology and digital image processing, giving birth to newer advances such as harmonic imaging, automated border detection and quantification, 3-dimensional (3D) imaging, and speckle tracking. In addition, miniaturization of instruments now allows physicians to examine patients at the bedside and render a more accurate diagnosis than that provided by physical examination. In this article, we will provide a brief discussion of some of these newer developments and their promising applications.

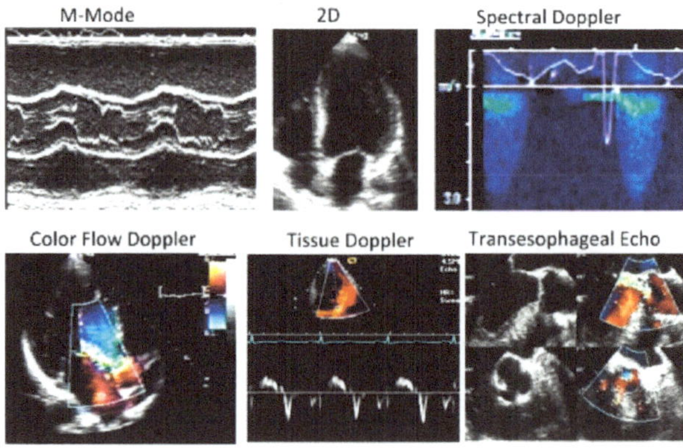

Fig.2.1 Images of the common echocardiography and Doppler modalities used in cardiac ultrasound

Advances in Image Quality and Border Detection

The quality of echocardiographic images is dependent on the expertise of the sonographer and also on the body size and habitus of the patient. Improvements in transducer technology, digital image acquisition, and computer processing are providing better image quality in the difficult patient. However, there is still a sizeable subgroup of patients with suboptimal images that do not allow accurate cavity measurements to be made. Certain ultrasound contrast agents consist of stable microbubbles that reflect ultrasound waves and are small enough to cross the pulmonary capillaries when injected intravenously. These agents, when administered intravenously, opacify the left ventricle (LV) and provide a clear delineation of the cavity-endocardial border, thus improving the accuracy of LV volumes and ejection fraction (EF) determination.1 Because microbubbles are easily destroyed by ultrasound energy, performance of contrast imaging requires optimization of several settings in the ultrasound machine and the use of a low mechanical index (the setting that controls ultrasound power). Newer pulse sequencing technology has been developed that recognizes and processes the unique nonlinear fundamental and high-order harmonic signals generated by the reflected microbubbles. This results in improved sensitivity and a stronger contrast signal that provides excellent recognition of the cavity-endocardial border .

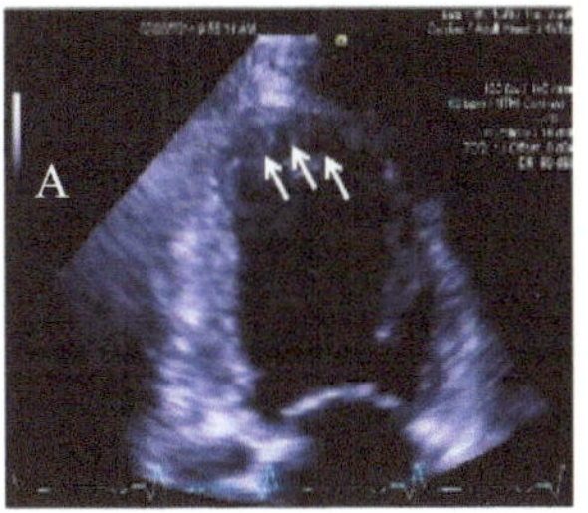

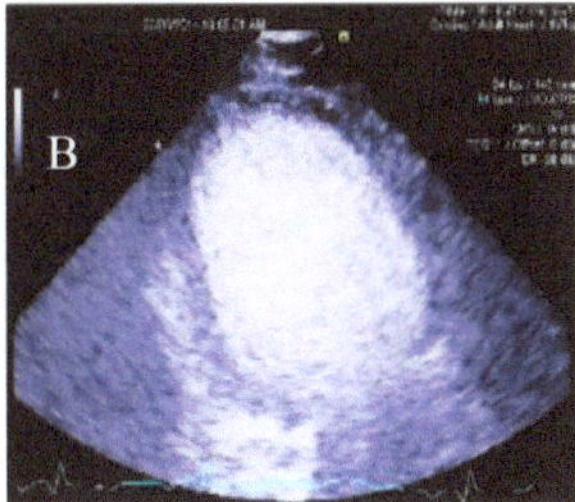

Fig 2.2 Contrast echocardiography using pulse sequencing technology performed in a patient with a dilated cardiomyopathy in whom there was suspicion of a thrombus at the apex (Panel A; arrows). Note in Panel B the excellent contrast effect that fills the entire LV cavity excluding the presence of a mass. Also note the contrast effect within the myocardium resulting from micro bubbles within the capillary circulation.

Automated gain control simplifies the process of acquiring images while optimizing gain settings for a particular window of examination. These improvements have facilitated detection of endocardial borders that, when combined with new pattern recognition technology, allow the system to automatically perform measurements of dimensions, area, and spectral Doppler velocities.When properly used, this improves the accuracy and reproducibility of measurements as well as patient flow in a busy clinical laboratory.

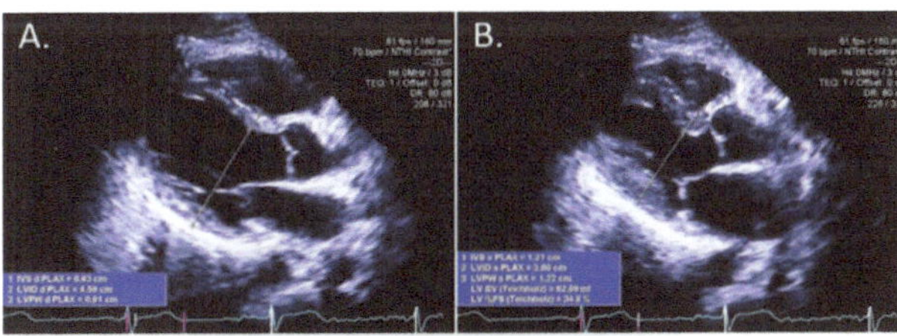

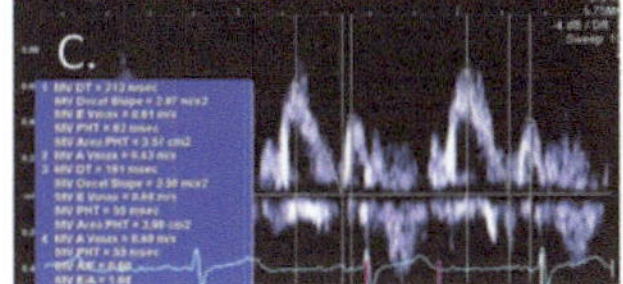

Fig 2.3 Panels A and B show end-diastolic and end-systolic frames, respectively, of a 2-dimensional echo parasternal view of the left ventricle, illustrating automatic measurements of left ventricular dimensions using a new pattern recognition technology. Panel C shows the same technology applied to pulsed-wave spectral Doppler

Advances in 3-Dimensional Echocardiography

Commercial ultrasound systems with 3D capability have been available for the past 8 to 10 years and have included both transthoracic and TEE transducers. Despite this, the modality has been slow to get incorporated into routine clinical use,, with the possible exception of 3D TEE, which has gained popularity in the evaluation of mitral valve pathology and in guiding complex interventional catheter procedures The promise of 3D was that it could shorten the time of an examination by taking one or two volumetric acquisitions from which multiple 2D and 3D views could be reconstructed. However, limitations in processing time reduce the size of the volumetric acquisition. Consequently, several acquisitions over multiple cardiac cycles have to be stitched together to construct a 3D image of the entire LV. This often results in image artifacts.. Furthermore, transducer technology has lagged behind image processing technology, thus limiting the quality of the images, particularly in patients with less than perfect image quality. This has also limited the quality of 3D color flow and has kept the technique from being routinely used to evaluate structural abnormalities and valve function. Despite these limitations, 3D provides automated quantification of LV volumes and EF. The results obtained can be quite accurate if the examination is properly performed and the patient has good image quality. However, in the absence of either of these, the results can be highly inaccurate and, if accepted by the interpreting physician, can lead to the wrong clinical decision.

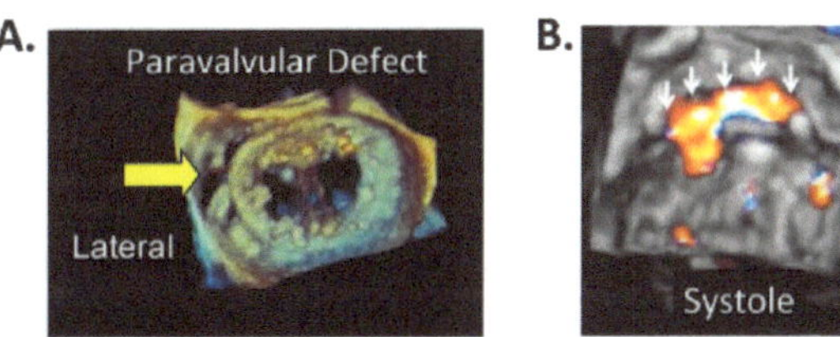

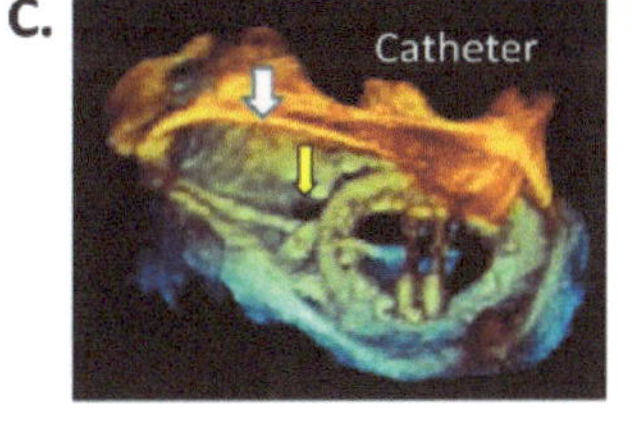

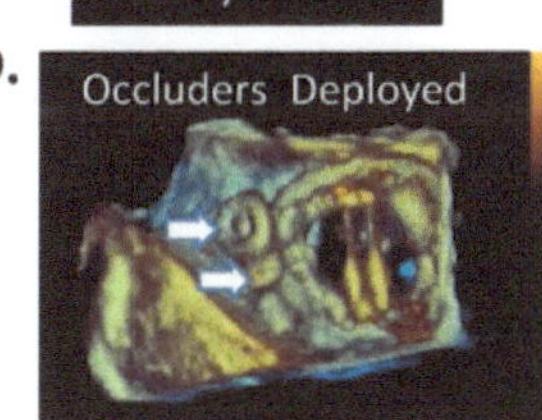

Fig 2.4 Three-dimensional echocardiography images obtained by TEE during an intervention to close a large paravalvular defect in a mechanical mitral prosthesis (yellow arrow). A reconstruction of the defect using 3D color Doppler is shown on panel B (arrows). Panel C illustrates placement of the guide wire (white arrow) across the defect (yellow arrow), which required making a loop in the left atrium and was guided by 3D. Panel D shows an image taken at the conclusion of the procedure demonstrating the two occluders in place. TEE: transthoracic echocardiogram; 3D: 3-dimensional

More recent advances in transducer technology combined with fast processors allow for a single 3D cardiac cycle acquisition with superior time resolution that should provide more reproducible and accurate quantification of LV volumes and EF.It should also improve the overall assessment of valvular structures.In addition to quantification of LV volumes, there are two other 3D applications that deserve mentioning. The first is quantifying the severity of mitral regurgitation (MR) by measuring the area of the vena contracta with 3D color flow, more often done with TEE . Studies from this institution suggest that this could provide a more accurate assessment of MR severity than current echocardiographic Doppler methods. With the technical improvements mentioned above, we may expect a greater application of this measurement with transthoracic 3D. The second application is to derive simultaneous and selected biplane orthogonal 2D images to facilitate and shorten the time of a TEE examination, especially during TEE-guided catheter interventions

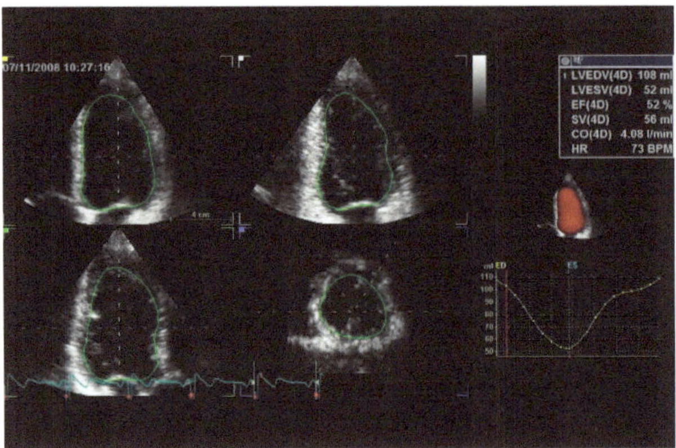

Fig.2.5 Quad view presentation of left ventricular using 4D auto LVQ software for measurement of left ventricular volumes and ejection fraction with three-dimensional echocardiography. Volume time-plot and quantitative analysis and three-dimensional model are presented in the right panel.

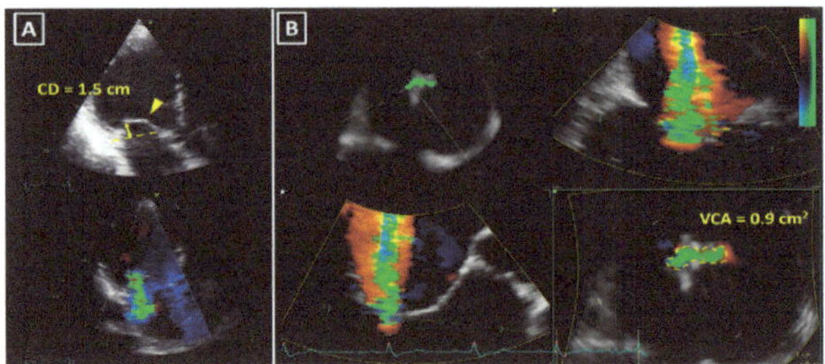

Fig 2.6 3D Vena Contracta Area in Secondary Mitral Regurgitation Full-volume color Doppler 3-dimensional (3D) transthoracic echocardiographic view obtained from a single heartbeat in functional mitral regurgitation (MR). The vena contracta is assessed by use of the cropping planes The frame rate for this single-beat acquisition is 20 volumes per second.

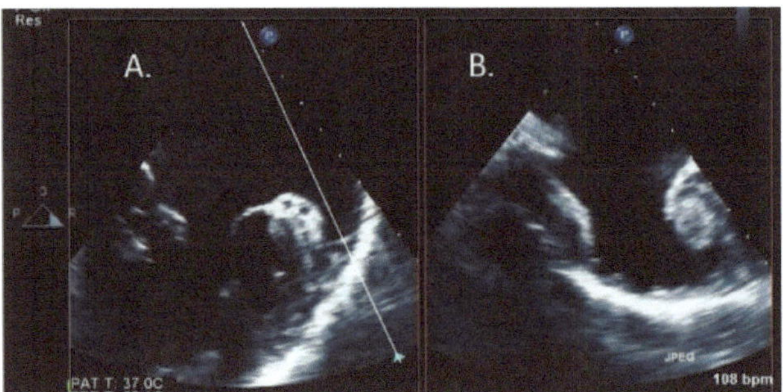

Fig.2.7 Biplane real-time images acquired simultaneously during a 3-dimensional transthoracic echocardiographic examination of the left atrial appendage. The image in Panel B is orthogonal to the plane outlined by the line in Panel A. A thrombus is seen in the left atrial appendage (Panel B).

In addition to quantification of LV volumes, there are two other 3D applications that deserve mentioning. The first is quantifying the severity of mitral regurgitation (MR) by measuring the area of the vena contracta with 3D color flow, more often done with TEE . Studies from this institution suggest that this could provide a more accurate assessment of MR severity than current echocardiographic Doppler methods.3 With the technical improvements mentioned above, we may expect a greater application of this measurement with transthoracic 3D. The second application is to derive simultaneous and selected biplane orthogonal 2D images to facilitate and shorten the time of a TEE examination, especially during TEE-guided catheter interventions

Advances in Strain Imaging

Strain (S) and strain rate (SR) imaging is one of the new promising technologies for the evaluation of cardiac function. Strain is the fractional shortening of two points within the myocardium (i.e., myocardial deformation) that could be aligned with a vector within the subendocardium, midwall, or subepicardium along a circumferential, radial, or longitudinal plane. In the past strain measurements were possible with tissue Doppler, but speckle tracking is now the preferred method due to less noisy signals and higher reproducibility. Speckle tracking is a recent development within the digital matrix of the reflected ultrasound.The system tracks minute speckles of reflected ultrasound throughout the cardiac cycle, measures the change in distance between them throughout systole and diastole, and creates strain and strain rate curve). Speckle tracking echocardiography (STE) is currently available on most ultrasound systems, and the accuracy of strain measurements has been validated in animal and clinical models. The analysis can be performed online as well as offline. Based on image quality and the experience of the analyst, reasonable levels of reproducibility can be attained. A more recent advancement combines 3D with strain imaging, allowing a 3D rendering of the strain vectors.

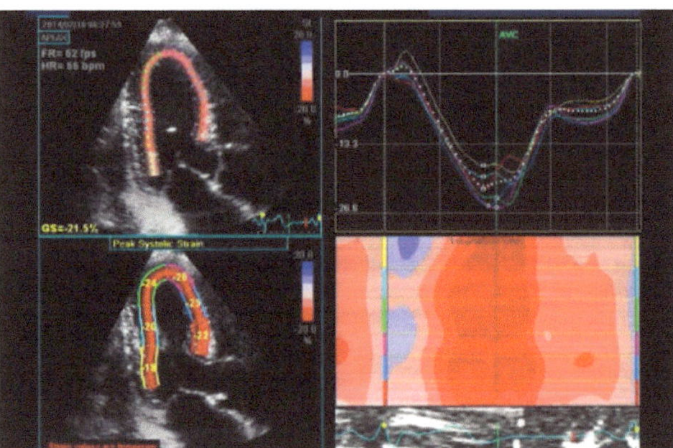

Fig 2.8 Longitudinal strain imaging derived with speckle tracking in an apical long-axis view. Strain is derived along six segments from base to apex. The individual regional strain curves are depicted in the right upper panel with the dotted white line indicating global strain in that view.

Over the past decade, strain measurements have moved from validation studies to clinical applications that include assessment of myocardial function in patients with coronary artery disease (CAD), hypertension, heart failure, valvular heart disease, and cardiomyopathy. Many of these studies have shown a decline in myocardial contractile function with these disorders despite normal EF and absence of symptoms.Furthermore, several studies are showing incremental prognostic value of strain measurements in these diseases. Measurements of strain and strain rate have also been applied to the right ventricle (RV) and left atrium (LA), as preliminary studies suggest they may provide a more accurate assessment of RV and LA function than that available by conventional measurements. Finally, integration of strain curves throughout the cardiac cycle from base to apex is providing insight into the mechanics of LV contraction, the importance of torsion, and the contribution of circumferential and longitudinal strain to LV function.

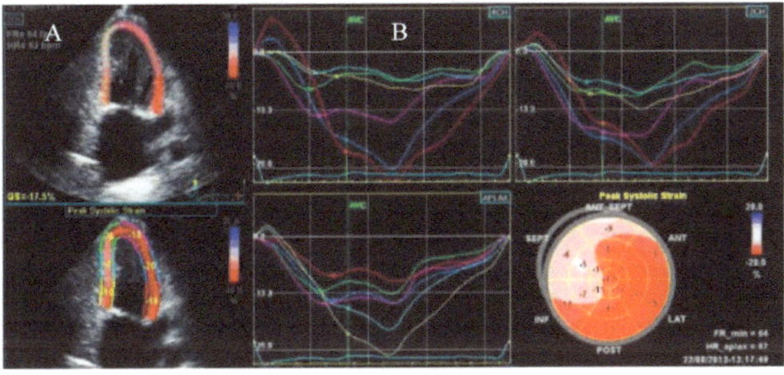

Fig 2.9 Longitudinal strain imaging obtained in a 45-year-old man with severe hypertension, concentric left ventricular hypertrophy, and normal ejection fraction (EF) (> 65%). Panel A shows strain imaging in the apical 2-chamber view. Regional strain curves from the apical 4-chamber, 2-chamber, and long-axis views are illustrated in panel B together with a "bulls-eye" depiction of peak systolic strain in all segments. Note that despite a normal EF, peak systolic strain is diminished in basal and mid septal, anteroseptal and inferior segments as well as in the apical inferior segment.

Several studies in animals and humans have shown abnormal systolic and diastolic deformation in the setting of acute ischemia. More recently, regional changes in diastolic strain were able to identify ischemia several minutes after the acute event. The detection of persistent abnormalities after relief of chest pain is particularly appealing in patients who present after pain resolution with abnormally elevated diastolic transverse strain in the risk area. This initial investigation opens the door for multicenter studies to evaluate which of the available S and SR parameters are the most accurate and reproducible. Notwithstanding the need for such studies, it is conceivable that measurements of S and SR will lead to greater objectivity and reproducibility in assessing regional function than what is currently available with subjective evaluation.Measurements of global longitudinal strain (as well as circumferential strain in some studies) have been shown to provide incremental prognostic information over clinical data,EF, and diastolic indices in patients with a variety of myocardial and valvular diseases. In addition, diastolic strain and strain rate measurements have been applied to assess LV relaxation and estimate filling pressures in patients with normal and depressed EF. LA strain has also been used to estimate LA pressures. Several studies have shown that myocardial imaging can detect abnormal cardiac function in patients with hypertrophic cardiomyopathy (HCM). In these studies, regional and global LV function were evaluated by myocardial S and SR. Reduced diastolic strain is often observed in these patients as well as profound abnormalities in septal and global LV longitudinal strain in the presence of preserved circumferential strain. Thus, it appears that LVEF is preserved by radial and circumferential deformation in HCM patients. Interestingly, the number of segments with abnormal longitudinal strain has been found to be a predictor of nonsustained ventricular tachycardia in this disease and is more accurate than maximum wall thickness and N-terminal pro-brain natriuretic peptide.

LV dysfunction has been increasingly detected with the administration of chemotherapy drugs. This can affect patient care as a drop in EF often influences the decision of whether or not to continue with a given medication. Recent studies in patients receiving chemotherapy have shown a reduction in peak longitudinal strain just before a fall in EF. Preliminary results suggest that the use of beta-blockers and ACE inhibitors during this early stage may prevent progression of LV dysfunction and clinical heart failure in these patients. Larger-scale trials will be needed to determine the role of strain imaging in the management of patients receiving chemotherapy agents.

Despite the promise of this new technology, there are still some limitations that are keeping strain imaging from becoming part of a routine clinical examination. First, acquisition of reliable strain curves requires echocardiographic images of good quality, training, and attention to meticulous technique without which the data loses accuracy and reproducibility. Second, measurements derived from these curves vary among different ultrasound vendors, which limit the establishment of normal ranges. Finally, data are currently lacking regarding how best to use strain measurements in the routine management of a cardiac patient.

Hand-Held Ultrasound Systems

With advancements in digital technology and digital image processing, ultrasound systems became smaller and lighter to where they could be hand-held and carried in a coat pocket. Current hand-held systems provide 2D images and color flow Doppler of diagnostic quality that allow physicians to examine patients at the bedside so they can rapidly assess ventricular and valvular function and screen for pericardial effusion and aortic root pathology. This type of focused examination can hasten the establishment of a cardiac diagnosis assess LV global and regional function, and streamline the selection of patients who will benefit from a comprehensive echocardiographic examination or a referral to another imaging modality. When properly applied, this approach should reduce cost and improve patient care in both the acute and outpatient settings. However, a hand-held instrument in the hands of an inexperienced physician increases the risk of an inaccurate diagnosis that can harm the patient or increase utilization of expensive imaging tests. Therefore, it is essential that any physician using this exciting new modality receives proper training. Preliminary studies suggest that such a level of training is feasible within a reasonable time period. It is not unreasonable to predict that we will soon see physicians trained to use these devices during their residency or even in medical school. In fact, there are some who predict that these instruments will become the "stethoscope of the future."

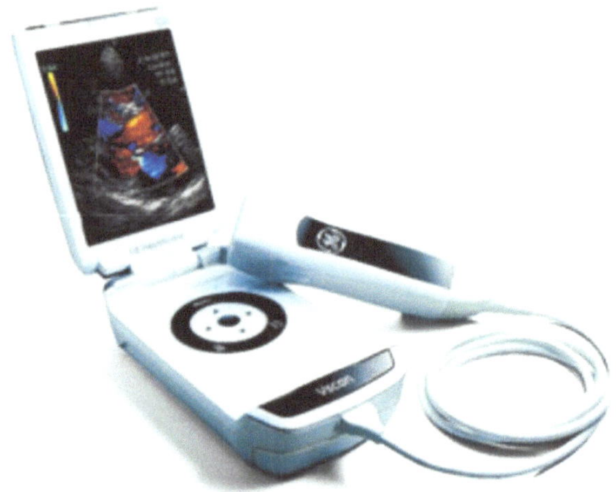

Fig.2.10 A bedside, focus examination of the heart is performed by a physician using a hand-held device.

Adaptive contrast enhancement

Conventional echocardiographic imaging is a hardware-based beamforming technique. After the probe sends out an acoustic beam and receives the returning signals, the beamformer amplifies and digitalizes the signals, and displays them in a horizontal line format. The adaptive contrast enhancement (ACE) algorithm is a software-based beamforming technique that acquires and temporarily stores multiple sequential datasets from each probe element before analyzing it with parallel processors . With the ACE algorithm, the image pixel is observed over a short period of time to determine whether or not data for this pixel originated from a real structure or noise/artifact. This software strengthens the image pixel from the real structure, and suppresses the image pixel from noise or artifact. Then, a high contrast resolution image is obtained When the researchers at the Mount Sinai Icahn School of Medicine, New York, compared echocardiographic images obtained using the ACE algorithm with images obtained using standard hardware-based beamforming techniques, they found that the software-based beamformer technique with ACE algorithm significantly improves the visualization of endocardial borders in the anteroseptal, anterolateral, inferolateral, inferior, anterior, and apical wall segments.They also found that this new technology can reduce medical costs by lessening the need for contrast usage and additional diagnostic testing .

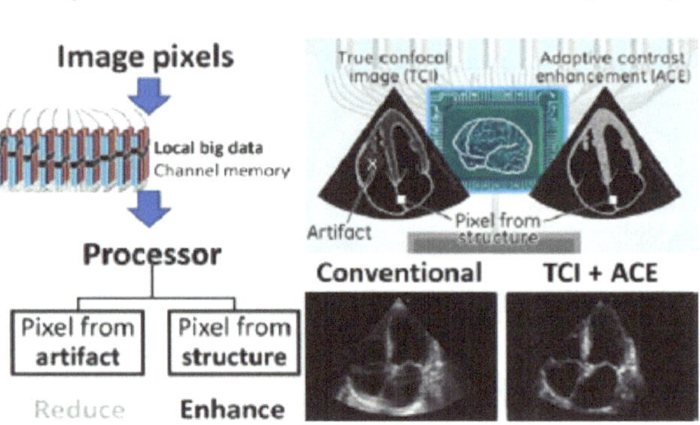

Fig.2.11 Adaptive contrast enhancement (ACE) is a software-based beamforming technique that acquires and temporarily stores multiple imaging datasets from each probe element before analyzing it. The processor determines the image pixel originated from a real structure or noise/artifact. By enhancing the pixel from a real structure and reducing the pixel from noise or artifact, a high contrast resolution image is obtained. TOI = true confocal image.

Automated 3D chamber quantification for left heart

Previous studies have demonstrated that 3D echocardiography is more accurate and reproducible than 2D echocardiography because direct measurement of volumes can be achieved without the need for geometrical assumptions and limitations associated with foreshortening .However, quantitative analysis of 3D volumetric data is more complex and time consuming than that of conventional 2D volumetric data. It is not easy to include 3D quantitative analysis in the daily workflow for routine examination.Heart ModelA.I. is a fully automated 3D transthoracic echocardiography analysis software that simultaneously detects left atrial and left ventricular endocardial borders throughout the cardiac cycle using an adaptive analytics algorithm that consists of knowledge-based identification of initial global shape and orientation followed by patient-specific adaptation .This technology reduces the tedious work for 3D quantitative analysis by simplifying the user interface and analytical steps, and simultaneously measures the 3D volumes and function of the left atrium and left ventricle Compared with the conventional 3D quantitative methods the new module (HeartModelA.I.) sharply reduces the time needed for 3D quantitative analysis

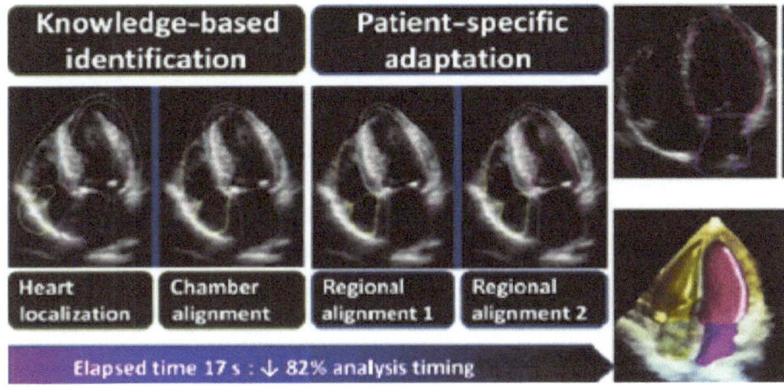

Fig. 2.12 HeartModelA.I. is a fully automated 3D chamber quantification module that simultaneously detects left atrial and left ventricular endocardial borders throughout the cardiac cycle, using an adaptive analysis algorithm that consists of knowledge-based identification of initial global shape and orientation followed by patient-specific adaptation. 3D = three dimensional; TTE = transthoracic echocardiography.

(from 148 seconds to 17 seconds, reducing analysis time by 82%) and obtains more accurate data with better reproducibility. By greatly reducing the analysis time, this technology dramatically increases the opportunity to incorporate 3D quantitative analysis into routine examinations.

OPEN-ACCESS ECHOCARDIOGRAPHY

Open access echocardiography is a diagnostic service for general practitioners (GPs) which enables them to obtain an echocardiogram for patients with suspected heart failure or valve disease, without referral to a cardiologis About 80% of requests are for suspected heart failure or a murmur. The role of open-access echocardiography is controversial, and the indications differ from those of hospital-based practice because patients who are ill are not suitable, even if they have an acceptable indication for echocardiography. They should instead undergo echocardiography as part of an emergency or out-patient assessment.

POINT OF CARE (POC) ECHOCARDIOGRAPHY

POC Echo is an echocardiographic study conducted by a physician at the patient's bedside. It can be categorised into focussed Echo and limited Echo. A broad spectrum of cardiovascular disorders can be detected and graded with bed-side inspection, palpation and auscultation. However, the PE skills required to diagnose abnormal cardiovascular findings have been declining. Studies assessing PE abilities have shown significant error and omission rates for physicians at all levels of training . This decline in PE skills has been attributed to the reliance on newer technological methods of diagnosis as well as decreasing availability of time for bedside teaching.

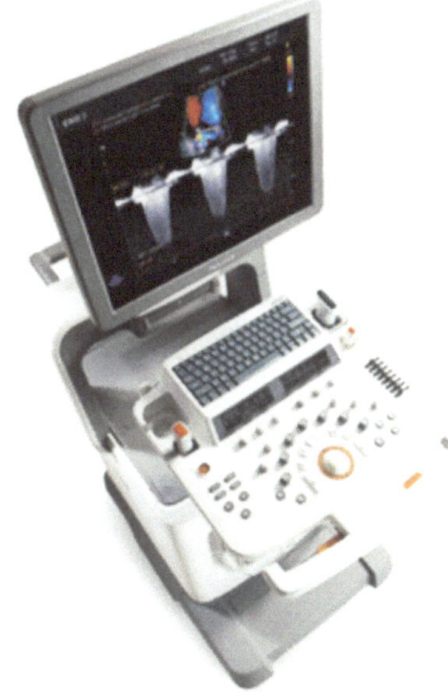

Fig.2.13 Showing photograph of a echocardiographic machine which is commonly used in point of care echocardiography.

Technological advances over the past 2 decades have made ultrasound equipment quite portable, with functionality and image quality similar to high-end ultrasound systems used in dedicated imaging laboratories. Echocardiography and vascular laboratories are using these portable ultrasound machines to perform studies on patients who are unable to travel to the imaging laboratory. The same equipment now enables other healthcare providers to perform ultrasound examinations at the point of care (POC), that is, ultrasound examinations performed and interpreted at the bedside in real time. At present, the most commonly used devices for POC ultrasonography include portable, cart-based machines that are smaller and lighter than traditional systems, while offering the same features as larger ultrasound systems. The cart-based machines are often equipped with batteries and have bootup times as short as 15 seconds. Although a wide range of cart-based ultrasound systems is currently available, these systems have demonstrated adequate image quality to answer focused POC questions, even in patients with obesity or chronic obstructive pulmonary disease.

More recently, pocket-size ultrasound devices have been developed by various vendors. These devices have sizes approaching those of smart phones and are equipped with a battery and a single transducer. Although these devices cur-rently do not have advanced features such as spectral or tissue doppler, they allow for gray-scale imaging (B-mode) and color-flow Doppler and are capable of recording both still images and video clips.

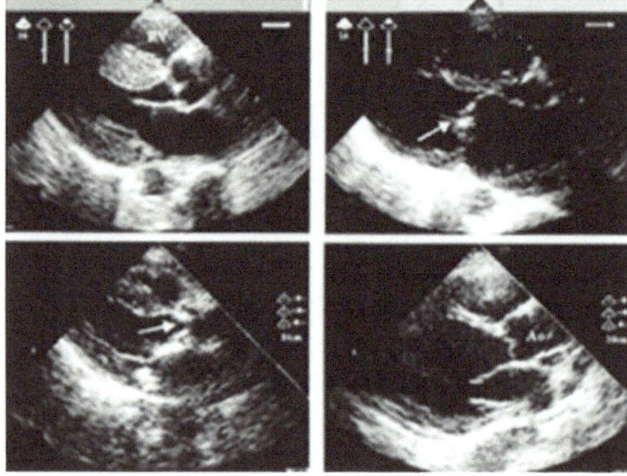

Fig.2.14 Examples of still-frames obtained from two-dimensional echocardiographic studies acquired using the miniaturized echocardiographic device. (A) Parasternal long-axis view obtained from a patient with hypertensive heart disease. (B) Parasternal long-axis view obtained from a patient with rheumatic mitral stenosis. (C) Parasternal long-axis view obtained from a patient with severe sclerocalcific aortic valve stenosis and calcification of the mitral valve. (D) Parasternal long-axis view obtained from a patient with a dilated cardiomyopathy. Ao = aorta; LA = left atrium; LV = left ventricle; RV = right ventricle.

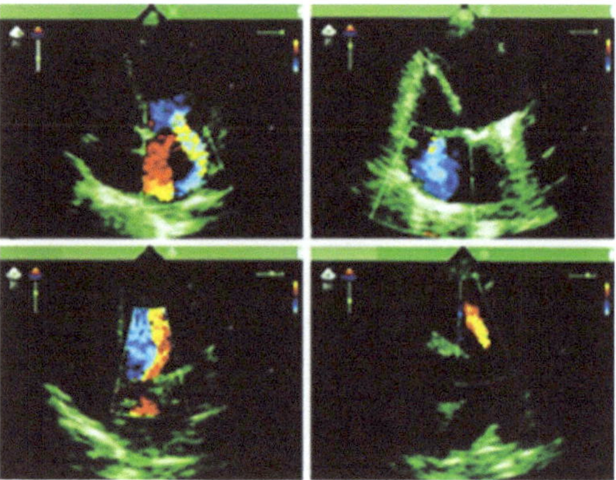

Fig.2.15 Examples of color Doppler still-frames acquired using the miniaturized echocardiographic device. (A) Apical four-chamber view depicting moderately severe mitral regurgitation. (B) Apical four-chamber view depicting moderate tricuspid regurgitation. (C) Apical four-chamber view depicting moderately severe aortic insufficiency. (D) Parasternal short-axis view depicting pulmonic insufficiency. Ao = aorta; LV = left ventricle; PA = pulmonary artery; RA = right atrium; RV = right ventricle.

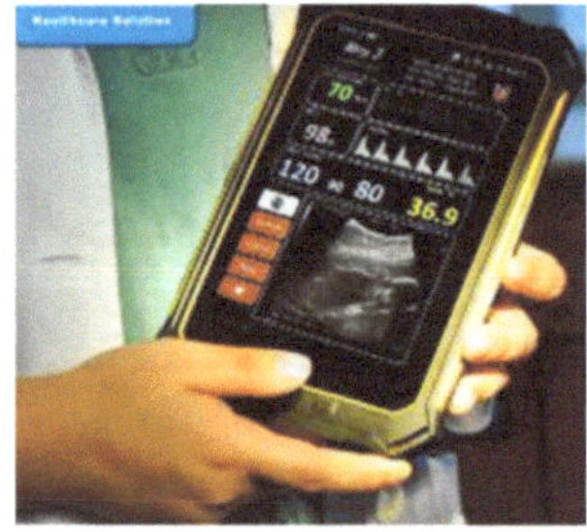

Fig 2.16. Pocket ultrasound used for point of care assessment of heart health.

POC ultrasonography has become an indispensable diagnostic tool for clinicians from various specialties in the assessment and management of patients in the acute care setting and is used to examine almost all organs of the body, including heart, lungs, intra abdominal organs, and blood vessels. For example, multiple studies have demonstrated that clinician-performed ultrasound is reliable in detecting free intraperitoneal fluid in trauma patients and has thus replaced diagnostic peritoneal lavage at many trauma centers. In central line placement, ultrasound guidance confers a significantly lower complication rate and is rapidly becoming standard of care. The latter is one of the reasons why portable ultrasound systems are now available throughout many hospitals. POC echocardiography has been proven equally beneficial, in the detection of pericardial effusions or the determination of cardiac activity in patients with pulseless electrical activity.In parallel with the improvement of image quality and pro-vider skills, more advanced assessments, including global LV function, right ventricular dilatation, and inferior vena cava diameter have been adopted.

VIRTUAL ECHOCARDIOGRAPHY

When it is not physically existing as such but made by software to appear to do so."virtual images"Evaluation of intracardiac anatomy from multiple two-dimensional echocardiographic images requires a mental conceptualisation process that is complicated by cardiac dynamics. Currently, real-time 3D echocardiographic images of the heart do no longer demand this difficult and individually variable conceptualisation processes, by offering an equivocal presentation of cardiac anatomy throughout the cardiac cycle. However, the full 3D potential of these imaging modalities cannot be appreciated, since the 3D data are presented on a flat 2D screen. Virtual dynamic systems, known as virtual reality, can assist with the interpretation of 3D data of the heart in space and makes it possible to 'dive' into the 3D model of the heart . This study is an attempt in the technological process of the future to evaluate whether virtual reality is feasible for 3D echocardiography and if 3D echocardiographic images in a virtual reality can advance to a clinically useful tool. The BARCO (Barco N.V., Kortrijk, Belgium) I-space installed at the ErasmusMC, is a so-called four-walled CAVE(tm)-like virtual reality system. In the I-space researchers are surrounded by computer-generated stereo images, which are projected by 4 high quality DLP-projectors on three walls and the floor of a small "room". The virtual reality system has a resolution of 1280 by 1024 pixels per projector. This is comparable to or greater than the resolution of the CRT monitors and LCD

TRANSMITRAL FLOW PROPAGATION VELOCITY (VP)

Echocardiographic Doppler assessment of left ventricular (LV) filling is the mainstay of our evaluation of myocardial diastolic function (DF) and dysfunction (DD). Due to its insight into LV filling, pulse wave Doppler (PWD) has been termed as the "clinician's Rosetta stone" for simplifying our understanding of this complex process(1). An understanding and appreciation of DF has introduced clinicians to a new paradigm of a comprehensive ventricular assessment", i.e., systolic as well as diastolic function. Traditional means of left ventricular (LV) DF assessment, i.e., PWD of the transmitral inflow (E,A waves and deceleration time) and the pulmonary venous inflow (S,D and atrial reversal waves) are highly load dependent and require significant post-acquisition manipula-tion for accurate diagnosis. Also, due to the unique history of DD (Impaired relaxation to Pseudo-normal to Restrictive Pat-tern), the clinicians are sometimes required to do "unmasking pre-load reduction maneuvers" to correctly identify the type of diastolic abnormality. Because of the aforementioned reasons, these parameters have limited application in the operating room. Transmitral flow propagation velocity (Vp) is a recently described parameter of the assessment of the rapid filling phase (Active Relaxation Component) of the diastole. It is obtained by a combination of color-flow Doppler and m-mode inter-rogation of the mitral inflow during diastole. The concept of Vp is based on the principle of the development of progressive negative intra-ventricular pressure gradients (suction force) during the active relaxation phase. The presence of a negative intra-ventricular pressure gradient has been validated in experimental studies to correlate with the invasively measured time constant (Tau) of relaxation i.e. –dP/dT.

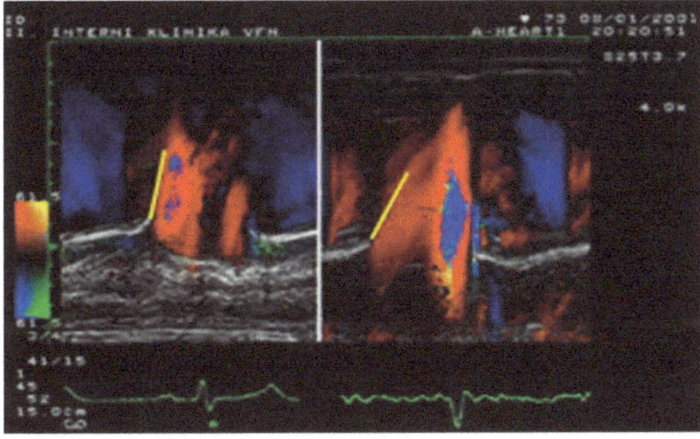

Fig.2.17 Representative examples of color M-mode recordings with the method of measuring Vp as the slope of the first aliasing velocity during early filling (yellow or white line). The subject with normal LV diastolic function (Vp> 0.5 ms-1) (left) and the patient with abnormal LV diastolic function (Vp<0.5 ms-1)) (right). Vp, flow propagation velocity.

Clinically, the vortex and slope of flow of blood from left atrium to LV is determined by this "suction force", which in turn depends upon the diastolic properties (Active Relaxation) of the left ventricle. The clinical application of Vp as a measure of DD was first described by Brun and Takatsuji et al. and was later validated by Garcia et al. by simultaneous Doppler and cardiac catheterization studies . Initially the slope between flow and no-flow in the LV was used to describe the filling pattern, but the slope of the "first aliasing velocity" obtained by adjustment of Nyquist limit to 30-40 cm/sec generated more reproduc-ible results. A value of Vp of < 0.45 m/sec was identified as diagnostic of "impaired relaxation".

DIGITAL ECHOCARDIOGRAPHY

The first efforts in digital echocardiography occurred in the early 1980s. Given storage capacity and processing speed limitation, digital echo was limited to stress testing and evaluation of coronary artery disease, using a quadscreen format and grayscale images. New technological advances in echocardiography today permit registering moving images in digital format, allowing logical archival; rapid data retrieval, copy, and transfer; off-line quantitative analysis; and side-by-side comparison with superior image resolution

The American Society of Echocardiography established a task force in 1992 to educate the echocardiographic community on the promise and pitfalls of digital echocardiography and advise the Digital Images and Communications in Medicine (DICOM) committee on a standard image format for echocardiography

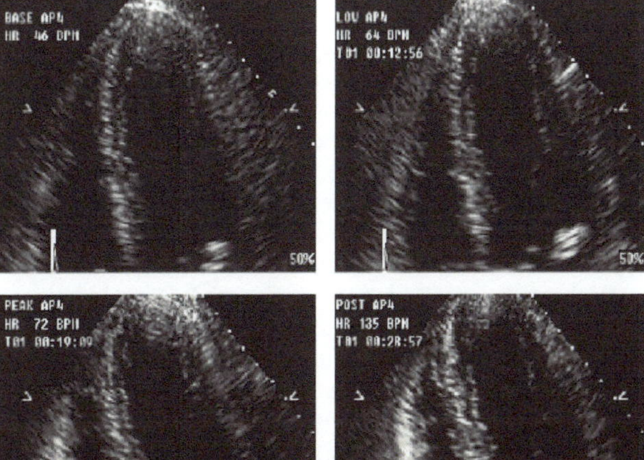

Fig.2.18 An example of an abnormal dobutamine stress echocardiogram. The fourchamber view is shown and demonstrates apical and lateral ischemia. The abnormality is apparent only at peak stress (lower right quad).

Artificial intelligence in echocardiography: detection, functional evaluation, and disease diagnosis (AI)

In light of the great progress in artificial intelligence, the ongoing trends toward high contrast resolution, high frame rate, and rapid and automated 3D analysis will facilitate the continued progress of echocardiography during the coming decade. Nowadays, the aforementioned two new technologies are currently owned by different companies. It would be great if these two technologies could be combined in the same platform.

Highlights

1. *Application of artificial intelligence (AI) in echocardiography is now widely studied, and AI technique has the potential to optimize the diagnostic potential of echocardiography.*
2. *Application of artificial intelligence in echocardiography is important in the following aspects: recognizing the standard section, cardiac cavity automatic segmentation, functional left ventricle assessment, and cardiac disease diagnosis.*
3. *Standardized data collection and image annotation are essential for artificial intelligence in echocardiography.*

Background

The application of artificial intelligence (AI) technology in cardiovascular imaging has become a research hotspot in recent years, as it may reduce treatment cost and help avoid unnecessary testing AI technology has been progressively applied for processing multiple modal images, such as auxiliary electrocardiograph diagnosis cardiac computerized tomography (CT) detection and radionuclide myocardial perfusion imaging In the diagnosis and treatment of heart diseases, AI techniques have been applied to electrocardiography, vectorcardiography, echocardiography, and electronic health records As a non-invasive imaging detection method for cardiac structure and functional evaluation, echocardiography technology has certain limitations. These include a long procedure time (more than 20 min, even if no abnormalities are detected), multiple measurement values that increase the duration complexity and user subjectivity, complex analyses during the evaluation, high standard of individualized assessments high operator subjectivity, and wide observation ranges and distinctions among observers that persist even under standardized conditions. These limitations also lead to a high demand for medical specialist training in the field of echocardiography. In recent years, the application of AI for diagnosis and treatment using echocardiography has been shown to have the potential to solve these problems.The integration of echocardiography and AI is not a brand new topic. Earlier cases of integrated application of echocardiography and machine learning can be traced back to 1978 when Fourier analysis was used to evaluate the waveform of anterior mitral leaflets via M-mode ultrasound. Studies have confirmed that this method had a remarkable impact on auxiliary diagnosis of mitral valve prolapse .

Machine learning is a significant AI method. Before deep learning was proposed in 2006, plenty of machine learning algorithms had been applied to echocardiographic evaluation of cardiac function, image optimization, and structural observation in the form of software or cutting edge technology, such as semi-automatic speckle tracking technology and the Simpson method. In early 2020, the Food and Drug Administration announced that it had authorized Caption Guidance software from Caption Health to be available for sale to collect data from echocardiographic images The development of novel technologies, such as deep learning and neural networks, has effectively improved the efficacy of echocardiography making standard section identification of cardiac anatomical structures, automatic recognition and segmentation of cardiac structures, cardiac functional evaluation, and auxiliary disease diagnosis faster and more accurate. Although a series of articles published in high-level journals positively affirm the role of AI technology in diagnosis of echocardiography, there are remaining concerns, such as insufficient standardization of echocardiography, poor robustness, and insufficient generalization of the models in clinical applications. This review summarizes the application and advantages of echocardiography integrated with AI, analyzes the associated limitations, and systematically investigates the future trends of AI technology in echocardiography from the perspective of practical applications

Functional left ventricle assessment with assistance from AI technology

Functional evaluation of the left ventricle is one of the most important and routine examination procedures in echocardiographic diagnosis. Functional evaluation indicators of the left ventricle systole include left ventricular ejection fraction (EF), left ventricular volume, left ventricular wall motion function, myocardial contractility and global longitudinal strain (GLS). EF is the most convenient and commonly used indicator for evaluating left ventricular systolic function. Since EF is a ratio when no segmental motion abnormality is present in the ventricular wall, EF can be determined using an M-mode chart by measuring the inside diameter ratio of the left ventricular end diastole to systole. A more precise approach for EF measurement is the biplane Simpson method, especially when segmental motion abnormalities such as myocardial infarction occur in the ventricular wall. The M-mode of certain left ventricular sections cannot represent the motion of the entire left ventricle. At this time, it is necessary to estimate the overall volume using the Simpson method. Regardless of the method

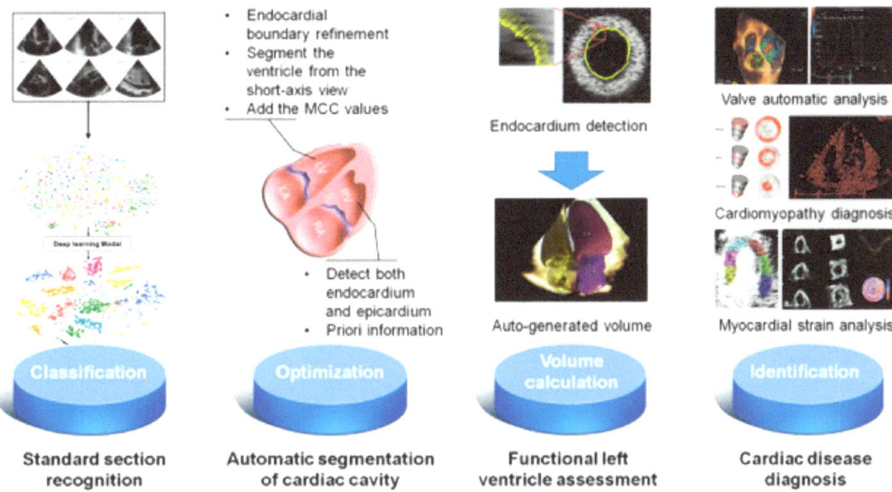

Fig.2.19 Application of artificial intelligence in echocardiography

employed, evaluations rely on visual observation and manual boundary tracing, while repeatability and accuracy depend on the physician's experience The inter- and intra-observer variability can also be substandard when the functional left ventricle assessment is performed by a person.Previous research on left ventricular function assessment with assistance of AI technology has been mainly based on automatic segmentation of the left ventricle and endocardial tracking technology At present, there are several commercial software packages that can achieve high-accuracy 2D and 3D echocardiography measurements, which further realize the automated assessment of the left heart function. One of the commonly used software is the Philips EPIQ series for transthoracic 3D echocardiography left ventricular cavity quantitative system HeartModel (Philips, Eindhoven, Netherlands), which utilizes an adaptive analysis algorithm AutoLV (TomTec Imaging System, Germany) is an additional standard tracking system for left ventricular ejection fraction and longitudinal strain. Various clinical studies have shown that automatic software used to assess the ventricular volume and ejection fraction can provide accuracy that is similar to manual methods, which has a good correlation with cardiac MRI In spite of this, boundary identification is still prone to errors limiting accuracy. With the development of automated technique, some researchers have tried to reduce these errors by using evaluation methods without volume measurements.These algorithms mimicked what an experienced human eye and brain can do, instead of tracing the endocardial borders and calculating employed, evaluations rely on visual observation and manual boundary tracing, while repeatability and accuracy depend on the physician's experience The inter- and intra-observer variability can also be substandard when the functional left ventricle assessment is performed by a person.Previous research on left ventricular function assessment with assistance of AI technology has been mainly based on automatic segmentation of the left ventricleand endocardial tracking technology At present, there are several commercial software packages that can achieve high-accuracy 2D and 3D echocardiography measurements, ventricular volumes Since the analyses of GLS are time consuming and demand expertise, AI technique can help identify the standard apical views, perform timing of cardiac events, trace the myocardium, perform motion estimation, and measure GLS in less than 15 s. It was prove to have highly significant correlation with a conventional speckle-tracking application. Furthermore, AI technology may help novices quickly acquire skills in quality diagnostic imaging to improve the inter- and intra-observer variability For the prognosis, a novel multicenter research demonstrated that AI-based LV analyses were significant predictors of mortality, which is better than manual measurement. It could minimize variability of quantification of LVEF and LVLS. AI can be a game-changer in this field, providing a reproducible LVEF evaluation that is independent of human observer.

Automatic segmentation of cardiac cavity with assistance of AI technology

The shape and function of the four chambers of the heart (left/right ventricle, left/right atrium) are observed following the determination of the cardiogram section. If the heart morphology is affected by certain disease-related factors, the standard pressure and volume will change, resulting in cardiac chamber enlargement, compensatory wall thickening, and cardiac remodeling .Therefore, it is important to obtain accurate segmentation of cardiac ultrasound images and understand the morphological changes for clinical diagnosis. Masses of echocardiography instruments are equipped with semi-automatic cardiac chamber segmentation software. Manual segmentation is tedious, time-consuming, and subjective. Hence, automatic and precise segmentation can decrease the occurrence of the above-mentioned problems and has favorable clinical values. At present, cardiac chambers are automatically segmented by recognizing the endocardial wall in 2D or three-dimensional (3D) images, which is common in segmentation of the left and right ventricles. During segmentation, the automatic evaluation and accurate measurement of parameters such as cardiac cavity size can also be accomplished.

Left ventricular segmentation

Left ventricular segmentation is popular in the automatic segmentation of the heart chamber. The accurate measurement of ejection fraction and evaluation of the movement in left ventricular myocardium can be achieved by segmenting the left ventricle. Two- and three-dimensional ultrasound methods are both widely used in the assessment of left ventricular segmentation. Compared to 2D ultrasound images, 3D-image resolution is lower. Manual processing and analysis are also extremely time-consuming. Fully automatic left ventricular segmentation based on ultrasound images remains a challenging task due to rapid and large-scale myocardial movements, respiratory interference, inconsistent motion between mitral valve opening and closing, in addition to inherent noise and artifacts in ultrasound imaging. Some methods have been proposed to address the above-mentioned issues.Compared to left ventricular segmentation, right

Right ventricular segmentation

ventricular segmentation presents a relatively difficult-to-resolveproblem. These problems are related to the characteristics of the right ventricle and its wall, including complex crescent-shaped structure, presence of trabecular myocardium, thinner and weaker right ventricular walls, irregular endocardium shapes and edges on cardiogram images, and relatively poor image quality due to its behind-sternum, location leading to lung gas irruption and shadow of the sternum. These cause blurred ventricular wall echo and even disappearance of entire lateral walls in some images. However, accurate evaluation of right ventricular function is significant for functional analysis of the circulatory system, surgery selection of congenital heart disease (CHD), and prediction and evaluation of heart failure.The precise identification and segmentation of right ventricular ultrasound images can quickly and efficiently capture the diameter, area, and volume of the right ventricle, myocardial thickness, fractional area changes, as well as other indicators to provide more information for auxiliary clinical diagnostics.. To overcome these issues, Qin et al. proposed an automatic segmentation framework based on the sparse matrix transform and introduced a wall thickness constraint feature. A positive segmentation result was acquired via detection of endocardium and epicardium at the same time when the lateral walls are blurred .

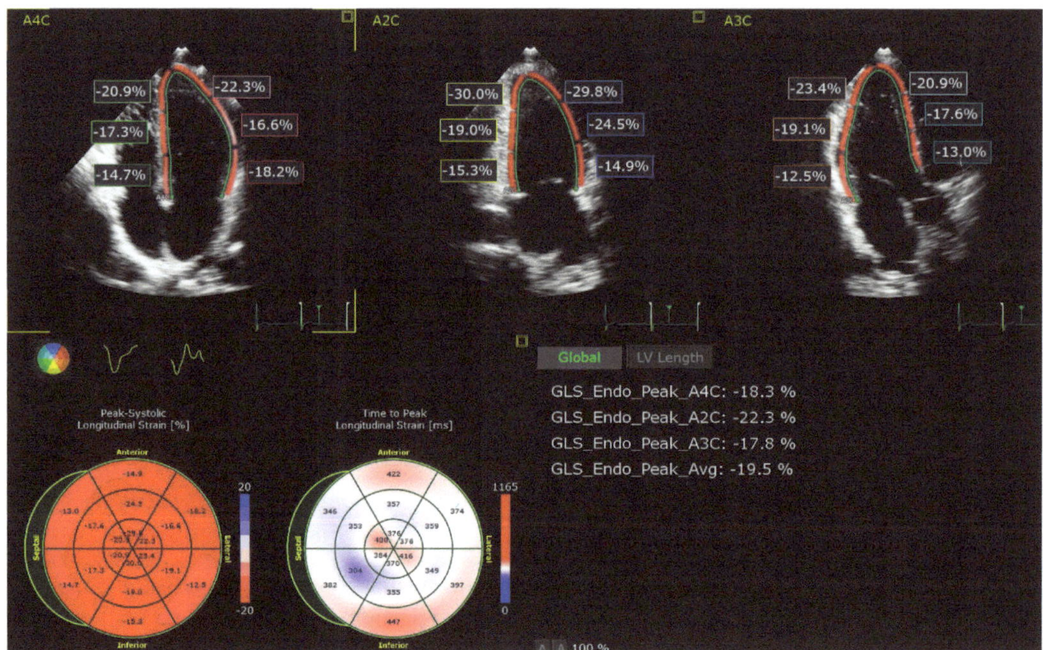

Fig 2.20 Automatic border detection and strain analysis from the three standard apical views calculating regional and global longitudinal strain. Image courtesy of Berthold Klas.

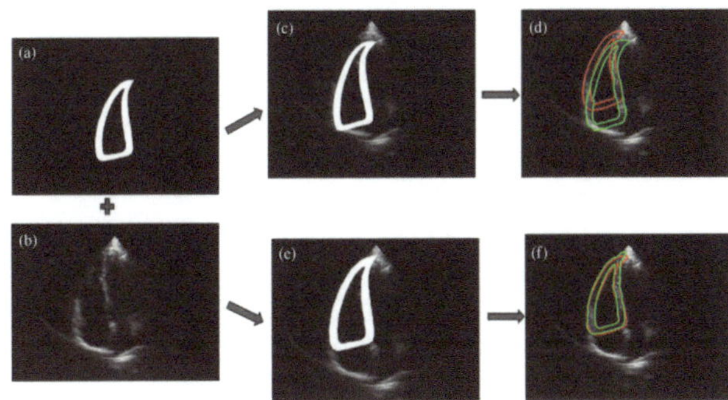

Fig 2.21 GA optimized initialization and segmentation results without and with SMT-based transform, where green lines are segmented results and red lines are the corresponding gold lines. (a) Mean shape of the training model. (b) Echocardiographic image to be segmented, where locations, rotations and scales of RV regions are usually changeable because of different imaging angles and different subjects. (c) GA optimized mask without SMT-based transform. (d) Segmented result based on mask (c). (e) GA optimized mask with SMT-based transform. (f) Segmented result based on mask (e).

Atrial and multi-chamber heart segmentation

Echocardiographic atrial segmentation has certain application values in minimally invasive interventional treatment of arrhythmia such as cardiac electrophysiology. For example, in radiofrequency ablation treatment of atrial fibrillation, 3D transesophageal echocardiography (3D-TEE) can be utilized to guide cardiac electrophysiological intervention (locating ablation points) in real time. However, there is a prerequisite that the changes in the atrial anatomical structure have to be real-time monitored for precise positioning Accordingly, Alexander et al. have applied an active shape model derived from computed tomography angiography (CTA) in a multi-chamber to segment the atrioventricle in a 3D-TEE image, improving segmentation accuracy in the left atrium, which previously had a poor segmentation performance. Furthermore, because 3D-TEE segmentation in the left atrium is vulnerable to scanning range restrictions, the team adopted fusion-imaging technology to merge the CTA and 3D-TEE images for construction of wide-view 3D-TEE images, which contributed to left atrial segmentation resolution and enhanced segmentation efficiency. This research has an important significance for cardiac surgery, where it can help to provide precise positioning for atrial fibrillation ablation Although AI technology can effectively segment atrioventricular structures in echocardiography, recognition and segmentation precision needs to be advanced further due to interference of lung gas, ribs, and artifacts. Algorithm updates, such as multiple iterations, efficient search methods, particle filters, and online collaborative training approaches, combined with deep learning algorithms and multiple dynamic models will further optimize echocardiographic segmentation performance

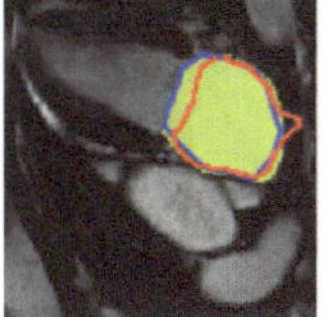
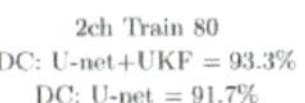

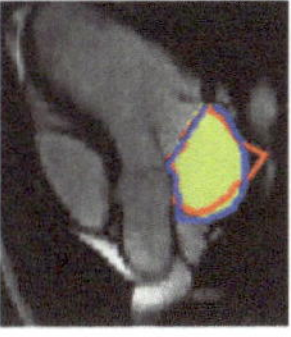

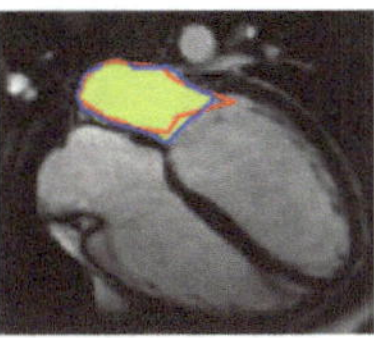

Fig.2.22 Fully automated left atrium segmentation from anatomical cine long-axis MRI sequences using deep convolutional neural network with unscented Kalman filter

Cardiac disease diagnosis with assistance of AI technology

Valvular heart disease

Routine echocardiography can visually investigate cardiac valve shapes and activities. Its repeatability is not reliable due to subtle valve structure variations and wide heart motion ranges, as well as the intra- and inter-observer differences in recognizing valve stenosis, prolapse, calcification, and valve insufficiency. The mitral and aortic valves are the objectives of AI technology in cardiac valve evaluation, especially focusing on observation of valve morphology and regurgitation. Similarly, AI technique is helpful in the assessment of valvular heart disease. For example, automatic evaluation software for proximal isovelocity surface area (PISA) of mitral insufficiency can conduct an automatic measurement of mitral valve regurgitant orifice area and regurgitant volume to evaluate the severity of valve regurgitation. PISA for 3D echocardiography has a superior accuracy compared to 2D image analysis software, which has excellent consistency with

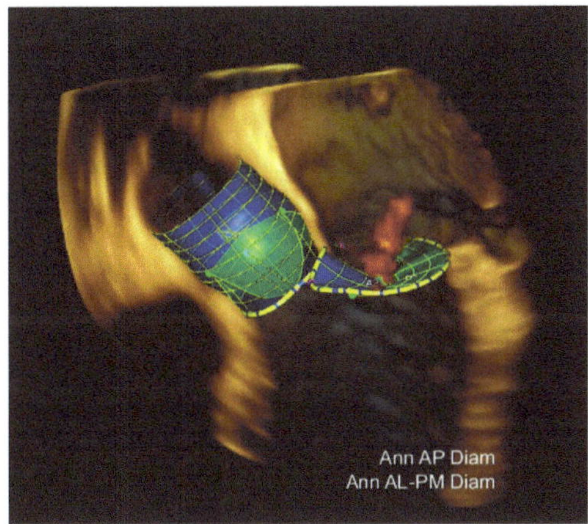

Fig 2.23 An example of automatic valve analysis with three-dimensional modeling of the aortic and mitral valves. A red jet of mitral regurgitation can be seen coming from the center of the valve into the left atrium. Image courtesy of Marti McCulloch.

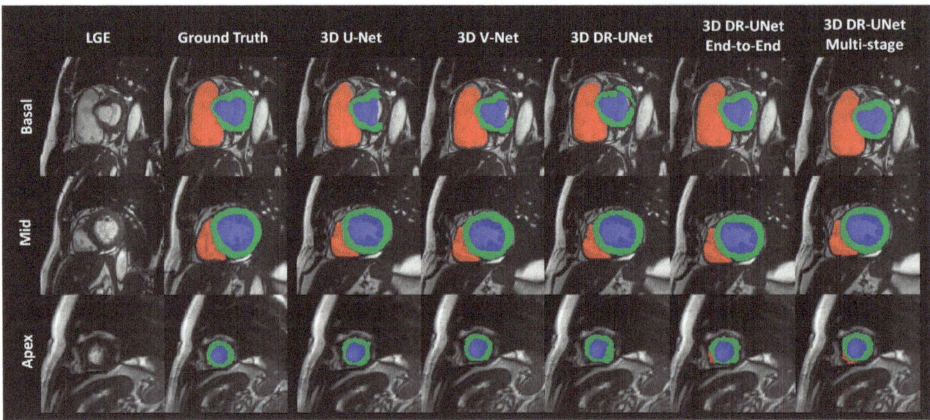

Fig.2.24 depicts segmentation of the RV, LV, and MYO at the ED phase, for a test sample from the ACDC dataset, generated using each network. Rows from top to bottom depict the basal, middle and apical slices, respectively. In all figures, red, blue and green represent the RV, LV, and MYO, respectively.

transesophageal ultrasound and MRI measurements Another study used real-time 3D volume color-flow Doppler technique to quantify valve regurgitation volume, which also achieved high consistency in MRI measurements. In addition, valve morphology can be automatically analyzed by implementing automated measurements of the morphological mitral valve parameters, including 3D ring length and height, 2D area, commissural width, overlap width, 3D leaflet area, anterior and posterior leaflet angle, non-planar angle, prolapse, valve height, and volume. Previous research has confirmed that there is no significant difference between automatic and manual measurements This type of semi-automatic software has a favorable diagnostic value for valve morphology-related diseases such as mitral valve prolapses. It also enhances the non-experts' accuracy in prolapse detection It can also be employed for intervalvular monitoring with advantages of consistency and repeatability

Structural abnormalities in the congenital aortic valve, senile aortic valve calcification, and rheumatic fever are the common causes of aortic stenosis (AS). The method of aortic valve replacement is crucial for severe AS. Before valve replacement surgery, valve diameter measurement and areas in 2D echocardiography have been manually detected to evaluate the level of valve stenosis and provide a sufficient basis to determine the size of artificial valves. However, because of the dynamic changes in the position of aortic valves in vivo, 2D static image-based assessment is not only subjective but also only reveals the measurement results of one or two frames during the cardiac cycle. Some research studies have adopted an automatic tracking algorithm based on anatomical affine optical flow for fast and automatic tracking of aortic valves and proximal end of the left ventricular outflow tract using 3D-TEE technology to optimize the measurement. It provides dynamic and accurate supporting information for preoperative planning of aortic valve replacement surgery, helping to improve the accuracy of valve evaluation and enhancing surgeon confidence.

Cardiomyopathy

Cardiomyopathy can be classified into two major categories of primary and secondary cardiomyopathy according to the cause. AI-assisted echocardiographic diagnosis of cardiomyopathy can be carried out via multiple imaging modes, such as 2D ultrasound, M-mode, and color Doppler. Based on accurate wall recognition and ventricular segmentation, automatic measurement of ventricular volume measurement, accurate assessment of cardiac function, and accurate visualization of myocardial movement through speckle tracking technology can be realized. The acquisition of these indicators helps to achieve rapid and precise detection of hypertrophic cardiomyopathy and cardiac amyloidosis. In the latest research, a human-interpretation-free machine learning pipeline based on the combination of ECG and echocardiography had been developed to detect cardiac amyloidosis. Multicenter study had confirmed that the artificial intelligence-enabled fully automated detection model outperformed interpretation by expert cardiologists in the diagnosis of cardiac amyloidosis On the other hand, speckle tracking imaging technology is widely used for the diagnosis of cardiomyopathy. Myocardial strain analysis is helpful for diagnosis of various types of cardiomyopathy .Sengupta et al. created a machine learning algorithm based on speckle tracking technology images to distinguish between constrictive pericarditis and restrictive cardiomyopathy using an associative memory classifier (AMC). As an additional challenge, both of the diseases have similar ultrasonographic features, such as enlarged left and right atrium, relatively small ventricle, pericardial effusion, and widening vena cava.Clinical diagnosis emphasizes the changes in myocardial strain parameters.

For example, strain values of left ventricular walls in constrictive pericarditis are significantly lower than those of ventricular septa, while restrictive cardiomyopathy does not have this feature. The study used AMC to demonstrate that analysis of the first 15 speckles tracking echocardiographic variables can classify diseases more accurately (area under the curve (AUC) of 89.2%). This method is better than the Doppler method alone (AUC of 82.1%) and the overall longitudinal strain (AUC of 63.7%), which obtained precision results. The study also used machine learning to automatically distinguish between male patients with hypertrophic cardiomyopathy and athlete cardiac physiological hypertrophy Due to the diversification of ventricular morphology in patients with dilated cardiomyopathy (DCM), segmentation of the left ventricular boundary (especially segmentation near the ventricle apex) is more complex than that of the normal left ventricle. To address the ventricular wall changes caused by DCM, Mahmood et al applied a support vector machine classifier to distinguish between normal and dilated left ventricles. Although the average classification accuracy of the study was only 77.8% (affected by cumulative errors), size evaluation accuracy of the left ventricle reached 87.2% and left ventricular boundary segmentation accuracy was 89.3%. The ROI region recognition accuracy was 92.5%, providing a research foundation for further development of reliable decision-making tools.

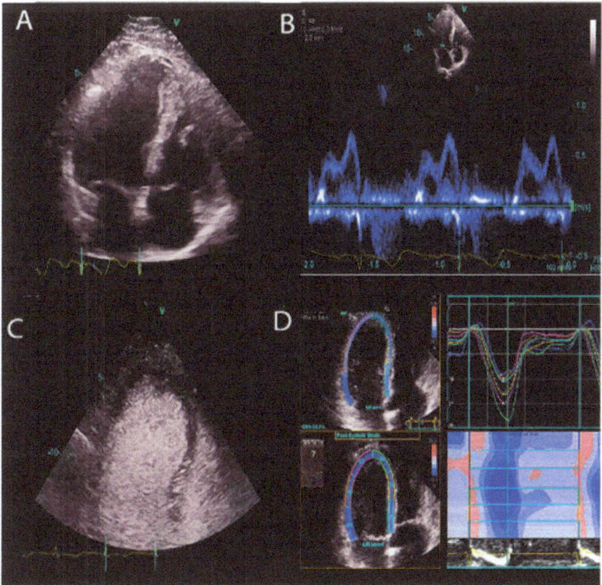

Fig.2.25 Sample US images showing different US modes. (A) B-mode image of the apical 4 chamber view of a heart. (B) Doppler image of mitral inflow. (C) Contrast enhanced ultrasound image of left ventricle. (D) Strain imaging of the left ventricle

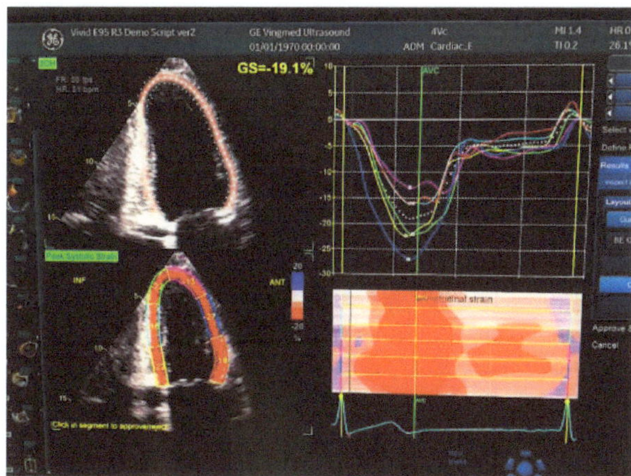

Fig.2.26 An example of artificial intelligence on the GE Healthcare Vivid E95 system shown at ASE 2019 where the AI automatically pulls in an exam, identifies the left ventricle and myocardial boards and then calculates all the strain measurements in less than 10 seconds. While AI automation can greatly speed workflow, there are questions about the accuracy of AI for the next step in making diagnoses.

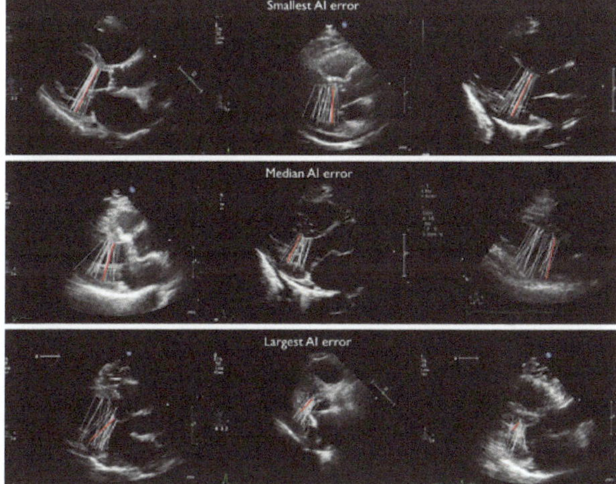

Fig.2.27 Nine examples of artificial intelligence (AI) measurements of left ventricular (LV) dimension, drawn from 200 frames, showing the range of AI performance, with expert consensus as the reference standard. Top: the 3 cases with the smallest AI error, Bottom: the 3 cases with the largest AI error. Middle: median cases when ranked by size of AI error, that is, showing typical performance. In each panel, AI measurements are in red, and 2×13=26 expert measurements in gray.

Coronaray atherosclerotic heart disease diagnosis with AI Technology

Coronary heart disease, also known as coronary atherosclerotic heart disease, is one of the most common coronary artery diseases, which is classified as a special type of cardiomyopathy. Echocardiography can assist in its diagnosis by visually observing myocardial movement and changes in cardiac morphology. AI technology can effectively improve subjectivity of conventional echocardiographic examination of coronary heart disease, increase detection systematicity, and help to better distinguish between normal and infarcted myocardial images For the ultrasound diagnosis of coronary heart disease combined with AI technology, experts have utilized the method of discrete wavelet transform and texture feature analysis , showing that the AI method using classifiers to automatically sort echocardiographic images can provide the characteristic parameters required for clinical diagnosis, as well as reduce the occurrence of complications. In terms of 3D ultrasound heart imaging, studies have constructed myocardial infarction models in pigs and sheep and applied the EchoPAC PC (GE, Andover, MA, USA) program to analyze results. This method is a semi-automatic assessment of left ventricular quality and local strain values. In addition to traditional ultrasound examinations, myocardial perfusion can diagnose coronary artery disease by quantifying the infarct area via examination of myocardial contrast ultrasound. The AI method can also perform an automatic calculation of myocardial perfusion parameters and reduce human error

Echocardiography can be integrated with machine learning to obtain a huge set of clinical data on echocardiographic changes. Machine learning can integrate these data into categories to assist physicians in accurately and rapidly diagnosing myocardial ischemia changes. In the prognosis of coronary heart disease, a previous research had develop a method based on texture parameters of native echocardiogram or contrast-enhanced acquisition to evaluate left ventricular function recovery 1 year after myocardial infarction. The highest rates of accurate prediction reached to 79%

Diagnosis of intracardiac masses

In addition to the auxiliary diagnosis of the above-mentioned conventional diseases, AI technology can be applied to classify and recognize intracardiac masses (like left atrium/ ear thrombosis, cardiac tumors and vegetation) For example, due to the complex and diverse anatomical structures of the left atrial appendage and the limited range of motion of the TEE probe, the resulting ultrasound artifacts may lead to misdiagnosis. Diagnosis through images of the left atrial (auricular) thrombosis depend on the patient's anticoagulant drug plan. Sun et al. performed transesophageal echocardiography on 130 patients with atrial fibrillation with image reconstruction. Subsequently, the study extracted the texture features of the gray-level co-occurrence image matrix and performed the classification using artificial neural networks. The model classification AUC was 0.932, which is much higher than sonographer's diagnosis, where AUC was0.834. The study demonstrated that the Artificial Neural Network model can significantly improve TEE diagnosis of the left atrium (ear) thrombosis in patients with atrial

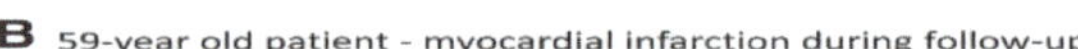

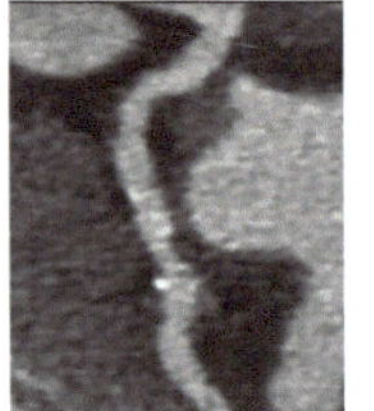

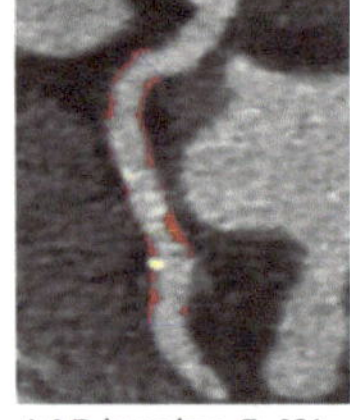

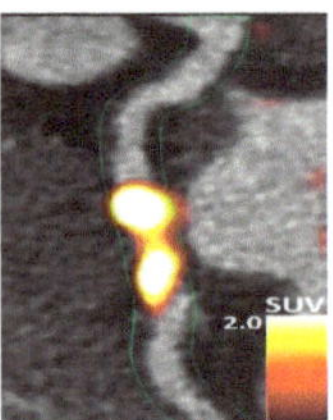

Fig.2.28 Case examples of quantitative plaque analysis on coronary CT angiography and 18F-NaF PET in patients with established coronary artery disease. Hybrid CT angiography and 18F-NaF PET of coronary arteries. (A) A 70-y-old male, who presented with diffused largely noncalcified disease (middle panel in red) in the LAD and demonstrated increased 18F-NaF uptake in the LAD on PET. (B) A 59-y-old male with mild LCX atherosclerosis, who presented with a high noncalcified plaque burden (middle panel in red) on CT angiography, significant 18F-NaF uptake and experienced a lateral non–ST-segment elevation myocardial infarction during follow-up. LAD = left anterior descending; LCX = left circumflex; LAP = low attenuation plaque. Credit: First author Jacek Kwiecinski and senior author Piotr Slomka, Cedars-Sinai, Los Angeles, Calif., in collaboration with Edinburgh University, UK.

fibrillation, which is conducive to early diagnosis and treatment

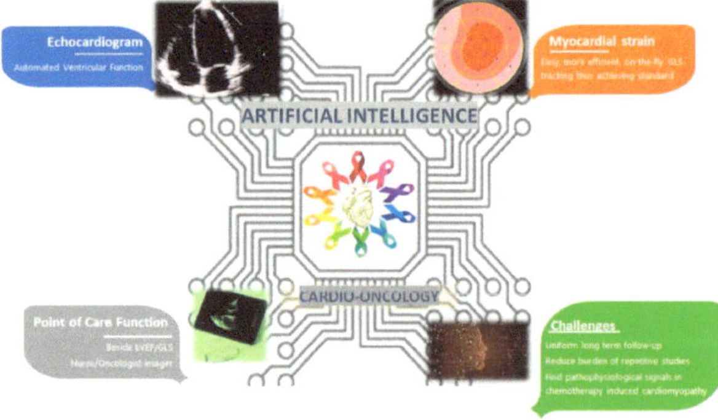

Fig.2.29 Opportunities for the application of artificial intelligence to echocardiography in CardioOncology include automation of left ventricular function assessment and strain, as well real-time AI-guided image acquisition particularly with point-of-care tools at the bedside, inthe examination room, or in low resource settings

Clinical application / limitations

In addition to black box effects, overfitting problems, ethical issues, and other common limitations associated with AI application in the medical field AI echocardiography limitations also exist. First, echocardiography is not a bloodless mechanical operation. Communication between physicians and patient plays an indispensable role in disease diagnosis, while the current AI technology has not been able to perform human–computer interactions. In the future, there is a possibility that clinical work performed by a physician will be gradually substituted by AI, which will not in favor of further model optimization and sustainable development Based on our experiences, echocardiography and AI-integrated application, standardized data collection, and image annotation are essential. Due to its complexities and rapid heartbeat, the echocardiographic section standardization is more difficult compared to other organ section standardization, which may not conducive to the data collection in multi-center studies Furthermore, the difference of physiological and anatomical structures of the heart among races can not be ignore. It means that the model with a high accuracy on one specific dataset may not be feasible on another data set. Therefore, while accepting the assistance of this technology, sonographers should also consider how to utilize its best functions and determine what outcomes need to be adapted for patients.

Conclusion and future outlook

Artificial intelligence is the next big revolution which is changing the world. As per " Forbes " the world is getting more intelligent day by day. The estimate is that the majority of the tasks will be performed by AI and machines by the year 2030. Artificial intelligence is a very powerful technology which is changing the world. It is one of the most exciting and promising technologies of the 21st century. Artificial intelligence is affecting various industries including transport, healthcare, ecommerce, etc. It is changing the world in so many ways. It is affecting each and every domain of life. It is one of the most powerful technologies. It is changing the world by making life easy for human beings.
Some of the limitations include:

- AI does not have the ability to understand context
- AI does not have the ability to learn new concepts.
- AI does not have the ability to understand the aesthetic or emotional value of an experience.
- AI cannot be creative.
- AI cannot generalize from a small amount of data.
- AI cannot be aware of its own existence

AI is making lots of progress in the scientific sector. Artificial Intelligence can handle large quantities of data and processes it quicker than human minds.

Bibliography And Acknowledgement

- Alexander H, Ben R, Harriet W, et al. Improved segmentation of multiple cavities of the heart in wideview 3-D transesophageal echocardiograms. Ultrasound Med Biol. 2015;41(7):1991–2000.
- Alsharqi M, Upton R, Mumith A, et al. Artificial intelligence: a new clinical support tool for stress echocardiography. Expert Rev Med Devices. 2018;15(8):513–5.
- Alsharqi M, Woodward WJ, Mumith JA, et al. Artificial intelligence and echocardiography. Echo Res Pract. 2018;5(4):115–25.
- Arbeille P, Provost R, Zuj K, et al. Teles-operated echocardiography using a robotic arm and an internet connection. Ultrasound Med Biol. 2014;40(10):2521–9.
- Asch FM, Mor-Avi V, Rubenson D, et al. Deep learning-based automated echocardiographic quantification of left ventricular ejection fraction: a point-of-care solution. Circ Cardiovasc Imaging. 2021;14(6):e012293.
- Asch FM, Poilvert N, Abraham T, et al. Automated echocardiographic quantification of left ventricular ejection fraction without volume measurements using a machine learning algorithm mimicking a human expert. Circ Cardiovasc Imaging. 2019;12(9):e009303.
- Bersvendsen J, Orderud F, Lie Ø, et al. Semiautomated biventricular segmentation in three-dimensional echocardiography by coupled deformable surfaces. J Med Imaging. 2017;4(2):024005.
  Brandt V, Emrich T, Schoepf UJ, et al. Ischemia and outcome prediction by cardiac CT based machine learning. Int J Cardiovasc Imaging. 2020.
- Carneiro G, Nascimento JC. Multiple dynamic models for tracking the left ventricle of the heart from ultrasound data using particle filters and deep learning architectures. In: 2010 IEEE Computer Society Conference on Computer Vision and Pattern Recognition. IEEE; 2010. p. 2815–2822.
- Chin CG, Chung FP, Lin YJ, et al. The application of novel segmentation software to create left atrial geometry for atrial fibrillation ablation: the implication of spatial resolution. J Chin Med Assoc. [published online ahead of print].
- Choi J, Hong GR, Kim M, et al. Automatic quantification of aortic regurgitation using 3D full volume color doppler echocardiography: a validation study with cardiac magnetic resonance imaging. Int J Cardiovasc Imaging. 2015;31:1379–89.
  Chu WK, Raeside DE. Fourier analysis of the echocardiogram. Phys Med Biol. 1978;23(1):100–5.
- de Agustin JA, Marcos-Alberca P, Fernandez-Golfin C, et al. Direct measurement of proximal isovelocity surface area by singlebeat three-dimensional color Doppler echocardiography in mitral regurgitation: a validation study. J Am Soc Echocardiogr. 2012;25:815–23.
- de Alexandria A, Cortez P, Bessa J, et al. pSnakes: a new radial active contour model and its application in the segmentation of the left ventricle from echocardiographic images. Comput Methods Programs Biomed. 2014;116(3):260–73.
- Dey D, Slomka PJ, Leeson P, et al. Artificial intelligence in cardiovascular imaging. J Am Coll Cardiol. 2019;73(11):1317–35.
- Gandhi S, Mosleh W, Shen J, et al. Automation, machine learning, and artificial intelligence in echocardiography: a brave new world. Echocardiography. 2018;35(9):1402–18.
- Goto S, Mahara K, Beussink-Nelson L, et al. Artificial intelligence-enabled fully automated detection of cardiac amyloidosis using electrocardiograms and echocardiograms. Nat Commun. 2021;12(1):2726.
- Haak A, Vegas-Sánchez-Ferrero G, Mulder H, et al. Segmentation of multiple heart cavities in 3-D transesophageal ultrasound images. IEEE Trans Ultrason Ferroelectr Freq Control. 2015;62(6):1179–89.
- Hannun AY, et al. Cardiologist- level arrhythmia detection and classification in ambulatory electrocardiograms using a deep neural network. Nat Med. 2019;25:65–9.
- Human vs AI-based echocardiography analysis as predictor of mortality in acute COVID-19 patients: WASE-COVID study. ACC Scientific Sessions, 2021.

- Jin CN, Salgo IS, Schneider RJ, et al. Using anatomic intelligence to localize mitral valve prolapse on three-dimensional echocardiography. J Am Soc Echocardiogr. 2016;29:938–45.
- Johnson KW, Jessica TS, Glicksberg BS, et al. Artificial intelligence in cardiology. J Am Coll Cardiol. 2018;71(23):2668–79.
- Kagiyama N, Toki M, Hara M, et al. Efficacy and accuracy of novel automated mitral valve quantification: three-dimensional transesophageal echocardiographic study. Echocardiography. 2016;33:756–63.
- Knackstedt C, Bekkers SCAM, Schummers G, et al. Fully automated versus standard tracking of left ventricular ejection fraction and longitudinal strain: the FAST-EFs multicenter study. J Am Coll Cardiol. 2015;66(13):1456–66.
- Krittanawong C, Johnson KW, Rosenson RS, et al. Deep learning for cardiovascular medicine: a practical primer. Eur Heart J. 2019;40(25):2058–73.
- Krittanawong C, Zhang H, Wang Z, Aydar M, Kitai T. Artificial intelligence in precision cardiovascular medicine. J Am Coll Cardiol. 2017;69(21):2657–64.
- Kuehn BM. Cardiac imaging on the cusp of an artificial intelligence revolution. Circulation. 2020;141(15):1266–7.
- Kumar S, Nilsen WJ, Abernethy A, et al. Mobile health technology evaluation: the health evidence workshop. Am J Prev Med. 2013;45:228–36.
- Kusunose K, Abe T, Haga A, et al. A deep learning approach for assessment of regional wall motion abnormality from echocardiographic images. JACC Cardiovasc Imaging. 2019;S1936–878X(19):30318–3.
- Kusunose K, Haga A, Abe T, et al. Utilization of artificial intelligence in echocardiography. Circ J. 2019;83(8):1623–9.
- Kusunose K, Haga A, Yamaguchi N, et al. Deep learning for assessment of left ventricular ejection fraction from echocardiographic images. J Am Soc Echocardiogr. 2020;33(5):632-635.e1.
- Li Y, Chahal N, Senior R, et al. Reproducible computer-assisted quantification of myocardial perfusion with contrast-enhanced ultrasound. Ultrasound Med Biol. 2017;43(10):2235–46.
- Li Y, Garson CD, Xu Y, Helm PA, Hossack JA, French BA. Serial ultrasound evaluation of intramyocardial strain after reperfused myocardial infarction reveals that remote zone dyssynchrony develops in concert with left ventricular remodeling. Ultrasound Med Biol. 2011;37(7):1073–86.
- Litjens G, Ciompi F, Wolterink JM, et al. State-of-the-art deep learning in cardiovascular image analysis. JACC Cardiovasc Imaging. 2019;12(8 Pt 1):1549–65.
- Liu CX, Jiao D, Liu Z. Artificial Intelligence (AI)-aided disease prediction. BIO Integration. 2020;1(3):130–6.
- Madani A, Arnaout R, Mofrad M, et al. Fast and accurate view classification of echocardiograms using deep learning. NPJ Digital Med. 2018;1:6.
- Mahmood R, Syeda-Mahmood T. Automatic detection of dilated cardiomyopathy in cardiac ultrasound videos. In: AMIA Annu Symp Proc. 2014. p. 865–871.
- Michael E, Jonathan T, Grace E, et al. Transesophageal echocardiography guidance for robot-assisted level III inferior vena cava tumor thrombectomy: a novel approach to intraoperative care. J Cardiothorac Vasc Anesth. 2018;32:S1053077018303495
- Nabi W, Bansal A, Xu B. Applications of artificial intelligence and machine learning approaches in echocardiography. Echocardiography. 2021;38(6):982–92.
- Narang A, Bae R, Hong H, et al. Utility of a deep-learning algorithm to guide novices to acquire echocardiograms for limited diagnostic use. JAMA Cardiol. 2021. [Epub ahead of print].
- Østvik A, Smistad E, Aase SA, et al. Real-time standard view classification in transthoracic echocardiography using convolutional neural networks. Ultrasound Med Biol. 2019;45(2):374–84.
- Qin X, Cong Z, Fei B, et al. Automatic segmentation of right ventricular ultrasound images using sparse matrix transform and a level set. Phys Med Biol. 2013;8(21):7609–24.
- Salte IM, Østvik A, Smistad E, et al. Artificial intelligence for automatic measurement of left ventricular strain in echocardiography. JACC Cardiovasc Imaging. 2021.
- Sanders WE Jr, Burton T, Khosousi A, et al. Machine learning: at the heart of failure diagnosis. Curr Opin Cardiol. 2021;36(2):227–33.
- Saris AE, Nillesen MM, Lopata RG, et al. Correlation-based discrimination between cardiac tissue and blood for segmentation of the left ventricle in 3-D echocardiographic images. Ultrasound Med Biol. 2014;40(3):596–610.
- Schneider M, Bartko P, Geller W, et al. A machine learning algorithm supports ultrasound-naïve novices in the acquisition of diagnostic echocardiography loops and provides accurate estimation of LVEF. Int J Cardiovasc Imaging. 2021;37(2):577–86.
- Seetharam K, Kagiyama N, Sengupta PP. Application of mobile health, telemedicine and artificial intelligence to echocardiography. Echo Res Pract. 2019;6(2):R41–52.
- Sengupta PP, Huang YM, Bansal M, et al. Cognitive machine-learning algorithm for cardiac imaging: a pilot study for differentiating constrictive pericarditis from restrictive cardiomyopathy. Circ Cardiovasc Imaging. 2016;9:e004330.
- Slomka PJ, Miller RJ, Isgum I, Dey D. Application and translation of artificial intelligence to cardiovascular imaging in nuclear medicine and noncontrast CT. Semin Nucl Med. 2020;50(4):357–66.
- Streiff C, Zhu M, Panosian J, et al. Comprehensive evaluation of cardiac function and detection of myocardial infarction based on a semi-automated analysis using full-volume real time three-dimensional echocardiography. Echocardiography. 2015;32(2):332–8.
- Strzelecki M, Materka A, Drozdz J, et al. Classification and segmentation of intracardiac masses in cardiac tumor echocardiograms. Comput Med Imaging Graph. 2006;30(2):95–107.
- Strzelecki M, Skonieczka S, Kasprzak JD, et al. Analysis of myocardial texture in resting echocardiographic images predicts recovery 1 year after myocardial infarction. In: 2016 Signal Processing: Algorithms, Architectures, Arrangements, and Applications (SPA) IEEE. 2016.
- Sudarshan V, Acharya UR, Ng EY, et al. Automated identification of infarcted myocardium tissue characterization using ultrasound images: a review. IEEE Rev Biomed Eng. 2015;8:86–97.
- Sun L, Li Y, Zhang YT, et al. A computer-aided diagnostic algorithm improves the accuracy of transesophageal echocardiography for left atrial thrombi. J Ultrasound Med. 2014;33(1):83–91.
- Tamborini G, Piazzese C, Lang RM, et al. Feasibility and accuracy of automated software for transthoracic three-dimensional left ventricular volume and function analysis: comparisons with two-dimensional echocardiography, three-dimensional transthoracic manual method, and cardiac magnetic resonance imaging. J Am Soc Echocardiogr. 2017;30(11):1049–58.
- Thavendiranathan P, Liu S, Datta S, et al. Quantification of chronic functional mitral regurgitation by automated 3-dimensional peak and integrated proximal isovelocity surface area and stroke volume techniques using real-time 3-dimensional volume color Doppler echocardiography: in vitro and clinical validation. Circ Cardiovasc Imaging. 2013;6:125–33.
- Tsang W, Salgo IS, Medvedofsky D, et al. Transthoracic 3D Echocardiographic Left Heart Chamber Quantification Using an Automated Adaptive Analytics Algorithm. JACC Cardiovasc Imaging. 2016;9(7):769–82.
- Ye Z, Kumar Y, Sing G, et al. Deep echocardiography: a first step toward automatic cardiac disease diagnosis using machine learning. J Internet Technol. 2020;21(6):1589–600.
- Zhang J, Gajjala S, Agrawal P, et al. Fully automated echocardiogram interpretation in clinical practice. Circulation. 2018;138:1623–35.
- Zhang Y, Gao Y, Jiao J, et al. Robust boundary detection and tracking of left ventricles on ultrasound images using active shape model and ant colony optimization. Biomed Mater Eng. 2014;24(6):2893–9.

Current Devices In Cardiac Rhythm Monitoring

CHAPTER 3

AMBULATORY ELECTROCARDIOGRAPHY (ECG)

began in 1949 when Norman "Jeff" Holter developed a monitor that could wirelessly transmit electrophysiologic data.1 His original device used vacuum tubes, weighed 85 pounds, and had to be carried in a backpack. Furthermore, it could send a signal a distance of only 1 block

At the time, it was uncertain if this technology would have any clinical utility. However, in 1952, Holter published the first tracing of abnormal cardiac electrical activity in a patient who had suffered a posterior myocardial infarction.By the 1960s, Holter monitoring systems were in full production and use.

Since then, advances in technology have led to small, lightweight devices that enable clinicians to evaluate patients for arrhythmias in a real-world context for extended times, often with the ability to respond in real time.Many ambulatory devices are available, and choosing the optimal one requires an understanding of which features they have and which are the most appropriate for the specific clinical context. This article reviews the features, indications, advantages, and disadvantages of current devices, and their best use in clinical practice

INDICATIONS FOR AMBULATORY ECG MONITORING

Several guidelines have been published to help practitioners understand the available ambulatory ECG devices and their uses in clinical practice.5,6 The latest, published in 2017 by the International Society for Holter and Noninvasive Electrocardiology and Heart Rhythm Society, divided indications for ambulatory cardiac monitoring into 3 broad categories: diagnosis, prognosis, and arrhythmia assessment.

Diagnosis

The most common diagnostic role of monitoring is to correlate unexplained symptoms, including palpitations, presyncope, and syncope, with a transient cardiac arrhythmia. Monitoring can be considered successful if findings on ECG identify risks for serious arrhythmia and either correlate symptoms with those findings or demonstrate no arrhythmia when symptoms occur.

A range of arrhythmias can cause symp toms. Some, such as premature atrial contractions and premature ventricular contractions, may be benign in many clinical contexts. Others, such as atrial fibrillation, are more serious, and some, such as third-degree heart block and ventricular tachycardia, can be lethal.

Arrhythmia symptoms can vary in frequency and cause differing degrees of debility. The patient's symptoms, family history, and baseline ECG findings can suggest a more serious or a less serious underlying rhythm. These factors are important when determining which device is most appropriate.

Ambulatory ECG can also be useful in looking for a cause of cryptogenic stroke, ie, an ischemic stroke with an unexplained cause, even after a thorough initial workup. Paroxysmal atrial fibrillation is a frequent cause of cryptogenic stroke, and because it is transient, short-term inpatient telemetry may not be sufficient to detect it. Extended cardiac monitoring, lasting weeks or even months, is often needed for clinicians to make this diagnosis and initiate appropriate secondary prevention.

Prognosis

In a patient with known structural or electrical heart disease, ambulatory ECG can be used to stratify risk. This is particularly true in evaluating conditions associated with sudden cardiac death.

For example, hypertrophic cardiomyopathy and arrhythmogenic right ventricular dysplasia or cardiomyopathy are 2 cardiomyopathies that can manifest clinically with ventricular arrhythmias and sudden cardiac death. Ambulatory ECG can detect premature ventricular contractions and ventricular tachycardia and identify their frequency, duration, and anatomic origin. This information is useful in assessing risk of sudden cardiac death and determining the need for an implantable cardioverter-defibrillator.

Similarly, Wolff-Parkinson-White syndrome, involving rapid conduction through an accessory pathway, is associated with increased risk of ventricular fibrillation and sudden cardiac death. Ambulatory ECG monitoring can identify patients who have electrical features that portend the development of ventricular fibrillation. Also associated with sudden cardiac death are the inherited channelopathies, a heterogeneous group of primary arrhythmic disorders without accompanying structural pathology. Ambulatory ECG monitoring can detect transient electrical changes and nonsustained ventricular arrhythmias that would indicate the patient is at high risk of these disorders.

Assessing arrhythmia treatment

Arrhythmia monitoring using an ambulatory ECG device can also provide data to assess the efficacy of treatment under several circumstances.

The "pill-in-the-pocket" approach to treating atrial fibrillation, for example, involves self-administering a single dose of an antiarrhythmic drug when symptoms occur. Patients with infrequent but bothersome episodes can use an ambulatory ECG device to detect when they are having atrial fibrillation, take their prescribed drug, and see whether it terminates the arrhythmia, all without going to the hospital

Ambulatory ECG also is useful for assessing pharmacologic or ablative therapy in patients with atrial fibrillation or ventricular tachycardia. Monitoring for several weeks can help clinicians assess the burden of atrial fibrillation when using a rhythm-control strategy; assessing the ventricular rate in real-world situations is useful to determine the success of a rate-control strategy. Shortly after ablation of either atrial fibrillation or ventricular tachycardia, ECG home monitoring for 24 to 48 hours can detect asymptomatic recurrence and treatment failure.Some antiarrhythmic drugs can prolong the QT interval. Ambulatory ECG devices that feature real-time monitoring can be used during drug initiation, enabling the clinician to monitor the QT interval without admitting the patient to the hospital.

Ultimately, ambulatory ECG monitoring is most commonly used to evaluate symptoms. Because arrhythmias and specific symptoms are unpredictable and transient, extended monitoring in a real-world setting allows for a more comprehensive evaluation than a standard 10-second ECG recording.

AMBULATORY ECG DEVICES

Numerous ambulatory ECG devices are available, each with various features . Which features are most important depends on the severity and frequency of the symptoms, the suspected diagnosis, and the risk that the patient will not adhere to recording instructions.

Continuous external monitoring: The Holter monitor

The traditional ambulatory ECG device is the Holter monitor, named after its inventor. This light, portable, battery-operated recorder can be worn around the neck or clipped to the belt . The recorder connects via flexible cables to gel electrodes attached to the patient's chest. The monitor may have 2, 3, or 12 channels. Recording is typically done continuously for 24 to 48 hours, although some newer devices can record for longer. Patients can press a button to note when they are experiencing symptoms, allowing for potential correlation with ECG abnormalities. The data are stored on a flash drive that can be uploaded for analysis after recording is complete.

Clinical Applications

Given its relatively short duration of monitoring, the Holter device is typically used to evaluate symptoms that occur daily or nearly daily. An advantage of the Holter monitor is its ability to record continuously, without requiring the patient to interact with the device. This feature provides "full disclosure," which is the ability to see arrhythmia data from the entire recording period.These features make Holter monitoring useful to identify suspected frequently occurring silent arrhythmias or to assess the overall arrhythmia burden. A typical Holter report can contain information on the heart rate (maximum, minimum, and average), ectopic beats, and tachy- and bradyarrhythmias, as well as representative samples.

The Holter device is familiar to most practitioners and remains an effective choice for ambulatory ECG monitoring. However, its use has largely been replaced by newer devices that overcome the Holter's drawbacks, particularly its short duration of monitoring and the need for postmonitoring analysis. Additionally, although newer Holter devices are more ergonomic, some patients find the wires and gel electrodes uncomfortable or inconvenient.

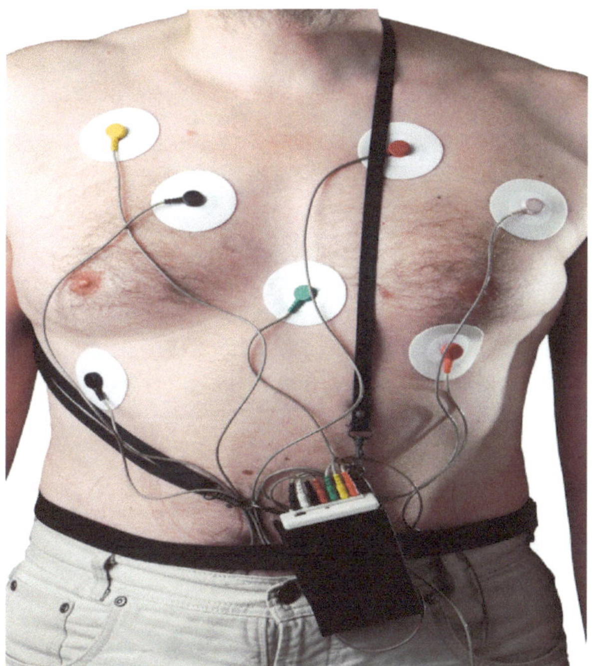

Fig.3.1 24-Hours Holter monitoring system showing placement of wires over the chest and recording apparatus is tied around the waist as shown in this fig.

Intermittent monitoring: Event recorders

Unlike the continuous monitors, intermittent recording devices (also called event recorders), capture and store tracings only during an event. Intermittent recording monitors are of 2 general types: post-event recorders and loop recorders. These devices can extend the overall duration of observation, which can be especially useful for those whose symptoms and arrhythmias are infrequent. Post-event recorders are small and self-contained, not requiring electrodes.The device is carried by the patient but not worn continuously. When the patient experiences symptoms, he or she places the device against the chest and presses a button to begin recording. These tracings are stored on the device and can be transmitted by telephone to a data center for analysis. Although post-event recorders allow for monitoring periods typically up to 30 days, they are limited by requiring the patient to act to record an event.

Clinical Application

These devices are best used in patients who have infrequent symptoms and are at low risk. Transient or debilitating symptoms, including syncope, can limit the possibility of capturing an event.

Intermittent monitoring: Loop recorders

Loop recorders monitor continuously but record only intermittently. The name refers to the device's looping memory: ie, to extend how long it can be used and make the most of its limited storage, the device records over previously captured data, saving only the most important data. The device saves the data whenever it detects an abnormal rhythm or the patient experiences symptoms and pushes a button. Data are recorded for a specified time before and after the activation, typically 30 seconds.

Loop recorders come in 2 types:

- External
- Implantable.

1.External loop recorders

External loop recorders look like Holter monitors . but they have the advantage of a much longer observation period—typically up to 1 month. The newest devices have even greater storage capacity and can provide "backward" memory, saving data that were captured just before the patient pushed the button.

In studies of patients with palpitations, presyncope, or syncope, external loop recorders had greater diagnostic yield than traditional 24-hour Holter monitors. This finding was supported by a clinical trial that found 30-day monitoring with an external loop recorder led to a 5-fold increase in detecting atrial fibrillation in patients with cryptogenic stroke

Disadvantages of external loop recorders are limited memory storage, a considerable reliance on patient activation of the device, and wires and electrodes that need to be worn continuously.

Clinical Application

External loop recorders are most effective when used to detect an arrhythmia or to correlate infrequent symptoms with an arrhythmia. They are most appropriately used in patients whose symptoms occur more often than every 4 weeks. They are less useful in assessing very infrequent symptoms, overall arrhythmia burden, or responsiveness to therapy

2.Implantable loop recorders

Implantable loop recorders are small devices that contain a pair of sensing electrodes housed within an outer shell. They are implanted subcutaneously, usually in the left parasternal region, using local anesthesia. The subcutaneous location eliminates many of the drawbacks of the skin-electrode interface of external loop recorders.

Similar to the external loop recorder, this device monitors continuously and can be activated to record either by the patient by pressing a button on a separate device, or automatically when an arrhythmia is detected using a preprogrammed algorithm.

In contrast to external devices, many internal loop recorders have a battery life and monitoring capability of up to 3 years. This extended monitoring period has been shown to increase the likelihood of diagnosing syncope or infrequent palpitations..Given that paroxysmal atrial fibrillation can be sporadic and reveal itself months after a stroke, internal loop recorders may also have a role in evaluating cryptogenic stroke

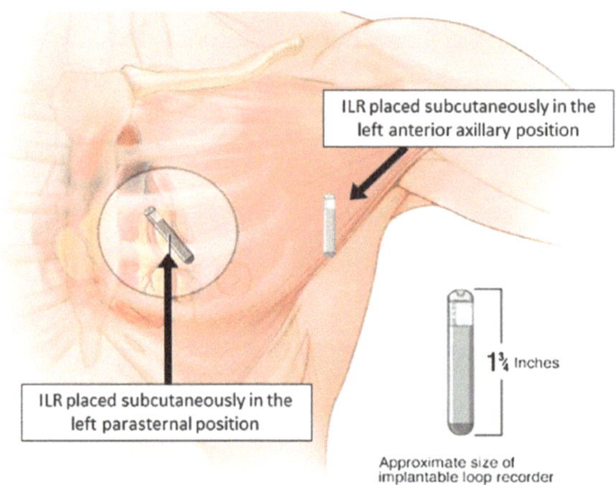

Fig.3.2 Implantable loop recorder (ILR) in the left parasternal and left anterior axillary positions. Both devices are placed subcutaneously

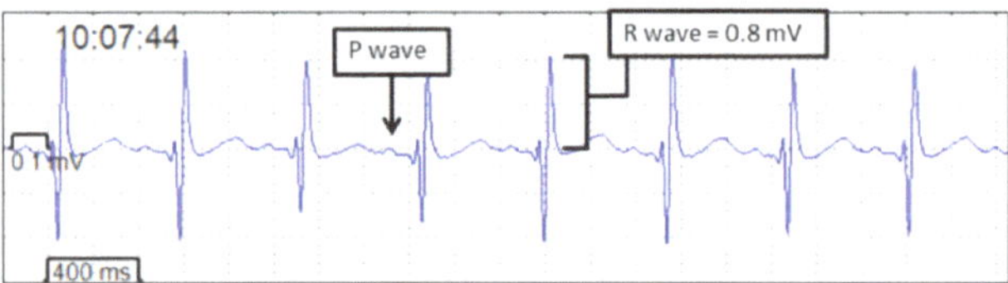

Fig.3.3 Electrocardiogram tracing from an ILR in the left anterior axillary position. R-wave measurement = 0.8 mV and p waves visible

The most important drawbacks of internal loop recorders are the surgical procedure for insertion, their limited memory storage, and high upfront cost. Furthermore, even though they allow for extended monitoring, there may be diminishing returns for prolonged observation.

Clinical Applications

For patients with palpitations, intermittent event monitoring has been shown to be cost-effective for the first 2 weeks, but after 3 weeks, the cost per diagnosis increases dramatically.16 As a result, internal loop recorders are reserved primarily for scenarios in which prolonged external monitoring has not revealed a source of arrhythmia despite a high degree of suspicion.

Mobile cardiac telemetry

Mobile cardiac telemetry builds on other ECG monitoring systems by adding real-time communication and technician evaluation. Physically, these devices resemble either hand-held event records, with a single-channel sensing unit embedded in the case, or a traditional Holter monitor, with 3 channels, wires, and electrodes

The sensor wirelessly communicates with a nearby portable monitor, which continuously observes and analyzes the patient's heart rhythm. When an abnormal rhythm is detected or when the patient marks the presence of symptoms, data are recorded and sent in real time via a cellular network to a monitoring center; the newest monitors can send data via any Wi-Fi system. The rhythm is then either evaluated by a trained technician or relayed to a physician. If necessary, the patient can be contacted immediately.

Mobile cardiac telemetry is typically used for up to 30 days, which allows for evaluation of less-frequent symptoms. As a result, it may have a higher diagnostic yield for palpitations, syncope, and presyncope than the 24-hour Holter monitor.Further, perhaps because mobile cardiac telemetry relies less on stored information and requires less patient-device interaction than external loop recorders, it is more effective at symptom evaluation.

Mobile cardiac telemetry also has a diagnostic role in evaluating patients with crypto-genic stroke. This is based on studies showing it has a high rate of atrial fibrillation detection in this patient population and is more effective at determining overall atrial fibrillation burden than loop recorders

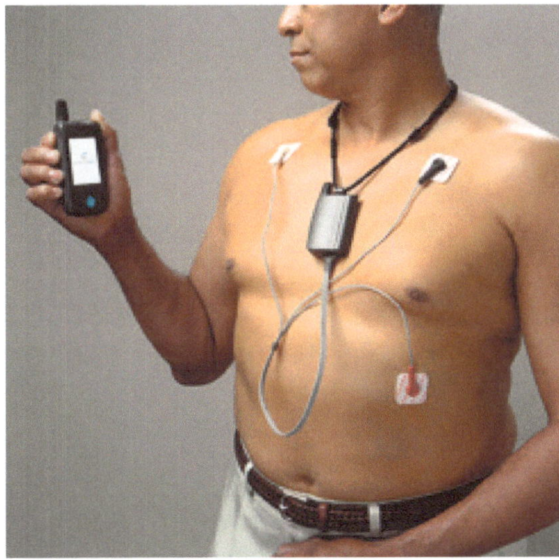

Fig.3.4 Mobile Cardiac Telemetry Systems Market

Clinical Uses

The key advantage of mobile cardiac telemetry is its ability to make rhythm assessments and communicate with technicians in real time. This allows high-risk patients to be immediately alerted to a life-threatening arrhythmia. It also gives providers an opportunity to initiate anticoagulation or titrate antiarrhythmic therapy in the outpatient setting without a delay in obtaining information. This intensive monitoring, however, requires significant manpower, which translates to higher cost, averaging 3 times that of other standard external monitors.

Patch monitors

These ultraportable devices are a relatively unobtrusive and easy-to-use alternative for short-term ambulatory ECG monitoring. They monitor continuously with full disclosure, outpatient telemetry, and post-event recording features.

Patch monitors are small, leadless, wireless, and water-resistant.They are affixed to the left pectoral region with a waterproof adhesive and can be worn for 14 to 28 days. Recording is usually done continuously; however, these devices have an event marker button that can be pressed when the user experiences symptoms. They acquire a single channel of data, and each manufacturer has a proprietary algorithm for automated rhythm detection and analysis.

Several manufacturers produce ECG patch monitors. Two notable devices are the Zio patch (iRhythm Technologies, San Francisco, CA) and the Mobile Cardiac Outpatient Telemetry patch (BioTelemetry, Inc, Malvern, PA).

The Zio patch is a continuous external monitor with full disclosure. It is comparable to the Holter monitor, but has a longer recording period. After completing a 2-week monitoring period, the device is returned for comprehensive rhythm analysis. A typical Zio report contains information on atrial fibrillation burden, ectopic rhythm burden, symptom and rhythm correlation, heart rate trends, and relevant rhythm strips.

The Mobile Cardiac Outpatient Telemetry patch collects data continuously and communicates wirelessly by Bluetooth to send its ECG data to a monitoring center for evaluation.

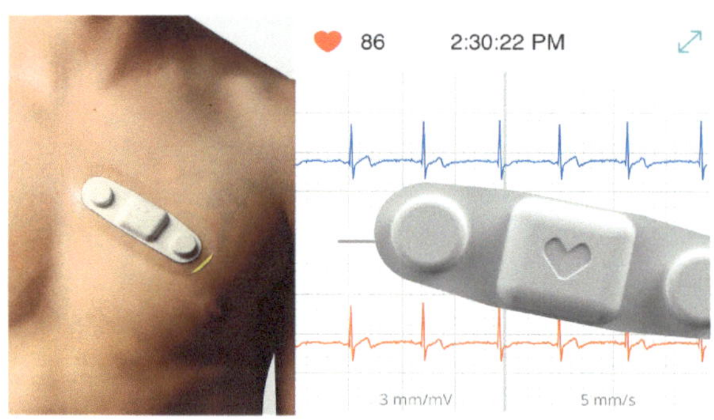

Fig.3.5 A small patch help monitor patients vital signs remotely (Photo courtesy of VivaLNK)

A principal advantage of patch monitors—and a major selling point for manufacturers—is their low-profile, ergonomic, and patient-friendly design. Patients do not have to manage wires or batteries and are able to shower with their devices. Studies show that these features increase patient satisfaction and compliance, resulting in increased diagnostic yield. Additionally, patch monitors have the advantage of a longer continuous monitoring period than traditional Holter devices (2 weeks vs 1 or 2 days), affording an opportunity to capture events that occur less frequently.

Validation studies have reinforced their efficacy and utility in clinical scenarios. In large part because of the extended monitoring period, patch monitors have been shown to have greater diagnostic yield than the 24-hour Holter monitor in symptomatic patients undergoing workup for suspected arrhythmia.

The role of patch monitors in evaluating atrial fibrillation is also being established. For patients with cryptogenic stroke, patch monitors have shown better atrial fibrillation detection than the 24-hour Holter monitor. Compared with traditional loop monitors, patch monitors have the added advantage of assessing total atrial fibrillation burden. Further, although screening for atrial fibrillation with a traditional 12-lead ECG monitor has not been shown to be effective, clinical studies have found that the patch monitor may be a useful screening tool for high-risk patients Nevertheless, patch monitors have drawbacks. They are not capable of long-term monitoring, owing to battery and adhesive limitations.20 More important, they have been able to offer only single-channel acquisition, which makes it more difficult to detect an arrhythmia that is characterized by a change in QRS axis or change in QRS width, or to distinguish an arrhythmia from an artifact. This appears to be changing, however, as several manufacturers have recently developed multi- lead ECG patch monitors or attachments and are attempting to merge this technology with fully capable remote telemetry

NEWER TECHNOLOGIES

The newest ambulatory ECG devices build on the foundational concepts of the older ones. However, with miniaturized electronic circuits, Bluetooth, Wi-Fi, and smartphones, these new devices can capture ECG tracings and diagnose offending arrhythmias on more consumer-friendly devices.

Smartphones and smartwatches have become increasingly powerful. Some have the ability to capture, display, and record the cardiac waveform. One manufacturer to capitalize on these technologies, AliveCor (Mountain View, CA), has developed 2 products capable of generating a single-lead ECG recording using either a smartphone (KardiaMobile) or an Apple watch (KardiaBand).

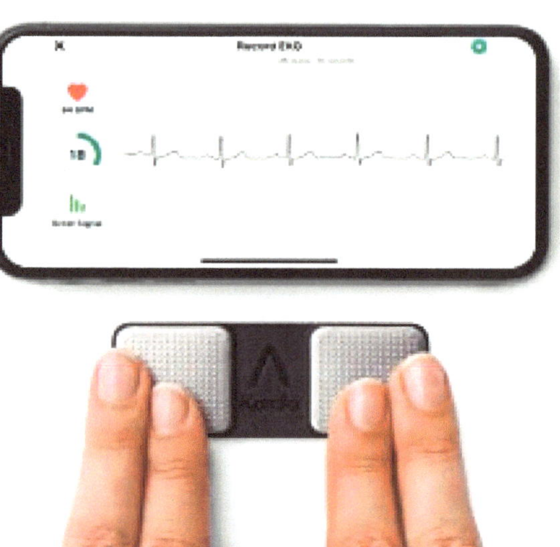

Fig.3.6 AliveCor Single Lead ECG Device - Fast & Accurate | US FDA Cleared & Clinically validated

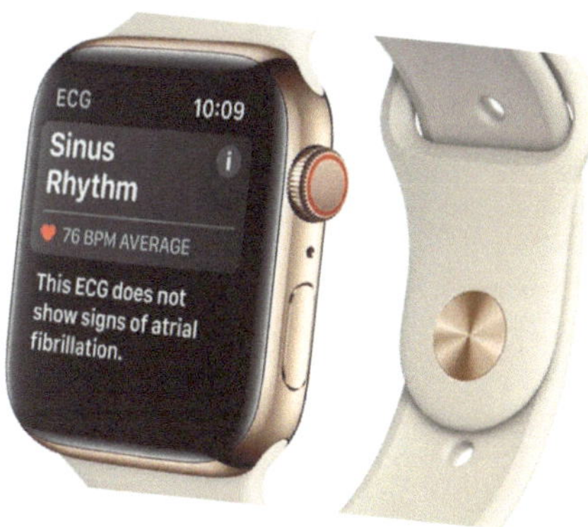

Fig.3.7 Apple Watch Series 4 tracks heart rhythm and call for help in case of a fall

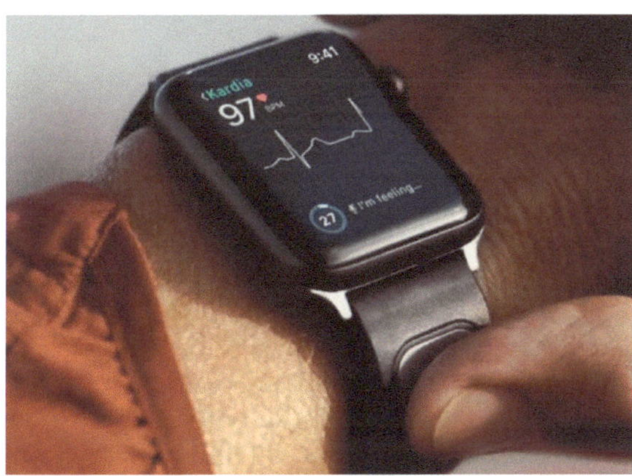

Fig.3.8 KardiaBand lets you monitor heart health from any Apple Watch While the Apple Watch Series 4 can take an ECG, earlier Apple Watch users are left out — which is where KardiaBand comes in. This seemingly ordinary watch band is solid black, resembling Apple's sport bands, but has a silver square located under the watch face. This simple square isn't decorative: it's a sensor, and pressing your thumb to it for 30 seconds will take medical-grade EKG.

Smartphones and smartwatches have become increasingly powerful. Some have the ability to capture, display, and record the cardiac waveform. One manufacturer to capitalize on these technologies, AliveCor (Mountain View, CA), has developed 2 products capable of generating a single-lead ECG recording using either a smartphone (KardiaMobile) or an Apple watch (KardiaBand).KardiaMobile has a 2-electrode band that can be carried in a pocket or attached to the back of a smartphone . The user places 1 or 2 fingers from each hand on the electrodes, and the device sends an ultrasound signal that is picked up by the smartphone's microphone. The signal is digitized to produce a 30-second ECG tracing on the phone's screen. A proprietary algorithm analyzes the rhythm and generates a description of "normal" or "possible atrial fibrillation." The ECG is then uploaded to a cloud-based storage system for later access or transmission. KardiaMobile is compatible with both iOS and Android devices.

The KardiaBand is a specialized Apple watch band that has an electrode embedded in it. The user places a thumb on the electrode for 30 seconds, and an ECG tracing is displayed on the watch screen.

The Kardia devices were developed (and advertised) predominantly to assess atrial fibrillation. Studies have validated the accuracy of their algorithm. One study showed that, compared with physician-interpreted ECGs, the algorithm had a 96.6% sensitivity and 94.1% specificity for detecting atrial fibrillation. They have been found useful for detecting and evaluating atrial fibrillation in several clinical scenarios, including discharge monitoring in patients after ablation or cardiac surgery. In a longer study of patients at risk of stroke, twice-weekly ECG screening using a Kardia device for 1 year was more likely to detect incident atrial fibrillation than routine care alone.

Also, the Kardia devices can effectively function as post-event recorders when activated by patients when they experience symptoms. In a small study of outpatients with palpitations and a prior nondiagnostic workup, the KardiaMobile device was found to be non-inferior to external loop recorders for detecting arrhythmias. Additional studies are assessing Kardia's utility in other scenarios, including the evaluation of ST-segment elevation myocardial infarction and QT interval for patients receiving antiarrhythmic therapy

Cardiio Inc. (Cambridge, MA) has developed technology to screen for atrial fibrillation using an app that requires no additional external hardware. Instead, the app uses a smartphone's camera and flashlight to perform photo plethysmography to detect pulsatile changes in blood volume and generate a waveform

Based on waveform variability, a proprietary algorithm attempts to determine whether the user is in atrial fibrillation. It does not produce an ECG tracing. Initial studies suggest it has good diagnostic accuracy and potential utility as a population-based screening tool, but it has not been fully validated.

Recently, Apple entered the arena of ambulatory cardiac monitoring with the release of its fourth-generation watch (Apple Watch Series 4 model). This watch has built-in electrodes that can generate a single-lead ECG on the watch screen. Its algorithm can discriminate between atrial fibrillation and sinus rhythm, but it has not been assessed for its ability to evaluate other arrhythmias. Even though it has been "cleared" by the US Food and Drug Administration, it is approved only for informational use, not to make a medical diagnosis.

Integration of ambulatory ECG technology with smartphone and watch technology is an exciting new wearable option for arrhythmia detection. The patient-centered and controlled nature of these devices have the potential to help patients with palpitations or other symptoms determine if their cardiac rhythms are normal.

This technology, however, is still in its infancy and has many limitations. For example, even though these devices can function as post-event recorders, they depend on user-device interactions. Plus, they cannot yet perform continuous arrhythmia monitoring like modern loop recorders.

Additionally, automated analysis has largely been limited to distinguishing atrial fibrillation from normal sinus rhythm. It is uncertain how effective the devices may be in evaluating other arrhythmias. Single-lead ECG recordings, as discussed, have limited interpretability and value. And even though studies have shown utility in certain clinical scenarios, large-scale validation studies are lacking. This technology will likely continue to be developed and its clinical value improved; however, its clinical use requires careful consideration and collaborative physician-patient decision-making.

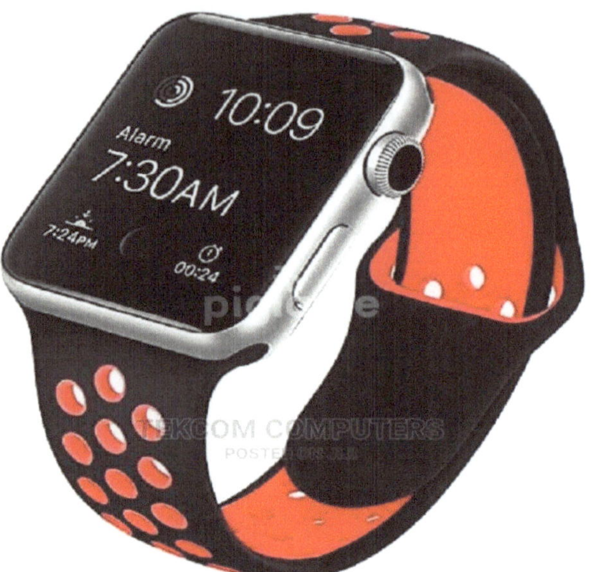

Fig.3.9 Ambulatory cardiac monitoring with the release of its fourth-generation watch (Apple Watch Series 4 model). This watch has built-in electrodes that can generate a single-lead ECG on the watch screen. Its algorithm can discriminate between atrial fibrillation and sinus rhythm, but it has not been assessed for its ability to evaluate other arrhythmias.

The Application of Artificial intelligence (AI) to the Electrocardiogram (ECG)

Key points

- The feasibility and potential value of the application of advanced artificial intelligence methods, particularly deep-learning convolutional neural networks (CNNs), to the electrocardiogram (ECG) have been demonstrated.
- CNNs developed with the use of large numbers of digital ECGs linked to rich clinical datasets might be able to perform accurate and nuanced, human-like interpretation of ECGs.
- CNNs have also been developed to detect asymptomatic left ventricular dysfunction, silent atrial fibrillation, hypertrophic cardiomyopathy and an individual's age, sex and race on the basis of the ECG alone.
- CNNs to detect other cardiac conditions, such as aortic valve stenosis and amyloid heart disease, are in active development.
- These approaches might be applicable to the standard 12-lead ECG or to data obtained from single-lead or multilead mobile or wearable ECG technologies.

- ·Evidence on patient outcomes, as well as the challenges and potential limitations from the real-world implementation of the artificial intelligence-enhanced ECG, continues to emerge.

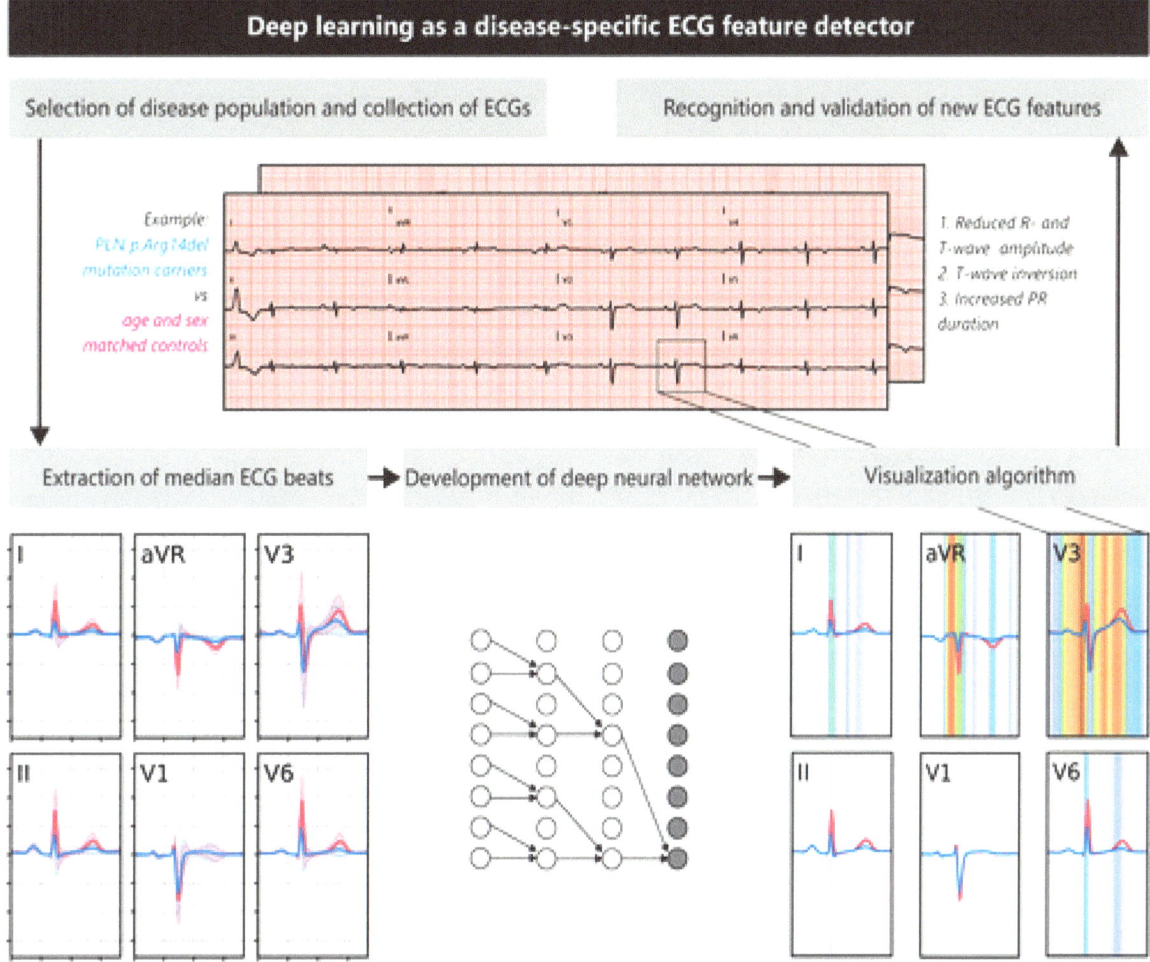

Fig.3.10 ECG interpretation requires expertise and is mostly based on physician recognition of specific patterns, which may be challenging in rare cardiac diseases. Deep neural networks (DNNs) can discover complex features in ECGs and may facilitate the detection of novel features which possibly play a pathophysiological role in relatively unknown diseases. Using a cohort of PLN (phospholamban) p.Arg14del mutation carriers, we aimed to investigate whether a novel DNN-based approach can identify established ECG features, but moreover, we aimed to expand our knowledge on novel ECG features in these patients.

Detection of silent AF from a sinus-rhythm ECG

To assess the likelihood of silent AF, a group of investigators from the Mayo Clinic developed a CNN to predict AF on the basis of a standard 12-lead ECG obtained during sinus rhythm

The algorithm was developed using nearly half a million digitally stored ECGs from 126,526 patients and was validated and tested in separate internal datasets. The model applied convolutions on a temporal axis and across multiple leads to extract morphological and temporal features during the training and validation processes. Patients with at least one ECG showing AF within 31 days after the sinus-rhythm ECG were classified as being positive for AF. In the testing dataset, the algorithm demonstrated an AUC of 0.87, sensitivity of 79.0%, specificity of 79.5% and an accuracy of 79.4% in detecting patients with documentation of AF using only information from the sinus-rhythm ECG. Therefore, the algorithm can detect nearly concomitant, unrecognized AF, rather than predict the long-term risk of AF. Conceptually, this AI tool converts a routine 10-s, 12-lead ECG into the equivalent of a prolonged rhythm-monitoring tool , although the duration of 'monitoring' and its yield require validation. Additionally, this tool can be applied retroactively to digitally stored ECGs from patients with a previous ESUS. This algorithm might facilitate targeted AF surveillance (such as using an ambulatory rhythm-monitoring patch or implantable loop recorder) in subsets of high-risk patients. This work is preliminary, but we are currently assessing the performance of this algorithm in identifying patients who might benefit from prospective AF screening or monitoring (with Holter or extended monitoring) and, ultimately, various stroke-prevention strategies. We also note that other groups have derived similar AF risk-prognostication tools that examine other electrophysiological parameters, such as signal-averaged ECG-derived P-wave analysis

ECGs are ubiquitously performed for a variety of screening, diagnostic and monitoring purposes, thereby providing ample opportunities for the application of this algorithm. The ultimate clinical utility of this approach will be determined by the observed positive and negative predictive values of the algorithm when applied to a given population and by the cost and downstream consequences, particularly for patient outcomes, related to follow-up diagnostic testing and therapies.Unlike the traditional risk-prediction models that comprise predefined variables, the CNN described above is agnostic, because we do not know what ECG features the CNN is 'seeing' and which factors drive its performance. The performance of the algorithm is likely to be based on a combination of ECG signatures that are known risk factors for AF (such as LV hypertrophy, , P-wave amplitude, atrial ectopy and heart rate variability) as well as others that are currently unknown or are not obvious to the human eye, in combination, in a non-linear manner34. The ECG is also likely to contain information that correlates with known clinical risk factors.

Antiarrhythmic drug management

Dofetilide and sotalol are commonly used for the treatment of AF. Their antiarrhythmic effect is exerted on the myocardium by prolonging the duration of the repolarization phase, meaning that QT prolongation is an anticipated effect of these drugs. Owing to the ensuing risk of substantial QT prolongation and potentially fatal ventricular proarrhythmia, patients require close monitoring with a continuous ECG in the hospital setting when these drugs are used, particularly for dofetilide. In addition, with the long-term use of these medications, the QT interval should be intermittently assessed because dose adjustments might be necessary in cases of substantial QT prolongation, concomitant medications with QT-prolonging effects and fluctuations in renal function (both sotalol and dofetilide are primarily metabolized through the kidneys).

Using serial 12-lead ECGs and linked information on plasma dofetilide concentrations in 42 patients who were treated with dofetilide or placebo in a crossover randomized clinical trial, a deep-learning algorithm predicted plasma dofetilide concentrations with good correlation (r = 0.85)50. By comparison, a linear model of the corrected QT interval correlated with dofetilide concentrations with a coefficient of 0.64 . This finding suggests that the QT interval might not accurately reflect the plasma dofetilide concentration in some patients and so might underestimate or overestimate the proarrhythmic risk.Machine-learning approaches, including supervised, unsupervised and reinforcement learning, have also been used to determine the optimal dosing regimen during dofetilide treatment In the future, patients treated with dofetilide, sotalol or other antiarrhythmic medications might avoid the need for hospitalization for drug loading or office visits for routinesurveillance ECGs by monitoring their own ECG using smartphone-using smartphone-based tools powered with AI capabilities to determine the plasma concentrations of the drug or the risk of drug-related toxic effects. The development of these AI algorithms applied to a single-lead ECG is still in progress.

Wearable and mobile ECG technologies

AI algorithms can be applied to wearable technologies, enabling rapid, point-of-care diagnoses for patients and consumers. Although many algorithms have been derived using 12-lead ECG data, some studies have demonstrated favourable performance even when algorithms are deployed on single-lead ECGs8. The performance of AI–ECG algorithms for the detection of HCM or the determination of serum potassium levels when applied to single-lead ECGs has been shown not to be significantly different from the performance when applied to 12-lead ECGs. Additionally, signals other than the ECG can also be analysed using AI approaches. For instance, a deep neural network has been developed to detect AF passively from photoplethysmography signals obtained from the Apple Watch. Newer iterations of the Apple Watch now allow users to confirm the presence of AF using electrophysiological signals obtained through a single bipolar vector

Implementation of AI–ECG

In contrast to data obtained through the clinical history, medical record review or imaging tests, the ease and consistency with which ECG data can be obtained and analysed for the development and implementation of AI models are likely to accelerate the uptake of the AI–ECG in clinical applications, with ensuing increases in workflow efficiency. The demonstrated capabilities of the AI–ECG described in the previous sections have the potential to influence the spectrum of patient care, including screening, diagnosis, prognostication, and personalized treatment selection and monitoring . The preliminary data on the performance of the AI–ECG algorithms are clearly promising, but these technologies will be meaningful only inasmuch as they improve our clinical practice and patient outcomes55. To this end, several AI technologies are currently being tested in various clinical applications.

Conclusions

The implementation of the AI–ECG is still in its infancy, but a continuously growing clinical investigation agenda will determine the added value of these AI tools, their optimal deployment in the clinical arena and their multifaceted and so-far largely unpredictable implications.

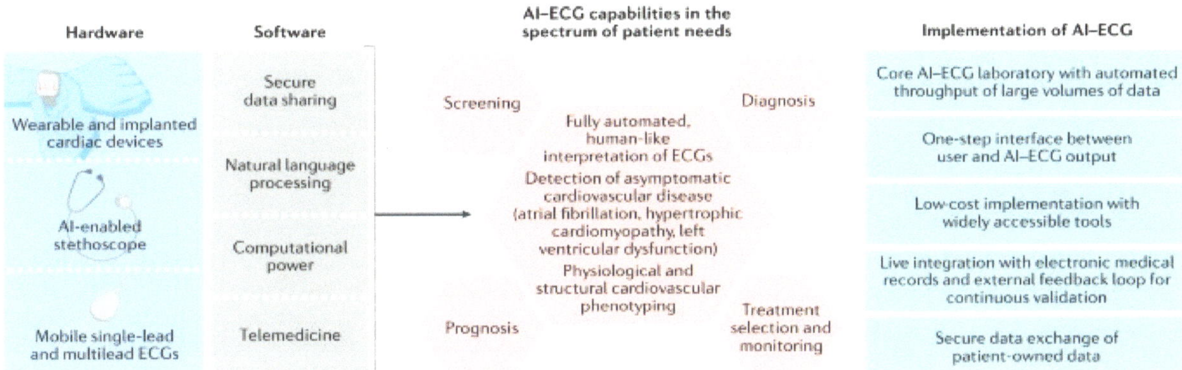

Fig.3.11 **Framework for AI–ECG applications in clinical practice.** Current, versatile electrocardiogram (ECG)-recording technologies (wearable and implantable devices, smartwatches and e-stethoscopes) coupled with the ability to store, transfer, process and analyse large amounts of digital data are increasingly allowing the deployment of artificial intelligence (AI)-powered tools in the clinical arena, addressing the spectrum of patient needs. The science of AI-enhanced ECG (AI–ECG) implementation, including the interface between patients and the AI–ECG output, integration of AI–ECG tools with electronic health records, patient privacy, and cost and reimbursement implications, is in its infancy and continues to evolve.

Bibliography And Acknowledgement

- Attia, Z. I. et al. An artificial intelligence-enabled ECG algorithm for the identification of patients with atrial fibrillation during sinus rhythm: a retrospective analysis of outcome prediction. Lancet 394, 861–867 (2019).
- Attia, Z. I. et al. Noninvasive assessment of dofetilide plasma concentration using a deep learning (neural network) analysis of the surface electrocardiogram: a proof of concept study. PLoS ONE 13, e0201059 (2018)
- Barbagelata A, Bethea CF, Severance HW, et al. Smartphone ECG for evaluation of ST-segment elevation myocardial infarction (STEMI): design of the ST LEUIS international multicenter study. J Electrocardiol 2018; 51(2):260–264
- Barrett PM, Komatireddy R, Haaser S, et al. Comparison of 24-hour Holter monitoring with 14-day novel adhesive patch electrocardiographic monitoring. Am J Med 2014; 127(1):95.e11–95.e17.
- Brignole M, Vardas P, Hoffman E, et alEHRA Scientific Documents Committee. Indications for the use of diagnostic implantable and external ECG loop recorders. Europace 2009; 11(5):671–687.
- Chan PH, Wong CK, Poh YC, et al. Diagnostic performance of a smartphone-based photoplethysmographic application for atrial fibrillation screening in a primary care setting. J Am Heart Assoc 2016; 5(7). pii:e003428.
- Christensen LM, Krieger DW, Hojberg S, et al. Paroxysmal atrial fibrillation occurs often in cryptogenic ischaemic stroke. Final results from the SURPRISE study. Eur J Neurol 2014; 21(6):884–889
- Cotter PE, Martin PJ, Ring L, Warburton EA, Belham M, Pugh PJ. Incidence of atrial fibrillation detected by implantable loop recorders in unexplained stroke. Neurology 2013; 80(17):1546–1550.
- Crawford MH, Bernstein SJ, Deedwania PC, et al ACC/AHA guidelines for ambulatory electrocardiography. A report of the American College of Cardiology/American Heart Association Task Force on Practice Guidelines (Committee to Revise the
- Guidelines for Ambulatory Electrocardiography). Developed in collaboration with the North American Society for Pacing and Electrophysiology. J Am Coll Cardiol 1999; 34(3):912–948
- Del Mar B The history of clinical Holter monitoring. Ann Noninvasive Elecrocardiol. 2005; 10(2):226–230.
- Dillon JJ, DeSimone CV, Sapir Y, et al. Noninvasive potassium determination using a mathematically processed ECG: proof of concept for a novel "blood-less, blood test". J Electrocardiol 2015; 48(1):12–18.
- Edvardsson N, Frykman V, van Mechelen R, et al PICTURE Study Investigators. Use of an implantable loop recorder to increase the diagnostic yield in unexplained syncope: results from the PICTURE registry. Europace 2011; 13(2):262–269
- Fung E, Jarvelin MR, Doshi RN, et al. Electrocardiographic patch devices and contemporary wireless cardiac monitoring. Front Physiol 2015; 6:149
- Garabelli P, Stavrakis S, Albert M, et al. Comparison of QT interval readings in normal sinus rhythm between a smartphone heart monitor and a 12-lead ECG for healthy volunteers and inpatients receiving sotalol or dofetilide. J Cardiovasc Electrophysiol 2016; 27(7):827–832
- Giada F, Gulizia M, Francese M, et al. Recurrent unexplained palpitations (RUP) study comparison of implantable loop recorder versus conventional diagnostic strategy. J Am Coll Cardiol 2007; 49(19):1951–1956.
- Gladstone DJ, Spring M, Dorian P, et al EMBRACE Investigators and Coordinators. Atrial fibrillation in patients with cryptogenic stroke. N Engl J Med 2014; 370(26):2467–2477
- Halcox JPJ, Wareham K, Cardew A, et al. Assessment of remote heart rhythm sampling using the AliveCor heart monitor to screen for atrial fibrillation: the REHEARSE-AF study. Circulation 2017; 136(19):1784–1794
- Holter NJ, Gengerelli JA Remote recording of physiological data by radio. Rocky Mt Med J 1949; 46(9):747–751.
- Joshi AK, Kowey PR, Prystowksy EN, et al. First experience with a mobile cardiac outpatient telemetry (MCOT) system for the diagnosis and management of cardiac arrhythmia. Am J Cardiol 2005; 95(7):878–881.
- Kennedy HL The history, science, and innovation of Holter technology. Ann Noninvasive Elecrocardiol 2006; 11(1):85–94.
- Lee SP, Ha G, Wright DE, et al. Highly flexible, wearable, and disposable cardiac biosensors for remote and ambulatory monitoring. npj Digital Medicine 2018
- Lobodzinski SS. ECG patch monitors for assessment of cardiac rhythm abnormalities. Prog Cardiovasc Dis 2013; 56(2):224–229.
- Locati ET, Moya A, Oliveira, et al. External prolonged electrocardiogram monitoring in unexplained syncope and palpitations: results of the SYNARR-Flash study. Europace 2016; 18(8):1265–1272
- Locati ET, Vecchi AM, Vargiu S, Cattafi G, Lunati M. Role of extended external loop recorders for the diagnosis of unexplained syncope, pre-syncope, and sustained palpitations. Europace 2014; 16(6):914–922.
- Locati ET. New directions for ambulatory monitoring following the 2017 HRS-ISHNE expert consensus. J Electrocardiol 2017; 50(6):828–832.
- Lowres N, Mulcahy G, Gallagher R, et al. Self-monitoring for atrial fibrillation recurrence in the discharge period post-cardiac surgery using an iPhone electrocardiogram. Eur J Cardiothorac Surg 2016; 50(1):44–51
- MacInnis H The clinical application of radioelectrocardiography. Can Med Assoc J 1954; 70(5):574–576
- Mitchell ARJ, Le Page P. Living with the handheld ECG. BMJ Innov 2015; 1:46–48.
- Monitoring in Patients with Stroke or TIA. Front Neurol 2015; 5:266
- Muhlestein JB, Le V, Albert D, et al. Smartphone ECG for evaluation of STEMI: results of the ST LEUIS pilot study. J Electrocardiol 2015; 48(2):249–259
- Narasimha D, Hanna N, Beck H, et al. Validation of a smartphone-based event recorder for arrhythmia detection. Pacing Clin Electrophysiol 2018; 41(5):487–494.
- Rothman SA, Laughlin JC, Seltzer J, et al.The diagnosis of cardiac arrhythmias: a prospective multi-center randomized study comparing mobile cardiac outpatient telemetry versus standard loop event monitoring. J Cardiovasc Electrophysiol 2007; 18(3):241–247.
- Rozen G, Vai J, Hosseini SM, et al. Diagnostic accuracy of a novel mobile phone application in monitoring atrial fibrillation. Am J Cardiol 2018; 121(10):1187–1191

- Schreiber D, Sattar A, Drigalla D, Higgins S. Ambulatory cardiac monitoring for discharged emergency department patients with possible cardiac arrhythmias. West J Emerg Med 2014; 15(2):194–198.
- Steinberg JS, Varma N, Cygankiewicz I, et al 2017 ISHNE-HRS expert consensus statement on ambulatory ECG and external cardiac monitoring/telemetry. Heart Rhythm 2017; 14(7
- Steinhubl SR, Waalen J, Edwards AM, et al. Effect of a home-based wearable continuous ECG monitoring patch on detection of undiagnosed atrial fibrillation: the mSToPS randomized clinical trial. JAMA 2018; 320(2):146–155.
- Tarakji KG, Wazni OM, Callahan T, et al. Using a novel wireless system for monitoring patients after the atrial fibrillation ablation procedure: the iTransmit study. Heart Rhythm 2015; 12(3):554–559
.
- Tayal AH, Tian M, Kelly KM, et al. Atrial fibrillation detected by mobile cardiac outpatient telemetry in cryptogenic TIA or stroke. Neurology 2008; 71(21):1696–1701
- Turakhia MP, Hoang DD, Zimetbaum P, Miller JD, Froelicher VF, Kumar UN, et al. Diagnostic utility of a novel leadless arrhythmia monitoring device. Am J Cardiol. (2013) 112:520–4
- Turakhia MP, Ullal AJ, Hoang DD, et al. Feasibility of extended ambulatory electrocardiogram monitoring to identify silent atrial fibrillation in high-risk patients: the Screening Study for Undiagnosed Atrial Fibrillation (STUDY-AF). Clin Cardiol 2015; 38(5):285–292
- William AD, Kanbour M, Callahan T, et al. Assessing the accuracy of an automated atrial fibrillation detection algorithm using smartphone technology: the iREAD study. Heart Rhythm 2018; 15(10):1561–1565.
- Zimetbaum P, Goldman A. Ambulatory arrhythmia monitoring: choosing the right device. Circulation 2010; 122(16):1629–1636
- Zimetbaum PJ, Kim KY, Josephson ME, Goldberger AL, Cohen DJ . Diagnostic yield and optimal duration of continuous-loop event monitoring for the diagnosis of palpitations: a cost-effectiveness analysis. Ann Intern Med 1998; 128(11):890–895

Clinical Application Of 3D Printing For Heart Diseases. (Review)

CHAPTER

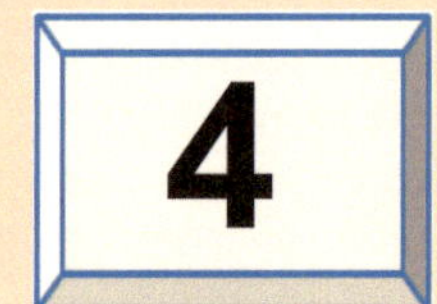

Cardiovascular diseases comprise the leading causes of death in all areas of the world and can be categorized as coronary artery disease, rheumatic heart disease, cardiomyopathy, congenital heart disease (CHD), valvular heart disease, carditis, and aortic aneurysms .As the population ages and progress continues in cardiovascular treatment options, cardiac surgeons and interventional cardiologists are confronted with complex and unpredictable anatomical challenges.Medical three-dimensional (3D) printing, also known as rapid prototyping or additive manufacturing, is the process of converting digital signals into physical models using 3D printers. It enables visual inspection and direct manipulation of models of human anatomy and pathology .It has been nearly 30 years since this technology was introduced into medicine. Three-dimensional printing was first used in orthopedics and maxillofacial surgery, especially in the manufacturing of surgical guides and personalized grafts involving the skull, mandible, dentures, and artificial joints .As 3D printing gained a foothold in other medical areas, evidence began to accumulate the usefulness of 3D-printed applications in the treatment of heart diseases, such as CHDs, valvular diseases, and hypertrophic cardiomyopathy .This review summarizes cardiac 3D printing workflow and discusses the clinical applications, current status, limitations, and future perspectives of cardiac 3D printing.

Basic Concepts Of Cardiac 3D Printing

Generating a 3D-printed heart model includes sequential stages of image acquisition, data postprocessing, and industrial-level manufacturing. Acquisition of 3D volumetric cardiovascular images from computed tomography (CT), magnetic resonance imaging (MRI), 3D transthoracic , or transesophageal echocardiography is the first step. Among these imaging modalities, CT angiography (CTA) is the one most frequently used, and CT images can be reconstructed ideally at about 1 mm thick. The second step in the 3D printing flowchart is image postprocessing with the aid of commercially available software programs (i.e., Materialise Mimics 21.0, Materialise, Leuven, Belgium), which discriminates between the anatomical area of interest and the adjacent tissues.During this process, DICOM (Digital Imaging and Communications in Medicine) cardiac images from radiology and cardiac imaging workstations are transformed and universally stored in standard tessellation language (STL) format. Computer-aided design software is used to refine the STL file by segmenting, wrapping, smoothing, and augmenting the model, manually or automatically, to exemplify anatomical and pathological areas and by adding connectors between separate anatomical structures of interest before printing. Afterward, a 3D printer (i.e., J750, Stratasys, Eden Prairie, MN, USA) interprets data in an STL file to manufacture a physical object. Material jetting technology, which can combine several materials within the same 3D-printed cast, thereby enabling the fabrication of models of human anatomy and pathology that contain different tissues, is the present ideal 3D printing technique. Finally, postprocessing by removal of support materials, ultraviolet curing, polishing, cleaning, sterilization, and labeling is also crucial to the quality of the models.

Applications Of Cardiac 3D Printing

Applications of 3D printing in the cardiac field range from CHDs, valvular heart diseases, left atrial appendage occlusion (LAAO), arrhythmia, to hypertrophic cardiomyopathy

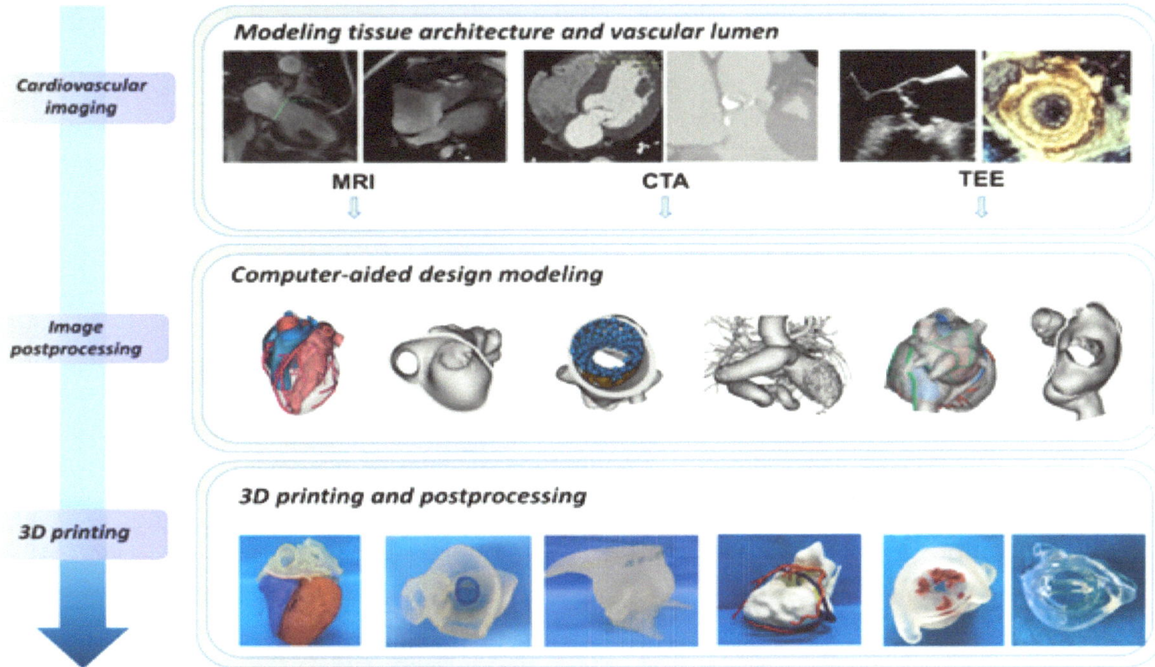

Fig.4.1 Three-dimensional printing flowchart of the cardiac system. MRI: magnetic resonance imaging, CTA: computed tomography angiography, TEE: transesophageal echocardiography, 3D: three-dimensional

Three-dimensional printing provides unparalleled tactile perception and true volumetric assessment of complex cardiovascular pathological conditions by offering unprecedented illustrations and spatial appreciation of cardiovascular structures. First, it can be used for patient education and doctor–patient communication .In the past, patient educational methods included using paper materials, watching videos, and engaging in patient–doctor dialogue. However, these methods can only target diseases, not individual cases.Moreover, individual differences exist in terms of patients' understanding of diseases, learning capacity, and compliance. Due to the advantage of 3D printing in facilitating patient education and doctor–patient communication, 3D printing-assisted perioperative educational intervention has been shown to effectively control the anxiety of patients with acute trauma, relieve pain, and improve sleep satisfaction Second, 3D printing plays a useful role in the study and application of investigational devices. For newly developed cardiac medical devices, using a 3D printing technique can reduce the cost and time of molding, thus optimizing the whole design process. Third, 3D printing acts as an ideal tool for simulating surgery and surgical planning. Cardiovascular physicians can carry out a computer-aided 3D virtual operation based on individualized medical image data to find the best surgical plan for individual patients by simulated analysis, which takes advantage of the characteristics of computer hemodynamics Through virtual surgical design and computational hemodynamic simulation, 3D printing technology can also be used to perform and predict quantitative changes in hemodynamic parameters and blood flow trajectories during the operation and reduce surgical risks by providing reliable information. One can measure in advance important parameters such as gradient, velocity, and volume using the 3D-printed model One can further use the physical 3D-printed model to practice cutting, stitching, and knotting skills. Meanwhile, strategy development including selection of device type, device size, and different approaches is crucial to the success of cardiovascular intervention; 3D-printed models can provide sufficient information to make appropriate choices Furthermore, careful planning before the operation or the intervention using the 3D models, including anticipation of complications such as annular rupture, paravalvular leak, the need for a pacemaker, and coronary artery occlusion, can further guarantee procedural success Lastly, 3D printing technology plays an important role in training medical professionals and students. Because the anatomical structure of the heart is delicate, complicated, and difficult for beginners to comprehend, the lack of satisfactory teaching tools presents an unavoidable obstacle. With the introduction of 3D printing technology, medical professionals can now practice with realistic anatomical models before the operation to improve the success rate and accuracy of the operation Not only can it help reduce costs, but it can also reduce radiation and procedural times. In particular, it provides an excellent model for teaching medical professionals and medical students to understand the changes that occur in the heart and its connection with surrounding vessels in different disease states

Three-dimensional printing and congenital heart disease

The incidence of CHDs is 0.8%–1.2%, and most patients with CHD need surgical or interventional treatment. CHD is characterized by a complex anatomical structure and great individual variability. Although dynamic 3D echocardiography, multislice spiral CT, MRI, and other imaging techniques have shown their advantages in the diagnosis of complex CHD, it is still difficult to obtain intuitive anatomical details. By transforming individual imaging data into physical models, 3D printing technology can reproduce the pathological structure and precisely represent the internal and external spatial structures of the heart, thereby providing the basis for an accurate diagnosis .Shi-Joon Yoo of Toronto Children's Hospital reported that 3D-printed models,such as those for a double outlet right ventricle and hypoplastic left heart syndrome, were better than imaging data for preoperative surgical

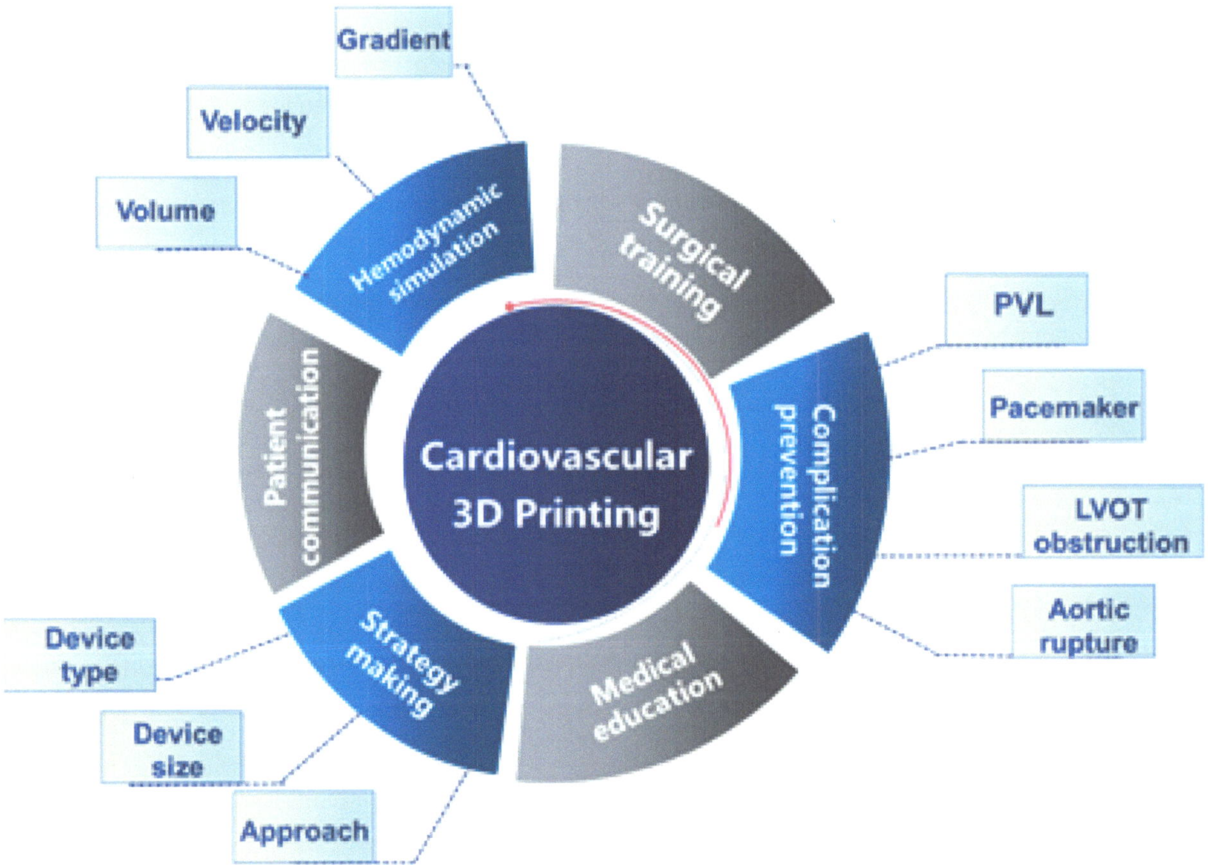

Fig.4.2 Function of three-dimensional printing in the cardiovascular field. 3D: three-dimensional, PVL: paravalvular leak, LVOT: left ventricular outflow tract

training and evaluation . Harikrishnan et al. at the Westchester Medical Center, New York, printed the heart model of a patient with pulmonary atresia combined with a single ventricle . With the help of this model, a one and half single ventricle corrective procedure was successfully completed. Israel Valverde et al. printed a 3D heart model for a child with transposition of the great arteries, ventricular septal defect, and severe pulmonary valve stenosis . The location and size of the ventricular septal defect and its spatial anatomical structure

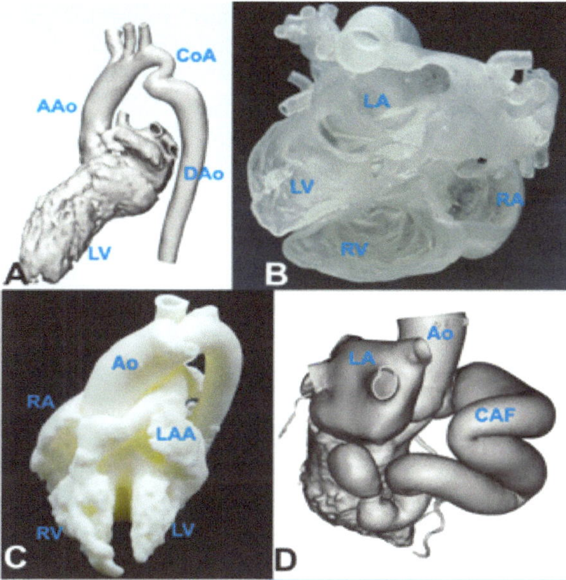

Fig.4.3 Three-dimensional (3D)-printed model of congenital heart diseases. a Computer modeling shows the internal structural profile of complex congenital heart diseases and coarctation of the aorta. The ascending aorta and descending aorta remain normal. b 3D-printed model of cor triatriatum. The left atrium of the patient is separated into false and true chambers by a septum; the structures of the left ventricle, the right atrium, and the right ventricle remain normal. c 3D-printed model of a double outlet right ventricle. The right ventricle of the patient is connected to both the aorta and the pulmonary artery. d 3D-printed model of a coronary fistula. A giant right coronary artery fistula drained to the left ventricle is shown. AAo: ascending aorta, CAF: coronary artery fistula, CoA: coarctation of the aorta, DAo: descending aorta, Ao: aorta, LAA: left atrial appendage, LA: left atrium, LV: left ventricle, RA: right atrium, RV: right ventricle. Image data, 3D computer reconstructions, and 3D-printed models are from the Department of Cardiovascular Surgery, Xijing Hospital

with the great artery were clearly displayed on the model. With the help of 3D models, the surgical staff of the Department of Cardiovascular Surgery at Xijing Hospital has performed more than 100 surgical procedures for patients with complex CHDs including pulmonary atresia, complete transposition of the great arteries, double outlet right ventricle, cor triatriatum, coarctation or disconnection of the aorta, vascular ring, abnormal coronary artery, and persistent truncus arteriosus . The models have helped the medical professionals to understand the internal spatial structure of the complex CHD and to formulate individual plans for surgical procedures. The operating time was greatly shortened, and the outcomes were good. The 3D-printed models were valuable for decision-making and intraoperative orientation.Doctors from the Department of Cardiovascular Surgery, West China Hospital, used 3D-printed models to mimic cardiac surgical procedures, thereby teaching and training young doctors and medical students. 3D models were printed before the operations, and the medical professionals could perform resections, suturing, and retraction and could simulate key steps of the operation using the individualized models

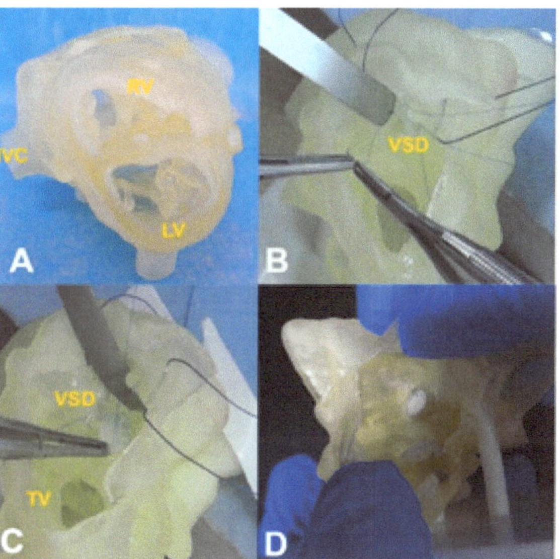

Fig.4.4 Three-dimensional (3D)-printed models of congenital heart diseases used for training. a 3D-printed model of a ventricular septal defect. b Training for the basic operative skills of suturing using a 3D-printed model. c Training young doctors and medical students using a 3D-printed model. d Evaluation of the

suture technique using a 3D-printed model. VSD: ventricular septal defect, IVC: inferior vena cava, LV: left ventricle, RV: right ventricle, TV: tricuspid valve. The 3D-printed models are from the Department of Cardiovascular Surgery, West China Hospital

Doctors from the Department of Cardiovascular Surgery, Xiangya Second Hospital of Central South University, used the 3D-printed heart model to mimic radiofrequency ablation of atrial fibrillation and mitral valve repair in a patient with mirror-image dextrocardia. By repeatedly practicing on the 3D model, the medical team became familiar with the special anatomical structure of the patient, which increased confidence and strengthened collaboration among the team members. The special rare case was successfully completed with a shortened procedural time and no complications

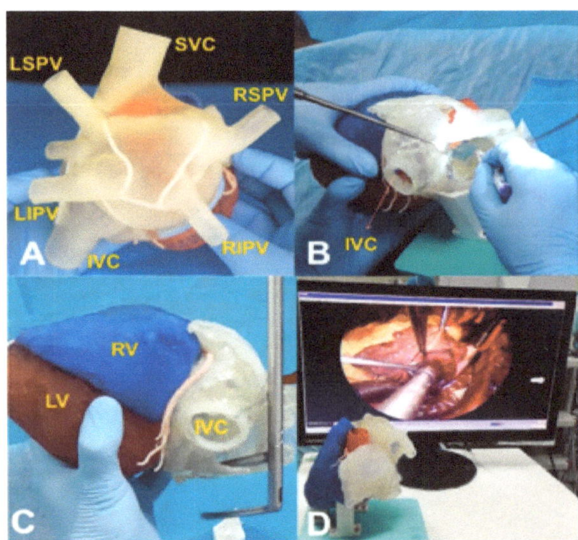

Fig.4.5 Three-dimensional (3D)-printed heart model to mimic the radiofrequency ablation of atrial fibrillation and a mitral valve repair operation in a patient with mirror-image dextrocardia. **a** 3D-printed heart model with planned ablation route; **b** surgical planning of the ablation route; **c** using the atrial fibrillation clamp to mimic the ablation procedure;d **3D** printing technique-guided radiofrequency ablation of atrial fibrillation and mitral valve repair operation. IVC: inferior vena cava, LSPV: left superior pulmonary vein, LIPV: left inferior pulmonary vein, LV: left ventricle, RIPV: right inferior pulmonary vein, RSPV: right superior pulmonary vein, RV: right ventricle, SVC: superior vena cava. Image data, 3D computer reconstruction, and 3D-printed model are from the Department of Cardiovascular Surgery, Xiangya Second Hospital of Central South University

Three-dimensional printing and transcatheter aortic valve replacement

Transcatheter aortic valve replacement (TAVR) is an emerging minimally invasive valve replacement operation to treat severe aortic valve disease. This type of operation does not require cardiopulmonary bypass and results in rapid postoperative recovery . Since its introduction, TAVR has been increasingly used and has benefited more than 500,000 patients . The effectiveness and safety of TAVR have been widely recognized in recent years, and the procedure was approved in 2020 by the U.S. Food and Drug Administration to use in low-risk patients with aortic stenosis. Although the TAVR operation is simpler than the traditional surgical procedure, its risks and complications should not be underestimated. Familiarity with and accurate positioning of the instruments comprise the core of the TAVR operation. Unlike that of traditional surgical procedures, the success of TAVR depends more on devices and imaging. Preprocedural evaluation, strategic planning, and complication prevention are of vital importance in the success of TAVR. 3D printing technology, as an emerging useful tool, plays a more and more important role in improving the success rate of TAVR .

Mimicking the transcatheter aortic valve replacement procedure

After nearly 20 years of development, approximately 50 kinds of devices are used in TAVR procedures worldwide. Many of them involve multiple steps and finely tuned operative procedures, and one careless move can have serious adverse consequences. Therefore, adequate training is needed to abbreviate the TAVR learning curve and to improve procedural safety and clinical success. Using the 3D model, the TAVR operation can be simulated in vitro, which helps the surgeon and the heart team become more familiar with the performance of the different TAVR devices, shortens the learning curve, improves the technical success rate of the team, and reduces mortality and complications among the patients. Figure 6 illustrates how to mimic the transapical TAVR procedure using a 3D-printed model and a J-valve system (Jiecheng Ltd., Suzhou, China). Due to the complexity of the system, physicians benefit from practicing and becoming familiar with each step of the releasing mechanism of the device, further improving the outcome of the TAVR procedure.

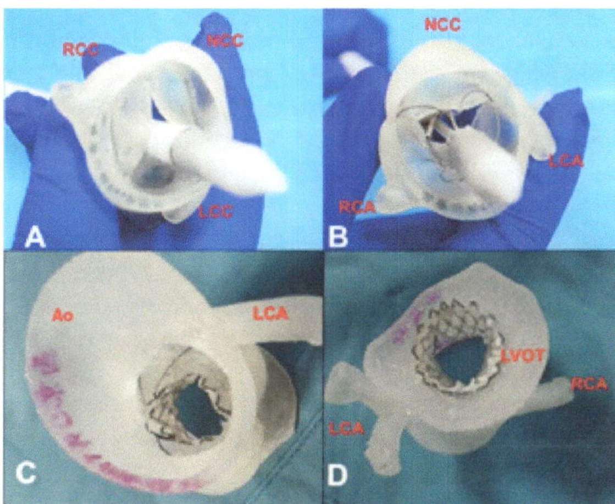

Fig.4.6 Three-dimensional (3D)-printed heart model to mimic the transcatheter aortic valve replacement (TAVR) procedure. a Transducing system across the valve; b releasing the step 1 button; c fully releasing the stented valve; d left ventricle view of the model to evaluate the results of the TAVR procedure. Ao: aorta, LCA: left coronary artery, LCC: left coronary cusp, LVOT: left ventricular outflow tract, NCC: non-coronary cup, RCA: right coronary artery, RCC: right coronary cups. Image data, 3D computer reconstruction, and 3D-printed model are from the Department of Cardiovascular Surgery, Xijing Hospital

Predicting the possibility of conduction block

Postoperative conduction block may be attributed to calcified plaque displacement, which causes sustained pressure on or permanent damage to the atrioventricular conduction system at the junction of the right coronary valve and the non-coronary valve. The ventricular end of the prosthetic valve may also damage the conduction system located at the ventricular septum. Researchers from the Georgia Institute of Technology and the Piedmont Heart Institute printed out a model of aortic stenosis with calcification and simulated the process of balloon dilation and valve releasing . The researchers were able to detect the direction of the deviation and observe the orientation of the stent valve affected by severe calcification, thus evaluating the probability of conduction block. The results suggested that severe calcification of the root and annulus can easily cause the valve to shift laterally, thereby causing conduction block. Through in vitro simulation and comparison of different valves, the study also found that the shorter valve rack may cause less conduction block.

Preventing coronary artery occlusion

Coronary artery occlusion after TAVR is a rare but extremely serious complication . The mortality rate of coronary artery occlusion after TAVR may be > 50%. The risk factors for acute or delayed coronary artery occlusion include (1) large calcification at the edge of the left and right coronary sinuses; (2) coronary height < 10 mm; (3) sinus diameter < 30 mm or a small aortic sinus; and (4) long aortic valve leaflets. It is extremely important to accurately predict the dynamic changes of the anatomical structure before beginning the operation.

In the Department of Cardiovascular Surgery, Xijing Hospital, doctors used the 3D-printed TAVR model to simulate the process of balloon dilation and the valve-releasing procedure to evaluate the possibility of coronary artery occlusion during TAVR and delayed coronary artery occlusion after surgery. If the patient is really at high risk, in vitro simulation would be helpful for the doctors to determine whether open surgery or a coronary-protecting strategy is indicated .

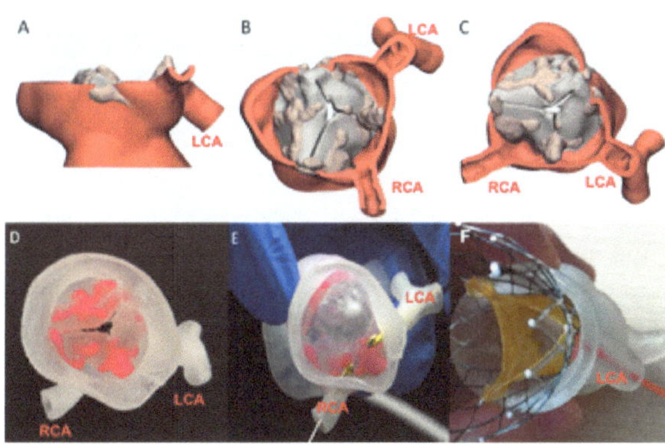

Fig.4.7Three-dimensional (3D) digital model to evaluate the risk of coronary artery occlusion during TAVR. a–c Computer 3D model shows the calcification of the valve

continued

leaflets and the height of the coronary artery in patients at risk of coronary artery occlusion. d 3D-printed model shows the calcification of the valve leaflets and the height of the coronary artery. e In vitro balloon dilation using the 3D-printed model to evaluate the possibility of coronary obstruction. f In vitro valve implantation using the 3D-printed model to evaluate the possibility of coronary obstruction. LCA: left coronary artery, RCA: right coronary artery. Image data, 3D computer reconstruction, and 3D-printed model are from the Department of Cardiovascular Surgery, Xijing Hospital

Predicting paravalvular leakage

Prediction of paravalvular leakage before TAVR is of great significance for developing a surgical strategy and selecting a valve. Researchers from the Georgia Institute of Technology and the Piedmont Heart Institute printed a multimaterial model of the aortic root . By controlling the "diameter and bending wavelength" of the printed material, the model was able to simulate the physiological characteristics of the aortic tissue. The model can even show the special conditions of valve leaflets, such as calcification deposition and leaflet thickening, and depict the anatomical information accurately and completely. The results suggest that the 3D model can show exactly which patients are likely to develop paravalvular leakage and even the location and severity of the complication. Qian et al. established a model to quantitatively predict postoperative leakage after TAVR using 3D printing technology, which has shown great value in predicting the incidence, severity, and location of paravalvular leakage after TAVR

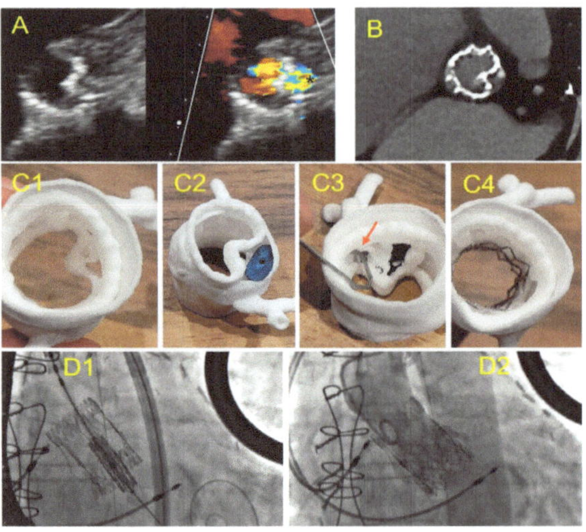

Caption Next Column

Fig. 4.8 PVL after Perceval Bio-prosthesis implantation. (A) Aortic TTE view: incomplete expansion of the prosthetic framework against the annular aortic wall (left) causing large PVL (*); (B) cardiac CT of the Perceval prosthesis showing an invagination of the prosthetic armature in a same view as (A); (C) 3D printed model in superior aortic view showing the gap between the aortic wall and the invaginated prosthetic armature (C1); testing of an Amplatzer Valvular Plug III 14 × 5 mm (C2) showing residual gap and obstruction of the left coronary ostium ((C3)-red arrow); simulation of a TAVI valve-in-valve which allowed complete apposition of the Perceval framework to the aortic wall (C4); (D) TAVI valve-in-valve procedure: implantation of an Edwards balloon expandable prosthesis (D1) into Perceval armature without residual leakage (D2).

Three-dimensional printing and left atrial appendage occlusion

Transcatheter LAAO is a new method to prevent thromboembolism in patients with non-valvular atrial fibrillation by fixing the occluder inside the left atrial appendage (LAA) to prevent blood from entering the LAA. Its clinical benefits and safety have been confirmed by many clinical studies, and it has become an alternative treatment to prevent stroke in patients with atrial fibrillation. At the same time, the complexity and variability of LAA make it difficult to place the occluding devices in suitable locations.The occluder often needs to be replaced many times, which may increase the risk of LAA injury, thrombosis, and pericardial tamponade. In 2015, Otton et al. reported the successful treatment of LAAO in a 74-year-old patient, guided by 3D printing .Transesophageal echocardiography examination showed that the diameter of the LAA opening was 15 and 18 mm. The LAA model was printed according to the data obtained from CTA. Three types of occluders, 21, 24, and 27 mm, were selected for test occlusion in vitro. They found that the 21-mm and the 27-mm occluders deployed in the 3D-printed model were either too small or too large; the 24-mm occluder was finally used during the operation to achieve complete occlusion. Currently, 3D printing technology can effectively assist decision-making related to LAAO .]. Scholars of the First Affiliated Hospital of Xi'an Jiaotong University use 3D-printed models to simulate LAAO and to choose the appropriate size and position, using the push–pull experiment to test the stability of the device .

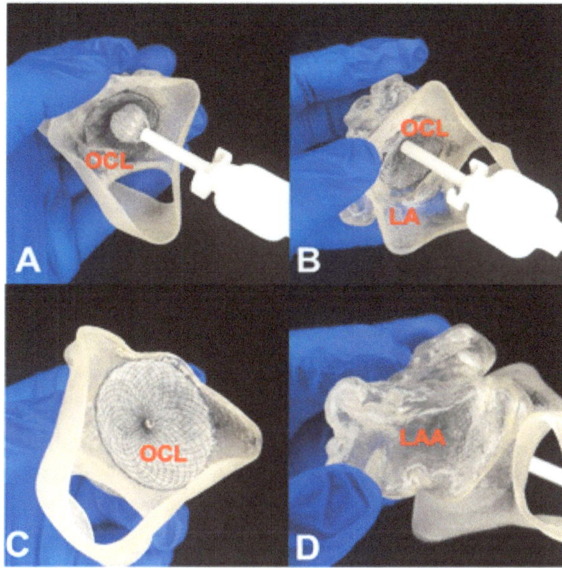

Fig.4.9 Three-dimensional (3D)-printed simulated left atrial appendage occlusion. a Partially released device using the 3D-printed left atrial appendage model; b push–pull experiment to test the stability of the device, c fully released device using the 3D-printed left atrial appendage model, d left atrial appendage view of the model to evaluate the results of the procedure. LAA: left atrial appendage, LA: left atrium, OCL: occluder. Image data, 3D computer reconstruction, and 3D-printed model are from the Department of Cardiovascular Surgery, the First Affiliated Hospital of Xi'an Jiaotong University

Three-dimensional printing and hypertrophic cardiomyopathy

Hypertrophic cardiomyopathy is a common inherited cardiac disease that is characterized by abnormal heart structure, asymmetrical cardiac hypertrophy, heart failure, and arrhythmia. Current treatment methods mainly include drug therapy, surgical treatment, and alcohol septal ablation.Surgicaltreatment requires thoracotomy, which may result in a left bundle branch block, whereas alcohol ablation is less invasive but does not relieve obstruction of the left ventricular outflow tract in some patients Dr. Liu Liwen, from the Department of Ultrasound, Xijing Hospital, has developed the Liwen procedure for hypertrophic obstructive cardiomyopathy, that is, percutaneous transmyocardial radiofrequency ablation under the guidance of ultrasound . It is guided by ultrasound through a percutaneous transepicardial puncture through the tip of the heart to the area affected by ventricular septal hypertrophy; high-frequency waves can create local hypertrophic myocardial coagulation necrosis to achieve the goal of widening the left ventricular outflow tract. The 3D printing technique can be used to observe the anatomy of the heart, especially that of the distribution of the coronary arteries, and to guide the surgical planning for and the risk assessment of the Liwen procedure. A real 3D model of the heart was constructed using preoperative CTA or MRI data of patients with obstructive hypertrophic cardiomyopathy.

The coronary artery was displayed in a computer 3D model or a 3D-printed model. To prevent the electrode from damaging the coronary artery and the conduction bundle and to ensure the safety of the operation, the anatomical structure of the patient's heart can be fully understood, the optimal puncture site can be determined, and the proper electrode needle path can be set .At the same time, a 3D model corresponding to the CTA two-dimensional image and the ultrasound image can effectively guide the operation and shorten the operating time.

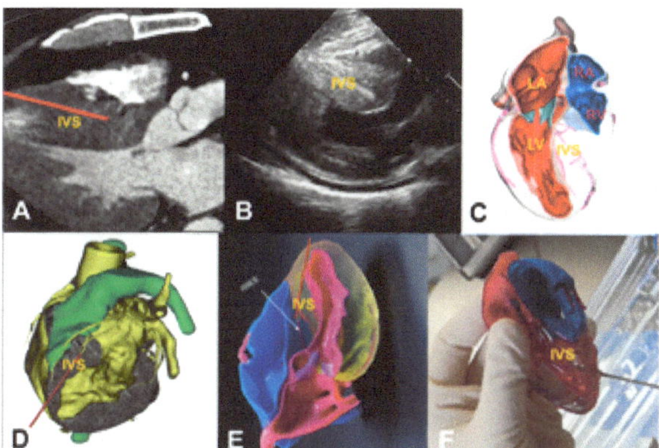

Fig 4.10 Ultrasound-guided percutaneous transluminal myocardial septal radiofrequency ablation (Liwen procedure) for the treatment of obstructive hypertrophic cardiomyopathy. a Computed tomography angiography (CTA) two-dimensional imaging display of the hypertrophic septum and the surgical path of radiofrequency ablation. The red line is a simulated electroacupuncture approach. The approach is shown to avoid the surface coronary artery and to ablate the septal branches during the operation. b Ultrasound images display the hypertrophic septum; the computer section shows the myocardium (continued next page)

c Digital three-dimensional (3D) model based on CTA images of the hypertrophic septum and the inner structure of the heart. d Digital 3D model based on CTA image display of the hypertrophic septum and the outer structure of the heart. e 3D cardiac printed model based on CTA images of the hypertrophic septum and the coronary artery branch. f Determination of the optimal puncture site and the proper electrode needle path using the 3D model. IVS: interventricular septum, LA: left atrium, LV: left ventricle, RA: right atrium, RV: right ventricle. Image data, computer 3D reconstruction, and 3D-printed models from the National Innovation Center for Additive Materials Manufacturing and the Department of Cardiovascular Surgery, Xijing Hospital

Limitations

Several factors limit the current wide clinical application of 3D printing in cardiac medicine. First, the model is usually printed during a single phase of the cardiac cycle, which limits the accurate representation of the dynamic heart function. Second, the currently available printing materials cannot truly replicate the physical and mechanical properties of human cardiovascular tissue in terms of several physical parameters, such as steadiness, tensile strength, elasticity, and memory capacity. Third, lack of robust data and standardization, lack of an accepted method to assess the accuracy of the produced models, and lack of large-scale studies and randomized clinical trials, all limit the wide promotion of cardiovascular 3D printing techniques. Fourth, image segmentation, computer-aided design, printing, and postprinting preparation for clinical use all require a strong and efficient team whose members have abundant anatomical knowledge and passion, which is hard to establish in the circumstances caused by the coronavirus disease 2019 pandemic. Last but not least, the cost-effectiveness and timeliness of this additive technology, the complexity of the workflow, and the lack of uniform financing models and of reimbursement structures are key issues making this technology currently mostly limited to teaching hospitals and research institutions. To solve these problems, we should choose the optimal phase of the cardiac cycle for 3D printing on the basis of the specific case under consideration; develop novel printing materials tobetter replicate the physical structureof the cardiovascular anatomy; teach and train young doctors and medical students to be familiar with the workflow of 3D printing; carry out large clinical trials to illustrate the advantages and disadvantages of 3D printing; and reduce the cost and price of 3D printing, therefore promoting its clinical application and benefiting more patients.

Future perspectives

With the rapid development of imaging and computer technology, the accuracy and simulation levels of cardiovascular 3D printing are constantly improving. 3D printing makes up for the inability of traditional image technology to precisely display complex structures, and computer 3D reconstruction helps cardiovascular physicians understand the pathological changes of human tissues more intuitively, which provides a new method for the precise treatment of patients with heart disease. Although the application of 3D printing in the cardiac field is still in its early stages, it can provide medical staff with in vitro visualization information and print individual 3D models to help doctors determine surgical procedures and promote communication between doctors and patients. It can also simulate surgical and interventional procedures, improve the success rate and safety of such procedures, and help train medical professionals and medical students. Meanwhile, new cardiovascular therapies might be developed based on 3D-printed models. With the further development of 3D printing technology, the advantages of customized and individualized manufacturing will help people to better understand cardiac diseases. In the future era of 3D +, developments in biological engineering technology, materials science, biology, computer science, and other disciplines will lead to the design of materials that can be implanted in the human body and result in new breakthroughs in the treatment of cardiac diseases. Meanwhile, the tissues and organs generated by biological 3D printing might also be applied in the treatment of cardiac diseases. 3D printing will constantly change the traditional treatment methods, improve the diagnosis and treatment of cardiac diseases, and better benefit patients with cardiac diseases.

Bibliography And Acknowledgement

- Batteux, C.; Azarine, A.; Karsenty, C.; Petit, J.; Ciobotaru, V.; Brenot, P.; Hascoet, S. Sinus Venosus ASDs: Imaging and Percutaneous Closure. Curr. Cardiol. Rep. 2021, 23, 138. [CrossRef]
- Batteux, C.; Meliani, A.; Brenot, P.; Hascoet, S. Multimodality fusion imaging to guide percutaneous sinus venosus atrial septal defect closure. Eur. Heart J. 2020, 41, 4444–4445. [CrossRef]
- Baumgartner H, Falk V, Bax JJ, De Bonis M, Hamm C, Holm PJ, Iung B, Lancellotti P, Lansac E, Munoz DR, Rosenhek R, Sjogren J, Tornos Mas P, Vahanian A, Walther T, Wendler O, Windecker S, Zamorano JL, Group ESCSD (2017) 2017 ESC/EACTS Guidelines for the management of valvular heart disease. Eur Heart J 38:2739–2791
- Calvert, P.A.; Northridge, D.B.; Malik, I.S.; Shapiro, L.; Ludman, P.; Qureshi, S.A.; Mullen, M.; Henderson, R.; Turner, M.; Been, M.; et al. Percutaneous Device Closure of Paravalvular Leak: Combined Experience From the United Kingdom and Ireland. Circulation 2016, 134, 934–944. [CrossRef]
- Chaowu Y, Hua L, Xin S (2016) Three-dimensional printing as an aid in transcatheter closure of secundum atrial septal defect with rim deficiency: in vitro trial occlusion based on a personalized heart model. Circulation 133:e608–e610
- Ciobotaru, V.; Combes, N.; Iriart, X.; Marijon, E.; Hascoet, S.; Nguyen, A.; Ternacle, J.; Defaye, P.; Jacon, P.; Lepillier, A.; et al. P2436Preliminary data from "LAA-Print French registry": A large national multi-centric prospective registry evaluating a new preoperative approach based on 3Dprinted simulation in LAAC procedures. Eur. Heart J. 2019, 40. [CrossRef]
- Ciobotaru, V.; Combes, N.; Martin, C.A.; Marijon, E.; Maupas, E.; Bortone, A.; Bruguière, E.; Thambo, J.-B.; Teiger, E.; Pujadas-Berthault, P.; et al. Left atrial appendage occlusion simulation based on three-dimensional printing: New insights into outcome and technique. EuroIntervention 2018, 14, 176–184. [CrossRef]
- Cruz-Gonzalez, I.; Barreiro-Pérez, M.; Valverde, I. 3D-printing in Preprocedural Planning of Paravalvular Leak Closure: Feasibility/ Proof-of-concept. Rev. Esp. Cardiol. 2019, 72, 342. [CrossRef] [PubMed]
- Cruz-Gonzalez, I.; Rama-Merchan, J.C.; Arribas-Jimenez, A.; Rodriguez-Collado, J.; Martin-Moreiras, J.; Cascon-Bueno, M.; Luengo, C.M. Paravalvular Leak Closure With the Amplatzer Vascular Plug III Device: Immediate and Short-term Results. Rev. Esp. Cardiol. 2014, 67, 608–614. [CrossRef]
- Dowling C, Bavo AM, El Faquir N, Mortier P, de Jaegere P, De Backer O, Sondergaard L, Ruile P, Mylotte D, McConkey H, Rajani R, Laborde JC, Brecker SJ (2019) Patient-specific computer simulation of transcatheter aortic valve replacement in bicuspid aortic valve morphology. Circ Cardiovasc Imaging 12:e009178
- El Sabbagh A, Eleid MF, Al-Hijji M, Anavekar NS, Holmes DR, Nkomo VT, Oderich GS, Cassivi SD, Said SM, Rihal CS, Matsumoto JM, Foley TA (2018) The various applications of 3D printing in cardiovascular diseases. Curr Cardiol Rep 20:47
- García, E.; Arzamendi, D.; Jimenez-Quevedo, P.; Sarnago, F.; Martí, G.; Sanchez-Recalde, A.; Lasa-Larraya, G.; Sancho, M.; Iñiguez, A.; Goicolea, J.; et al. Outcomes and predictors of success and complications for paravalvular leak closure: An analysis of the SpanisH real-wOrld paravalvular LEaks closure (HOLE) registry. EuroIntervention 2017, 12, 1962–1968. [CrossRef] [PubMed]
- Giannopoulos AA, Mitsouras D, Yoo SJ, Liu PP, Chatzizisis YS, Rybicki FJ (2016) Applications of 3D printing in cardiovascular diseases. Nat Rev Cardiol 13:701–718
- Giannopoulos AA, Steigner ML, George E, Barile M, Hunsaker AR, Rybicki FJ, Mitsouras D (2016) Cardiothoracic applications of 3-dimensional Printing. J Thorac Imaging 31:253–272.
- Gittard SD, Narayan RJ, Lusk J, Morel P, Stockmans F, Ramsey M, Laverde C, Phillips J, Monteiro-Riviere NA, Ovsianikov A, Chichkov BN (2009) Rapid prototyping of scaphoid and lunate bones. Biotechnol J 4:129–134
- Haghiashtiani G, Qiu K, Zhingre Sanchez JD, Fuenning ZJ, Nair P, Ahlberg SE, Iaizzo PA, McAlpine MC (2020) 3D printed patient-specific aortic root models with internal sensors for minimally invasive applications. Sci Adv 6:eabb4641.
- Harb SC, Rodriguez LL, Vukicevic M, Kapadia SR, Little SH (2019) Three-dimensional printing applications in percutaneous structural heart interventions. Circ Cardiovasc Imaging 12:e009014
- Hascoet, S.; Smolka, G.; Bagate, F.; Guihaire, J.; Potier, A.; Hadeed, K.; Lavie-Badie, Y.; Bouvaist, H.; Dauphin, C.; Bauer, F.; et al. Multimodality imaging guidance for percutaneous paravalvular leak closure: Insights from the multi-centre FFPP register. Arch. Cardiovasc. Dis. 2018, 111, 421–431. [CrossRef]
- Houeijeh, A.; Petit, J.; Isorni, M.-A.; Sigal-Cinqualbre, A.; Batteux, C.; Karsenty, C.; Fraisse, A.; Fournier, E.; Ciobotaru, V.; Hascoet, S. 3D modeling and printing in large native right ventricle outflow tract to plan complex percutaneous pulmonary valve implantation. Int. J. Cardiol. Congenit. Heart Dis. 2021, 4, 100161. [CrossRef]
- Iriart, X.; Ciobotaru, V.; Martin, C.; Cochet, H.; Jalal, Z.; Thambo, J.B.; Quessard, A. Role of cardiac imaging and three-dimensional printing in percutaneous appendage closure. Arch. Cardiovasc. Dis. 2018, 111, 411–420. [CrossRef] [PubMed]
- Isorni, M.-A.; Monnot, S.; Kloeckner, M.; Gerardin, B.; Hascoet, S. Innovative multi-modality imaging to assess paravalvular leak. Postepy Kardiol Interwencyjnej 2019, 15, 120–122. [CrossRef]
- Kong, F.; Wilson, N.; Shadden, S. A deep-learning approach for direct whole-heart mesh reconstruction. Med. Image Anal. 2021, 74, 102222. [CrossRef]
- McGurk M, Amis AA, Potamianos P, Goodger NM (1997) Rapid prototyping techniques for anatomical modelling in medicine. Ann R Coll Surg Engl 79:169–174. PMCID: PMC2502901
- Motwani, M.; Burley, O.; Luckie, M.; Cunnington, C.; Pisaniello, A.D.; Hasan, R.; Malik, I.; Fraser, D.G. 3D-printing assisted closure of paravalvular leak. J. Cardiovasc. Comput. Tomogr. 2020, 14, e66–e68. [CrossRef]
- Nicholls M (2017) Three-dimensional imaging and printing in cardiology. Eur Heart J 38:230–231.
- O'Neill, A.C.; Martos, R.; Murtagh, G.; Ryan, E.R.; McCreery, C.; Keane, D.; Quinn, M.; Dodd, J.D. Practical tips and tricks for assessing prosthetic valves and detecting paravalvular regurgitation using cardiac CT. J. Cardiovasc. Comput. Tomogr. 2014, 8, 323–327. [CrossRef]
- Onorato, E.M.; Muratori, M.; Smolka, G.; Malczewska, M.; Zorinas, A.; Zakarkaite, D.; Mussayev, A.; Christos, C.P.; Bauer, F.; Gandet, T.; et al. Midterm procedural and clinical outcomes of percutaneous paravalvular leak closure with the Occlutech Paravalvular Leak Device. EuroIntervention 2020, 15, 1251–1259. [CrossRef] [PubMed]

Newer Cardio-vascular CT Technology For Diagnosis OF Cardiovascular Diseases

CHAPTER

There have been a few big, recent advancements in cardiac computed tomography angiography (CCTA) imaging technology. The biggest of these was the introduction of two CT systems aimed specifically at the coronary imaging market — the GE Healthcare Cardiographe dedicated cardiac CT scanner and the Canon (formerly Toshiba) Aquilion Precision.The Cardiographe was developed by Israeli start-up company Arineta with input from several luminary physicians. It incorporates numerous technologies that are specifically aimed at improving coronary CT angiography, without concerns about using the machine for general radiology imaging. The company partnered with GE Healthcare to commercialize the scanner, which gained U.S. Food and Drug Administration (FDA) clearance in 2017. GE incorporated many of its latest CT advances for dose reduction, iterative reconstruction, metal artifact reduction and other features from its Revolution CT system. The Cardiographe was built to be very compact so it can fit into a physician's office, or utilize a smaller room than a standard 64-slice scanner. It offers 140 mm of anatomical coverage to scan the entire heart in one rotation without stitching. Its gantry rotation speed is 0.24 seconds, enabling very fast scans that freeze cardiac motion. Examples of CTA scans on the system presented in sessions were performed at 2 mSv of dose or below.The Aquilion Precision was unveiled for the first time at the 2017 Radiological Society of North America (RSNA) meeting and was cleared by the FDA in April 2018. It is unique in that it is the first CT system to offer a 0.25 mm resolution, rather that the standard 0.5 mm resolution on most of today's scanners. It is capable of resolving coronary anatomy as small as 150 microns, providing CT image quality with resolution typically seen only in cath lab angiography

This enables better visualization of tiny structures, such as the composition of coronary plaques, stent struts and smaller coronary vessels that are generally difficult to see on CTA scans. The resolution may aid in better plaque assessments, including clearer identification of vulnerable plaques, visualizing broken stent struts, and identification of a specific vendor's stents based on strut design in vessels.

The Precision uses a newly designed detector to provide more than twice the resolution of 0.5 mm systems. The scanner offers dose efficiency with detector channels that are only 0.25 mm thick. It also has improvements in scintillator quantum efficiency, detector circuitry and other components. The system features the industry's smallest focal spot tube, at 0.4 x 0.5 mm, and the industry's first routine 1,024 x 1,024 reconstruction matrix.

Key Specifications for CT Cardiac Imaging

Here is a list of some key technologies that should be considered when evaluating new CT scanners for cardiac imaging.

1. Speed — The faster the temporal resolution a scanner has, the faster its gantry can rotate around a patient. Some of the newest scanners move fast enough to capture images that freeze cardiac motion and prevent motion blur or the need to stitch images from several heartbeats to reconstruct a complete cardiac image.

2. Motion correction algorithms — This software can help compensate for cardiac motion to provide clearer images. This can help reduce the need for retakes and help reduce patient dose.

3. Cardiac metal artifact reduction software — Many cardiac patients have implanted hardware from previous procedures, including stents, surgical staples, sternum wires, septal or left atrial appendage (LAA) occluders, and pacemaker or implantable cardioverter defibrillator (ICD) leads. Any of these metal implants can cause metal artifact blooming or streaking artifacts that compromise the diagnostic quality of the images. The latest generation software offered by most vendors can largely compensate the photon starvation behind the metal or can reduce and cut through glare to see the underlying anatomy. Some newer software can increase image quality enough to visualize plaques or clots inside stents.

4. Calcium scoring software — Data continues to mount that calcium scoring is a good predictor of a patient's risk for future coronary events. It is also being advocated for screenings of patients who are on the fence about going on statin therapy.

5.Plaque assessment software:-This software is offered by all of the top CT system vendors and most of the third-party advanced visualization vendors. As more research accumulates and image resolution on CT scanners improves, quantifying the types of plaques seen in the coronary arteries on CT will likely play a bigger role. These CT assessments can help determine if an intervention is needed and help guide those interventions.

6. CT perfusion:-This software tracks the iodine contrast concentration levels in the myocardium. The software reconstructs color coded maps showing areas of low concentration (areas of poor blood flow caused by ischemia), similar to nuclear myocardial perfusion exams that show areas of poor metabolic activity due to ischemia. The data from these exams is available almost immediately, whereas nuclear scans may require the patient to be admitted overnight.

7. TAVR / structural heart planning software

CT systems with workflows optimized for transcatheter aortic valve replacement (TAVR) or other structural heart exams will be helpful as these procedures continue to see rapidly increasing volumes. Software for TAVR, mitral valve assessments, LAA and septal defect occlusion planning should be considered in health systems offering these procedures.

8. FFR-CT assessment capability As fractional flow reserve computed tomography (FFR-CT) gains reimbursement it is expected to see wider adoption. It can help definitively assess chest pain patients and either rule out coronary artery ischemia, or pinpoint the culprit lesions and the severity of blood flow obstruction, which can help better guide interventions. Invasive catheter-based FFR uses blood flow pressure readings before and after a coronary lesion to determine if a stenosis is hemodynamically significant and requires stenting. FFR-CT is noninvasive and uses super-computing, computational fluid dynamics to assess a virtual FFR, which may help eliminate the need for diagnostic catheterization. For more insights on what to look for in cardiac CT scanners,

Other New CT Scanners on the Market

GE unveiled a premium CT with similar specs, the Revolution Frontier, which has cleared the FDA and is expected to begin shipping in 2Q 2018. It is built around the company's Gemstone Clarity detector and Performix HD Plus X-ray tube. The super-premium CT can visualize structures to a resolution of 0.23 mm with 25 percent less electronic noise, according to GE. It also features spectral imaging.Siemens extended the concept of patient-centric mobile workflow with two new members of its "go" family – the Somatom go.All (64 slices per rotation) and go.Top (128 slices per rotation). The systems use a tablet device and remote controls, to eliminate the need for a traditional control room and enable more time with the patient scanner side. The 64-slice go.All can scan up to 100 mm in one second. The 128-slice go.Top can cover up to 175 mm per second with a range of 200 cm, enough to scan the length of a patient more than 6 and a half feet tall. The X-ray tube can be adjusted in 10-kilovolt increments. The go.Top also offers TwinBeam Dual Energy imaging. This splits the X-ray beam into two energy spectra before it reaches the patient, enabling providers to simultaneously examine the same body region at two different energy levels.

FFR-CT Can Identify Lesions Requiring Stenting

One of the new add-on advanced visualization technologies for CCTA that vendors are now offering is fractional flow reserve computed tomography (FFR-CT). It offers a completely a noninvasive FFR assessment of not just a coronary segment, but the entire coronary tree.

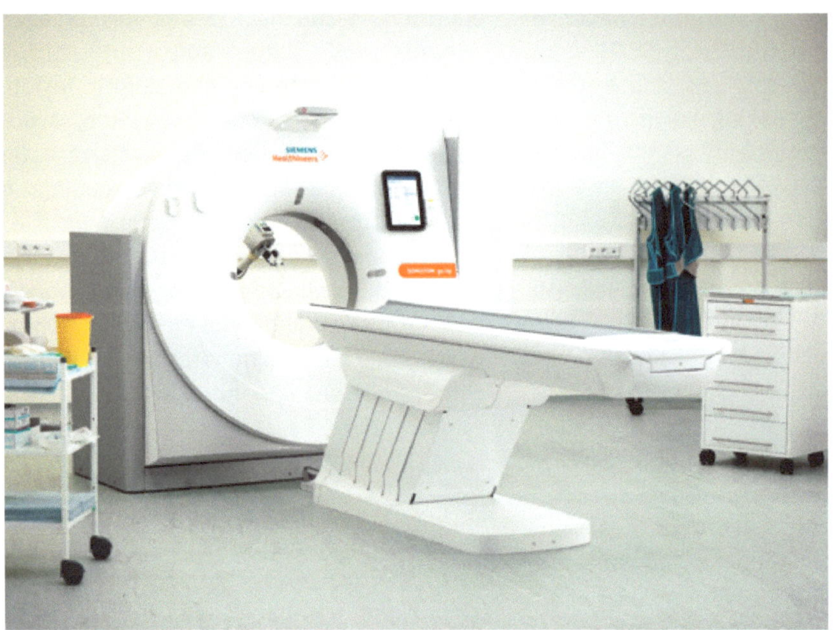

Fig. 5.1 Vendors introduce a dedicated CCTA scanner, the first high-resolution CT system

Invasive catheter-based FFR uses blood flow pressure readings before and after a coronary lesion to determine if a stenosis is hemodynamically significant and requires stenting. Traditionally CTA has been great at showing anatomical detail, including the percentage obstruction a lesion presents. But in the cath lab, it is often the case where a significant blockage seen on CT does not greatly impact blood flow. To avoid the need for a diagnostic catheterization for confirmation, FFR-CT uses super-computing computational fluid dynamics to assess a virtual FFR, which studies have shown has an 80 percent correlation with invasive FFR. This may be the key in making CT a true gatekeeper to the cath lab and for EDs to more quickly discharge chest pain patients where coronary blockages can be ruled out. Several vendors have recently created partnerships with HeartFlow, which offers FFR-CT technology that is cleared by the FDA.As CCTA sees wider adoption in emergency departments for quicker evaluation of chest pain patients, FFR-CT will likely see an increasing role to verify patients requiring percutaneous coronary intervention (PCI) and help reduce or eliminate the need for invasive diagnostic angiograms.

New Technologies Take Cardiac CT to the Next Level

CTA advances now enable physiological evaluation, lower dose scans using AI and photo-realistic imagerendering Here is an overview of a few of the biggest technology advances in cardiovascular computed tomography (CT). These are helping push CT angiography (CTA) to become a primary imaging modality with the ability to push beyond anatomical imaging to allow physiological imaging similar to the information offered by nuclear imaging and MRI.

Other advances include the ability to greatly lower dose and improve image quality using artificial intelligence (AI) image reconstruction and being able to show photo-realistic anatomical imaging that is helpful in explaining conditions to patients or surgeons.

CT Myocardial Perfusion Imaging

In March 2020, the Society of Cardiovascular Computed Tomography (SCCT) released a new expert consensus document on CT myocardial perfusion (CTP) imaging. The recommendations outline the use of both coronary anatomy and .

myocardial perfusion to help identify those patients who might most benefit from further invasive procedures to treat their coronary artery disease"CT perfusion has been developed and significantly validated over the last decade; however, its adoption into clinical practice has been limited by the lack of standardization and other factors. This international expert consensus group was comprised of a diverse group of individuals with significant experience in CT perfusion imaging and were tasked to identify some of the key principles that unify the various approaches to CTP," said writing group co-chair Amit Patel, M.D., FSCCT of University of Chicago.CT perfusion has been available for several years, but clinical study evidence was needed to show correlation between the analysis software, real-world disease and the gold-standard technologies of MRI and nuclear perfusion imaging. SCCT said the growing body of evidence has established the diagnostic accuracy and incremental value of myocardial CTP over coronary CTA. In single center studies, myocardial CTP imaging has demonstrated high accuracy when compared with single photon emission computed tomography (SPECT), cardiovascular magnetic resonance (CMR), invasive coronary angiography (ICA), positron emission tomography (PET) and invasive fractional flow reserve (FFR). Multicenter studies have also established the accuracy of combining myocardial CTP with coronary CTA. These studies suggest that CTP is particularly accurate when interpreted in the context of coronary CTA findings. The new consensus statement provides expert consensus regarding the performance and interpretation of CTP, including patient selection, image acquisition, post-processing and interpretation of CTP results."The combination of coronary CTA and CTP can be used to detect both coronary atherosclerosis as well as its physiological consequences. While further studies will continue to refine the capabilities of CTP, the current expert consensus statement will be useful for clinicians and researchers who are interested in adopting this technique," says writing group co-chair Ron Blankstein, M.D., MSCCT, of Brigham and Women's Hospital and SCCT president.

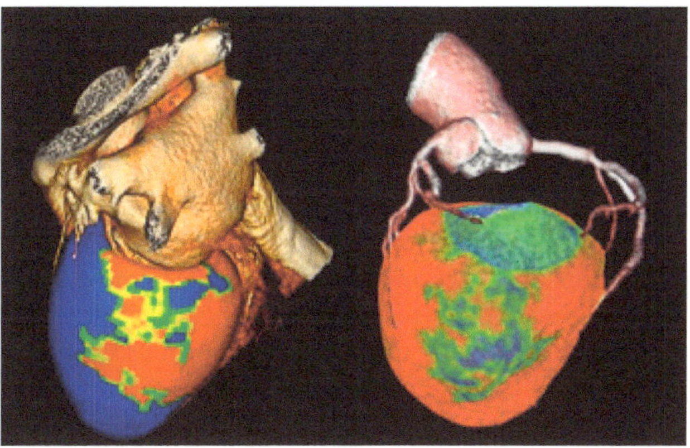

Fig. 5.2 Two examples of CT myocardial perfusion (CTP) imaging assessment software. Canon is on the left and GE Healthcare is on the right. Both of these technologies have been around for a few years, but there has been an increasing amount of clinical data from studies showing the accuracy of the technology compared to nuclear imaging, the current standard of care for myocardial perfusion imaging, and cardiac MRI.

Noninvasive CT-based FFR and Planning Interventional Procedures

A key diagnostic tool to determine if a stent is needed in a coronary lesion in the cath lab is pressure wire based FFR. However, the technology requires the use of pharmacological stress agent adenosine and a wire pull back in the vessel, taking additional procedure time and adding cost to the procedure limiting adoption. Expanded use of FFR would likely take place if the technology was less expensive and easier to use CT-based FFR (FFR-CT) is now being use by many larger hospitals to assess patients presenting with chest pain faster than traditional troponin testing, keeping patients overnight for morning nuclear scans or sending them to the Cath lab for invasive angiograms. FFR-CT is also starting to be used at some centers to help plan procedures.The CT imaging is sent to an outside vendor so it can be run through a computational fluid dynamics algorithm using a supercomputer to create a 3-D coronary tree with FFR ratios for all the vessel segments. It can take up to a couple hours to process the results, but it is fast enough to clear most patients to go home if there are no clear blockages anatomically or physiologically. "CT has advanced amazingly over the past 20 years," James Udelson, M.D., chief of the division of cardiology, Tufts Medical Center. "There is a 99 percent predictive value that if you see severe disease that you will find severe disease in the cath lab. The problem has been with moderate lesions, such as a 60 percent stenosis in the mid-LAD — is that physiologically significant? Patients who get CT are often cathed at a high rate, likely because a physician sees the moderate stenosis and are worried about it and they do a cath. Now, with FFR-CT, you can interrogate using just a resting CT dataset to see if that 60 percent stenosis is or is not physiologically significant."

Using this technology, Tufts has been able to reduce the number of diagnostic catheterizations for moderate stenosis patients, now only sending patients to the cath lab who are confirmed through the CT-FFR that they need revascularization.

revascularization conditions.

HeartFlow Planner is a non-invasive, real-time virtual modeling tool for coronary artery disease (CAD) intervention. It enables interventional cardiologists to virtually model clinical scenarios vessel-by-vessel, explore treatment strategies before a procedure."The information provided by the HeartFlow technology is powerful and will not only help us efficiently diagnose coronary artery disease, but help us better understand different treatment options," said Victor Marinescu, M.D., cardiologist Advocate Health Midwest Heart Specialists and member of the medical staff, Edward-Elmhurst Health. "The visual nature of the HeartFlow Planner also makes it a great tool to explain to patients what will happen during their procedure."

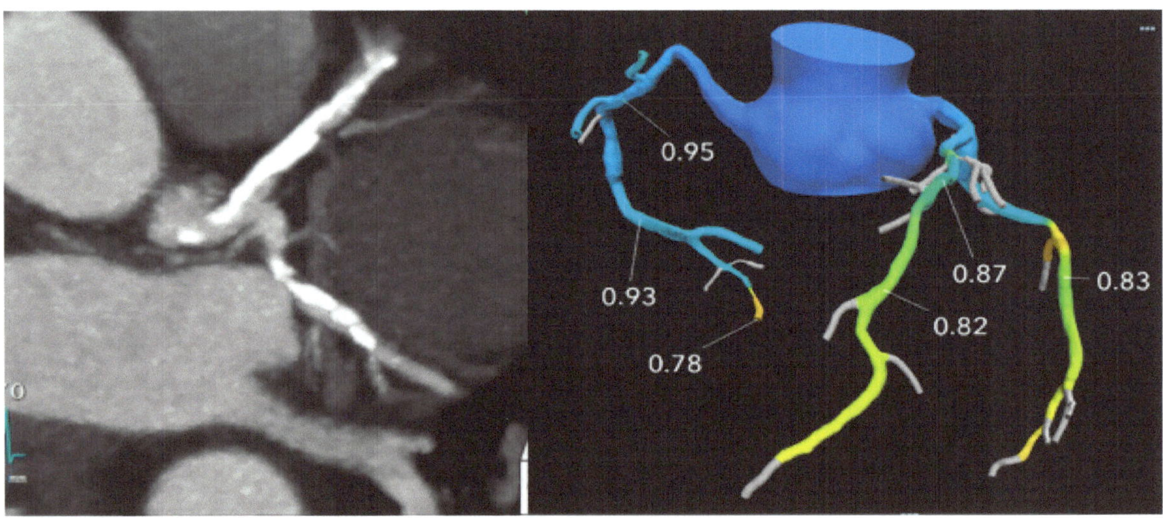

Fig. 5.3 A HeartFlow FFR-CT example showing comparison with a CT scan of heavily calcified coronary arteries. The lesion looks severe anatomically on CT, but it not significant enough to qualify for stenting according to the FFR-CT

Predicting Outcomes of Stent Procedures Using FFR-CT Modeling

The most recent iteration of the Heartflow FFR-CT technology that gained U.S. Food and Drug Administration (FDA) approval in September 2019 allows the user to virtually stent a vessel segment to determine the FFR value if the vessel was opened to its native lumen size.This serves as a planning tool to assess patients prior to entering the cath lab and predicting what their coronary flow might be under optimal

Artificial Intelligence Enters CT Image Reconstructions

CT vendors are developing new AI algorithms to reconstruct CT images better than conventional iterative or model-based reconstruction methods. Both Canon Medical Systems and GE Healthcare now have deep-learning CT image reconstruction software, both of which gained FDA clearance in the spring of 2019 In deep learning, you feed the system the answers (in the case of CT, what ideal clinical images

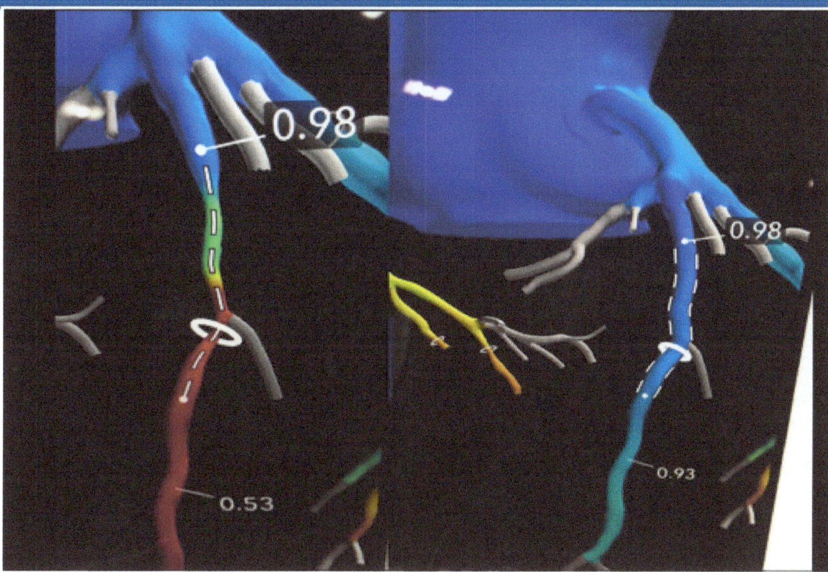

Fig. 5.4 HeartFlow Planner is a non-invasive, real-time virtual modeling tool for coronary artery disease (CAD) intervention. The HeartFlow Planner will enable interventional cardiologists to virtually model clinical scenarios vessel-by-vessel, explore treatment strategies for patients with CAD before each procedure, review cases with colleagues and ensure everyone has a clear picture of the initial treatment plan.

and resolution should look like) and the machine figures out what needs to be done with input image data to make it look like the ideal reference image, explained Jeannie Yu, M.D., FACC, FSCCT, director of cardiovascular imaging, Long Beach VA Health System. In this way, she said deep learning can be used to help in image resolution recovery that has better noise reduction and resolution than iterative reconstruction images. Her center is using Canon Medical Systems' AiCE deep learning reconstruction (DLR) software for the Precision CT system. The technology uses 10 convolutional neuro network (CNN) algorithms with different kernel sizes to reconstruct the images. Yu illustrated that this AI-driven software takes a lot of computing power, with the system operating using 71.2 teraflops. A teraflop is a unit of computing speed equal to one million floating-point operations per second. For comparison, Yu said IBM Watson AI software operates at 80 teraflops, a Playstation 4 game console at 1.8, Xbox One X gaming console at 6 and the iPhone X runs at 5 teraflops. GE Healthcare developed its Deep Learning Image Reconstruction (DLIR) software for the Revolution Apex CT system.This next-generation image reconstruction option uses a dedicated deep neural network (DNN) to generate what GE calls TrueFidelity CT Images.Compared to current iterative reconstruction technology, TrueFidelity CT images can elevate everyevery image to offer better image quality, image sharpness and noise texture, according to GE.

Photo-realistic and Surgical View Imaging

A few CT vendors now offer advanced visualization software offering realistic, photo-quality, surgical view image renderings. Canon Medical offers its Global Illumination photo-realistic rendering and Siemens Healthineers offers its cinematic image reconstruction. Vendors who offer this technology say it is not used for diagnostics, but can be helpful when explaining things to the patient and their family, educating physicians and staff, and for surgeons. It offers a realistic view of the anatomy that is easier for most people to understand who are not familiar with cardiac anatomy as it appears in traditional CT multiplanar reconstruction (MPR) images. Here are two examples of the technology: Canon example and Siemens example

ESC Guidelines Give Coronary CTA a Class 1 Recommendation

In September 2019, the European Society of Cardiology (ESC) published new guidelines on the diagnosis and management of chronic coronary syndromes (CCS), which classifies (CTA) as a Class 1 recommendation for diagnosing CAD in symptomatic

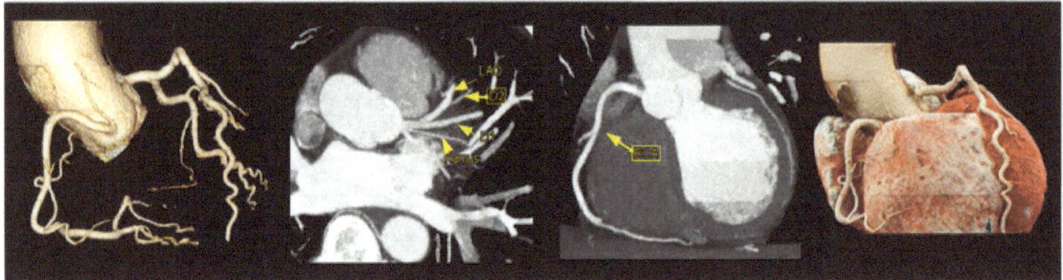

Fig. 5.5 Example of a normal CTA scan (no stenosis or plaque in any coronary artery) in a 43-year-old woman with family history of coronary artery disease. Heart rate was 65 beats/min for CTA. Effective dose for this axial prospectively ECG-triggered scan acquired with 100 kVp, was 1.5 mSv [dose length product (DLP) 107.1 mGy cm]

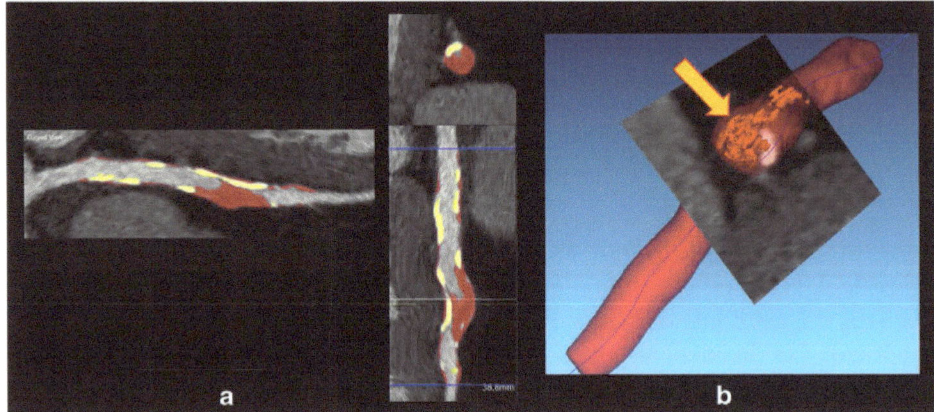

Fig. 5.6 High-risk coronary plaque quantification in the proximal left anterior descending artery by semi-automated software. a Curved MPR and straightened views showing NCP in red and CP in yellow. b 3D arterial view with arrow showing low-density noncalcified plaque (surrogate marker for the lipid core)

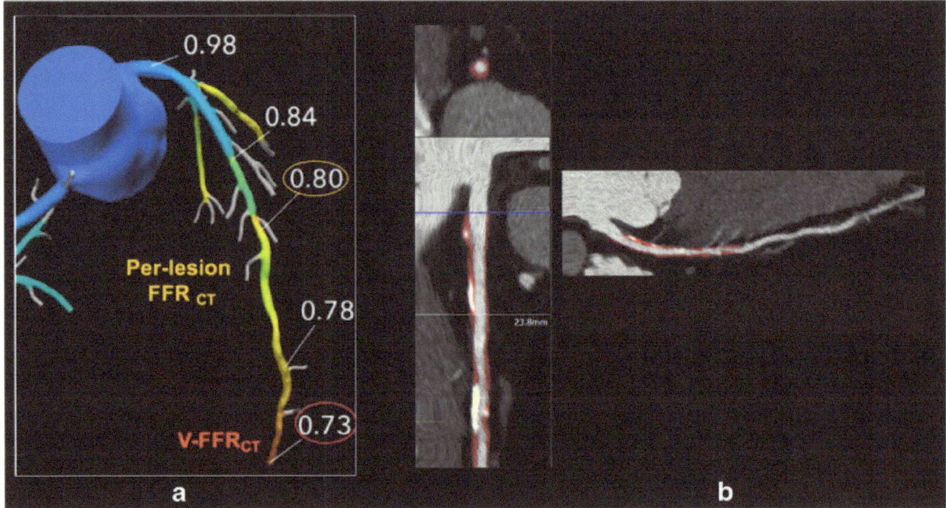

Fig. 5.7. (a) FFR-CT in left anterior descending artery with nonobstructive stenosis for a 52-year-old male with cardiovascular risk factors, showing progressively decreasing noninvasive FFR. (b) Quantitative plaque analysis showed diffuse atherosclerotic plaque with extensive noncalcified plaque (760 mm3, red), calcified plaque (67 mm3, yellow), maximum contrast density difference of 30% and maximum diameter stenosis of 47%

patients. The document, which is a continuation of the 2013 stable coronary artery disease (CAD) guidelines, updates the term to CCS to emphasize the dynamic nature of the disease.

Per the guideline, unless obstructive CAD can be excluded based on clinical evaluation alone, either non-invasive functional imaging or anatomical imaging using coronary CTA should be used as the initial test to rule out or establish the diagnosis of CCS.The new guideline suggests that "Coronary CTA is the preferred test in patients with a lower range of clinical likelihood of CAD, no previous diagnosis of CAD and characteristics associated with a high likelihood of good image quality."

"Depending on patient characteristics, local expertise and availability, as well as patient-specific considerations, physicians should decide between coronary CTA and ischemia testing," said ESC President-elect Stephan Achenbach, M.D., FSCCT. "This is a recognition of the numerous trials that have been performed to establish the usefulness and reliability of CT angiography as a first-line examination."

"The guideline recommendations are based on data that shows that the use of coronary CTA leads to accurate identification of coronary artery disease, which if treated appropriately, can lead to improved patient outcomes." added Blankstein. "The guidelines recognize that there are multiple factors that should be used in test selection, but that for many, a coronary CTA-first approach is beneficial."

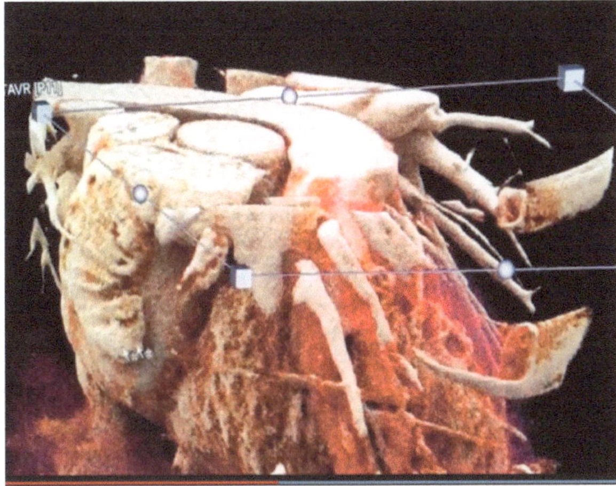

Fig. 5.8 showing Photo-realistic and Surgical View Imaging

Machine Learning with 18F-Sodium Fluoride PET and Quantitative Plaque Analysis on CT Angiography for the Future Risk of Myocardial Infarction

In everyday clinical practice, prediction of myocardial infarction is challenging and is typically based on cardiovascular risk factors and scores, especially in subjects with suspected coronary artery disease . However, in patients with established coronary artery disease, the performance of risk scores is limited, with c-statics ranging from 0.60 to 0.68 .Recently, advanced imaging techniques have demonstrated considerable promise in refining risk stratification in patients with established coronary artery disease. We have demonstrated that assessment of disease activity in the coronary arteries with 18F-sodium fluoride (18F-NaF) PET outperforms clinical variables and risk scores for the prediction of myocardial infarction in patients with a high burden of coronary artery disease.Similarly, in observational studies and a subanalysis of the SCOT-HEART trial, quantitative plaque analysis investigating both plaque type and burden on contrast enhanced CT angiography has emerged as a major predictor of adverse outcomes.To date, no study has investigated whether these 2 promising methods (which can be obtained during a single imaging session on a hybrid PET/CT scanner) are interchangeable or can provide superior predictive performance when used in combination.

CT Angiography and 18F-Sodium Fluoride PET

Acquisition and Reconstruction Patients underwent 18F-NaF PET on hybrid PET/CT scanners (128-slice Biograph mCT, Siemens Medical Systems; or Discovery 710, GE Healthcare) 60 min after intravenous administration of 18F-NaF (250 MBq). We acquired a noncontrast CT attenuation correction scan followed by a 30-min PET emission scan in list mode, a low-dose noncontrast ECG-gated CT for calculation of the coronary calcium, and a contrast-enhanced ECG-gated coronary CT angiogram, which was obtained in mid-diastole and end-expiration on the same PET/CT system without repositioning the patient. The ECG-gated PET list-mode dataset was reconstructed using harmonized protocols as described previously (supplemental materials)

Coronary Microcalcification Activity (CMA) Quantification Image analysis was performed in FusionQuant (Cedars-Sinai Medical Center) . We used a recently described measure of coronary 18F-NaF uptake, CMA, that quantifies PET activity across the entire coronary vasculature . CMA is a highly reproducible and robust measure of disease activity predicting both disease progression and myocardial infarction . We calculated the per-vessel and per-patient CMA maximum coronary SUV, and target-to-background ratio (TBR) as described previously (supplemental materials)

CT The coronary artery calcium score was measured in Agatston units (AU) using clinical software (NetraMD, Sclmage) on noncontrast CT scans. The presence, extent, and severity of coronary artery disease were evaluated on contrast-enhanced CT angiography by defining the segment involvement score, DUKE coronary artery disease index, and the number of vessels with >50% luminal stenosis . Multivessel coronary artery disease was defined as at least 2 major epicardial vessels with any combination of either >50% stenosis, or previous revascularization.

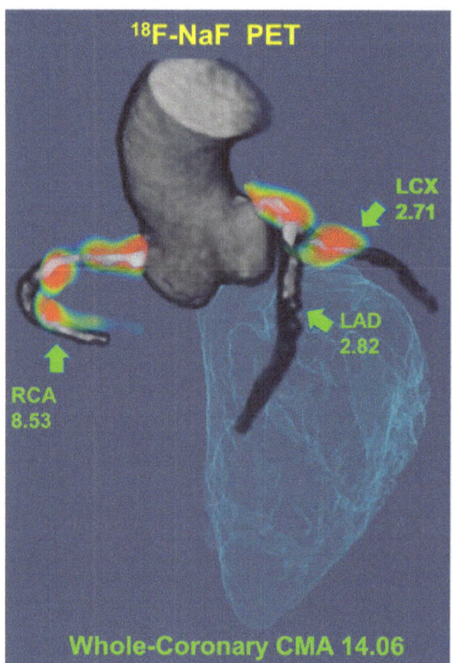

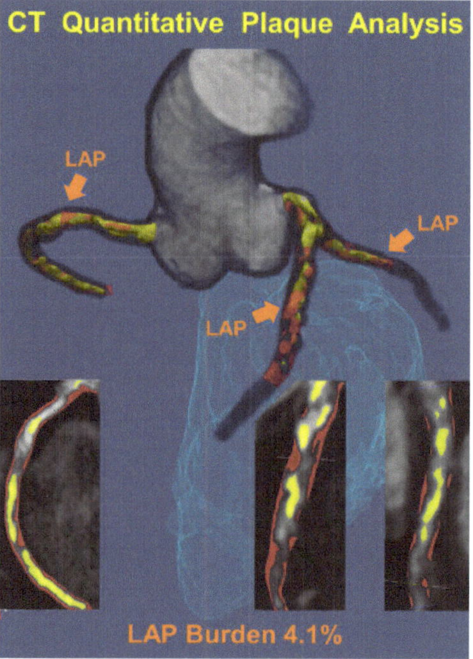

Fig. 5.9 Measuring disease activity across the coronary vasculature with 18F-NaF CMA and the low-attenuation plaque burden with quantitative plaque analysis. Three-dimensional (3D) rendering of coronary CT angiography coregistered with PET for evaluation of 18F-NaF uptake (blue and red; left panel). The CMA is a summary measure of 18F-NaF activity across the entire coronary vasculature as it includes all counts originating from the coronary artery 3D rendering of CT angiography–based quantitative plaque analysis with orange low-attenuation plaque (LAP) and yellow calcified plaque. The low-attenuation plaque burden was defined as the LAP volume × 100%/vessel volume. LAD = left anterior descending; LCX = left circumflex; RCA = right coronary artery.

Quantitative Plaque Analysis of CT Angiography We performed quantitative plaque analysis of all coronary segments with a lumen diameter greater than 2 mm using semiautomated software (AutoPlaque, version 2.0, Cedars-Sinai Medical Center). Proximal and distal limits of lesionswere manually marked by an experienced reader after examination of coronary CT angiographyimages in multiplanar format.

Subsequent plaque quantification was fully automated using adaptive scan-specific thresholds. Total, calcified, noncalcified as well as low attenuation plaque volumes were calculated. The plaque burden was calculated according to the following equation (plaque volume × 100%/vessel volume). The contrast density difference was the maximal difference in contrast density (mean Hounsfield unit/cross-sectional area) in the plaque and the reference proximal vessel cross section.

Machine Learning

Machine learning was used to derive a joint score for myocardial infarction by incorporating the key clinical variables, quantitative CT variables, and 18F-NaF PET findings. Model Building XGBoost is a recent implementation of a gradient boosting algorithm, which iteratively trains a set of weak learners (simple decision trees) using a given set of patient data, to build a combined strong classifier to identify an outcome . For every patient, the XGBoost algorithm computes an individualized probability of outcome, considering all input variables.

We applied XGBoost for prediction of myocardial infarction by building 3 models. First, a clinical model with baseline clinical characteristics: age, sex, comorbidities, medication, biomarkers, past medical history, and coronary calcium score (model 1). The second model was derived from quantitative plaque analysis variables (including low attenuation plaque burden and the contrast density difference). A final model incorporated clinical, CT and 18F-NaF PET data in combination. Model Testing Given the limited number of cases, we refrained from performing data-specific hypertuning and applied fixed XGBoost parameters established in our previous studies.Furthermore, to avoid biased results and limit overfitting, we tested all of our models using repeated 10-fold cross-testing, which separates training and testing data .The dataset was randomly split into 10-folds with similar myocardial infarction rates in each fold (stratified 10-folds). Ten models were created each from 90% of the data, and each tested in held-out test sample (10% of the data). These 10 held-out samples containing nonoverlapping test results were subsequently concatenated to evaluate the average performance of XGBoost in unseen data.Feature Importance To elucidate the influence of each of the variables included in the machine-learning model, we provided machine-learning feature importance scores. Importance is the relative amount that each attribute improves the XGBoost performance measure The variable importance was determined directly from the XGBoost model separately in each fold and returned from the XGBoost model for each variable. The variable importance represents the relative improvement in the log loss objective function of the XGBoost

All 293 study participants (65 ± 9 y; 84% male) had established coronary artery disease and were on guideline-recommended medical treatments (Table 1). Two-hundred thirty-seven (81%) patients had a history of revascularization, 191 (65%) had multivessel obstructive coronary artery disease, and the median coronary calcium score was 334 (76 to 804) AU. Over the 53 (40–59) months of follow-up, 22 subjects experienced a fatal (n = 3) or nonfatal (n = 19) myocardial infarction. The high burden of atherosclerosis was reflected in the quantitative plaque analysis derived from coronary CT angiography. The median total plaque volume was 1,174 (716 to 1,772) mm3 and consisted largely of noncalcified plaque (1,099 [647 to 1,574] mm3) with a substantial volume of low-attenuation plaque (88 [44 to 167] mm3). Over half of the study population (166 [56%]) had a low-attenuation plaque burden exceeding 4%. On PET, 109 (37.2%) patients presented with a high 18F-NaF CMA (>1.56; Fig. 2).

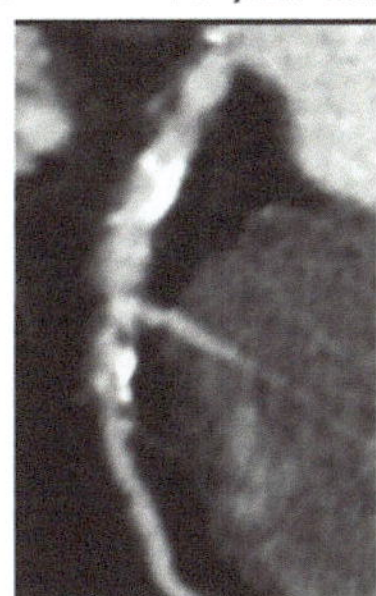
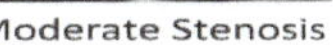

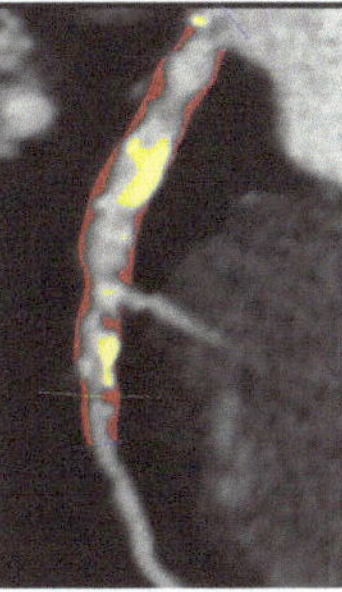

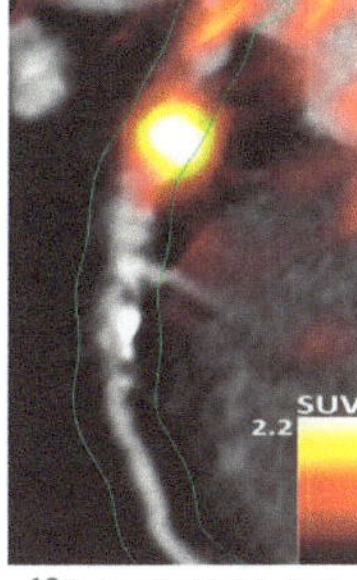

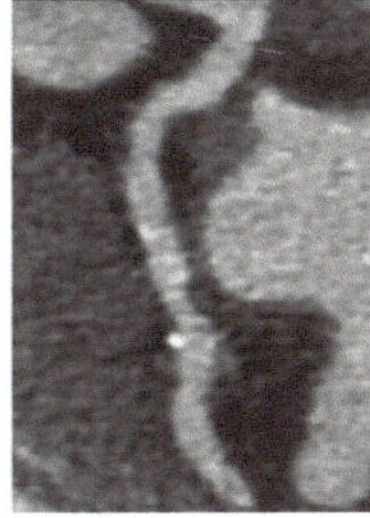

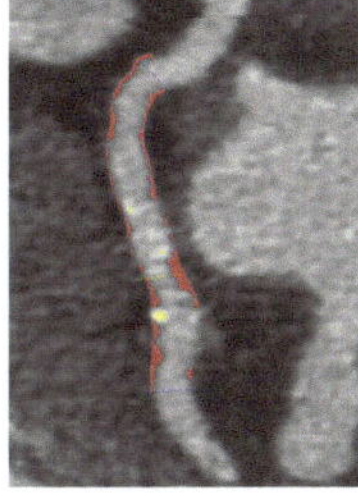

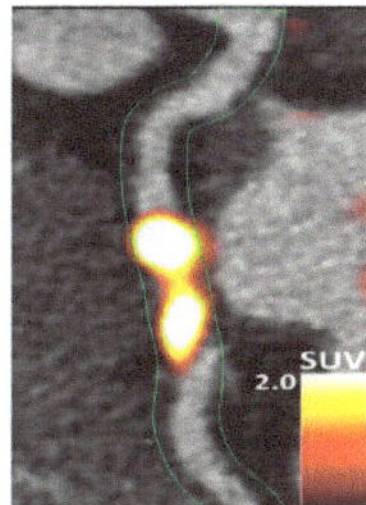

Fig. 5.10 Case examples of quantitative plaque analysis on coronary CT angiography and 18F-NaF PET in patients with established coronary artery disease. Hybrid CT angiography and 18F-NaF PET of coronary arteries. (A) A 70-y-old male, who presented with diffused largely noncalcified disease (middle panel in red) in the LAD and demonstrated increased 18F-NaF uptake in the LAD on PET. (B) A 59-y-old male with mild LCX atherosclerosis, who presented with a high noncalcified plaque burden (middle panel in red) on CT angiography, significant 18F-NaF uptake and experienced a lateral non–ST-segment elevation myocardial infarction during follow-up. LAD = left anterior descending; LCX = left circumflex; LAP = low attenuation plaque.

18F-NaF PET provides an assessment of vascular injury and disease activity across a wide spectrum of cardiovascular conditions including aortic stenosis, mitral annular calcification, abdominal aortic aneurysm, erectile dysfunction, bioprosthetic valve degeneration and coronary artery disease . Indeed, baseline 18F-NaF PET is consistently associated with future disease progression and adverse events in each of these conditions. On the other hand, quantitative assessment of atherosclerotic plaque on contrast-enhanced CT angiography allows us to measure the burden of different types of plaque across the coronary arteries.We recently demonstrated that the low-attenuation plaque burden provides powerful prediction of myocardial infarction, outperforming cardiovascular risk scores, Agatston coronary artery calcium scoring, or the presence and severity of obstructive coronary artery disease . Whether these 2 exciting developments can be used in combination to further advance risk prediction was previously unknown. Using the information from these approaches and by leveraging machine learning, we were able to build an integrated model for prediction of events in patients with established coronary artery disease, a group of patients in whom risk prediction is currently challenging. The XGBoost algorithm has been successfully implemented for risk prediction in a wide range of clinical scenarios It enables the incorporation of numerous predictors into the model even when these variables are correlated a major limitation with conventional regression analyses. Although we have previously shown that 18F-NaF uptake is associated with quantitative plaque analysis indices, our current analysis highlights the complementary prognostic information that PET and quantitative CT plaque assessments provide together.Indeed, our machine-learning model incorporating the information from these 2 modalities alongside clinical factors outperformed the individual components analyzed separately with a high c-statistic of 0.85. Importantly, our study also underscores that in patients with advanced coronary artery disease, markers of disease activity, plaque type and plaque burden provide risk prediction superior to clinical risk scores and conventional coronary calcium CT analyses.According to societal guidelines, patients with clinically manifest atherosclerotic arterial disease are considered to be at very high risk of a recurrent cardiovascular events and cardiovascular mortality. However, in everyday clinical practice, it is apparent that there is a wide distribution of actual risk for recurrent vascular events in patients with clinically established arterial disease. Although the population of subjects with manifested coronary artery disease is rapidly growing, accurate risk prediction in this important population remains challenging. The guideline-recommended SMART risk score was shown to have only a moderate c-statistic (0.64–0.68), and there is a paucity of data regarding the role imaging could play in this cohort.In our study we have targeted this important high-risk population. We have demonstrated that quantitative plaque analysis measures and the coronary microcalcification activity considerably improve stratification of patients' risk (c-statistic 0.85). In a conservative 10-fold cross testing machine-learning model, we showed that CT and PET data need to be used together for optimal stratification.

Conclusion

Both 18F-NaF uptake and quantitative plaque analysis measures from contrast CT are strong predictors of outcome in patients with established coronary artery disease. Optimal risk stratification can be achieved by combining these imaging assessments of plaque type, burden, and activity with clinical variables in a machine-learning model.

Bibliography And Acknowledgement

- Abbara S, Blanke P, Maroules CD, Cheezum M, Choi AD, Han BK, et al. SCCT guidelines for the performance and acquisition of coronary computed tomographic angiography: a report of the society of cardiovascular computed tomography guidelines committee: Endorsed by the North American Society for Cardiovascular Imaging (NASCI). J Cardiovasc Comput Tomogr. 2016;10:435–49. [PubMed] [Google Scholar]
- Achenbach S, Ropers U, Kuettner A, Anders K, Pflederer T, Komatsu S, et al. Randomized comparison of 64-slice single-and dual-source computed tomography coronary angiography for the detection of coronary artery disease. J Am Coll Cardiol Cardiovascular Imaging. 2008;1:177–86. [PubMed] [Google Scholar]
- Agatston A. S., Janowitz W. R., Hildner F. J., Zusmer N. R., Viamonte M., Jr., Detrano R. Quantification of coronary artery calcium using ultrafast computed tomography. Journal of the American College of Cardiology. 1990;15(4):827–832. doi: 10.1016/0735-1097(90)90282-T
- Agatston AS, Janowitz WR, Hildner FJ, Zusmer NR, Viamonte M Jr, Detrano R. Quantification of coronary artery calcium using ultrafast computed tomography. J Am Coll Cardiol. 1990;15: 827–32.
- Aikawa E., Nahrendorf M., Figueiredo J. L., et al. Osteogenesis associates with inflammation in early-stage atherosclerosis evaluated by molecular imaging in vivo. Circulation. 2007;116(24):2841–2850. doi: 10.1161/CIRCULATIONAHA.107.732867.
- Arad Y, Goodman KJ, Roth M, Newstein D, Guerci AD. Coronary calcification, coronary disease risk factors, C-reactive protein, and atherosclerotic cardiovascular disease events: the St Francis Heart Study. J Am Coll Cardiol. 2005;46:158–65.
- Arad Y, Spadaro LA, Goodman K, Newstein D, Guerci AD. Prediction of coronary events with electron beam computed tomography. J Am Coll Cardiol. 2000;36:1253–60. [
- Barreto M, Schoenhagen P, Nair A, Amatangelo S, Milite M, Obuchowski NA, et al. Potential of dual-energy computed tomography to characterize atherosclerotic plaque: ex vivo assessment of human coronary arteries in comparison to histology. J Cardiovasc Comput Tomogr. 2008;2:234–42.
- Becker A, Knez A, Becker C, Leber A, Anthopounou L, Boekstegers P, et al. Prediction of serious cardiovascular events by determining coronary artery calcification measured by multi-slice computed tomography. Dtsch Med Wochenschr. 2005;130: 2433–8.
- Beheshti M., Saboury B., Mehta N. Detection and global quantification of cardiovascular molecular calcification by fluoro18-fluoride positron emission tomography/computed tomography--a novel concept. Hellenic Journal of Nuclear Medicine. 2011;14(2):114–120.
- Bellinge J. W., Francis R. J., Majeed K., Watts G. F., Schultz C. J. In search of the vulnerable patient or the vulnerable plaque: 18F-sodium fluoride positron emission tomography for cardiovascular risk stratification. Journal of Nuclear Cardiology. 2018;25(5):1774–1783. doi: 10.1007/s12350-018-1360-2. -
- Berman DS, Hachamovitch R, Shaw LJ, Friedman JD, Hayes SW, Thomson LE, et al. Roles of nuclear cardiology, cardiac computed tomography, and cardiac magnetic resonance: noninvasive risk stratification and a conceptual framework for the selection of noninvasive imaging tests in patients with known or suspected coronary artery disease. J Nucl Med. 2006;47:1107–18.
- Blau M., Ganatra R., Bender M. A. 18F-fluoride for bone imaging. Seminars in Nuclear Medicine. 1972;2(1):31–37. doi: 10.1016/S0001-2998(72)80005-9.
- Boll DT, Merkle EM, Paulson EK, Fleiter TR. Coronary stent patency: dual-energy multidetector CT assessment in a pilot study with anthropomorphic phantom. Radiology. 2008;247:687–95
- Boll DT, Merkle EM, Paulson EK, Mirza RA, Fleiter TR. Calcified vascular plaque specimens: assessment with cardiac dual-energy multidetector CT in anthropomorphically moving heart phantom. Radiology. 2008;249:119–26.
- Budoff M. J., Young R., Burke G., et al. Ten-year association of coronary artery calcium with atherosclerotic cardiovascular disease (ASCVD) events: the Multi-Ethnic Study of Atherosclerosis (MESA) European Heart Journal. 2018;39(25):2401–2408. doi: 10.1093/eurheartj/ehy217.
- Callister T, Cooil B, Raya S, Lippolis N, Russo D, Raggi P. Coronary artery disease: improved reproducibility of calcium scoring with an electron-beam CT volumetric method. Radiology. 1998;208:807–14.
- Chen W., Dilsizian V. Targeted PET/CT imaging of vulnerable atherosclerotic plaques: microcalcification with sodium fluoride and inflammation with fluorodeoxyglucose. Current Cardiology Reports. 2013;15(6) doi: 10.1007/s11886-013-0364-4.
- ClinicalTrials gov. National Library of Medicine (U.S.). Dual Antiplatelet Therapy to Reduce Myocardial Injury. June 2020 ClinicalTrials gov. National Library of Medicine (U.S.). Effect of Evolocumab on Coronary Artery Plaque Volume and Composition by CCTA and Microcalcification by F18-NaF PET. June 2020
- ClinicalTrials gov. National Library of Medicine (U.S.). Study Prediction of Recurrent Events With 18F-Fluoride. June 2020
- Creager M. D., Hohl T., Hutcheson J. D., et al. 18F-fluoride signal amplification identifies microcalcifications associated with atherosclerotic plaque instability in positron emission tomography/ computed tomography images. Circulation. Cardiovascular Imaging. 2019;12(1):p. e007835. doi: 10.1161/CIRCIMAGING.118.007835
- Czernin J., Satyamurthy N., Schiepers C. Molecular mechanisms of bone 18F-NaF deposition. Journal of Nuclear Medicine. 2010;51(12):1826–1829. doi: 10.2967/jnumed.110.077933.
- Deseive S, Chen MY, Korosoglou G, Leipsic J, Martuscelli E, Carrascosa P, et al. Prospective randomized trial on radiation dose estimates of CT angiography applying iterative image reconstruction: the PROTECTION V study. J Am Coll Cardiol Img. 2015;8: 888–96.
- Detrano R, Guerci AD, Carr JJ, Bild DE, Burke G, Folsom AR, et al. Coronary calcium as a predictor of coronary events in four racial or ethnic groups. N Engl J Med. 2008;358:1336–45
- Doris M. K., Otaki Y., Krishnan S. K., et al. Optimization of reconstruction and quantification of motion-corrected coronary PET-CT. Journal of Nuclear Cardiology. 2020;27(2):494–504. doi: 10.1007/s12350-018-1317-5.
- Dweck M. R., Chow M. W., Joshi N. V., et al. Coronary arterial 18F-sodium fluoride uptake: a novel marker of plaque biology. Journal of the American College of Cardiology. 2012;59(17):1539–1548. doi: 10.1016/j.jacc.2011.12.037.
- Dweck M. R., Jenkins W. S. A., Vesey A. T., et al. 18F-sodium fluoride uptake is a marker of active calcification and disease progression in patients with aortic stenosis. Circulation-Cardiovascular Imaging. 2014;7(2):371–378. doi: 10.1161/circimaging.113.001508.

- Eisentopf J, Achenbach S, Ulzheimer S, Layritz C, Wuest W, May M, et al. Low-dose dual-source CT angiography with iterative reconstruction for coronary artery stent evaluation. J Am Coll Cardiol Img. 2013;6:458–65.
- Erbel R., Möhlenkamp S., Moebus S., et al. Coronary risk stratification, discrimination, and reclassification improvement based on quantification of subclinical coronary atherosclerosis: the Heinz Nixdorf Recall Study. Journal of the American College of Cardiology. 2010;56(17):1397–1406. doi: 10.1016/j.jacc.2010.06.030
- Ferreira M. J. V., Oliveira-Santos M., Silva R., et al. Assessment of atherosclerotic plaque calcification using F18-NaF PET-CT. Journal of Nuclear Cardiology. 2018;25(5):1733–1741. doi: 10.1007/s12350-016-0776-9.
- Fiz F., Morbelli S., Piccardo A., et al. 18F-NaF uptake by atherosclerotic plaque on PET/CT imaging: inverse correlation between calcification density and mineral metabolic activity. Journal of Nuclear Medicine. 2015;56(7):1019–1023. doi: 10.2967/jnumed.115.154229.
- Forsythe R. O., Dweck M. R., McBride O. M. B., et al. 18F-Sodium Fluoride Uptake in Abdominal Aortic Aneurysms: The SoFIA. J Am Coll Cardiol. 2018;71(5):513–523. doi: 10.1016/j.jacc.2017.11.053
- Fuchs TA, Stehli J, Bull S, Dougoud S, Clerc OF, Herzog BA, et al. Coronary computed tomography angiography with model-based iterative reconstruction using a radiation exposure similar to chest X-ray examination. Eur Heart J. 2014;35:1131–6
- Fuchs TA, Stehli J, Fiechter M, Dougoud S, Sah B-R, Gebhard C, et al. First in vivo head-to-head comparison of high-definition versus standard-definition stent imaging with 64-slice computed tomography. Int J Card Imaging. 2013;29:1409–16
- Greenland P, LaBree L, Azen SP, Doherty TM, Detrano RC. Coronary artery calcium score combined with Framingham score for risk prediction in asymptomatic individuals. JAMA. 2004;291: 210–5
- Greenland P., Blaha M. J., Budoff M. J., Erbel R., Watson K. E. Coronary calcium score and cardiovascular risk. Journal of the American College of Cardiology. 2018;72(4):434–447. doi: 10.1016/j.jacc.2018.05.027.
- Han J. H., Lim S. Y., Lee M. S., Lee W. W. Sodium [18F]fluoride PET/CT in myocardial infarction. Molecular Imaging and Biology. 2015;17(2):214–221. doi: 10.1007/s11307-014-0796-2.
- Hausleiter J, Meyer T, Hadamitzky M, Zankl M, Gerein P, DorrLer K, et al. Non-invasive coronary computed tomographic angiography for patients with suspected coronary artery disease: the coronary angiography by computed tomography with the use of a submillimeter resolution (CACTUS) trial. Eur Heart J. 2007;28:3034–41.
- Hell MM, Bittner D, Schuhbaeck A, Muschiol G, Brand M, Lell M, et al. Prospectively ECG-triggered high-pitch coronary angiography with third-generation dual-source CT at 70 kVp tube voltage: feasibility, image quality, radiation dose, and effect of iterative reconstruction. J Cardiovasc Comput Tomogr. 2014;8: 418–25.
- Hou Y, Xu S, Guo W, Vembar M, Guo Q. The optimal dose reduction level using iterative reconstruction with prospective ECG-triggered coronary CTA using 256-slice MDCT. Eur J Radiol. 2012;81:3905–11
- Huet P., Burg S., Le Guludec D., Hyafil F., Buvat I. Variability and uncertainty of 18F-FDG PET imaging protocols for assessing inflammation in atherosclerosis: suggestions for improvement. The Journal of Nuclear Medicine. 2015;56(4):552–559. doi: 10.2967/jnumed.114.142596
- Irkle A., Vesey A. T., Lewis D. Y., et al. Identifying active vascular microcalcification by 18F-sodium fluoride positron emission tomography. Nature Communications. 2015;6(1):p. 7495. doi: 10.1038/ncomms8495.
- Jadvar H., Desai B., Conti P. S. Sodium 18F-Fluoride PET/CT of Bone, Joint, and Other Disorders. Seminars in Nuclear Medicine. 2015;45(1):58–65. doi: 10.1053/j.semnuclmed.2014.07.008.
- Janssen T., Bannas P., Herrmann J., et al. Association of linear 18F-sodium fluoride accumulation in femoral arteries as a measure of diffuse calcification with cardiovascular risk factors: a PET/CT study. Journal of Nuclear Cardiology. 2013;20(4):569–577. doi: 10.1007/s12350-013-9680-8
- Jaskowiak C. J., Bianco J. A., Perlman S. B., Fine J. P. Influence of reconstruction iterations on 18F-FDG PET/CT standardized uptake values. Journal of Nuclear Medicine. 2005;46:424–428
- Johson R. C., Leopold J. A., Loscalzo J. Vascular calcification: pathobiological mechanisms and clinical implications. Circulation Research. 2006;99(10):1044–1059. doi: 10.1161/01.RES.0000249379.55535.21.
- Joshi N. V., Vesey A. T., Williams M. C., et al. 18F-fluoride positron emission tomography for identification of ruptured and high-risk coronary atherosclerotic plaques: a prospective clinical trial. Lancet. 2014;383(9918):705–713. doi: 10.1016/S0140-6736(13)61754-7.
- Kondos GT, Hoff JA, Sevrukov A, Daviglus ML, Garside DB, Devries SS, et al. Electron-beam tomography coronary artery calcium and cardiac events: a 37-month follow-up of 5635 initially asymptomatic low- to intermediate-risk adults. Circulation. 2003;107:2571–6.
- Kwiecinski J., Adamson P. D., Lassen M. L., et al. Feasibility of coronary 18F-Sodium fluoride Positron-Emission Tomography assessment with the utilization of previously acquired Computed Tomography angiography. Circ Cardiovasc Imaging. 2018;11(12):p. e008325. doi: 10.1161/CIRCIMAGING.118.008325.
- Kwiecinski J., Berman D. S., Lee S. E., et al. Three-hour delayed imaging improves assessment of coronary 18F-sodium fluoride PET. Journal of Nuclear Medicine. 2019;60(4):530–535. doi: 10.2967/jnumed.118.217885. 10.2967/jnumed.118.217885
- LaMonte MJ, FitzGerald SJ, Church TS, Barlow CE, Radford NB, Levine BD, et al. Coronary artery calcium score and coronary heart disease events in a large cohort of asymptomatic men and women. Am J Epidemiol. 2005;162:421–9
- Lassen M. L., Beyer T., Berger A., et al. Data-driven, projection-based respiratory motion compensation of PET data for cardiac PET/CT and PET/MR imaging. Journal of Nuclear Cardiology. 2019
- Lassen M. L., Cadet S., Massera D., et al. Aortic valve imaging using 18F-sodium fluoride: implications of triple motion correction on test-retest reproducibility. Journal of Nuclear Medicine. 2020;61(supplement 1):9–9.

- Lassen M. L., Kwiecinski J., Cadet S., et al. Data-driven gross patient motion detection and compensation: implications for Coronary18F-NaF PET imaging. The Journal of Nuclear Medicine. 2019;60(6):830–836.
- Lassen M. L., Kwiecinski J., Dey D., et al. Triple-gated motion and blood pool clearance corrections improve reproducibility of coronary 18F-NaF PET. Eur J NuclMedMol Imaging. 2019;46(12):2610–2620. doi: 10.1007/s00259-019-04437-x. Lassen M. L., Kwiecinski J., Slomka P. J. Gating Approaches in Cardiac PET Imaging. PET Clinics. 2019;14(2):271–279..
- Leipsic J, Labounty TM, Heilbron B, Min JK, Mancini GB, Lin FY, et al. Estimated radiation dose reduction using adaptive statistical iterative reconstruction in coronary CT angiography: the ERASIR study. AJR Am J Roentgenol. 2010;195:655–60.
- Maeda E, Tomizawa N, Kanno S, Yasaka K, Kubo T, Ino K, et al. The feasibility of forward-projected model-based iterative reconstruction SoluTion (FIRST) for coronary 320-row computed tomography angiography: a pilot study. J Cardiovasc Comput Tomogr. 2017;11:40–5
- Marchesseau S., Seneviratna A., Sjöholm A. T., et al. Hybrid PET/CT and PET/MRI imaging of vulnerable coronary plaque and myocardial scar tissue in acute myocardial infarction. Journal of Nuclear Cardiology. 2018;25(6):2001–2011. doi: 10.1007/s12350-017-0918-8.
- Massera D., Doris M. K., Cadet S., et al. Analytical quantification of aortic valve 18F-sodium fluoride PET uptake. Journal of Nuclear Cardiology. 2020;27(3):962–972. doi: 10.1007/s12350-018-01542-6
- Massera D., Trivieri M. G., Andrews J. P. M., et al. Disease activity in mitral annular calcification. Circulation: Cardiovascular Imaging. 2019;12(2):p. e008513. doi: 10.1161/ circimaging.118.008513. -
- McClelland R. L., Jorgensen N. W., Budoff M., et al. 10-year coronary heart disease risk prediction using coronary artery calcium and traditional risk factors: derivation in the MESA (Multi-Ethnic Study of Atherosclerosis) with validation in the HNR (Heinz Nixdorf Recall) Study and the DHS (Dallas Heart Study) Journal of the American College of Cardiology. 2015;66(15):1643–1653. doi: 10.1016/j.jacc.2015.08.035.
- McCollough CH, Leng S, Yu L, Fletcher JG. Dual-and multi-energy CT: principles, technical approaches, and clinical applications. Radiology. 2015;276:637–53.
- McCollough CH, Ulzheimer S, Halliburton SS, Shanneik K, White RD, Kalender WA. Coronary artery calcium: a multi-institutional, multimanufacturer international standard for quantification at cardiac CT. Radiology. 2007;243:527–38.
- McKenney-Drake M. L., Territo P. R., Salavati A., et al. 18F-NaF PET imaging of early coronary artery calcification. Journal of the American College of Cardiology. 2016;9(5):627–628. doi: 10.1016/j.jcmg.2015.02.026.
- Meijboom WB, van Mieghem CAG, Mollet NR, Pugliese F, Weustink AC, van Pelt N, et al. 64-Slice computed tomography coronary angiography in patients with high, intermediate, or low pretest probability of significant coronary artery disease. J Am Coll Cardiol. 2007;50:1469–75. [PubMed] [Google Scholar]
- \Meyer M, Haubenreisser H, Schoepf UJ, Vliegenthart R, Leidecker C, Allmendinger T, et al. Closing in on the K edge: coronary CT angiography at 100, 80, and 70 kV—initial comparison of a second-versus a third-generation dual-source CT system. Radiology. 2014;273:373–82
- Miller JM, Rochitte CE, Dewey M, Arbab-Zadeh A, Niinuma H, Gottlieb I, et al. Diagnostic performance of coronary angiography by 64-row CT. N Engl J Med. 2008;359:2324–36.
- Morsbach F, Desbiolles L, Plass A, Leschka S, Schmidt B, Falk V, et al. Stenosis quantification in coronary CT angiography: impact of an integrated circuit detector with iterative reconstruction. Investig Radiol. 2013;48:32–40.
- New S., Goettsch C., Aikawa M., et al. Macrophage-derived matrix vesicles: an alternative novel mechanism for microcalcification in atherosclerotic plaques. Circulation Research. 2013;113(1):72–77.
- Obaid DR, Calvert PA, Gopalan D, Parker RA, West NE, Goddard M, et al. Dual-energy computed tomography imaging to determine atherosclerotic plaque composition: a prospective study with tissue validation. J Cardiovasc Comput Tomogr. 2014;8:230–7.
- Park R, Detrano R, Xiang M, Fu P, Ibrahim Y, LaBree L, et al. Combined use of computed tomography coronary calcium scores and C-reactive protein levels in predicting cardiovascular events in nondiabetic individuals. Circulation. 2002;106:2073–7.
- Plonek T., Berezowski M., Kurcz J., et al. The evaluation of the aortic annulus displacement during cardiac cycle using magnetic resonance imaging. BMC Cardiovascular Disorders. 2018;18(1):154–156.
- Raggi P, Callister TQ, Cooil B, He ZX, Lippolis NJ, Russo DJ, et al. Identification of patients at increased risk of first unheralded acute myocardial infarction by electron-beam computed tomography. Circulation. 2000;101:850–5
- Rubeaux M., Joshi N. V., Dweck M. R., et al. Motion correction of 18F-NaF PET for imaging coronary atherosclerotic plaques. Journal of Nuclear Medicine. 2016;57(1):54–59.
- Ruzsics B, Lee H, Zwerner PL, Gebregziabher M, Costello P, Schoepf UJ. Dual-energy CT of the heart for diagnosing coronary artery stenosis and myocardial ischemia-initial experience. Eur Radiol. 2008;18:2414–24.
- Sánchez-Gracián CD, Pernas RO, López CT, Armentia ES, Liste AV, Caamaño MV, et al. Quantitative myocardial perfusion with stress dual-energy CT: iodine concentration differences between normal and ischemic or necrotic myocardium. Initial experience. Eur Radiol. 2016;26:3199–207
- Schwarz F, Nance JW Jr, Ruzsics B, Bastarrika G, Sterzik A, Schoepf UJ. Quantification of coronary artery calcium on the basis of dual-energy coronary CT angiography. Radiology. 2012;264: 700–7.
- Shaw L, Raggi P, Schisterman E, Berman D, Callister T. Prognostic value of cardiac risk factors and coronary artery calcium screening for all-cause mortality. Radiology. 2003;228:826–33
- Shemesh J, Morag-Koren N, Goldbourt U, Grossman E, Tenenbaum A, Fisman EZ, et al. Coronary calcium by spiral computed tomography predicts cardiovascular events in high-risk hypertensive patients. J Hypertens. 2004;22:605–10.
- Stehli J, Fuchs TA, Bull S, Clerc OF, Possner M, Buechel RR, et al. Accuracy of coronary CT angiography using a submillisievert fraction of radiation exposure: comparison with invasive coronary angiography. J Am Coll Cardiol. 2014;64:772–80.

- Taylor AJ, Bindeman J, Feuerstein I, Cao F, Brazaitis M, O'Malley PG. Coronary calcium independently predicts incident premature coronary heart disease over measured cardiovascular risk factors: mean three-year outcomes in the Prospective Army Coronary Calcium (PACC) project. J Am Coll Cardiol. 2005;46:807–14.
- Taylor AJ, Cerqueira M, Hodgson JM, Mark D, Min J, O'Gara P, et al. ACCF/SCCT/ACR/AHA/ASE/ASNC/NASCI/SCAI/SCMR 2010 appropriate use criteria for cardiac computed tomography: a report of the American College of Cardiology Foundation Appropriate Use Criteria Task Force, the Society of Cardiovascular Computed Tomography, the American College of Radiology, the American Heart Association, the American Society of Echocardiography, the American Society of Nuclear Cardiology, the North American Society for Cardiovascular Imaging, the Society for Cardiovascular Angiography and Interventions, and the Society for Cardiovascular Magnetic Resonance. J Am Coll Cardiol. 2010;56:1864–94.
- Tomizawa N, Nojo T, Akahane M, Torigoe R, Kiryu S, Ohtomo K. Adaptive iterative dose reduction in coronary CT angiography using 320-row CT: assessment of radiation dose reduction and image quality. J Cardiovasc Comput Tomogr. 2012;6:318–24.
- Trivieri M. G., Dweck M. R., Abgral R., et al. 18F-sodium fluoride PET/MR for the assessment of cardiac amyloidosis. Journal of the American College of Cardiology. 2016;68(24):2712–2714. doi: 10.1016/j.jacc.2016.09.953.
- Tzolos E., Kwiecinski J., Lassen M. L., et al. Observer repeatability and interscan reproducibility of 18F-sodium fluoride coronary microcalcification activity. Journal of Nuclear Cardiology. 2020 doi: 10.1007/s12350-020-02221-1.
- Tzolos E., Lassen M. L., Pan T., et al. Respiration-averaged CT versus standard CT attenuation map for correction of 18F-sodium fluoride uptake in coronary atherosclerotic lesions on hybrid PET/CT. Journal of Nuclear Cardiology. 2020 doi: 10.1007/s12350-020-02245-7.
- Tzolos E., Lassen M. L., Pan T., et al. Respiration-averaged CT versus standard CT attenuation map for correction of 18F-sodium fluoride uptake in coronary atherosclerotic lesions on hybrid PET/CT. Journal of Nuclear Cardiology. 2020 doi: 10.1007/s12350-020-02245-7.
- Uotani K, Watanabe Y, Higashi M, Nakazawa T, Kono AK, Hori Y, et al. Dual-energy CT head bone and hard plaque removal for quantification of calcified carotid stenosis: utility and comparison with digital subtraction angiography. Eur Radiol. 2009;19:2060–5.
- Vliegenthart R, Oudkerk M, Hofman A, Oei HH, van Dijck W, van Rooij FJ, et al. Coronary calcification improves cardiovascular risk prediction in the elderly. Circulation. 2005;112:572–7
- Von Spiczak J, Morsbach F, Winklhofer S, Frauenfelder T, Leschka S, Flohr T, et al. Coronary artery stent imaging with CT using an integrated electronics detector and iterative reconstructions: first in vitro experience. J Cardiovasc Comput Tomogr. 2013;7:215–22.
- Weininger M, Schoepf UJ, Ramachandra A, Fink C, Rowe GW, Costello P, et al. Adenosine-stress dynamic real-time myocardial perfusion CT and adenosine-stress first-pass dual-energy myocardial perfusion CT for the assessment of acute chest pain: initial results. Eur J Radiol. 2012;81:3703–10.
- Wong ND, Hsu JC, Detrano RC, Diamond G, Eisenberg H, Gardin JM. Coronary artery calcium evaluation by electron beam computed tomography and its relation to new cardiovascular events. Am J Cardiol. 2000;86:495–8
- Yang WJ, Zhang H, Xiao H, Li JY, Liu Y, Pan ZL, et al. High-definition computed tomography for coronary artery stents imaging compared with standard-definition 64-row multidectector computed tomography: an initial in vivo study. J Comput Assist Tomogr. 2012;36:295–300.

Transformative Technology Of 3D Printing In Congenital Heart Disease

CHAPTER

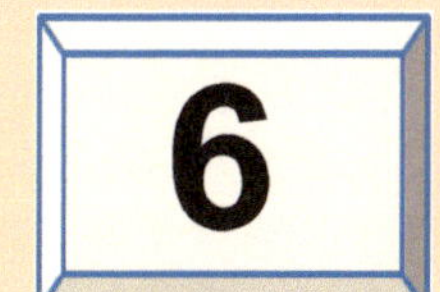

Survival in congenital heart disease has steadily improved since 1938, when Dr. Robert Gross successfully ligated for the first time a patent ductus arteriosus in a 7-year-old child. To continue the gains made over the past 80 years, transformative changes with broad impact are needed in management of congenital heart disease. Three-dimensional printing is an emerging technology that is fundamentally affecting patient care, research, trainee education, and interactions among medical teams, patients, and caregivers. This paper first reviews key clinical cases where the technology has affected patient care. It then discusses 3-dimensional printing in trainee education. Thereafter, the role of this technology in communication with multidisciplinary teams, patients, and caregivers is described. Three-dimensional (3D) printing is an additive manufacturing technique with increasing use in health care. As a fabrication technique 3D printing was recently listed by the McKinsey Global Institute as a "disruptive technology that will transform life, business and the global economy,"

1. Scope of Congenital Heart Disease and the Need for Transformative Care

The prevalence of CHD is approximately 9 in 1,000 live births. Survival rates vary by disease complexity, with long-term survival (>20 years) at approximately 95% for simple CHD, 90% for moderate complexity, and 80% for severe, complex CHD . Overall survival rates have steadily increased for even the most complex CHD , although survival alone is not a sufficient outcome measure in the current era.Other important metrics include the following: long-term morbidity; reintervention rates; length of hospitalization; neurodevelopmental outcomes; cost to the health care system; and patient or caregiver satisfaction. Obtaining the best outcomes requires an impact at multiple levels, including patients and caregivers, individual clinicians, the medical team and the health care system. 3D printing is a disruptive technology that is affecting each of these key areas in CHD.

The earliest papers on cardiovascular 3D printing were published in the early 2000s. Binder et al. showed feasibility from echocardiographic data in 2000, and Pentacost et al. produced 3D models replicating cardiac embryology from photomicrographic data in 2001. Soon thereafter, datasets from computed tomography (CT) or magnetic resonance imaging (MRI) were used to produce 3D cardiac models of increasing complexity , with a steady rise in publications in the past decade shows the applications of 3D printing in medicine, broadly categorized as surgical planning, education, and manufacturing of custom parts. Given that a 3D model is a replica of a patient's anatomy, models may be used for precise pre-surgical planning and simulation . Patient-specific pre-surgical planning may potentially reduce time spent in the operating room (OR) and result in fewer complications. In turn, this may lead to shorter post-operative stays, decreased reintervention rates, and lower health care costs. Given the relatively recent use of 3D printing in CHD, there are currently no data supporting these presumed outcomes. Most of the evidence in published reports is qualitative, through case reports and series. Emerging reports from other surgical subspecialties appear promising. Recent data from craniofacial reports suggest that 3D printing can improve outcomes, including saving time in the OR and thus translating to direct cost savings .

3D Printing Technology and Options for Cardiovascular Printing

Several recent publications have described the process of medical 3D ., summarized as these key steps:-

- Acquisition of a high-resolution 3D imaging dataset
- Segmentation of the anatomy using specialized post-processing software
- Computer-aided design to refine the design, add cut-planes, or include elements required for model stability
- Creation of a 3D file in a format recognized by the 3D printer, usually in the Surface Tessellation Language or stereolithography (STL) file format
- Printing of the physical model

3D printing technologies may be categorized as photopolymeric (the use of light to harden a deposited photopolymer), thermoplastic (extruding melted thermoplastics in layers to build up a model), or powder fusion (a process that fuses ceramic or metal powder by using an adhesive or laser beam to create a 3D object).. Printer resolution for higher-end medical-grade printers is in the order of micrometers, well within the resolution needed to print cardiac structures.

Principally, there are 2 main types of cardiac models: **"blood-pool" and "hollow"** models. Blood pool models are solid 3D representations of the blood pool within the cardiac chambers and vessels . They are created by segmenting the blood pool signal, usually from contrast-enhanced CT or MRI, after which the 3D object is printed. Noncardiovascular structures such as airways or soft tissue may also be included for printing. These models provide excellent visualization of the great vessels, extracardiac vasculature, and surrounding structures such as airways or the esophagus. The drawback of these types of models is their limited views of intracardiac anatomy.

Hollow models are created by applying a mesh representing myocardium and vessel walls around the blood pool signal and then digitally removing the blood pool signal to show the intracardiac cavities. The end result is a hollow model showing the intracardiac anatomy in detail. These models are usually sectioned along a pre-determined cut-plane with 2 or more sections showing the intracardiac anatomy.

A subtype of the hollow models consists of intact hollow models. These models also show the intracardiac anatomy but are printed intact (i.e., without a cut-plane), thereby resulting in the most accurate representation of the heart as it sits in the chest. When printed in a flexible material, these models allow cardiothoracic surgeons to use standard surgical approaches and see the anatomy from a "surgeon's perspective," as they would for the actual case. Thus, these models are ideal for surgical simulation, especially when they are printed in materials that can be cut, can hold suture, and can allow engraftment of foreign materials (e.g., patch, cannula).

Applications of 3D Printing in CHD

Several publications have described the use of 3D printing in CHD, spanning the spectrum from atrial or ventricular septal defects (ASDs, VSDs) to the most complex cardiac lesions . Published reports have been summarized in a recent textbook on cardiac 3D printing .

A selection of cases is now reviewed to show the main applications of 3D printing in CHD. These cases were selected from a cohort of pediatric and adult patients with CHD at our institution who underwent 3D printing. Most of these cases were printed for surgical planning and simulation; others with unique or rare anatomy were printed for trainee education. The majority of cases had complex CHD, with a median complexity score of 3 (simple = 1, moderate = 2, great = 3) . Most of the cases printed for surgical planning were high-risk surgical candidates, and the median Society of Thoracic Surgeons-European Association for Cardio-Thoracic Surgery mortality category (1 to 5) was 4.

Planning complex intracardiac repair

Three of 1,000 patients born with CHD require catheter-based or surgical intervention early in life . Outcomes are significantly affected by the complexity of the underlying anatomy and perioperative factors, including cardiopulmonary bypass time, ischemic time, or circulatory arrest time .3D models allow the visualization and understanding of complex spatial relationships and enable precise pre-surgical planning.

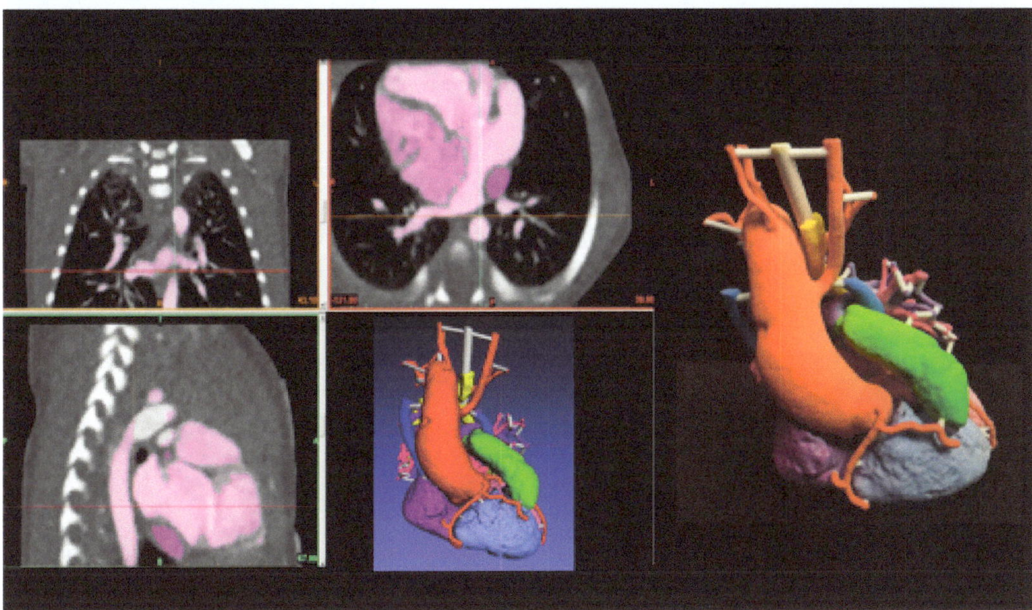

Fig.6.1 Blood Pool Cardiac 3D Model images on the left show the segmented blood pool signal. The model is shown on the right.

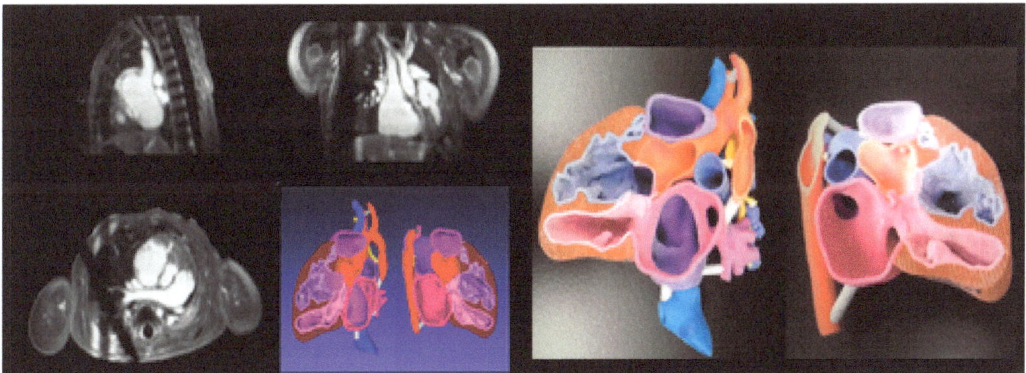

Fig.6.2 Hollow Cardiac 3D Model Showing Intracardiac Anatomy

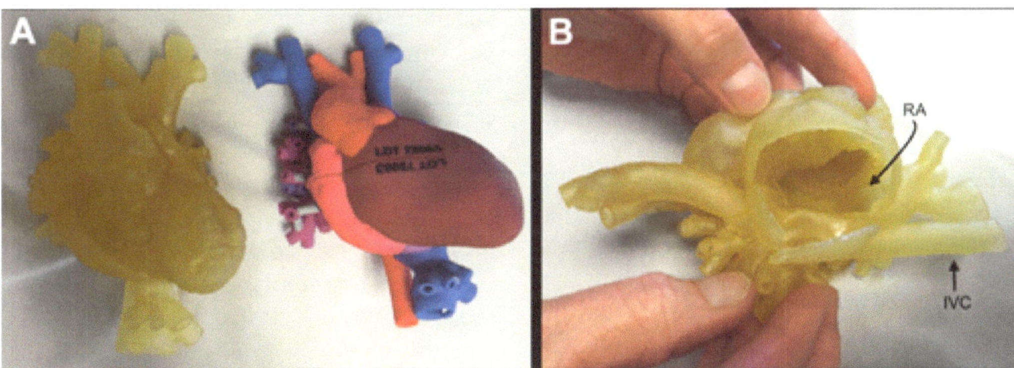

Fig.6.3 Models for Surgical Planning (A) Flexible hollow model printed intact with corresponding rigid multicolor model. (B) The "surgeon's view" through a right atriotomy. IVC = inferior vena cava; RA = right atrium.

A common application in CHD is planning repair of a double-outlet right ventricle (DORV) requiring a complex intracardiac baffle. This is typically a high-risk operation, Society of Thoracic Surgeons-European Association for Cardio-Thoracic Surgery category Several other groups have reported the use of 3D printing to plan complex intracardiac repairs in patients with multiple VSDs or DORV

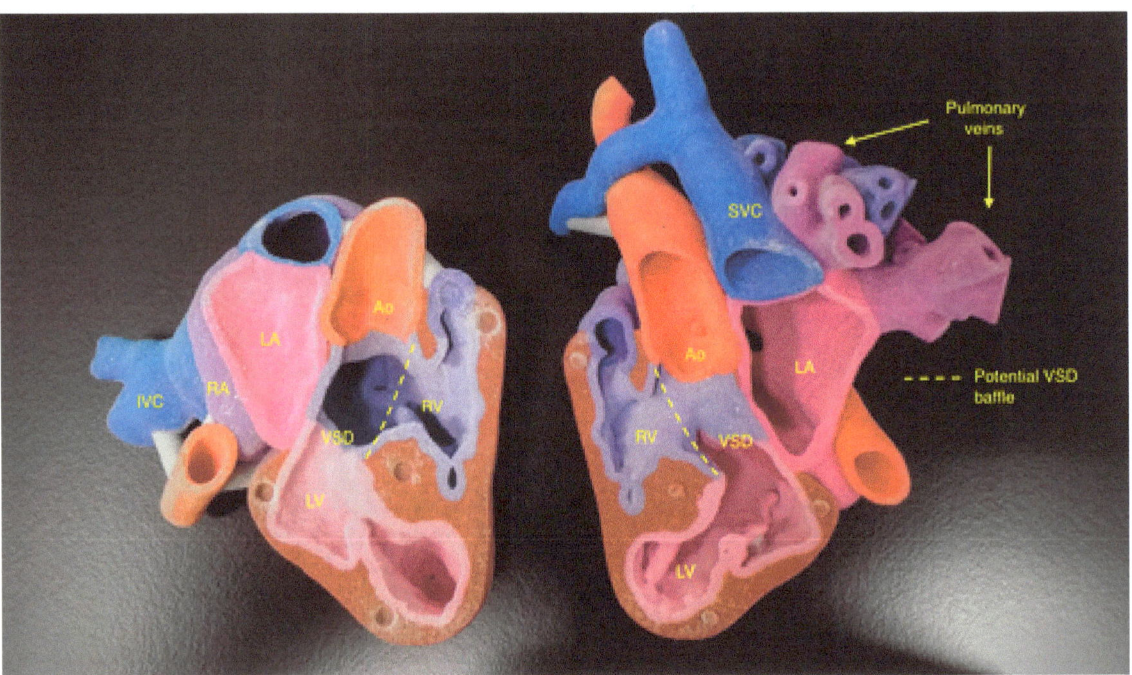

Fig.6.4 3D Model of Double-Outlet RV Showing Relationships Among Ventricles, VSD, and Outflows The dashed line indicates the potential ventricular septal defect (VSD) baffle pathway to achieve a 2-ventricle repair. Ao = aorta; LA = left atrium; LV = left ventricle; RV = right ventricle; SVC = superior vena cava;

Surgical simulation

The ultimate in pre-surgical planning using 3D models is one in which a "simulated surgery" is performed, as illustrated by the next case. The patient was a 3 1/2-year-old male child with heterotaxy, asplenia syndrome with complex single ventricle anatomy, and abnormal systemic and pulmonary venous connections (Figure 7). He had previously undergone bilateral bidirectional superior cavopulmonary connections (bilateral Glenn procedure) as part of single ventricle palliation. 3D printing was performed to plan his next surgery, a total cavopulmonary connection (aka Fontan). Two 3D models were printed; 1 multicolor with an axial cut-plane and a second flexible intact-heart model (no cut-plane) for surgical simulation. The internal anatomy of both models was identical. By using the models, detailed pre-surgical planning was performed. Specifically, the models were used to plan placement of the Fontan conduit (intracardiac or extracardiac) and to evaluate its relationship with systemic veins and impact on pulmonary veins. The model was also used to simulate "plan A," "plan B," or "bailout" scenarios, each with a unique surgical plan. This level of detailed surgical simulation is not feasible with current standard of care (e.g., 3D volumetric rendering), and it shows the added value of 3D printed models.

Extracardiac and vascular surgery

3D printing can be a valuable tool to plan extracardiac and vascular surgery in patients with CHD. 3D models are helpful for planning high-risk unifocalization surgery, . The 3D models show spatial relationships among the aorta, aortopulmonary collaterals (APCs), pulmonary veins, and airways that enabled detailed pre-surgical planning. Precise visualization of the complex relationships between APCs and surrounding structures enables easier identification and surgical manipulation during the case, thereby reducing operative time and potentially improving the surgical outcome. This patient underwent a right modified Blalock-Taussig-Thomas shunt to the right-sided APCs . followed by a left modified Blalock-Taussig-Thomas shunt and, ultimately, successful unifocalization . 3D printing for pulmonary atresia and MAPCAs offers significant benefits over current standard of care, also described in prior publications .

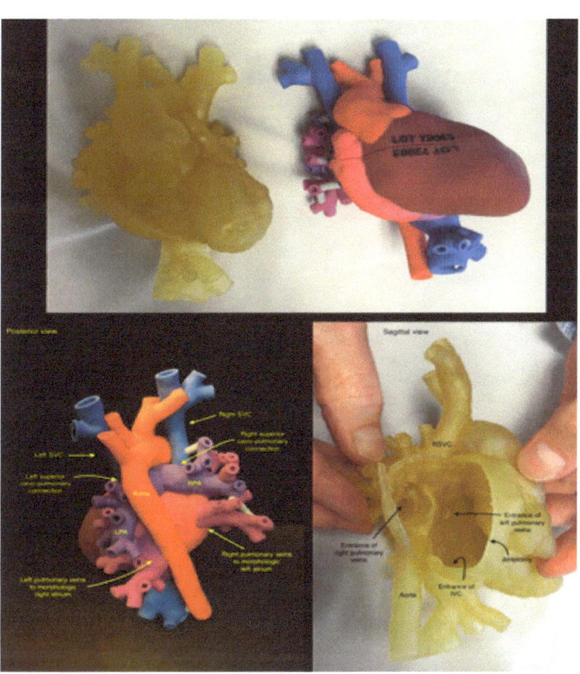

Fig.6.5 Simulated Surgery for Complex Total Cavopulmonary Connection Planning Using Flexible, Intact-Heart Model LPA = left pulmonary artery; RPA = right pulmonary artery; RSVC = right superior vena cava;

Ventricular assist device and heart transplant

An endpoint of many patients with CHD is heart failure requiring a ventricular assist device or heart transplant. 3D printing can aid in ventricular assist

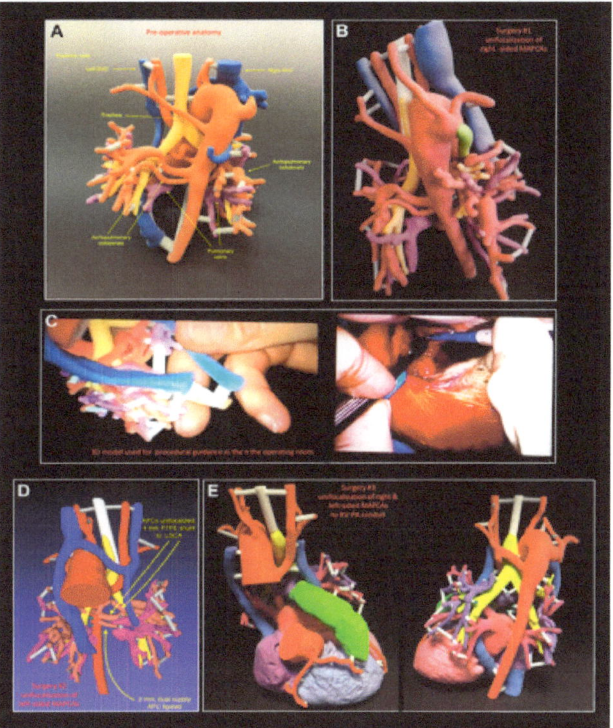

Fig.6.6 Staged Repair of Tetralogy of Fallot, Pulmonary Atresia, and MAPCAs

(A) Pre-operative anatomy. (B) Unifocalization of right-sided major aortopulmonary collateral arteries (MAPCAs) and small right pulmonary artery (PA)–to–right modified Blalock-Taussig-Thomas shunt. (C) Use of 3D model in the operating room for procedural guidance. (D) Unifocalization of left-sided major aortopulmonary collateral arteries–to–left modified Blalock-Taussig-Thomas shunt. (E) Right ventricular (RV)–to–pulmonary artery conduit placement (green) to unifocalized major aortopulmonary collateral arteries and takedown of bilateral modified Blalock-Taussig-Thomas shunts. APC = aortopulmonary collateral; LSCA = left subclavian artery; PTFE = polytetrafluoroethylene; SVC = superior vena cava.

device placement and optimizing function in complex CHD, as recently described by Farooqi et al and Saeed et al. . 3D printing can also assist with transplant planning for recipients with complex CHD More recently, a Melody valve was placed in a left ventricular–to–left superior vena cava conduit for conduit stenosis. 3D printing was performed to plan key components of the transplant, including thoracic entry,cannulation options, conduct of bypass, and graft-donor connections. 3D printing for transplant planning has been previously described for patients with complex pre-transplant anatomy .

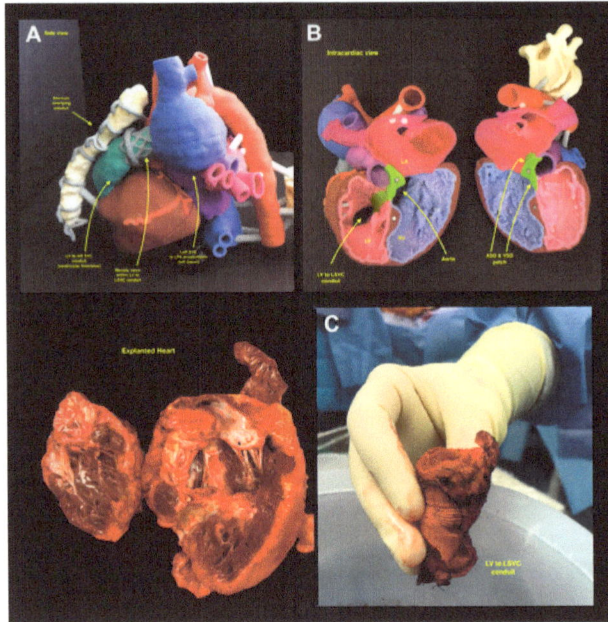

Fig.6.7 Heterotaxy, Unbalanced Atrioventricular Canal, Ventricular Inversion, Modified Fontan

(A) 3D model showing a left ventricle (LV)–to–left superior vena cava (LSVC) conduit and left-sided Glenn procedure that complicates transplantation of a normal donor heart. (B) Intracardiac anatomy. (C) Intraoperative findings: explanted heart and a left ventricle–to–left superior vena cava conduit, showing accuracy of the 3D model. ASD = atrial septal defect;

Airway abnormalities

In CHD cases, the airways may be involved in the pathophysiology or need to be accounted for in surgical planning, as demonstrated earlier in the case with tetralogy of Fallot with pulmonary atresia and MAPCAs. In some CHD lesions, airways may be directly affected by the cardiovascular disease. Examples include vascular rings (Figure 10A), where aberrant vessels cause airway compression, or compression from dilated pulmonary arteries in tetralogy of Fallot with absent pulmonary valve.Airway compression or tracheobronchomalacia can significantly add to morbidity of patients with CHD from prolonged ventilator dependence. 3D printing recently led to a momentous breakthrough in the management of these patients with the use of 3D printed bioresorbable airway splints. In this series 3D printed splints were implanted without complications and resulted in patency of the airway. If successful in larger cohorts, this application of 3D printing will dramatically change the management and outcomes for these challenging patients. Other applications of 3D printing in otolaryngology and airway abnormalities were recently reviewed by VanKoevering et al.

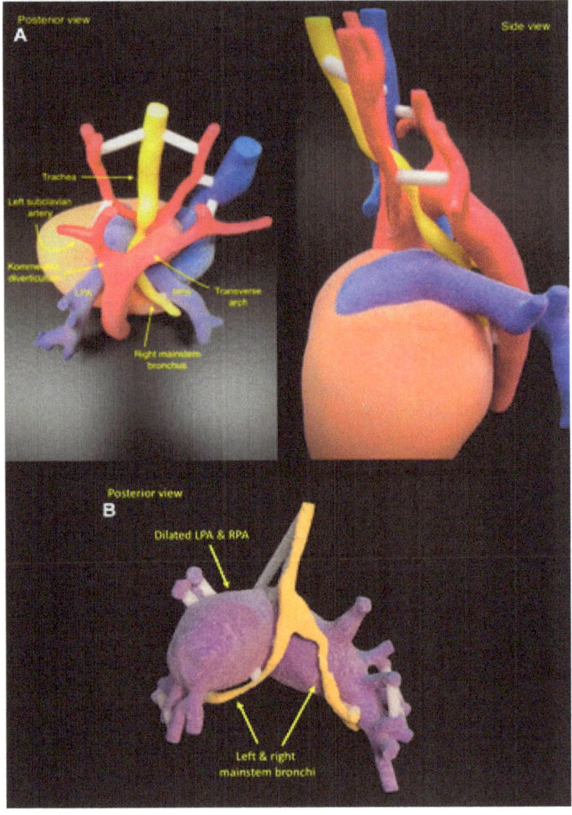

Fig.6.8 Airway Abnormalities in Congenital Heart Disease

(A) Vascular ring with posterior compression of trachea by a circumflex transverse arch coursing behind the aorta. (B) Severe branch pulmonary artery dilation in tetralogy of Fallot with absent pulmonary valve with compression and malacia of bilateral mainstem bronchi

Airway compression or tracheobronchomalacia can significantly add to morbidity of patients with CHD from prolonged ventilator dependence. 3D printing recently led to a momentous breakthrough in the management of these patients with the use of 3D printed bioresorbable airway splints.In this series 3D printed splints were implanted without complications and resulted in patency of the airway. If successful in larger cohorts, this application of 3D printing will dramatically

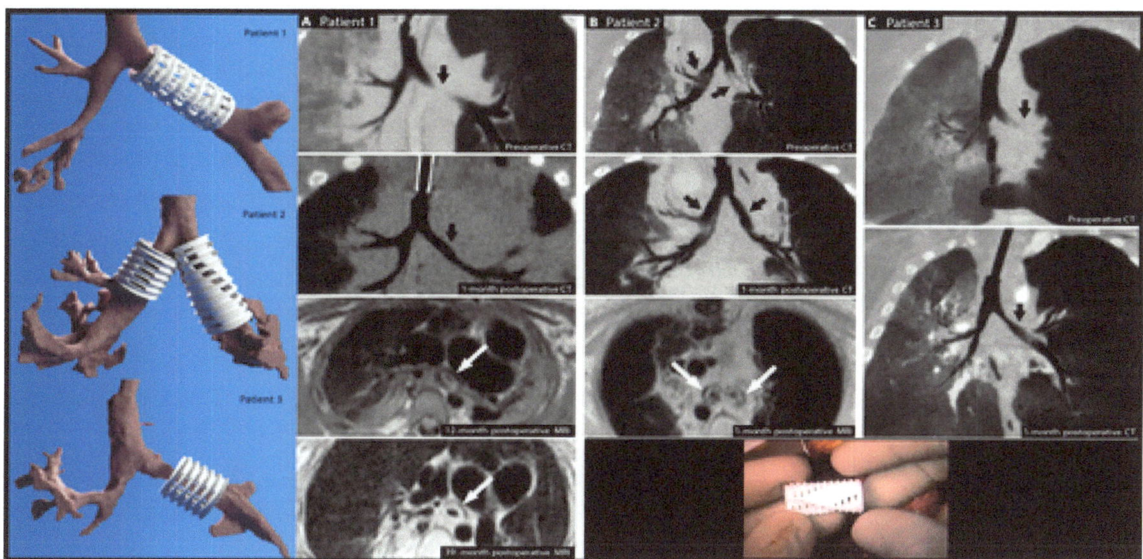

Fig.6.9 Bioresorbable Airway Splint Manufactured From Polycaprolactone With a Bellowed Design to Promote Expansion and Growth Over Time

change the management and outcomes for these challenging patients. Other applications of 3D printing in otolaryngology and airway abnormalities were recently reviewed by VanKoevering et al.

Catheter-based interventions

3D printing has been used for catheter-based interventions in CHD, although to a lesser degree compared with cardiothoracic surgery. Some noteworthy applications include the following: percutaneous pulmonary valve implantation, reported as early as 2007 ; coarctation procedures ; and stenting for aortic arch hypoplasia. Other reported applications include transcatheter ASD closure, double-lobed left atrial appendage closure , caval valve implantation , and stenting of Mustard baffle obstruction 3D printing is of particular interest in noncongenital structural heart disease, including transcatheter mitral and aortic valve interventions.. Potential benefits in interventional cardiology include visualization of complex anatomy that leads to decreased radiation and contrast from fluoroscopy and angiography and improved procedural outcome. Other benefits may include device development and testing in models that replicate abnormal anatomy . Finally, a key benefit may be feasibility testing for complex or borderline cases, as in the case of this 15-year-old male patient from our institution with repaired tetralogy of Fallot who met the criteria for pulmonary valve replacement.MRI measurements indicated that his right ventricular outflow tract dimensions were borderline large for transcatheter pulmonary valve replacement; thus, a 3D model was made in flexible material to trial pre-stenting as a precursor to transcatheter pulmonary valve replacement. The 3D model showed feasibility of the catheter-based strategy, and the procedure was carried out, with subsequent successful implantation of a transcatheter pulmonary valve, thereby avoiding surgery.

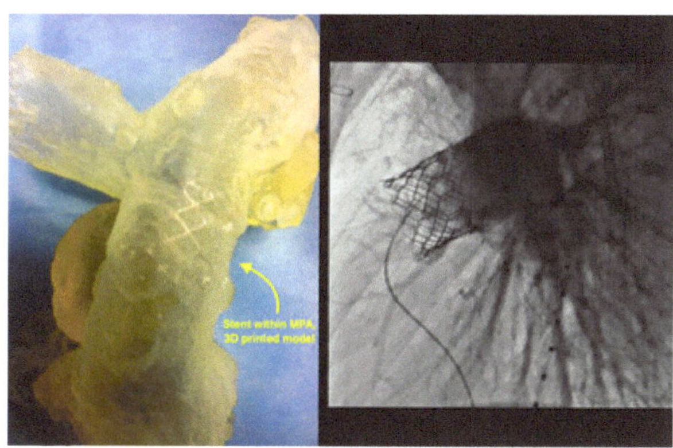

Fig.6.10 3D Printed Model in a Case of TOF With Borderline Large PA Measurements
Image on the left shows a stent within main pulmonary artery (MPA). Image on the right is an angiogram taken after successful transcatheter implantation of pulmonary valve. PA = pulmonary artery; TOF = tetralogy of Fallot.

Impediments to greater use of 3D models incatheter-based procedures include tissue characteristics of the models that do not respond to balloons and stents in the same way as native tissue. Moreover, current models do not reflect the physiological environment encountered during catheterization, with nonpulsatility a major limitation of static models. Both these limitations may be overcome with future iterations of 3D models,

Adults with congenital heart disease

Approximately 85% of children with CHD now survive into adulthood , and adults with CHD (ACHD) now outnumber children . There are an estimated 5 million adult survivors in the United States alone . Over the past few decades the proportion of all deaths in patients with CHD has shifted from infants to the ACHD population . Similar to their pediatric counterparts, risk factors that worsen ACHD outcomes include complex anatomy, prior surgeries, and length of time spent on cardiopulmonary bypass . Although the challenges involving complex ACHD are considerable, 3D printing may help in their management by applications described

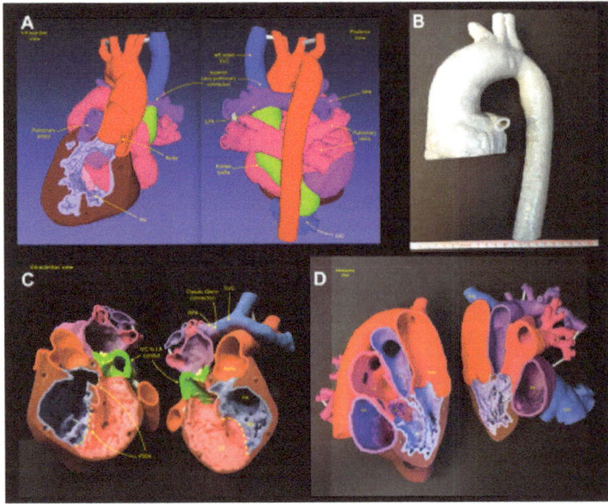

Fig 6.11 3D Models of Adults With Congenital Heart Disease (continued)

(A) A 31-year-old patient with dextrocardia, a double-outlet right ventricle (DORV), and a Fontan procedure. (B) A 19-year-old patient with a bicuspid aortic valve (not shown) and a severely dilated aortic root and ascending aorta. (C) A 40-year-old patient with a double-outlet right ventricle, 2 VSDs, and classic Glenn and modified Mustard procedures (conduit from inferior vena cava [IVC] to left atrium [LA], in green). (D) A 45-year-old patient with a left dominant unbalanced atrioventricular canal, a double-outlet right ventricle, and right ventricular outflow tract obstruction.

Accuracy and Quality Assurance in Cardiac 3D Printing

Accuracy in medical 3D printing is of paramount importance, although published reports on this topic are limited. Accuracy is defined by comparison with a gold standard, and in the case of 3D printed models, 1 metric of accuracy is comparison with operative findings. At our institution, the quality assurance process is driven by feedback from our surgical colleagues and findings in the OR. Between February 2015 and May 2017, the average accuracy score for 21 3D printed models at our institution was 4 of a possible 5 points when the surgeon compared model anatomy with findings in the OR. A similar quality assurance process was described by Hermsen et al. for surgical models of hypertrophic obstructive cardiomyopathy. We have found that direct and ongoing communication among the imaging, modeling, and surgical teams is essential for maintaining high levels of accuracy. In addition, model accuracy may be diminished if there is a significant delay between acquisition of source images and time of surgery. In infants and young children somatic growth and evolution of the pathophysiology can produce relatively large changes to the anatomy as time passes; thus, the pre-operative imaging and 3D modeling should be performed close to the time of anticipated surgery.Besides direct comparison with OR findings, other metrics of accuracy include comparison with source images and user feedback. Olivieri et al. reported that 3D printed models from echocardiographic data were comparable in measurements of VSDs when compared with source images. Yoo et al. reported data from 50 surgeons after undergoing a Hands-on Surgical Training course using 3D models.The majority of cardiothoracic surgeons reported that the 3D models were of "excellent" or "good" quality for surgical simulation . Finally, accuracy of 3D models may be judged in terms of their ability to recreate native physiology, not just anatomy. The innovative work of Vukicevic et al. has shown the ability to recreate "hemodynamics" of abnormal aortic valves in 3D models, with Doppler characteristics nearly identical to those of the patient's own diseased valve

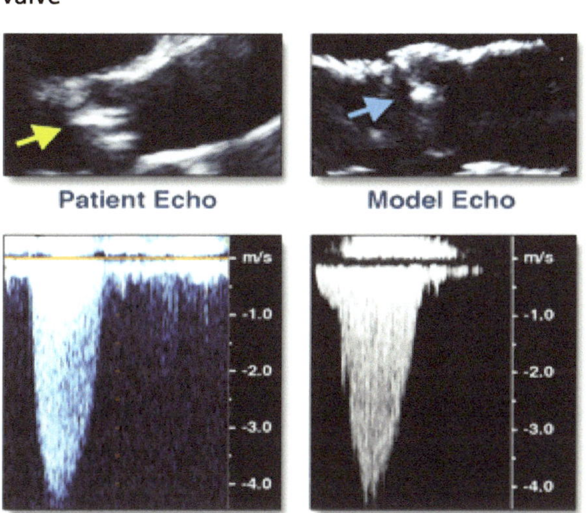

Fig.6.12 **Patient and Model Doppler Comparisons** Doppler profile of a patient's echocardiogram on the left, compared with the Doppler image from the 3D printed model on the right. Arrows point towards the aortic valve from the patient's echocardiogram (left) and model (right).

3D Printing for Trainee Education and Surgical Simulation

Another arena where 3D printing can bring about transformative change is in the education and training of the next generation of physicians. This is an established practice in neurosurgery) and otolaryngology , with more recent application in cardiology . Although medical training has long followed the practice of "see 1, do 1, teach 1," use of 3D models in education represents a paradigm shift from an apprenticeship model to a simulator-based learning method that complements traditional mentored training .3D models in CHD can reduce the learning curve for cardiac trainees in 3 key areas:

- Understanding complex 3D anatomy
- High-fidelity simulation experiences
- Exposure to rare cases

As a tool for surgical simulation, 3D printing has been applied toward septal myectomy for hypertrophic obstructive cardiomyopathy , vascular procedures, and complex congenital procedures, as described by Yoo et al.

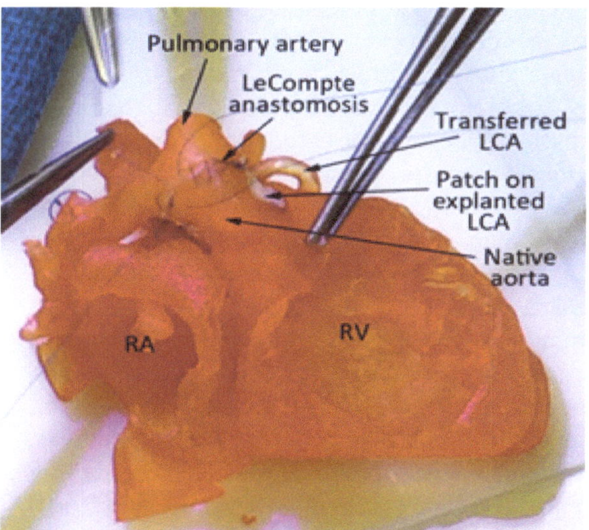

Fig.6.13 **Simulated Arterial Switch Operation From a Hands-on Surgical Training Course for Cardiothoracic Surgeons** Reproduced with permission from Yoo et al. LCA = left coronary artery.

In addition to allowing practice on highly accurate simulators, the 3D models expose trainees to pathological features they may rarely encounter. This shifts the practice of surgery from an "opportunity-based"to a "curriculum-based" experience. For experienced practitioners, models may be used for lifelong learning, for maintenance of certification, or for practice before challenging cases. Thus, a repository of 3D printed cardiovascular models with the spectrum of CHD would be an ideal educational resource The 3D print Heart Library at the National Institutes of Health is a good example of this concept. Electronic 3D models may supplement traditional learning methods. Finally, virtual reality displays may be used as complementary platforms to interact with electronic 3D models, with several robust options currently available

3D Printing to Facilitate Communication Within theMedicalTeamandfor Counseling Patients and Families

Cardiac surgery and perioperative care are conducted in a multidisciplinary setting requiring highly skilled and specialized teams. Communication among specialists is essential for avoiding errors and optimizing patient outcomes . 3D models provide clarity, and they are cornerstones around which multiple subspecialists can gather to discuss the pathological condition, surgical plan, anticipated outcomes, and perioperative care. In so doing, they may reduce medical errors, a postulate that deserves further investigation.

In addition to facilitating communication among medical team members, 3D models enable better communication between the medical team and patients or their caregivers . The models can help the patient or caregiver better understand the disease process, risks, benefits, and alternatives. Anecdotally, our institutional practice is to counsel patients and families by using 3D models if a model has been printed for a case. Eleven caregivers who completed a questionnaire for cardiac models between 2014 and 2017 reported that the models were "very helpful" (score 5 of 5) to improve understanding of the anatomy.

Similarly, Biglino et al. reported that 3D models could help improve the family's experience with medical care when models were used for counseling. More data are needed on the potentially powerful impact of 3D printing in patient and family education and shared decision making.

Advanced Applications and Future Directions

3D printing is rapidly evolving in medicine, with technical improvements in printers and software fueling new and exciting applications in patient care, innovation, and research. In cardiovascular medicine, a major limitation is high-resolution printing of structures currently not well resolved by CT or MRI, such as atrioventricular valves or the atrial septum. 3D printing from 3D echocardiography could potentially overcome these limitations, with some promising early results.3D printing from angiographic imaging could expand options, currently largely unexplored . The next evolution in 3D printing would be "multimodality" printing, with a model created by combining key elements of the anatomy from different imaging modalities. True co-registration of a highly accurate dataset is a technical challenge, and there are some early feasibilitydata.

In addition to advances in 3D dataset acquisition and post-processing, the next major step forward in 3D printing will likely be driven by improvements in printer technology and print materials. "Tissue mimicking" materials currently under development would enable the creation of more life-like models that replicate the patient's unique anatomy and physiology. Currently there are highly accurate noninvasive methods to assess cardiac function and blood flow , including methods to assess 3D information over the cardiac cycle, thereby providing "4D" function and flow. These multivariate datasets could be integrated into 3D models to build holistic models to advance our understanding of cardiac disease. As 3D models achieve more realistic states, they may be used to study pathophysiology, predict long-term outcomes, and choose optimal treatment plans or surgical repairs. Recent studies have analyzed blood flow in deformable models , including flow characteristics in patients with hypoplastic left heart syndrome following Norwood arch reconstruction.Finally, bioprinting offers the potential to make the leap from printing "life-like" to living tissue itself. This revolutionary technology is in its infancy; however, several techniques now exist that can deposit bioinks in precise locations to build up complex tissue constructs . Bioprinting has been applied to print anatomically shaped cartilage structures , skin , implants for bone growth , and even a 3D printed "bionic ear" Within cardiology, researchers have reported techniques to print vasculature, myocardium, and valves . These applications and bioprinting techniques were recently reviewed by Duan . Although current and future applications of 3D printing are exciting and potentially game-changing, broad adoption is currently hampered by the costs of modeling and printing. The cost of a 3D printing center to a medical program is considerable, and at minimum it includes the cost of segmentation software, a medical-grade 3D printer, material costs, and personnel with 3D printing expertise. Some of the costs may be lowered by printing off-site through commercial vendors, although with inherent trade-offs in long-term costs and turn-around time. These are evolving issues, and the ultimate viability of medical 3D printing will in large part depend on the impact it has on improving patient care.

2. 3D Printing Applications For Percutaneous Structural Interventions In Congenital Heart Disease

The past several decades have seen remarkable advancements in percutaneous interventions for treatment of congenital heart disease (CHD). These advancements have been significantly aided by improvements in noninvasive diagnostic imaging. The use of three-dimensional (3D) printed models for planning and simulation of catheter-based procedures has been demonstrated for numerous cardiac defects and has been shown to reduce complications, procedure times, and limit radiation exposure. This paper reviews the process by which patient-specific 3D cardiac models are produced, as well as numerous applications of these models for use in percutaneous interventions in CHD.

Image postprocessing

Prior to creating a 3D model, a volumetric imaging dataset is acquired. CT and MRI are the most commonly used modalities for creating 3D reconstructions, although echocardiography and rotational angiography have also been used. Preference of one modality over another depends largely on the experience of the center, the structure of interest, and age of patient. CT has been shown to be the easiest modality for model creation as it allows for particularly detailed segmentation of great vessels and intracardiac anatomy due to high spatial resolution Alternatively, MRI or contrast-enhanced magnetic resonance angiography offers whole heart 3D datasets while avoiding radiation exposure, which is preferred in younger patients. More recently, there have been several reports on the use of 3D echocardiography in creating 3D reconstructions.

Novel echocardiographic transducers as well as advancements in software and hardware have enhanced echocardiographic images, making them more suited for 3D modeling The use of echocardiography is beneficial as it is more widely available and avoids both radiation exposure and the necessity of radiocontrast administration. This modality, however, has an inferior tissue-to-blood pool contrast, which makes image segmentation significantly more challenging. Echocardiography is also the preferred means by which to visualize cardiac valves and the atrial septum, which are poorly delineated in both CT and MRI. Hybrid imaging techniques have also been developed, which combine cross-sectional datasets with ultrasound in order to create complete heart models with embedded valve leaflets for more comprehensive visualization of intracardiac anatomy.

Following the acquisition of the imaging dataset, a 3D rendering is created through a process known as segmentation[8]. The files are first uploaded as a DICOM (Digital Imaging and Communications in Medicine) dataset into 3D visualization software, such as Mimics (Materialise, Belgium), or open-source software, such as 3D Slicer (Slicer Wiki). Pixel-intensity-based thresholding is then employed to highlight the blood pool within the desired region. Subsequently, regions of interest are isolated through manual or semi-automatic techniques. The process of segmentation is the most time-consuming step of creating a 3D reconstruction. Accuracy of the model is largely determined by blood pool-to-tissue contrast, spatial resolution of the imaging technique, motion artifact of the image, and the technician's understanding of anatomic relationships]. The 3D rendering is then imported as a stereolithography (stl) file into a 3D visualization software, such as 3-Matic (Materialise, Belgium), or open source programs, such as Blender or Owlet, for postprocessing to establish a print-compatible model.This process involves converting the object into a meshed surface file, hollowing the model, smoothing surfaces, and trimming vessels or chamber walls in order to visualize the area of interest[5]. The 3D rendered object is converted into a computer-aided design format that can be converted into a physical object using a 3D printer.

Once complete, the 3D rendering undergoes rapid prototyping on a 3D printer. Capabilities of 3D printers vary based on build volume, layer resolution, materials, and colors available. The print technology utilized should be chosen based on the specific goal of the heart model. In making this decision, the material needed, level of detail, and turnaround time are all taken into consideration. Options for 3D printing include fused deposition modeling (FDM), Colorjet, Polyjet printing, and selective laser sintering. In FDM, a thermoplastic filament is extruded in a specified pattern that immediately hardens. This process typically has a shorter turnaround time and comes at a significantly lower cost. Colorjet printing is an additive manufacturing technology in which a core material is spread in thin layers and solidified by extrusion of a color binder. This technology allows for recreation of highly complex geometries in relatively short production times[. Polyjet printing, in contrast, allows for higher resolution printing of multiple materials in different colors, but it is much more costly and thus less often employed for routine modeling. This technique enables the use of flexible, translucent materials, which are optimal for rehearsing surgical procedures as they can be cut, retracted, and sutured in order to effectively simulate procedures. Additionally, selective laser sintering utilizes a high-power laser to fuse metal or ceramic powder, resulting in a highly accurate model. This method, however, is often cost prohibitive in comparison to other techniques. For each technique, the print material is sequentially layered, and the final model is encased in support material, which can be removed manually or by soaking in a solution.

Clinical applications

The use of 3D printed models has been described widely for numerous percutaneous interventions for the treatment of CHD. One of the most well described interventions in which 3D models play a role is transcatheter valve implantation. These procedures represent the fastest growing area of innovation in the field of pediatric interventional cardiology, with numerous devices developed in the last decade. Transcatheter valve replacements are beneficial because they enable proceduralists to correct valve regurgitation or stenosis without the need for repeat surgical interventions over the course of the patient's life. Among these procedures, pulmonary valve replacement in repaired cases of Tetralogy of Fallot and aortic valve replacement for aortic stenosis or regurgitation are the most widely described. Poterucha et al. described a case of repaired tetralogy of Fallot in which the native right ventricular outflow tract (RVOT) was deemed to be unfavorable for percutaneous intervention. A 3D model of the RVOT was then developed using 3D rotational angiography, which helped the interventionalist identify a landing zone for implantation of a Melody Valve (Medtronic, Fridley, Minnesota). A study by Shievano and colleagues showed that the use of 3D printed models allowed for more accurate selection of candidates for successful percutaneous pulmonary valve implantation (PPVI) than 3D MRI reconstructions alone. Qian et al. demonstrated the use of 3D printed models of the left ventricular outflow tract (LVOT) and aortic root of patients with aortic stenosis. The models approximated the precise anatomy and flexibility of the LVOT, which had substantial tissue calcifications, and were used to test valve implantation prior to the procedure. This permitted the proceduralists to assess the feasibility of the intervention and predict paravalvular leak after transcatheter aortic valve replacement. To test paravalvular leak, the models underwent analysis of strain distribution using a maximum bulge index, which aided in prediction of the degree of leakage following percutaneous valve implantation. This technique ultimately assisted in identifying ideal candidates for percutaneous rather than surgical intervention Along the same lines, Ripley et al. studied the use of 3D models to replicate patient-specific aortic root anatomy prior to transcatheter aortic valve replacement and they found that the models provide insight into how the patient anatomy will interact with implanted medical devices. This enables interventionalists to predict potential challenges in device placement and complications during or following the procedure

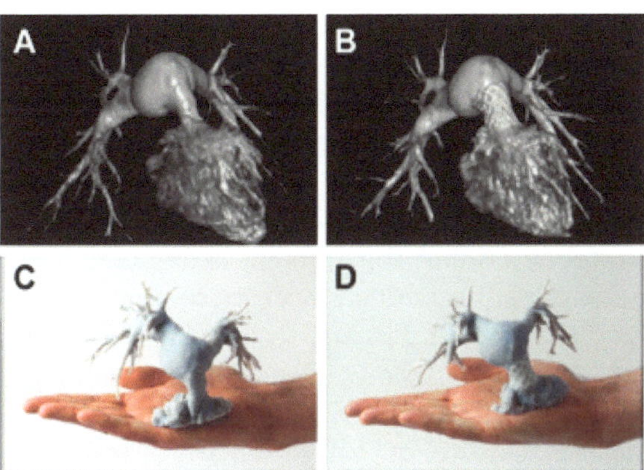

Fig.6.14 3D DynaCT reconstruction and 3D printed models: pre-Melody valve implantation in the RVOT (A, C); and post-Melody valve implantation in the RVOT (B, D). Reprinted with permission from Poterucha et al.. 3D: three-dimensional; RVOT: right ventricular outflow tract

An increasing number of devices have become available for atrioventricular valve repair using a percutaneous approach. Little et al. reported a case in which a 3D printed model was used to aid in procedural planning for a patient undergoing mitral valve repair with Mitraclip (Abbott, Abbott Park, Illinois). This group printed a multi-material 3D model in order to produce more realistic, deformable valve leaflets and recreate subvalvular calcium deposits within the adjacent myocardium. The model was then used to aid in the selection and sizing of the specific clip It enabled more accurate determination of a landing point for the device that avoided adjacent calcified tissue, and provided direct visualization of the effect of the implant on surrounding valve morphology and function Scanlan and colleagues performed a study in which patient-specific pediatric atrioventricular valves were modeled from 3D echocardiography[. The valves were printed and molded using custom software. The molded silicone valves were shown to be significantly more realistic for cutting and suturing, thus enhancing pre-procedural simulation. The technique is presently too time and labor intensive for widespread implementation

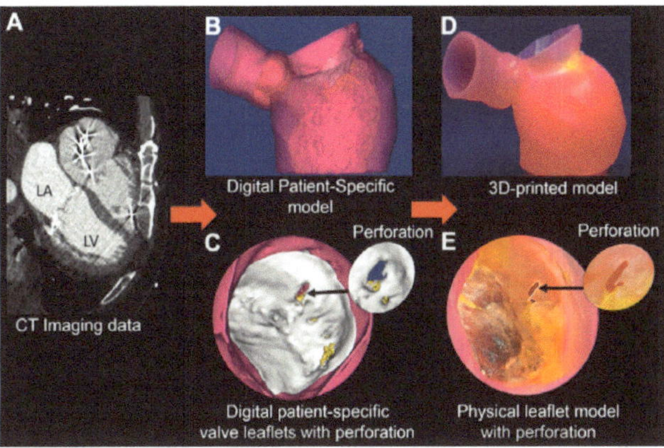

Fig.6.15 CT images (A) are used to create a digital model (B) and to assign tissue properties (C); the multi-material patient-specific 3D model (D, E) is then printed to replicate the mitral valve leaflet geometry, regional calcium deposition, and pathology. Reprinted with permission from Little et al. CT: computed tomography; 3D: three-dimensional

3D printed models are commonly used as guides for percutaneous closure of complicated atrial and ventricular septal defects. Velasco Forte et al. described a case in which a flexible, translucent 3D model was developed from a cardiac MRI in order to simulate the correction of a sinus venosus atrial septal defect (ASD). The model in this case allowed the interventionalists to accurately assess the anatomy and precise spatial relationships among the superior vena cava (SVC), left atrium (LA), and an anomalous pulmonary vein (PV). The model was also used to determine the length of the stent required to close the defect and assess the positioning of the stent necessary to redirect blood flow from the anomalous PV to the LA without obstructing flow from other vessels. Ultimately, a custom stent was successfully implanted into the SVC to close the sinus venosus ASD and commit the anomalous PV drainage correctly to the LA.

Another technically challenging percutaneous intervention that has the potential to be enhanced by patient-specific 3D printed models is endovascular stenting of the aorta in cases of aortic hypoplasia or coarctation. Placement of a stent within the aorta can result in many complications including stent migration, stroke, and occlusion of head and neck vessels by the stent itself. Valverde et al. presented a case in which a 3D model of a hypoplastic transverse aortic arch was created that closely mimicked the distensibility of the native vasculature and its response to stent delivery. In the case described, the endovascular stenting procedure was simulated on the printed model under fluoroscopic guidance prior to the percutaneous intervention. This simulation provided the proceduralists the opportunity to devise an optimal interventional approach, as well as determine the appropriate stent size, length, and position within the aorta3D printed models have recently been described for use in patients undergoing left atrial appendage (LAA) closure. Occlusion of the LAA in patients with atrial fibrillation significantly reduces thromboembolic risk in those who have contraindications to systemic anticoagulation. Given the variable dimensions and morphology of the LAA, accurately sizing and positioning an occluder device in the orifice of the LAA can be challenging. Additionally, implanting a sub-optimally sized device to occlude the orifice can result in complications such as peri-device leakage, thrombus formation, device migration, and cardiac injury. Fan et al. conducted a study assessingthe utility of 3D printed models created from 3D trans-esophageal echocardiography to aid in the selection of an appropriately sized device . They found that device sizing based on 3D-printed models was associated with higher implantation success, shorter procedural times, and fewer complications. Iriart et al. described their technique of printing the entire left atrium and atrial septum in addition to the LAA in order to determine the optimal orientation for transseptal puncture during device placement. They also found that the models are invaluable in training physicians and fellows and augmenting communication with patients.

Percutaneous closure of patent ductus arteriosus (PDA) is another intervention that has the potential to benefit from the use of 3D printed models. Particularly in adult cases, the PDA can be long, tortuous, and calcified, which

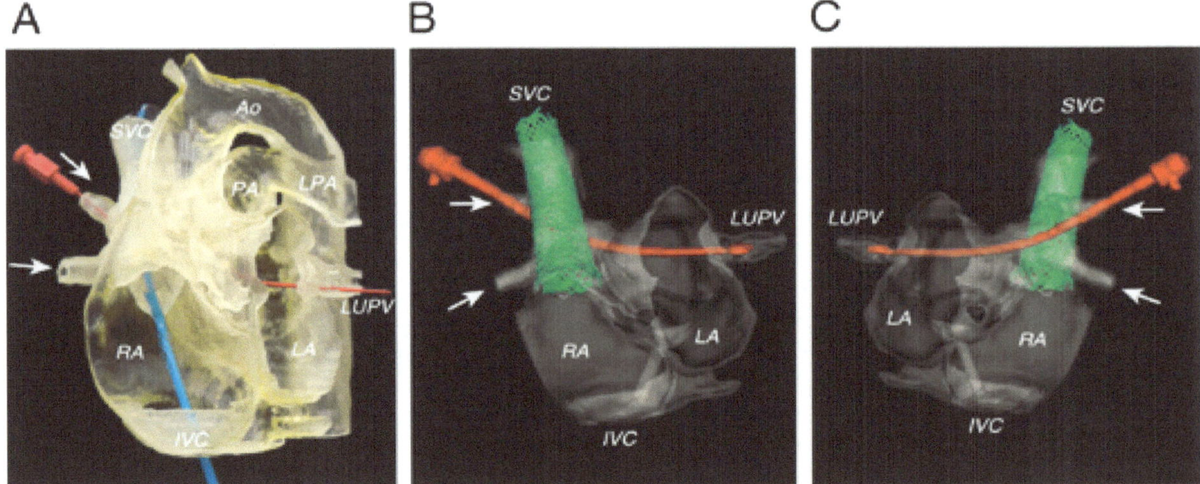

Fig.6.16 The flexible, translucent model (A) was examined to assess the relationship of the anomalous PVs (arrows) to the SVC and LA. A balloon-mounted stent catheter was placed in the SVC to RA junction (blue catheter), while a dilator (red) was passed from the anomalous right upper PV to the left upper PV. This model allowed for calculation of the length of the stent required to close the defect and redirect the flow of the partial anomalous pulmonary venous drainage toward the LA. CT of the model was performed using 3D rotational X-ray acquisition, shown from anteroposterior (B) and postero-anterior views (C) (dilator in red; stent in green). Reprinted with permission from Velasco Forte et al.[18]. PV: pulmonary vein; SVC: superior vena cava; LA: left atrium; RA: right atrium; CT: computed tomography; 3D: three-dimensional

makes catheter-based device placement challenging. Matsubara and colleagues presented a case in which patient-specific 3D printed models were created to detail the precise anatomy of the proximal aorta, aortic arch, PDA, and pulmonary artery.These models allowed for selection of a particular device and exact size. They also allowed the interventionalists to simulate and practice device deployment within the models themselves, thereby decreasing fluoroscopic and procedural times.

3D models can be instrumental in decision making to determine feasibility of transcatheter intervention. A recent case at our center involved a 78-year-old patient with a sinus venosus atrial septal defect with partial anomalous pulmonary venous return of the right upper pulmonary vein (RUPV) to the superior vena cava. A 3D model was created from a cardiac CT to demonstrate the relationship between the anomalous pulmonary venous return, atrial communication, and left atrium for potential use of a covered stent toreroute the RUPV flow. Although the cross-sectional imaging was helpful in delineating the pulmonary venous anatomy, the 3D model provided a much clearer picture of the spatial relationship among the RUPV, superior vena cava, and the left atrium. It was determined that use of a covered stent would result in occlusion of the RUPV in the position needed to ensure stent stability and avoid embolization. The patient will undergo surgical intervention for this congenital heart defect.Finally, We described a case in which a large fistula, arising from the left coronary artery to the right atrium, was modeled in order to devise an approach for interventional closure.The 3D printed model enabled the interventionalists to consider several different approaches to transcatheter closure of the fistula . Practicing the device closure on the 3D model demonstrated the feasibility of using a venous approach to access the fistula and provided insight on the optimal device to use for the procedure, with the goal of ultimately limiting procedure time and thereby reducing radiation exposure

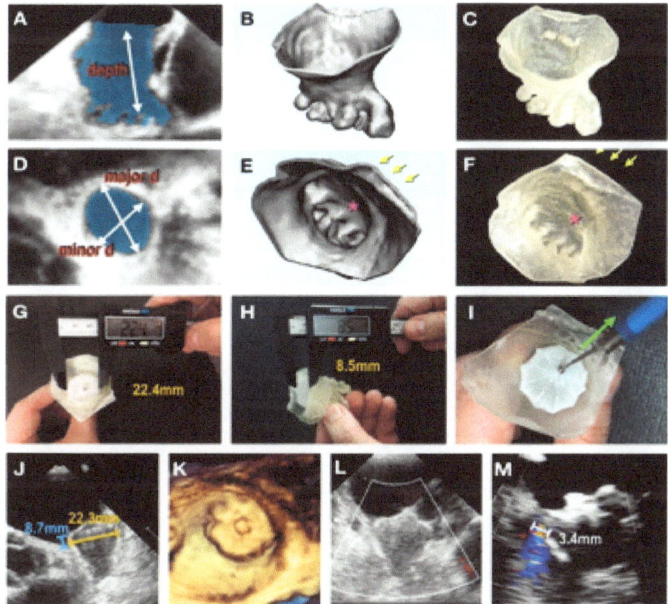

Fig.6.17 Echocardiography-based 3D printing of patient-specific models. Segmentation of LAA (shaded area) from 3D TEE data (A, D) is turned into a digital object (B, E), and printed using tissue-mimicking material (C, F). The major and minor ostial diameters and depth of the LAA are measured. Arrows denote pulmonary vein ridge; stars denote appendicular trabeculations. Closure devices are then sized and placed within the 3D model (G-I), and device compression and (H) protrusion are measured using a digital caliper. Device stability is assessed using the tug-test (I). Device placement visualized on TEE (J-L), and color Doppler assessment showing no peri-device leak (M). Reprinted with permission from Fan et al. LAA: left atrial appendage; TEE: trans-esophageal echocardiogram; CT: computed tomography; 3D: three-dimensional

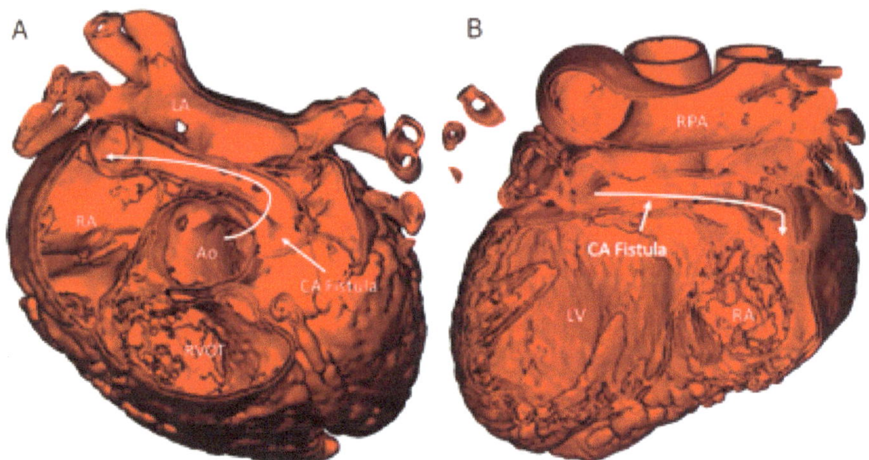

Fig. 6.18 The course of the coronary fistula (CAF) is viewed from a short axis view of the heart. From the leftward aspect of the aortic root, it courses posterior to the aorta (Ao) and rightward to drain into the right atrium (RA) (A); coronal view of the heart, as viewed from the posterior aspect, reveals the course of the CA fistula, almost parallel to the right pulmonary artery (RPA) from left to right to drain into the right atrium (B). CA: coronary artery; LA: left atrium; RVOT: right ventricular outflow tract

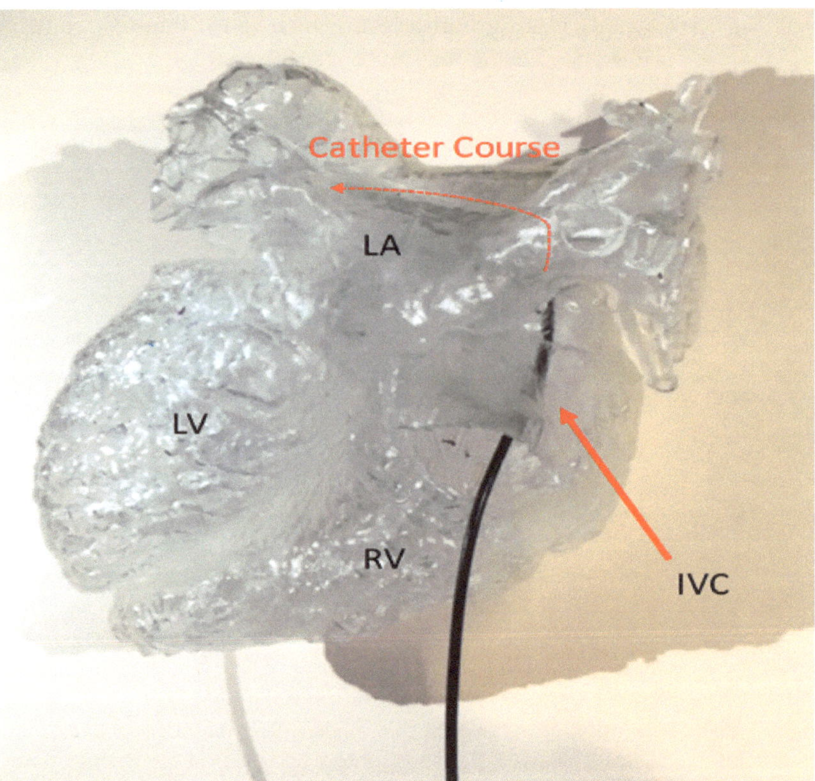

Fig. 6.19 3D printed model of the CA printed in a clear resin (Formlabs, Somerville, MA) allows planning of the transcatheter approach to closure of the fistula as viewed from the posterior aspect. A catheter courses from the inferior vena cava through the fistula (red dotted line). 3D: three-dimensional; CA: coronary artery; LA: left atrium; LV: left ventricular; RV: right ventricular; IVC: inferior vena cava

Limitations

There are numerous limitations to creating and using 3D printed models that have prevented widespread adoption in most programs. A major consideration is that the creation of 3D models is a time-intensive process requiring familiarity with segmentation and computer automated design software, as well as an in-depth understanding of cardiac morphology. There is no standardized approach to creating these models, which can ultimately result in a wide variation in the quality of models produced. This was evidenced by Burkhardt et al. in an article evaluating the inter-operator variability in modeling the RVOT based on the threshold chosen for the initial segmentation. Another limitation is that rigid, or even flexible, 3D printed models only provide a snapshot of the cardiac structure at a specific point in the highly dynamic cardiac cycle, thus limiting our understanding of how these structures will change over the course of one heartbeat. Finally, creation of these models, while helpful in procedural planning, is not reimbursed by most insurance companies, and the prohibitively high cost of the software and 3D printing equipment significantly limits their utility on a routine basis. More studies are required to further assess the cost-effectiveness and diagnostic accuracy of these models prior to widespread implementation in the field of pediatric cardiology.

Future directions

Recently, there has been movement toward developing materials that more closely mimic the feel and behavior of myocardium, valve leaflets, and vessel walls. Novel materials combined with the use of multiple imaging modalities could also aid in enhanced identification of valve tissue, chordae tendineae, and other structures that are less well defined with current methods. Developing models that accurately mimic both healthy and pathologic tissue would be invaluable in implementing these models routinely. This advancement would not only allow for more accurate procedural planning but also be invaluable in training surgeons and interventionalists[2]. Further advances in imaging techniques and software to ease the burden of segmentation would allow for more widespread implementation of this technology to a broader range of conditions. Finally, 3D printing has the potential to aid in the design and construction of patient-specific catheter-based devices for numerous percutaneous interventions, which would further help to decrease procedural complications and improve long-term outcomes.

Conclusion

3D printed models have become increasingly invaluable tools in the field of pediatric cardiology. These models improve diagnostic ability, guide perioperative planning, and have thereby ushered in a vast array of new surgical and interventional approaches and techniques. Interventional cardiology has particularly benefitted from the advancement of 3D modeling, as the models can be used to devise and adjust procedural approaches and practice percutaneous procedures, which has the potential to drastically reduce complications, decrease procedure times, and significantly limit radiation exposure. Ultimately, the use of 3D models has significantly improved our ability to practice personalized medicine and has helped to enhance the care of patients with cardiac defects through percutaneous procedures.

3. 3D Printing in Medicine of Congenital Heart Dseases

Congenital heart diseases causing significant hemodynamic and functional consequences require surgical repair. Understanding of the precise surgical anatomy is often challenging and can be inadequate or wrong. Modern high resolution imaging techniques and 3D printing technology allow 3D printing of the replicas of the patient's heart for precise understanding of the complex anatomy, hands-on simulation of surgical and interventional procedures, and morphology teaching of the medical professionals and patients. CT or MR images obtained with ECG-gating and breath-holding or

Table 6.1 Imaging techniques applicable for 3D Tprinting of heart models

Imaging Modality	Imaging Techniques
Computed tomography (CT)	• ECG-gated breath-held contrast-enhanced angiography • Non-ECG-gated contrast-enhanced angiography
Magnetic resonance (MR)	• Non-contrast 3D SSFP (steady state free precession) imaging • Non-ECG-gated 3D FLASH (fast low angle shot) angiography using gadolinium-based extracellular contrast agent • ECG-gated respiration-navigated 3D IR (inversion recovery) FLASH angiography using gadolinium-based blood pool contrast agent (Gadofoveset: ABLAVAR®, Lantheus Medical Imaging, Inc. MA, USA) • ECG-gated respiration-navigated 4D MUSIC (multiphase steady-state imaging with contrast enhancement) using ultra-small supermagnetic iron oxide (USPIO: Ferumoxyol, AMAG Pharmaceuticals, Lexington, MA, USA)
Ultrasound	• 3D grey-scale echocardiography • 3D color or power Doppler echocardiography
X-ray angiography	• Rotational CT angiography

respiration navigation are best suited for 3D printing. 3D echocardiograms are not ideal but can be used for printing limited areas of interest such as cardiac valves and ventricular septum. Although the print materials still require optimization for representation of cardiovascular tissues and valves, the surgeons find the models suitable for practicing closure of the septal defects, application of the baffles within the ventricles, reconstructing the aortic arch, and arterial switch procedure. Hands-on surgical training (HOST) on models may soon become a mandatory component of congenital heart disease surgery program. 3D printing will expand its utilization with further improvement of the use of echocardiographic data and image fusion algorithm across multiple imaging modalities and development of new printing materials. Bioprinting of implants such as stents, patches and artificial valves and tissue engineering of a part of or whole heart using the patient's own cells will open the door to a new era of personalized medicine

Applicable medical imaging techniques

Any medical images acquired in 3D demonstrating the blood pool distinct from the myocardium and vessel wall can be used for 3D printing . Ideally, electrocardiographic (ECG) gating and breath-holding or respiration navigation is required to avoid artifact from cardiac and respiratory motion. However, the images obtained without ECG-gating and/or free breathing are still applicable for 3D printing if it is not aimed to show small structures such as coronary arteries. The volume data with isotropic resolution is preferred.ECG-gated CT angiograms provide a spatial resolution of 0.3–0.7 mm and are the most commonly used images among currently applicable imaging modalities in 3D printing of cardiovascular structures. In CT angiography, it is important to time the scanning when all cardiac chambers are homogeneously enhanced. It is also important to inject a generous amount of saline chaser to minimize the artifact from undiluted contrast medium remaining in the superior or inferior vena cava and its tributaries. Although MR angiograms may provide <1 mm spatial resolution, high resolution imaging is at the expense of significant compromise in signal-to-noise ratio. If there is no significant stenotic lesion or valvular regurgitation that cause artifact from turbulent flow, non-contrast 3D SSFP (steady state free precession) imaging provides the images of sufficient quality. However, contrast-enhanced angiography is required in most cases with congenital heart disease. In conventional MR angiography using an extracellular contrast agent

ECG-gating is hardly applicable and a degree of artifact from cardiac motion is unavoidable. ECG-gated and respiration-navigated 3D FLASH (fast low angle shot) angiography using blood-pool contrast agent (Gadofoveset: ABLAVAR®, Lantheus Medical Imaging, Inc. MA, USA) provides excellent images with homogeneous distribution of contrast medium and no significant artifact from turbulent flow Most recently, ultrasmall superparamagnetic iron oxide (USPIO: Ferumoxyol, AMAG Pharmaceuticals, Lexington, MA, USA) that is used for treatment of iron deficiency anemia has been tried for angiography in children with excellent results and can certainly be applied for 3D printing.

Ultrasound is not an ideal imaging modality for 3D printing because of the limited access windows for imaging and abundant artifacts from bones and air. However, certain parts of the heart such as atrial and ventricular septa can be imaged appropriately for 3D printing . Although the results are not satisfactory, cardiac valve leaflets can also be imaged and printed with ultrasound data. Lastly, rotational CT angiograms obtained from modern x-ray angiographic equipment can be used for 3D printing

Postprocessing of image data

The postprocessing procedure includes: 1) segmentation, 2) conversion of the DICOM (Digital Imaging and Communication in Medicine) file to the STL (Stereolithography or Standard Tessellation Language) or other file fomat for 3D printing, and 3) computer aided design (CAD)

The blood pool is segmented using thresholding algorithm with manual adjustment (Fig. 2). The better the image quality, the easier the segmentation process. When the boundary between the blood pool and the myocardium or vessel wall is not readily recognizable by automated thresholding, extensive manual work using drawing, erasing and regional thresholding tools and interpolation of the data between the slices are required. The manual work requires in depth understating of normal and pathological anatomy as well as its appearance on cross-sectional imaging. Once segmentation is completed, the 3D volume data is converted to a file format for 3D printing

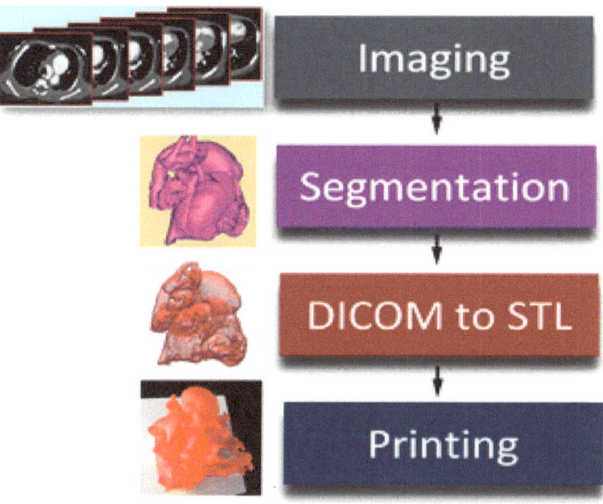

Fig.6.20 Diagram showing the steps in data processing for 3D printing. DICOM, digital imaging and communication in medicine; STL, stereolithography, standard tessellation language or standard triangle language

The file format conversion process includes a user-defined number of iterations for smoothing of the surface of the object. The lower number of iteration provides the models that are close to what are in the original image data, while the surface of the model may appear rough. The higher number of iteration provides a smoother surface of the model, while the detail of the surface anatomy is compromised to a certain extent. The operator needs to define the optimum number of iteration and smoothing factor according to the purposes of 3D printing. As the current imaging technologies do not provide good images of the cardiac valves, it is advisable to demarcate the annuli of the cardiac valves on the model. By marking a few points on the attachment of the valves to the wall using CAD program, an interpolated line of valve insertion is created and assigned a thickness (Figs. 2b and 3). The graphically designed annuli of the cardiac valves are then added to the model.

For the assessment of congenital heart diseases, two types of heart models are valuable: cast models of blood pool and wall models for endocardial surface representation. Cast models provide an excellent overview of the anatomy. Wall models provide detailed information regarding the endocardial surface anatomy. It is ideal to have the entire wall of the heart and vessels represented in the 3D print models

To achieve this goal, both inner and outer boundaries of the cardiac cavities and vessels (endocardial and epicardial surfaces for the heart) should be delineated. Although achievable, it is a time consuming process to delineate the outer boundary of the wall as the signal intensities of the myocardium and vessels are not distinctively different from those of the adjacent mediastinal tissues. Furthermore, a complete wall model requires a large amount of expensive print material, while it is stiff and heavy. As the surgeons operate mostly on the inside of the heart, it is generally sufficient if the endocardial surface anatomy is accurately shown on the models.

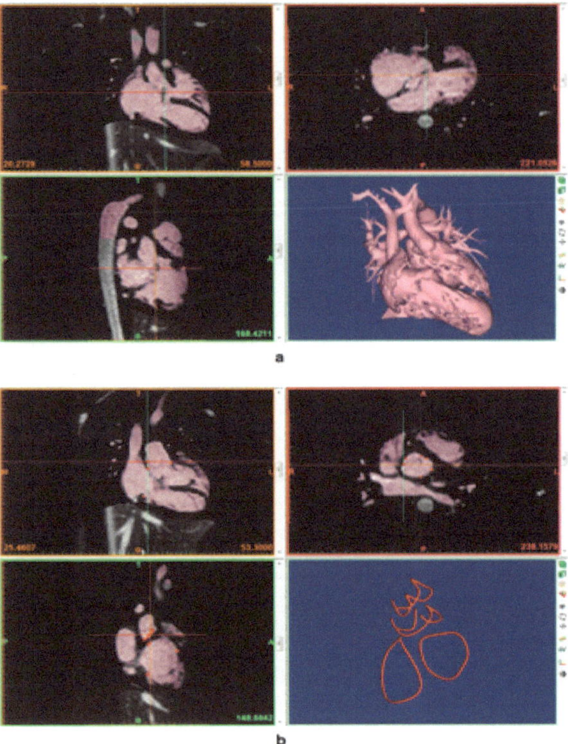

Fig.6.21 Segmentation process in a commercially available software program (Mimics®, Materialise, Leuven, Belgium) using magnetic resonance angiograms from a patient with congenitally corrected transposition of the great arteries with a ventricular septal defect. a Segmentation using thresholding and manual edition with a volume rendered image on the right lower panel. b Linear representation of the cardiac valvar attachments. A few points of attachment sites of each cardiac valve were marked and connected using a tool called "spline"

The endocardial surface anatomy can be represented by graphically adding a shell on the surface of the cavity cast that is clearly and distinctly definable. The result is a negative of the cast model with a wall of an arbitrary thickness . In order to visualize the inner surfaces of the heart and vessels, a few windows are made on the shell. For surgical practice, the entry window for surgical procedure is opened and the model is mounted on the plate to provide a stable position and to restrict movement of the model during the procedure . However, such shelling process is not applicable for representation of the lumens of small and tightly packed vessels such as peripheral pulmonary arteries and veins.

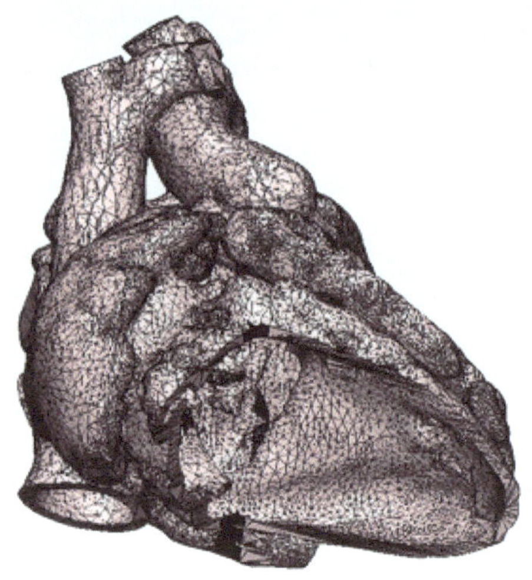

Fig.6.22 Surface geometry in STL (Stereolithography or Standard Tessellation Language) . The surface of the object is divided into a number of triangles without any gap and overlap

3D printing process

The STL files are loaded to the software program of the 3D printer and the materials are assigned to the files for printing. Most commercially available 3D printers are designed for building rigid plastic models, while a few printers are capable of building models with soft rubber-like materials. Ideally, the printing material should have the physical properties such as consistency, elasticity, tensile strength,tear resistance and memory capacity are similar to those of human soft tissue.

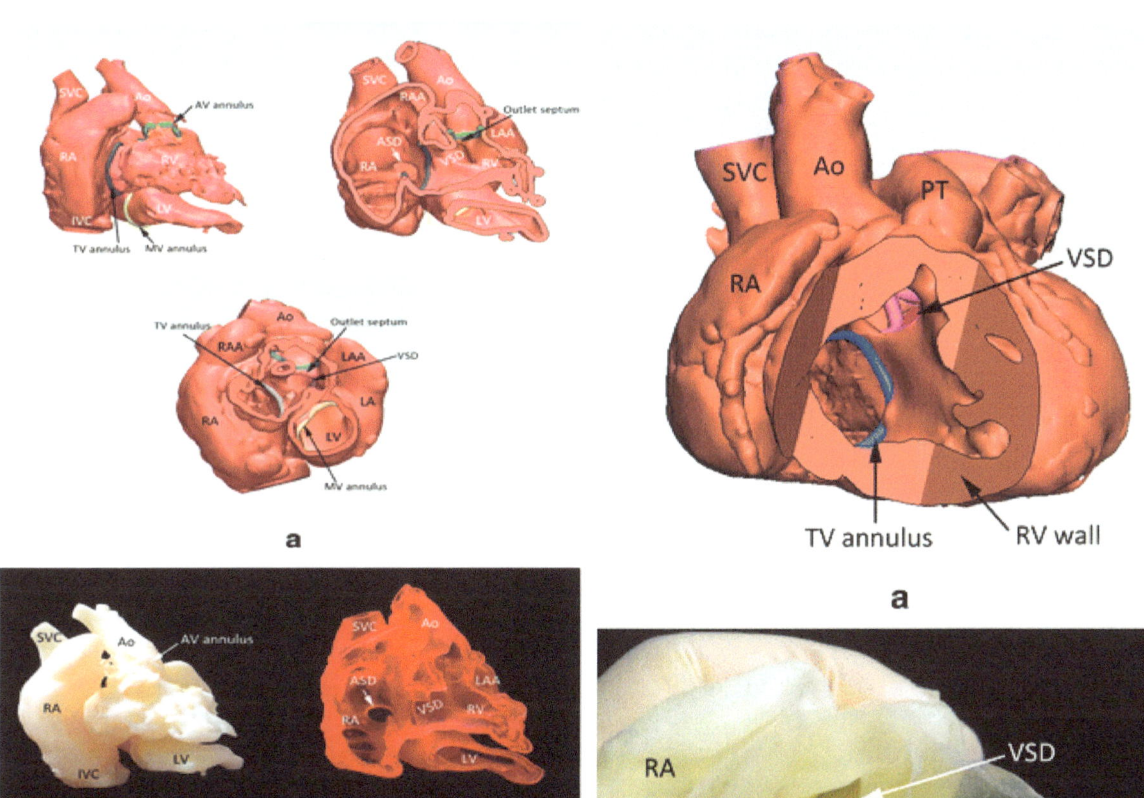

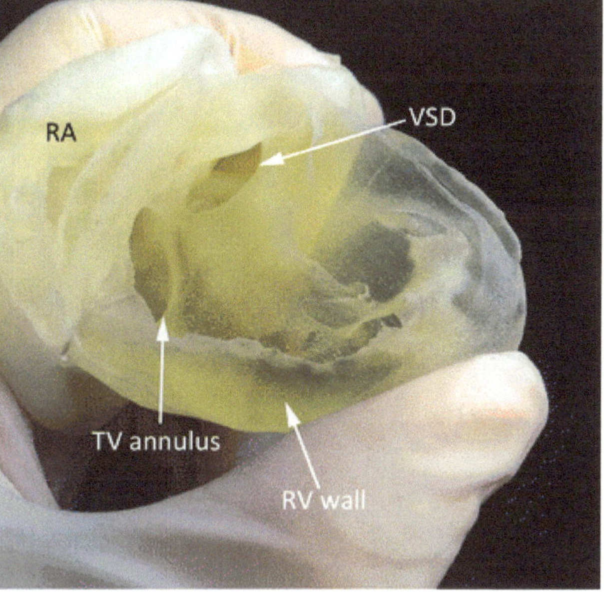

Fig.6.23 Screen-display of the STL files (a) and photographs of the corresponding models (b) in a case with so-called twisted or criss-cross heart with transposition of the great arteries and a ventricular septal defect (VSD). Cast model (top left), wall model after removal of the anterior free wall of the right atrium and right and left ventricles (top right), and wall model with the apical two thirds of the ventricles removed (bottom) are shown. The cardiac valve annuli are marked by the spline curves that were graphically designed as shown in Fig. 2B. Ao, aorta; ASD, atrial septal defect; AV, aortic valve; IVC, inferior vena cava; LA, left atrium; LAA, left atrial appendage; LV, left ventricle; MV, mitral valve; SVC, superior vena cava; TV, tricuspid valve

Fig.6.24 Screen-display (a) and photograph (b) of the 3D print model of the heart with tetralogy of Fallot. The full thickness of the myocardium was carefully segmented with both endocardial and epicardial boundaries delineated by thresholding and manual editing. Although it is considered ideal, the postprocessing was time consuming and the model is stiff to be used for surgical simulation. Ao, aorta; PT, pulmonary trunk; SVC, superior vena cava; TV, tricuspid valve; RA, right atrium; RV, right ventricle; VSD, ventricular septal defect

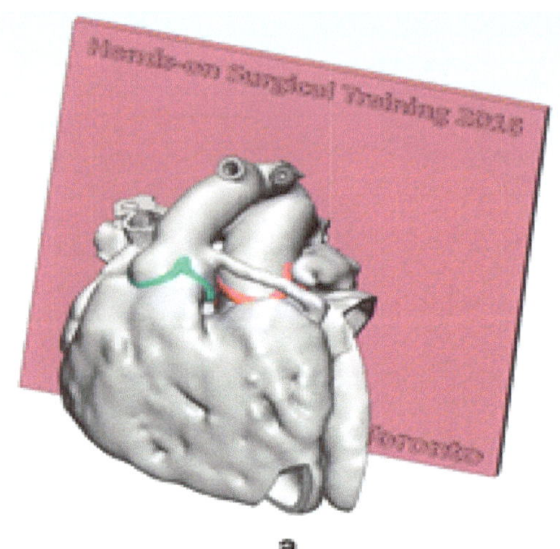

a

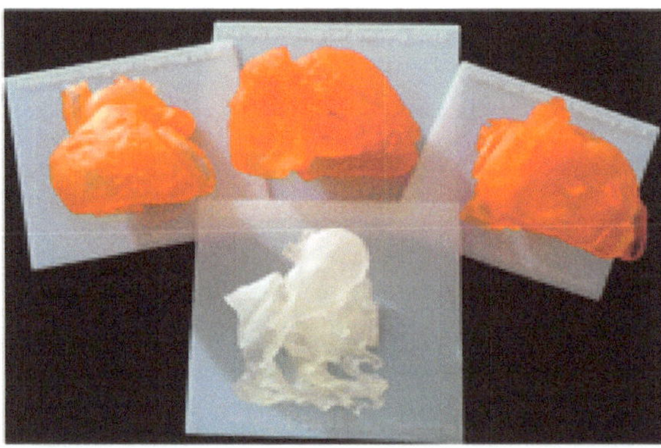

b

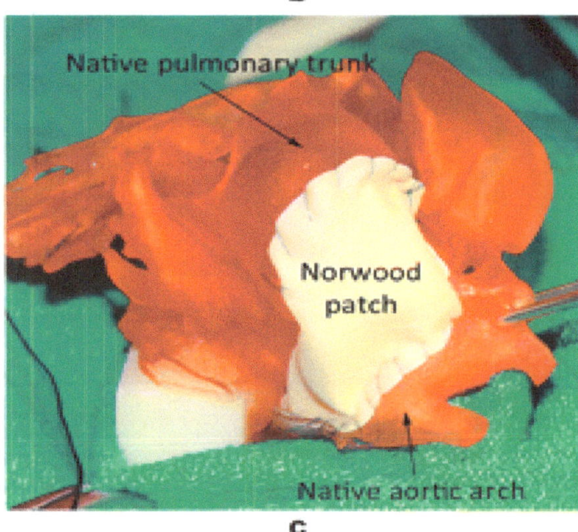

c

Fig.6.25 Models for surgical practice or training. a Screen-display of the STL file shows the heart mounted on a graphically designed platform. b Four example models for surgical training. c A 3D print model with hypoplastic left heart syndrome on which a surgeon underwent a Norwood procedure

Among the existing 3D printers, the printers using polyjet technology and photopolymer resin materials (Objet Connex Series printer and TangoPlus FullCure resin, Stratasys Ltd, Minnesota, USA, and Projet 5500X printer and Visijet CE NT-Elastomeric Natural resin, 3DSystems, Rockhill, USA) provide the physical properties of the printed models closest to those of human soft tissue, allowing simulated surgical and interventional procedures. If the purpose of 3D printing is for demonstration of the anatomy of the heart, any commercially available printer with an acceptable print resolution can be used.

With current 3D printing technology, 3D printing typically takes 3–10 hours to build a single piece of the heart model depending on its size. After the model is completely built, it is harvested and the supporting material and/or the unused print materials are washed out with a waterjet, blown away with an airjet or melted down with chemicals and water. Depending on the materials used and the complexity of the geometry, this cleaning process takes a few minutes to an hour. Powder-based models require curing with chemicals and heat. Although some printers build the models with multiple colors, others provide limited color options. When the printed model is white or faintly colored, one may want to dye the model with a slightly dark color for improved perceptual representation of the complex surface anatomy.

Current applications

Planning and simulation for surgical and interventional procedures.

Preoperative assessment with 3D print models reduces the degree of uncertainty as regards to the patient's specific anatomy. In selected cases, 3D printing can contribute to an improved outcome as precise preoperative understanding of the complex anatomy may obviate or shorten lengthy exploration, and therefore operation and cardiopulmonary bypass time can be reduced . Surgical procedure on a patient with congenital heart disease is usually performed through a midline sternotomy or lateral thoracotomy and a small incision in the wall of an atrium, an arterial trunk or, rarely, a ventricle. As the patient's thorax and heart sizes are small in children the actual surgical scene is difficult to inspect especially from the assistant's position during the surgery. If the sterilized models showing the important surgical anatomy of the patient's heart.were given to the surgical team, the primary operator's procedure would be facilitated with precise and streamlined assistance from the assistants. In addition, 3D print models made of flexible material can be used for practice surgery before the real operation.

For preoperative assessment of congenital heart diseases, we typically make three models for each case: a cast model of blood pool for the overview, a wall model with the atrial and ventricular free wall partly removed for the atrial and ventricular septal anatomy, and a wall model with the apical halves to two thirds of the ventricles removed for the anatomy of the bases of the ventricles . As discussed, a model mounted on a plate can be provided for preoperative surgical practice The most common indication was double outlet right ventricle where the feasibility of intraventricular baffling procedure should be accurately assessed before undergoing biventricular repair . In this regard, 3D print models certainly provide the surgeons with clear and undisputable information. Although it is rare, so-called twisted or criss-cross heart is an important indication for 3D printing . In these cases, the spatial relationship of the cardiac chambers and great arteries and overall intracardiac anatomy are difficult to understand and explain.

With the 3D print models in the observer's hands, complex anatomy can be understood instantaneously and requires no explanation using ambiguous terminology introduced in the description of this particular pathology

For the surgical simulation, the print materials are still far from ideal and the representation of the cardiac valves is limited. The print material does not represent tissue properties of myocardium and enocardial and epicardial linings, limiting assessment of the tissue response to the surgical procedure or deployment of medical devices. In our limited experience, however, the surgeons find the models suitable for practicing surgical simulation procedures such as closure of the septal defects, application of the baffles within the ventricles, reconstructing the aortic arch, and arterial switch procedure (Fig. 6). 3D print models are also used for interventional procedures to test whether the size and shape of the device would fit the patient's specific anatomy and to practice the intended procedure

Contemporary morphology teaching with 3D print models

Traditionally, pathological specimens removed from the patients during autopsy or heart transplantation are used for cardiac morphology teaching. Although the specimens are valuable

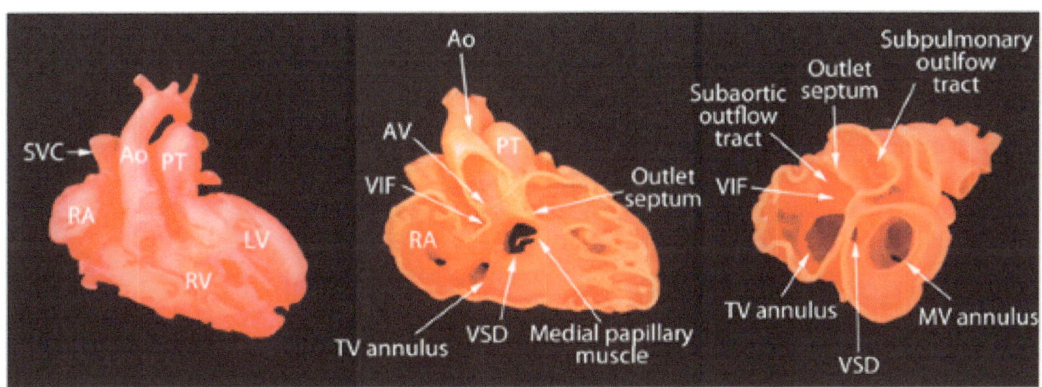

Fig.6.26 Photographs of the 3D print models of a case with double outlet right ventricle. Although echocardiograms showed that the ventricular septal defect (VSD) is remote from both arterial valves, 3D models show that the VSD is able to be routed to the aortic valve allowing biventricular repair. Ao, aorta; AV, aortic valve; LA, left atrium; LV, left ventricle; MV, mitral valve; SVC, superior vena cava; TV, tricuspid valve; VIF, ventriculoinfundibular fold

educational resources, they are scarce and do not represent the whole spectrum of pathology. With improvement of the surgical and medical management of congenital heart diseases and changing concept on human right issues regarding retention of the removed human organs in the pathology laboratory, fewer specimens will be available. On the other hand, the existing specimens are exposed to wear and tear. 3D print models are great educational resources . By using the living patients' imaging data, almost entire varieties of congenital heart diseases can be covered with 3D print models. The pathological features can be demonstrated in any desired planes or views. Any number of models can be reproduced and shared, and access to the models is not limited. With current technology, however, the valve tissues and myocardial pathology are hardly reproducible. Despite such a limitation, contemporary morphology teaching sessions using 3D printed educational model sets have increasingly been introduced in international and national meetings in the last few years.

3D print models are helpful in education of the patients and their parents. The patient's cardiovascular pathology and the intended or previously performed surgical or interventional procedures are easy to understand when they are explained using 3D print models.

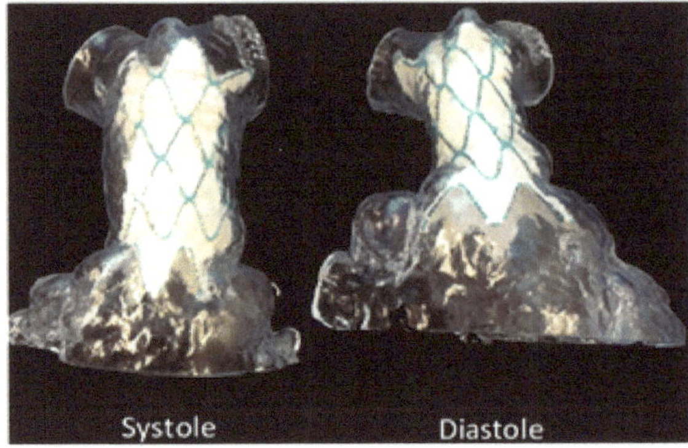

Fig.6.27 Photographs of the 3D print models of right ventricular outflow tract obtained in systole and diastole from a patient with severe pulmonary regurgitation after repair of tetralogy of Fallot. The fitness of the stent in the outflow tract was tested for both systole and diastole before the procedure

Hands-on surgical training (HOST)

Learning surgical techniques in congenital heart disease is challenging. As discussed, the size of the heart in children is usually small and the access routes for the procedure are limited for observation. In addition, the rarity of certain congenital heart diseases further limits the opportunity to learn and to improve the surgical skills. 3D printed models are great resources for surgical training . The supervisors can take unlimited time in showing their procedures. The trainees can take enough time in learning and practicing surgical procedures and repeat the procedures until they feel confident. To the experienced surgeons, 3D print models can be used for development of the new procedures or to improve their surgical skills for rare diseases. In a personal communication, one of our senior surgeons commented that it usually takes a few years for the surgeons to learn how to do the Norwood operation in hypoplastic left heart syndrome and that he should have been able to learn the procedure overnight if 3D print models of a few cases with different pathologic variations would have been available for practice. We organized or supported three HOST courses in the last 12 months. All three courses were successful with high audience satisfaction [Yoo SJ, Spray T, Austine E, van Arsdell GS, et al. Hands-on surgical training (HOST) on congenital heart surgery using 3D print models. In preparation]. We strongly advise the surgeons and trainees to practice their surgical skills on 3D print models first before performing the specific operation on the patients.

Current limitations

The limitations of 3D printing occur in all stages, during imaging, postprocessing and printing. Precise representation of any moving anatomical structures requires high spatial and temporal resolutions. With currently available imaging technologies, it is difficult to image the fine moving structures such as valve leaflets and chordae tendinae with the image quality sufficient enough for 3D printing. These fine structures are important as the abnormalities in these structures are usually associated with significant hemodynamic functional consequences and require delicate surgical repair. As discussed, 3D printing has significant limitations in using the data from ultrasound which is the primary and cheapest imaging technology in cardiac imaging.

Segmentation of the required structures in postprocessing software programs primarily relies on thresholding of signal intensities. When the adjacent structures do not have distinctly different signal intensities allowing automatic boundary detection, extensive time-consuming manual editing is required and the accuracy is significantly compromised.

It is ideal to print the heart using flexible materials with the physical properties similar to that of the human myocardium and valve tissues, especially when practice procedures were to be performed on the models. There are only a few flexible print materials, each of them being able to be used on a specific type of printer only. The surgeons find the models made of flexible material are more difficult to be sewn and easily torn or cut through as compared to real human myocardium or vessels.

The most important limiting factor in applications of 3D printing in patient care and teaching medical professionals is its high cost rather than its utility. The available software programs, printers and printing materials are expensive. Postprocessing is labor-intensive and often requires the hands of experienced imagers. Although 3D printing is also called rapid prototyping, it is fundamentally a time consuming process to build any object by adding numerous layers. The expenses per case can be unbearably high for small programs.

Although most 3D printers are provided with the company's own specification regarding print resolution, reports on its reproducibility and accuracy in human applications are scarce and prospective studies in larger cohorts are required. Nonetheless, it is of no doubt that 3D models are very helpful in understanding the complex morphology and spatial relationship among the structures. However, the models should be carefully reviewed in conjunction with the standard imaging findings as certain degrees of distortion and abbreviation of the information are inevitable during postprocessing and printing.

As have been the cases for any other procedures in their early developing phases when the objective data are lacking or scarce, it will take time for the insurance and its governing organizations to recognize 3D printing as a standard medical procedure and provide reimbursement for the service. In this respect, prospective clinical trials on use of 3D printing in congenital heart disease surgery and surgical training are crucially important to prove the cost-benefit of this newly developing technology.

Future direction

Of little doubt, 3D printing will be widely used in the medicine of congenital heart diseases. Hands-on surgical training will gradually become an essential component in the surgical training programs. For rare and complex surgical procedures, hands-on training on the 3D print models will be the prerequisite requirement for performing the procedure on the patients.

Currently available print materials are not satisfactory for surgical practice. High quality silicone appears closest to the myocardial tissue and best suited for surgery. Currently, silicon models can be made using injection molding technology where silicone is infused into the 3D printed mold . Shiraishi et al used urethane to produce models with rubber-like consistency using molding technique . Although 3D printers using silicon as the printing material are not available, a few commercial companies have recently announced the plans for release of silicone-based printer in the near future

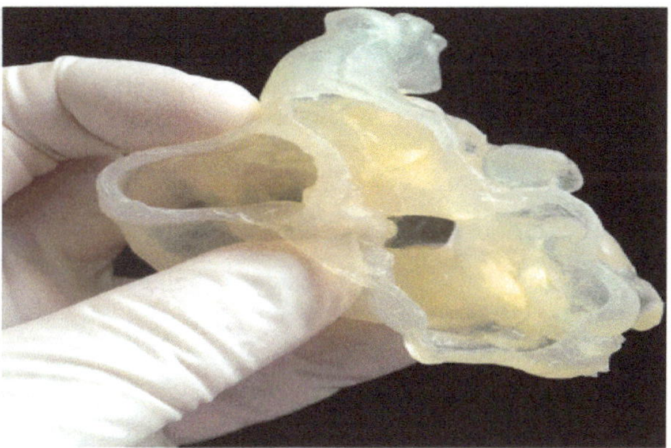

Fig 6.28 Photograph of a model made of silicone using injection molding technique

As discussed, each imaging modality has its own strengths and weaknesses. Both contrast-enhanced CT and MR are excellent in visualization of the blood pool, while ultrasound is far superior to CT and MR in the demonstration of the anatomy and function of the cardiac valves and chordae tendinae. Image fusion is to improve the image content by combining useful information from multiple imaging modalities . The process requires precise image registration process for spatial coordination between the images from different imaging modalities and mathematical algorithm for combining data from different sources. Image fusion technology will certainly enhance the image quality by compensating the weaknesses of each imaging modality and reduce the extent of artifact. 3D printing can be used for personalized implants such as stents, surgical patches and artificial valves . 3D printing has also been experimentally used for tissue engineering such as cardiac valves. Using 3D printing, a scaffold is printed and the cardiac progenitor cells are laid down with matrix for growth . While a clinically viable product has not yet been fabricated, tissue printing eventually will allow fabrication of the implants made of the patient's own stem cells and possibly obviate drug testing on animals by testing on bioprinted human tissues or organs

Conclusions

3D printing has found its niche applications in the medicine of congenital heart diseases. 3D print models allow instantaneous understanding of any complex anatomy and simulation or hands-on training of surgical and interventional procedures. It has made a small revolution in teaching and surgical practice. We expect that Hands-on surgical training (HOST) will soon become a mandatory component of the congenital heart disease surgery programs. 3D printing will expand its utilization with further improvement of imaging and printing technologies and development of new printing materials. Bioprinting and tissue engineering will open the door to the new era of personalized medicine.

Bibliography And Acknowledgement

- Anwar S., Singh G.K., Petrucci O., Eghtesady P., Woodard P.K. and Billadello J.J. : Adult congenital heart disease. In: Rapid Prototyping in Cardiac Disease . Edited by Farooqi K.M. . Cham, Switzerland: Springer International Publishing2017: 99.
  Anwar S., Singh G.K., Varughese J.et al. : "3D printing in complex congenital heart disease: across a spectrum of age, pathology, and imaging techniques". J Am Coll Cardiol Img 2017; 10: 953.
- Armillotta A, Bonhoeffer P, Dubini G, Ferragina S, Migliavacca F, Sala G, et al. Use of rapid prototyping models in the planning of percutaneous pulmonary valved stent implantation. Proc Inst Mech Eng H. 2007;221(4):407–16.
- Armillotta A, Bonhoeffer P, Dubini G, et al. Use of rapid prototyping models in the planning of percutaneous pulmonary valved stent implantation. Proc Inst Mech Eng H 2007;221:407-16.
- Barach P., Johnson J.K., Ahmad A.et al. : "A prospective observational study of human factors, adverse events, and patient outcomes in surgery for pediatric cardiac disease". J Thorac Cardiovasc Surg 2008; 136: 1422.
- Bernhard J.-C., Isotani S., Matsugasumi T.et al. : "Personalized 3D printed model of kidney and tumor anatomy: a useful tool for patient education". World J Urol 2016; 34: 337.
- Bhatla P., Tretter J.T., Ludomirsky A.et al. : "Utility and scope of rapid prototyping in patients with complex muscular ventricular septal defects or double-outlet right ventricle: does it alter management decisions?". Pediatr Cardiol 2017; 38: 103.
- Biglino G, Capelli C, Wray J, Schievano S, Leaver LK, Khambadkone S, et al. 3D-manufactured patient-specific models of congenital heart defects for communication in clinical practice: feasibility and acceptability. BMJ Open. 2015;5(4):e007165.
- Biglino G., Capelli C., Taylor A.M. and Schievano S. : 3D printing cardiovascular anatomy: a single-centre experience. In: New Trends in 3D Printing . Edited by Shishkovsky I.V. . London, United Kingdom: InTechOpen2016: 1.
- Biglino G., Capelli C., Wray J.et al. : "3D-manufactured patient-specific models of congenital heart defects for communication in clinical practice: feasibility and acceptability". BMJ Open 2015; 5. e007165–5.
- Binder T.M., Moertl D., Mundigler G.et al. : "Stereolithographic biomodeling to create tangible hard copies of cardiac structures from echocardiographic data: in vitro and in vivo validation". J Am Coll Cardiol 2000; 35: 230.
- Binder TM, Moertl D, Mundigler G, Rehak G, Franke M, Delle-Karth G, et al. Stereolithographic biomodeling to create tangible hard copies of cardiac structures from echocardiographic data: in vitro and in vivo validation. J Am Coll Cardiol. 2000;35:230–7.
- Boneva R.S., Botto L.D., Moore C.A., Yang Q., Correa A. and Erickson J.D. : "Mortality associated with congenital heart defects in the United States". Circulation 2001; 103: 2376.
- Burkhardt BEU, Brown NK, Carberry JE, et al. Creating three dimensional models of the right ventricular outflow tract: infuence of contrast, sequence, operator, and threshold. Int Journal Cardiovasc Imaging 2019;35:2067-76.
- Borrello J. and Backeris P. : Rapid prototyping technologies. In: Rapid Prototyping in Cardiac Disease . Edited by Farooqi K.M. . Cham, Switzerland: Springer International Publishing2017: 41.
  Botto L.D., Correa A. and Erickson J.D. : "Racial and temporal variations in the prevalence of heart defects". Pediatrics 2001; 107

- Boneva R.S., Botto L.D., Moore C.A., Yang Q., Correa A. and Erickson J.D. : "Mortality associated with congenital heart defects in the United States". Circulation 2001; 103: 2376.
- Borrello J. and Backeris P. : Rapid prototyping technologies. In: Rapid Prototyping in Cardiac Disease . Edited by Farooqi K.M. . Cham, Switzerland: Springer International Publishing2017: 41.
- Botto L.D., Correa A. and Erickson J.D. : "Racial and temporal variations in the prevalence of heart defects". Pediatrics 2001; 107. e32–2.
- Bramlet M, Dori Y, Olivieri LJ. NIH 3D Print Exchange. Bethesda, MD: National Institutes of Health. Available at: https://3dprint.nih.gov/collections/heart-library. Accessed June 28, 2017.
- Bramlet M, Olivieri L, Farooqi K, Ripley B, Coakley M. Impact of three-dimensional printing on the study and treatment of congenital heart disease. Circ Res 2017;120:904-7.
- Brown K.L., Ridout D.A., Goldman A.P., Hoskote A. and Penny D.J. : "Risk factors for long intensive care unit stay after cardiopulmonary bypass in children". Crit Care Med 2003; 31: 28.
- Bucher K. : "New frontiers of medical illustration". JAMA 2016; 316: 2340.
- Byrne N., Velasco Forte M., Tandon A., Valverde I. and Hussain T. : "A systematic review of image segmentation methodology, used in the additive manufacture of patient-specific 3D printed models of the cardiovascular system". JRSM Cardiovascular Disease 2016; 5. 2048004016645467.
- Cantinotti M, Valverde I, Kutty S. Three-dimensional printed models in congenital heart disease. Int J Card Imaging 2017;33:137-44.
- Chaowu Y., Hua L. and Xin S. : "Three-dimensional printing as an aid in transcatheter closure of secundum atrial septal defect with rim deficiency: in vitro trial occlusion based on a personalized heart model". Circulation 2016; 133: e608.
- Chepelev L, Wake N, Ryan J, et al. Radiological Society of North America (RSNA) 3D printing Special Interest Group (SIG): guidelines for medical 3D printing and appropriateness for clinical scenarios. 3D Print Med 2018;4:1-38.
- Cheung DY, Duan B, Butcher JT. Current progress in tissue engineering of heart valves: multiscale problems, multiscale solutions. Expert Opin Biol Ther. 2015;15(8):1155–72.
- Conti A., Pontoriero A., Iatì G.et al. : "3D-printing of arteriovenous malformations for radiosurgical treatment: pushing anatomy understanding to real boundaries". Cureus 2016; 8: e594.
- Costello J.P., Olivieri L.J., Su L.et al. : "Incorporating three-dimensional printing into a simulation-based congenital heart disease and critical care training curriculum for resident physicians". Congenit Heart Dis 2015; 10: 185.
- Costello JP, Olivieri LJ, Krieger A, Thabit O, Marshall MB, Yoo SJ, et al. Utilizing three-dimensional printing technology to assess the feasibility of high fidelity synthetic ventricular septal defect models for simulation in medical education. World J Pediatr Congenit Heart Surg. 2014;5(3):421–6
- Costello JP, Olivieri LJ, Su L, Krieger A, Alfares F, Thabit O, et al. Incorporating three-dimensional printing into a simulation-based congenital heart disease and critical care training curriculum for resident physicians. Congenit Heart Dis. 2015;10(2):185–90.
- Dearani J.A., Connolly H.M., Martinez R., Fontanet H. and Webb G.D. : "Caring for adults with congenital cardiac disease: successes and challenges for 2007 and beyond". Cardiol Young 2007; 17: 87.
- Deferm S., Meyns B., Vlasselaers D. and Budts W. : "3D-printing in congenital cardiology: from flatland to spaceland". J Clin Imaging Sci 2016; 6. 8–5.
- Dolk H, Loane M, Garne E. Congenital heart defects in Europe: prevalence and perinatal mortality, 2000 to 2005. Circulation. 2011;123:841–9.
- Duan B. : "State-of-the-art review of 3D bioprinting for cardiovascular tissue engineering". Ann Biomed Eng 2017; 45: 195.
- Duan B., Hockaday L.A., Kang K.H. and Butcher J.T. : "3D bioprinting of heterogeneous aortic valve conduits with alginate/gelatin hydrogels". J Biomed Mater Res A 2013; 101: 1255.
- Erikssen G., Liestøl K., Seem E.et al. : "Achievements in congenital heart defect surgery: a prospective, 40-year study of 7038 patients". Circulation 2015; 131: 337.
- Fan Y., Kwok K.W., Zhang Y. and Cheung G. : "Three-dimensional printing for planning occlusion procedure for a double-lobed left atrial appendage". Circ Cardiovasc Interv 2016; 9: e003561
- Fan Y, Yang F, Cheung GSH, et al. Device sizing guided by echocardiography-based three-dimensional printing is associated with superior outcome after percutaneous left atrial appendage occlusion. J Am Soc Echocardiogr 2019;32:708-19.
- Farooqi K.M., Nielsen J.C., Uppu S.C.et al. : "Use of 3-dimensional printing to demonstrate complex intracardiac relationships in double-outlet right ventricle for surgical planning". Circ Cardiovasc Imaging 2015; 8. e003043–3.
- Farooqi K.M., Saeed O., Zaidi A.et al. : "3D printing to guide ventricular assist device placement in adults with congenital heart disease and heart failure". J Am Coll Cardiol HF 2016; 4: 301.
- Farooqi K.M., Uppu S.C., Nguyen K.et al. : "Application of virtual three-dimensional models for simultaneous visualization of intracardiac anatomic relationships in double outlet right ventricle". Pediatr Cardiol 2015; 37: 90.
- Farooqi KM, Nielsen JC, Uppu SC, Srivastava S, Parness IA, Sanz J, et al. Use of 3-dimensional printing to demonstrate complex intracardiac relationships in double-outlet right ventricle for surgical planning. Circ Cardiovasc Imaging. 2015;8(5):e003043.
- Farooqi KM, Sengupta PP. Echocardiography and three-dimensional printing: sound ideas to touch a heart. J Am Soc Echocardiogra. 2015;28(4):398–404.
- Farooqi KM, Cooper C, Chelliah A, et al. 3D printing and heart failure: the present and the future. JACC Heart Fail 2019;7:132-42.
- Fleming M., Smith S. and Slaunwhite J. : "Investigating interpersonal competencies of cardiac surgery teams". Can J Surg 2006; 49: 22.
- Garekar S., Bharati A. and Chokhandre M. : "Clinical application and multidisciplinary assessment of three dimensional printing in double outlet right ventricle with remote ventricular septal defect". World J Pediatr Congenit Heart Surg 2016; 7: 344.
- Gaynor J.W., Mahle W.T. and Cohen M.I. : "Risk factors for mortality after the Norwood procedure". Eur J Cardiothorac Surg 2002; 22: 82.

- Gentles T.L., Mayer J.E. and Gauvreau K. : "Fontan operation in five hundred consecutive patients: factors influencing early and late outcome". J Thorac Cardiovasc Surg 1997; 114: 376.
- Giamberti A., Chessa M., Abella R.et al. : "Morbidity and mortality risk factors in adults with congenital heart disease undergoing cardiac reoperations". Ann Thorac Surg 2009; 88: 1284.
- Giannopoulos A.A., Mitsouras D., Yoo S.-J., Liu P.P., Chatzizisis Y.S. and Rybicki F.J. : "Applications of 3D printing in cardiovascular diseases". Nat Rev Cardiol 2016; 13: 701.
- Gilon D, Cape EG, Handschumacher MD, Song JK, Solheim J, VanAuker M, et al. Effect of three-dimensional valve shape on the hemodynamics of aortic stenosis: three-dimensional echocardiographic stereolithography and patient studies. J Am Coll Cardiol. 2002;40(8):1479–86.
- Giroud J.M., Jacobs J.P., Fricker F.J. and Spicer D. : "Web based "global virtual museum of congenital cardiac pathology."". Prog Pediatr Cardiol 2012; 33: 91.
- Giroud JM, Jacobs JP, Spicer D, Backer C, Martin GR, Franklin RC, et al. Report from the international society for nomenclature of paediatric and congenital heart disease: creation of a visual encyclopedia illustrating the terms and definitions of the international pediatric and congenital cardiac code. World J Pediatr Congenit Heart Surg. 2010;1(3):300–13.
- Gosnell J., Pietila T., Samuel B.P., Kurup H.K.N., Haw M.P. and Vettukattil J.J. : "Integration of computed tomography and three-dimensional echocardiography for hybrid three-dimensional printing in congenital heart disease". J Digit Imaging 2016; 29: 665.
- Grant E.K. and Olivieri L.J. : "The role of 3-D heart models in planning and executing interventional procedures". Can J Cardiol 2017; 33: 1074.
- Green A. : "Outcomes of congenital heart disease: a review". Pediatr Nurs 2004; 30: 280.
- Greil GF, Kuettner A, Flohr T, Grasruck M, Sieverding L, Meinzer HP, et al. High-resolution reconstruction of a waxed heart specimen with flat panel volume computed tomography and rapid prototyping. J Comput Assist Tomogr. 2007;31(3):444–8.
- Greil GF, Wolf I, Kuettner A, Fenchel M, Miller S, Martirosian P, et al. Stereolithographic reproduction of complex cardiac morphology based on high spatial resolution imaging. Clin Res Cardiol. 2007;96(3):176–85
- Hadeed K., Dulac Y. and Acar P. : "Three-dimensional printing of a complex CHD to plan surgical repair". Cardiol Young 2016; 26: 1432.
- Han F, Rapacchi S, Khan S, Ayad I, Salusky I, Gabriel S, et al. Four-dimensional, multiphase, steady-state imaging with contrast enhancement (MUSIC) in the heart: a feasibility study in children. Magn Reson Med. 2015;74(4):1042–9
- Hermsen J.L., Burke T.M., Seslar S.P.et al. : "Scan, plan, print, practice, perform: Development and use of a patient-specific 3-dimensional printed model in adult cardiac surgery". J Thorac Cardiovasc Surg 2017; 153: 132.
- Hoffman J. and Kaplan S. : "The incidence of congenital heart disease". J Am Coll Cardiol 2002; 39: 1890
- Holst K.A., Dearani J.A., Burkhart H.M.et al. : "Risk factors and early outcomes of multiple reoperations in adults with congenital heart disease". Ann Thorac Surg 2011; 92: 122.
- Hu A., Wilson T., Ladak H., Haase P. and Fung K. : "Three-dimensional educational computer model of the larynx: voicing a new direction". Arch Otolaryngol Head Neck Surg 2009; 135: 677.
- Iriart X, Ciobotaru V, Martin C, et al. Role of cardiac imaging and three-dimensional printing in percutaneous appendage closure. Arch Cardiovasc Dis 2018;111:411-20.
- Jacobs C.A. and Lin A.Y. : "A new classification of three-dimensional printing technologies: systematic review of three-dimensional printing for patient-specific craniomaxillofacial surgery". Plast Reconstr Surg 2017; 139: 1211
- Jacobs S, Grunert R, Mohr FW, Falk V. 3D-Imaging of cardiac structures using 3D heart models for planning in heart surgery: a preliminary study. Interact Cardiovasc Thorac Surg. 2008;7(1):6–9.
- Jana S. and Lerman A. : "Bioprinting a cardiac valve". Biotechnol Adv 2015; 33: 1503.
- Javan R., Herrin D. and Tangestanipoor A. : "Understanding spatially complex segmental and branch anatomy using 3D printing: liver, lung, prostate, coronary arteries, and circle of Willis". Acad Radiol 2016; 23: 1183.
- Jonas R.A. : "Training fellows in paediatric cardiac surgery". Cardiol Young 2016; 26: 1474.
- Kang SL, Benson L. Recent advances in cardiac catheterization for congenital heart disease. F1000Res 2018;7:1-13.
- Kappetein A.P. and Windecker S. : The heart team in acute cardiac care. In: The ESC Textbook of Intensive and Acute Cardiovascular Care . Edited by Tubaro M. and Vranckx P. . Oxford, United Kingdom: Oxford University Press2015: 87.
- Kapur K.K. and Garg N. : "Echocardiography derived three-dimensional printing of normal and abnormal mitral annuli". Ann Card Anaesth 2014; 17: 283.
- Khairy P., Ionescu-Ittu R., Mackie A.S., Abrahamowicz M., Pilote L. and Marelli A.J. : "Changing mortality in congenital heart disease". J Am Coll Cardiol 2010; 56: 1149.
- Kim MS, Hansgen AR, Carroll JD. Use of rapid prototypingin the care of patients with structural heart disease. Trends Cardiovasc Med. 2008;18(6):210–6.
- Kim MS, Hansgen AR, Wink O, Quaife RA, Carroll JD. Rapid prototyping: a new tool in understanding and treating structural heart disease. Circulation. 2008;117(18):2388–94.
- Kiraly L, Tofeig M, Jha NK, Talo H. Three-dimensional printed prototypes refine the anatomy of post-modified Norwood-1 complex aortic arch obstruction and allow presurgical simulation of the repair. Interact Cardiovasc Thorac Surg. 2016;22(2):238–40.
- Kiraly L., Tofeig M., Jha N.K. and Talo H. : "Three-dimensional printed prototypes refine the anatomy of post-modified Norwood-1 complex aortic arch obstruction and allow presurgical simulation of the repair". Interact Cardiovasc Thorac Surg 2016; 22: 238.
- Kirklin J.W., Blackstone E.H., Tchervenkov C.I. and Castaneda A.R. : "Clinical outcomes after the arterial switch operation for transposition: patient, support, procedural, and institutional risk factors. Congenital Heart Surgeons Society". Circulation 1992; 86: 1501.

- Kolli K.K., Min J.K., Ha S., Soohoo H. and Xiong G. : "Effect of varying hemodynamic and vascular conditions on fractional flow reserve: an in vitro study". J Am Heart Assoc 2016; 5. e003634–14.
- Kossivas F, Angeli S, Kafouris D, Patrickios CS, Tzagarakis V, Constantinides C. MRI-based morphological modeling, synthesis and characterization of cardiac tissue-mimicking materials. Biomed Mater. 2012;7(3):035006
- Kotsis S.V. and Chung K.C. : "Application of the "see one, do one, teach one" concept in surgical training". Plast Reconstr Surg 2013; 131: 1194
- Kung E.O., Les A.S., Figueroa C.A.et al. : "In vitro validation of finite element analysis of blood flow in deformable models". Ann Biomed Eng 2011; 39: 1947.
- Kurup HK, Samuel BP, Vettukattil JJ. Hybrid 3D printing: a game-changer in personalized cardiac medicine? Expert Rev Cardiovasc Ther. 2015;13(12):1281–4.
- Lee J.M., Sing S.L., Tan E. and Yeong W.Y. : "Bioprinting in cardiovascular tissue engineering: a review". Int J Bioprinting 2016; 2: 27.
- Lee W., Debasitis J.C., Lee V.K.et al. : "Multi-layered culture of human skin fibroblasts and keratinocytes through three-dimensional freeform fabrication". Biomaterials 2009; 30: 1587.
- Little S.H., Vukicevic M., Avenatti E., Ramchandani M. and Barker C.M. : "3D printed modeling for patient-specific mitral valve intervention: repair with a clip and a plug". J Am Coll Cardiol Intv 2016; 9: 973.
- Lloyd-Jones D., Adams R., Carnethon M.et al. : "Heart disease and stroke statistics—2009 update: a report from the American Heart Association Statistics Committee and Stroke Statistics Subcommittee". Circulation 2009; 119: e21.
- Ma XJ, Tao L, Chen X, Li W, Peng ZY, Chen Y, et al. Clinical application of three-dimensional reconstruction and rapid prototyping technology of multislice spiral computed tomography angiography for the repair of ventricular septal defect of tetralogy of Fallot. Genet Mol Res. 2015;14(1):1301–9
- Mahle W.T., Spray T.L., Wernovsky G., Gaynor J.W. and Clark B.J. : "Survival after reconstructive surgery for hypoplastic left heart syndrome". Circulation 2000; 102 Suppl 3: III136.
- Mahmood F., Owais K., Taylor C.et al. : "Three-dimensional printing of mitral valve using echocardiographic data". J Am Coll Cardiol Img 2015; 8: 227.
- Mannoor M.S., Jiang Z., James T. and Kong Y.L. : "3D printed bionic ears". Nano Lett 2013; 13: 2634.
- Manyika J, Chui M, Bughin J, Dobbs R, Bisson P. Disruptive Technologies: Advances That Will Transform Life, Business, and the Global Economy. McKinsey Global Institute, 2013.
- Maragiannis D., Jackson M.S., Igo S.R.et al. : "Replicating patient-specific severe aortic valve stenosis with functional 3D modeling". Circ Cardiovasc Imaging 2015; 8: e003626.
- Markert M., Weber S. and Lueth T.C. : "A beating heart model 3D printed from specific patient data". Conf Proc IEEE Eng Med Biol Soc 2007; 2007: 4472.
- Markstedt K., Mantas A., Tournier I., Martínez Ávila H., Hägg D. and Gatenholm P. : "3D bioprinting human chondrocytes with nanocellulose-alginate bioink for cartilage tissue engineering applications". Biomacromolecules 2015; 16: 1489.
- Mashari A., Montealegre-Gallegos M., Knio Z.et al. : "Making three-dimensional echocardiography more tangible: a workflow for three-dimensional printing with echocardiographic data". Echo Res Pract 2017; 3: R57.
- Matsubara D, Kataoka K, Takahashi H, Minami T, Yamagata T. A patient-specific hollow three-dimensional model for simulating percutaneous occlusion of patent ductus arteriosus: Its clinical usefulness. International Heart Journal 2019;60:100-7.
- Matsumoto JS, Morris JM, Foley TA, Williamson EE, Leng S, McGee KP, et al. Three-dimensional physical modeling: applications and experience at mayo clinic. Radiographics. 2015;35(7):1989–2006.
- Meier L.M., Meineri M., Hiansen J.Q. and Horlick E.M. : "Structural and congenital heart disease interventions: the role of three-dimensional printing". Neth Heart J 2017; 25: 65.
- Messina M, Rigsby C, Deng J, Bi X, McNeal G (2013) 3D navigator-gated inversion recovery FLASH (Nav_IR_Flash) with blood pool contrast agent. Magnetom Flash 3/2013.
- Michael S., Sorg H., Peck C.-T.et al. : "Tissue engineered skin substitutes created by laser-assisted bioprinting form skin-like structures in the dorsal skin fold chamber in mice". PLoS One 2013; 8: e57741.
- Mitsouras D, Liacouras P, Imanzadeh A, Giannopoulos AA, Cai T, Kumamaru KK, et al. Medical 3D printing for the radiologist. Radiographics. 2015;35(7):1965–88.
- Mitsouras D. and Liacouras P.C. : 3D Printing Technologies, Vol. 3 . Cham, Switzerland: Springer International Publishing2017.
- Moons P., Bovijn L., Budts W., Belmans A. and Gewillig M. : "Temporal trends in survival to adulthood among patients born with congenital heart disease from 1970 to 1992 in Belgium". Circulation 2010; 122: 2264.
- Moore T., Madriago E.J., Renteria E.S.et al. : "Co-registration of 3D echo and MR data to create physical models of congenital heart malformations". J Cardiovasc Magn Resonan 2015; 17: P198.
- Moore RA, Riggs KW, Kourtidou S, et al. Three-dimensional printing and virtual surgery for congenital heart procedural planning. Birth Defects Res 2018;110:1082-90.
- Morrison R.J., Hollister S.J., Niedner M.F.et al. : "Mitigation of tracheobronchomalacia with 3D-printed personalized medical devices in pediatric patients". Sci Transl Med 2015; 7. 285ra64–4.
- Mosadegh B, Xiong G, Dunham S, et al. Current progress in 3D printing for cardiovascular tissue engineering. Biomed Mater. 2015;10(3):034002
- Mottl-Link S, Boettger T, Krueger JJ, Rietdorf U, Schnackenburg B, Ewert P, et al. Images in cardiovascular medicine. Cast of complex congenital heartmalformation in a living patient. Circulation. 2005;112:e356–7.
- Mottl-Link S, Hübler M, Kühne T, Rietdorf U, Krueger JJ, Schnackenburg B, et al. Physical models aiding in complex congenital heart surgery. Ann Thorac Surg. 2008;86(1):273–7.

- Muraru D., Veronesi F., Maddalozzo A.et al. : "3D printing of normal and pathologic tricuspid valves from transthoracic 3D echocardiography data sets". Eur Heart J Cardiovasc Imaging 2017; 18: 802.
- Ngan E.M., Rebeyka I.M., Ross D.B.et al. : "The rapid prototyping of anatomic models in pulmonary atresia". J Thorac Cardiovasc Surg 2006; 132: 264.
- Ngan EM, Rebeyka IM, Ross DB, Hirji M, Wolfaardt JF, Seelaus R, et al. The rapid prototyping of anatomic models in pulmonary atresia. J Thorac Cardiovasc Surg. 2006;132:264–9.
- Noecker A.M., Chen J.-F., Zhou Q.et al. : "Development of patient-specific three-dimensional pediatric cardiac models". ASAIO J 2006; 52: 349.
- Noecker AM, Chen JF, Zhou Q, White RD, Kopcak MW, Arruda MJ, et al. Development of patient-specific three-dimensional pediatric cardiac models. ASAIO J. 2006;52(3):349–53.
- O'Brien S.M., Clarke D.R., Jacobs J.P. and Jacobs M.L. : "An empirically based tool for analyzing mortality associated with congenital heart surgery". J Thorac Cardiovasc Surg 2009; 138: 1139.
- O'Neill B., Wang D.D., Pantelic M.et al. : "Transcatheter caval valve implantation using multimodality imaging". J Am Coll Cardiol Img 2015; 8: 221.
- Olivieri L., Krieger A., Chen M.Y., Kim P. and Kanter J.P. : "3D heart model guides complex stent angioplasty of pulmonary venous baffle obstruction in a Mustard repair of D-TGA". Int J Cardiol 2014; 172: e297.
- Olivieri L.J., Krieger A., Loke Y.-H., Nath D.S., Kim P.C.W. and Sable C.A. : "Three-dimensional printing of intracardiac defects from three-dimensional echocardiographic images: feasibility and relative accuracy". J Am Soc Echocardiogr 2015; 28: 392.
- Olivieri LJ, Krieger A, Loke YH, Nath DS, Kim PC, Sable CA. Three-dimensional printing of intracardiac defects from three-dimensional echocardiographic images: feasibility and relative accuracy. J Am Soc Echocardiogr. 2015;28(4):392–7.
- Olivieri LJ, Krieger A, Loke YH, et al. Three-dimensional printing of intracardiac defects from three-dimensional echocardiographic images: feasibility and relative accuracy. J Am Soc Echocardiogr 2015;28:392-7.
- Pentecost J.O., Sahn D.J., Thornburg B.L., Gharib M., Baptista A. and Thornburg K.L. : "Graphical and stereolithographic models of the developing human heart lumen". Comput Med Imaging Graph 2001; 25: 459.
- Poterucha J.T., Foley T.A. and Taggart N.W. : "Percutaneous pulmonary valve implantation in a native outflow tract". J Am Coll Cardiol Intv 2014; 7: e151.
- Poterucha JT, Foley TA, Taggart NW. Percutaneous pulmonary valve implantation in a native outflow tract: 3-dimensional DynaCT rotational angiographic reconstruction and 3-dimensional printed model. JACC Cardiovasc Interv. 2014;7(10):e151–2.
- Qian Z, Wang K, Liu S, et al. Quantitative prediction of paravalvular leak in transcatheter aortic valve replacement based on tissue-mimicking 3D Printing. JACC Cardiovasc Imaging 2017;10:719-31.
- Rapid Prototyping in Cardiac Disease . Edited by Farooqi K.M. . Cham, Switzerland: Springer International Publishing2017.
- Rehder R., Abd-El-Barr M., Hooten K., Weinstock P., Madsen J.R. and Cohen A.R. : "The role of simulation in neurosurgery". Childs Nerv Syst 2016; 32: 43..
- Ripley B., Kelil T., Cheezum M.K.et al. : "3D printing based on cardiac CT assists anatomic visualization prior to transcatheter aortic valve replacement". J Cardiovasc Comput Tomogr 2016; 10: 28.
- Ripley B, Kelil T, Cheezum MK, et al. 3D printing based on cardiac CT assists anatomic visualization prior to transcatheter aortic valve replacement. J Cardiovasc Comput Tomogr 2016;10:28-36.
- Ryan J.R., Moe T.G., Richardson R., Frakes D.H., Nigro J.J. and Pophal S. : "A novel approach to neonatal management of tetralogy of Fallot, with pulmonary atresia, and multiple aortopulmonary collaterals". J Am Coll Cardiol Img 2015; 8: 103.
- Saeed O., Farooqi K.M. and Jorde U.P. : Assessment of ventricular assist device placement and function. In: Rapid Prototyping in Cardiac Disease . Edited by Farooqi K.M. . Cham, Switzerland: Springer International Publishing2017: 133
- Samuel B.P., Pinto C., Pietila T. and Vettukattil J.J. : "Ultrasound-derived three-dimensional printing in congenital heart disease". J Digit Imaging 2014; 28: 459.
- Samuel BP, Pinto C, Pietila T, Vettukattil JJ. Ultrasound-derived three-dimensional printing in congenital heart disease. J Digit Imaging. 2015;28(4):459–61.
- Schievano S, Migliavacca F, Coats L, Khambadkone S, Carminati M, Wilson N, et al. Percutaneous pulmonary valve implantation based on rapid prototyping of right ventricular outflow tract and pulmonary trunk from MR data. Radiology. 2007;242:490–7.
- Schievano S., Migliavacca F., Coats L.et al. : "Percutaneous pulmonary valve implantation based on rapid prototyping of right ventricular outflow tract and pulmonary trunk from MR data". Radiology 2007; 242: 490
- Tack P., Victor J., Gemmel P. and Annemans L. : "3D-printing techniques in a medical setting: a systematic literature review". Biomed Eng Online 2016; 15: 115.
- U, Wolf I, Schnackenburg B, Ewert P, Huebler M, et al. The practical clinical value of three-dimensional models of complex congenitally malformed hearts. J Thorac Cardiovasc Surg. 2009;138(3):571–80
- Valverde I, Gomez G, Coserria JF, Suarez-Mejias C, Uribe S, Sotelo J, et al. 3D printed models for planning endovascular stenting in transverse aortic arch hypoplasia. Catheter Cardiovasc Interv. 2015;85(6):1006–12
- Warnes C.A., Bhatt A.B., Daniels C.J., Gillam L.D. and Stout K.K. : "COCATS 4 Task Force 14: training in the care of adult patients with congenital heart disease". J Am Coll Cardiol 2015; 65: 1887.
- Yoo S.-J., Thabit O., Kim E.K.et al. : "3D printing in medicine of congenital heart diseases". 3D Printing Med 2016; 2: 1
- Zopf D.A., Hollister S.J., Nelson M.E., Ohye R.G. and Green G.E. : "Bioresorbable airway splint created with a three-dimensional printer". N Engl J Med 2013; 368: 2043.

AI In Cardiovascular Imaging for Risk Stratification In CAD

CHAPTER 7

Artificial intelligence (AI) describes the use of computational techniques to perform tasks that normally require human cognition. Machine learning and deep learning are subfields of AI that are increasingly being applied to cardiovascular imaging for risk stratification. Deep learning algorithms can accurately quantify prognostic biomarkers from image data. Additionally, conventional or AI-based imaging parameters can be combined with clinical data using machine learning models for individualized risk prediction. The aim of this review is to provide a comprehensive review of state-of-the-art AI applications across various noninvasive imaging modalities (coronary artery calcium scoring CT, coronary CT angiography, and nuclear myocardial perfusion imaging) for the quantification of cardiovascular risk in coronary artery disease

- Artificial intelligence (AI) is increasingly being applied to noninvasive cardiovascular imaging modalities for risk stratification in coronary artery disease.
- Deep learning algorithms can perform automated measurements of prognostic biomarkers directly from image data.
- Conventional or AI-based imaging parameters can be integrated with clinical data using machine learning models for per-patient risk prediction.
- The objective ranking of variables in individualized machine learning prediction models increases the explainability of AI findings.

Various Techniques used for Risk Stratification In CAD

AI is a field of computer science that aims to mimic human cognition in performing tasks such as object or pattern recognition, planning, and problem-solving. The term big data refers to large and heterogeneous data sets that require computational techniques such as AI for their analysis and interpretation In health care, this includes data from the omics fields (eg, genomics, metabolomics, proteomics, lipidomics), tabular data from electronic health records, and imaging data. Within big data exist individual measurable characteristics or datapoints known as features. In imaging, this could be represented by voxel intensity, the spatial distribution of voxels, a vector of motion, or conventional metrics used in clinical practice. The quality, accuracy, and richness of features in data are key determinants of AI model performance.

Machine learning (ML), a subfield of AI, enables computer algorithms to automatically learn and improve from experience through exposure to vast amounts of data While many different algorithmic approaches—or models—exist within ML, they all aim to achieve one of two tasks. The first is supervised learning, in which a labeled data set is used to predict a known outcome. This involves the iterative selection and weighting of individual features to learn the underlying patterns within the data that best fit the outcome.Examples of supervised learning algorithms include linear regression, support vector machines, and random forest. The second task is unsupervised learning, whereby unlabeled data are used to predict unknown associations. These models attempt to capture relationships inherent to the structure of the features themselves; examples include clustering and principal component analysis Deep learning (DL) is a specific form of ML that uses multilayered artificial neural networks to make predictions directly from input data. The most commonly used DL networks for image analysis are convolutional neural networks (CNNs). These contain many layers stacked on top of each other,

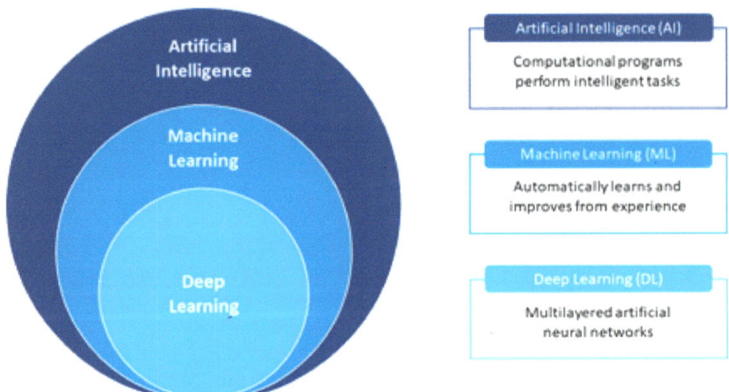

Fig.7.1 Basics of artificial intelligence (AI), machine learning (ML), and deep learning. Artificial intelligence describes the use of computational techniques to perform tasks characteristic of human intelligence. ML is a subfield of AI that enables computers to automatically learn by being exposed to large amounts of data. Deep learning is a specific form of ML that uses multilayered artificial neural networks to make predictions directly from input data.

including one or more convolutional layers that create a feature map summarizing the presence of detected features in the input (6). In health care, some of the greatest successes of DL have been in the field of computer vision, which handles tasks such as object classification, detection, and segmentation from digital images or videos (6). Raw image data are typically transformed to features prior to input into the CNNs. Another emerging application of DL has been for processing of tabular data contained in electronic health records for per-patient predictions. This includes structured data such as laboratory results, diagnostic codes, and demographics, as well as unstructured data that requires standardization and sequencing.

Radiomics is the process of extracting thousands of computational quantitative features (most of which are invisible to the human eye) from medical images. These features capture the complex spatial relationship between voxels by describing textural patterns or geometric properties within a given imaging region of interest. ML techniques can then be applied to these data sets to identify imaging biomarkers of significant clinical value.In cardiovascular imaging, AI algorithms can be used to both identify new imaging biomarkers and integrate data from many different sources to provide patient-tailored risk prediction.

1.Noncontrast Cardiac CT

Coronary Artery Calcium Scoring

Coronary artery calcium (CAC), a specific marker of coronary atherosclerosis, is a powerful predictor of angiographically significant obstructive CAD (26) and incident cardiovascular events . Incremental prognostic value over standard clinical risk scores has also been consistently reported . In current clinical practice, CAC scoring from noncontrast electrocardiographically gated cardiac CT requires manual interaction by a human operator. Using commercially available software, the reader identifies and labels all voxels above a threshold of 130 HU to quantify the Agatston score (30) or volume score . This approach can be labor-intensive and time-consuming; thus, a more automated workflow that reduces the need for human interaction is highly desirable.

ML approaches for the rapid and automated quantification of CAC from dedicated noncontrast cardiac CT have shown promising results. Wolterink et al trained a random forest classifier comprising numerous individual decision trees to distinguish between true calcifications and other candidate calcifications based on size, shape, position, and intensity features. The resultant per-patient Agatston and volume scores demonstrated a strong correlation (r = 0.94) with expert manual measurements

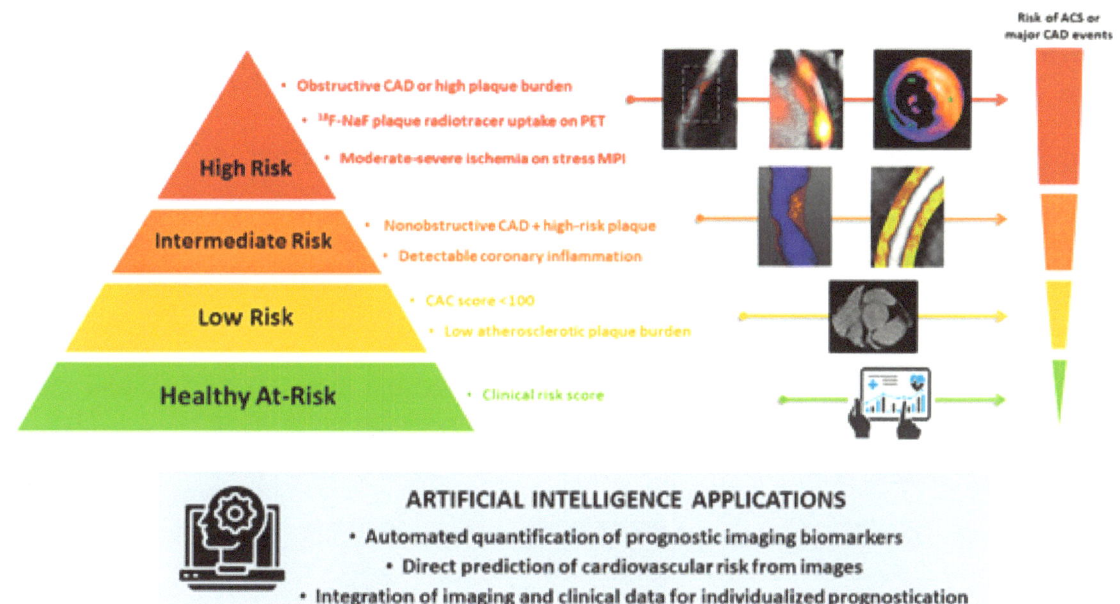

Fig.7.2 Artificial intelligence (AI) in cardiovascular imaging for risk stratification. Clinical risk stratification based on anatomic and functional imaging assessment of coronary artery disease (CAD). The image case examples (from left to right) correspond to the descriptions (from top to bottom) adjacent to the risk pyramid. AI algorithms can perform automated measurements of prognostic biomarkers from image data. Additionally, conventional or AI-based imaging parameters can be combined with clinical data using machine learning models for individualized risk prediction. ACS = acute coronary syndrome, CAC = coronary artery calcium, 18F-NaF = fluorine 18 sodium fluoride, MPI = myocardial perfusion imaging. Overview of AI Applications for Risk Stratification in Cardiovascular Imaging Studies

In an extension of this work, the authors introduced a multiclass classification of candidate coronary calcifications to detect CAC per artery, along with an ambiguity detection system that flagged difficult cases for expert review (8). Intraclass correlation coefficients between automatic and fully manual CAC volume scores improved with expert review of difficult cases that had been flagged by the algorithm: left anterior descending artery (0.98 vs 1.00), left circumflex artery (0.69 vs 0.95), and right coronary artery (0.95 vs 0.99). No ambiguous candidates were identified in close to half of all CT scans. Automatic scoring combined with expert review led to a faster processing time of 45 seconds, compared with 128 seconds per scan for fully manual scoring.CAC scores can also be derived from chest CT performed for other indications, such as lung cancer screening, thus paving the way for application of AI algorithms in large sets of screening data. Fully automated ML- and DL-based quantification of CAC has been evaluated in large data sets of low-dose, ungated CT scans from national lung cancer screening trials in Europe and the United States, demonstrating feasibility and high reliability compared with manual measurements. Similar results were observed for a CAC scoring DL algorithm trained using radiation therapy–planning CT scans of patients with breast cancer acquired during free breathing Recently, van Velzen et al (9) sought to validate a DL method for automated CAC scoring using multiple cardiac and chest CT protocols. In 7240 patients who underwent various types of noncontrast chest CT scans, the investigators used two consecutive CNNs to quantify the Agatston score. The first CNN detected candidate calcifications on each image and assigned them to a coronary artery, and the second CNN classified these calcifications as true positive or false positive (Fig 3, A). The DL algorithm was trained and tested on three separate data sets stratified by scan type

Compared with manual CAC scoring, the DL algorithm produced reliable measurements, with intraclass correlation coefficients of 0.79–0.97 across the range of scan types. In cardiovascular risk categorization according to the Agatston score, DL had excellent agreement with manual CAC scoring (κ = 0.90 for all test scans). These findings lend support to the use of such a DL method to aid clinicians in CAC scoring across a wide range of noncontrast chest CT images.While AI enables direct computation of CAC measures from CT images, the Agatston score quantified by conventional methods can either suspected of having CAD or with established CAD. An ML model incorporating clinical variables (age, sex, risk factors, and cholesterol levels) yielded an area under the receiver operating characteristic curve (AUC) of 0.77 for predicting the presence of obstructive CAD at CCTA. The addition of CAC score to the ML model resulted in a significantly higher AUC (0.88), which also outperformed a statistical model containing the CAC score and CAD consortiumclinical score (AUC, 0.86) and the CAD consortium clinical score alone (AUC, 0.73; $P < .05$ for all comparisons). Hence, integration of the CAC

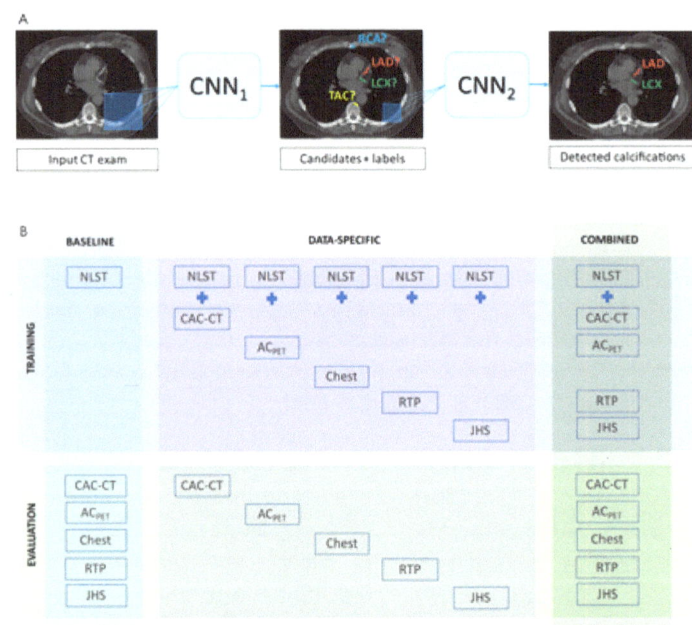

Fig.7.3 Automatic coronary artery calcium scoring. A, The deep learning algorithm consists of two convolutional neural networks (CNNs). The first CNN (CNN1) detects candidate calcifications (voxels) with attenuation of greater than 130 HU and assigns them to a coronary artery, and the second CNN (CNN2) detects true calcified voxels among candidates detected by the first CNN. B, The baseline algorithm was trained with National Lung Screening Trial (NLST) scans, and its performance was evaluated in each CT protocol type. Five data-specific algorithms were trained, according to CT protocol type, and evaluated in the respective CT type. The combined algorithm was trained and evaluated using all available CT protocol types. CT types used for training were NLST CT scans, coronary artery calcium scoring CT (CAC-CT), PET attenuation correction CT (ACPET), diagnostic chest (Chest) CT, radiation therapy treatment planning (RTP) CT, and Jackson Heart Study (JHS) CT scans. exam = examination, LAD = left anterior descending artery, LCX = left circumflex artery, RCA = right coronary artery, TAC = thoracic aorta calcification. (Reprinted, with permission)

also be used as an input into AI models for risk prediction.Al'Aref et al trained an ML algorithm with extreme gradient boosting (XGBoost; https://xgboost.ai/) using clinical data from 35 281 patients score and clinical data with ML could potentially be adopted in clinical practice to enhance risk stratification and inform referral for downstream testing such as CCTA

In 66 636 asymptomatic individuals from the CAC Consortium, Nakanishi et al developed a LogitBoost-based ML model incorporating 20 CAC measures (total and per-vessel Agatston, volume, and density scores), non-CAC metrics (including thoracic and aortic calcium scores), and 46 clinical variables for the prediction of CAD-related death at 10-year follow-up. The ML model (AUC, 0.86) provided superior risk prediction compared with either the atherosclerotic cardiovascular disease (ASCVD) risk score (AUC, 0.83) or the CAC score (AUC, 0.82; P < .001 for both). This comprehensive ML approach also outperformed ML with clinical data alone or CT data alone. Hence, an ML model that can use all available information has the potential to become a routine risk assessment tool, especially as electronic health records are widely adopted in clinical practice and their platforms enable increasingly seamless integration of clinical and imaging data.

2.Epicardial Adipose Tissue Quantification

Epicardial adipose tissue is a metabolically active fat depot located between the myocardium and visceral pericardium that modulates coronary arterial function.Epicardial adipose tissue volume, which traditionally has been quantified from routine CAC scoring CT using manual or semiautomated techniques , has been shown to associate with coronary atherosclerosis and incident cardiac events.Recently, Commandeur et al developed a fully automated DL-based method for epicardial adipose tissue quantification., which was tested in a large multicenter study and showed a strong correlation with expert manual measurements (r = 0.97; P < .001). DL computation was rapid, with a time of approximately 6 seconds per case, compared with a time of 15 minutes per case for experts. Epicardial adipose tissue measures derived using this DL algorithm were subsequently used for prognostication in 2068 asymptomatic participants from the Early Identification of Subclinical Atherosclerosis by Noninvasive Imaging Research (EISNER) trial . In that study, DL-based epicardial adipose tissue volume was independently associated with increased risk of major adverse cardiovascular events (MACEs) (hazard ratio, 1.35 [95% CI: 1.07, 1.68] per case for experts. Epicardial adipose tissue measures derived using this DL algorithm were subsequently used for prognostication. in 2068 asymptomatic participants from the Early Identification of Subclinical Atherosclerosis by Noninvasive Imaging Research (EISNER) trial . In that study, DL-based epicardial adipose tissue volume was independently associated with increased risk of major adverse cardiovascular events (MACEs) (hazard ratio, 1.35 [95% CI: 1.07, 1.68] per doubling; P = .009), following adjustment for ASCVD risk score and CAC score Epicardial adipose tissue attenuation by this method was inversely associated with MACE risk (hazard ratio, 0.83 [95% CI: 0.72, 0.96] per 5 HU increase; P = .01). Such rapid, automated measurements of epicardial adipose tissue have the potential for integration into routine reporting of calcium scoring CT, providing real-time, complementary information on cardiovascular risk.

In addition, Commandeur et al combined DL-based epicardial adipose tissue metrics with clinical variables and the CAC score using an XGBoost algorithm for risk stratification in a separate EISNER substudy. The ML risk score (AUC, 0.82) outperformed the ASCVD risk score or CAC score alone (AUC, 0.77 for both; P < .05) for long-term prediction of MACE. A major advantage of this ML approach is its ability to explicitly describe the influence of each variable for individualized prediction and provide so-called explainable AI.This is particularly important given that many ML algorithms are considered “black boxes” with no clear justification for their decision-making. Further, such stratification of significant clinical and imaging parameters could potentially guide therapy targeted at the specific factors affecting cardiovascular outcomes.

3.Coronary CT Angiography

Coronary Artery Stenosis Detection and Grading

The prognostic value of anatomic assessment of CAD with CCTA is well established, with coronary stenosis detection and quantification being the cornerstone of routine clinical reporting. Currently, these tasks rely on visual assessment and are therefore subject to substantial interobserver variability A number of AI approaches have been able to automatically

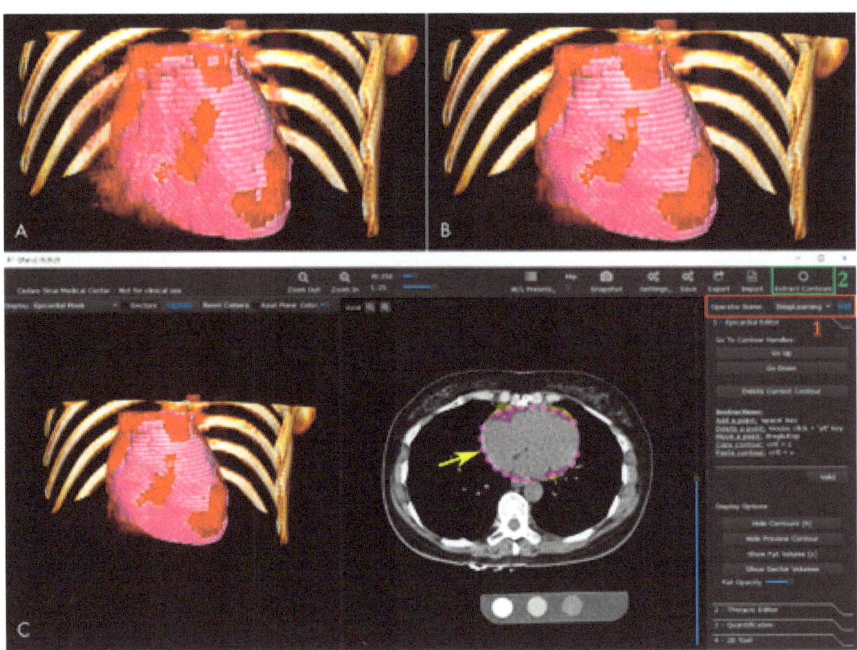

Fig.7.4 Deep learning–based quantification of epicardial adipose tissue. A, Three-dimensional rendering of epicardial adipose tissue (pink overlay) derived from coronary artery calcium scoring CT, B, as manually measured by an expert, and C, as automatically quantified by a deep learning algorithm embedded in research software (QFAT [version 2.0; Cedars-Sinai Medical Center]). (Reprinted, with permission)

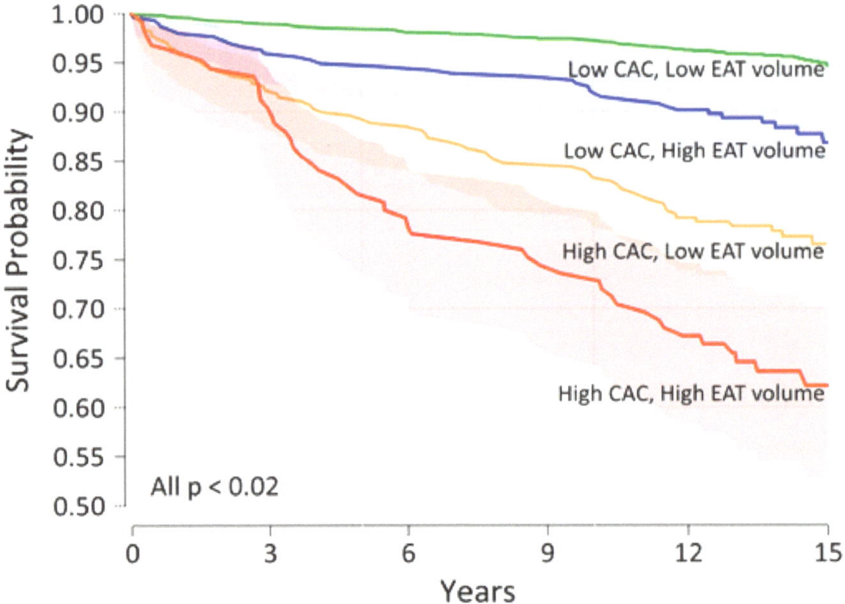

Fig.7.5 Risk stratification by coronary artery calcium (CAC) score and deep learning–based epicardial adipose tissue (EAT) volume. Kaplan-Meier curves of MACE-free survival in asymptomatic individuals from the Early Identification of Subclinical Atherosclerosis by Noninvasive Imaging Research trial stratified by low (< 100) versus high (≥ 100) CAC score and low (< 113 cm3) versus high (≥ 113 cm3) EAT volume. Risk was highest in individuals with a high CAC score and high EAT volume. (Reprinted, with permission)

determine the degree of coronary stenosis directly from image data. Kang et al used a support vector machine incorporating geometric and plaque features to detect coronary artery lesions with at least 25% stenosis in a data set of 42 patients, yielding high sensitivity (93%) and specificity (95%) compared with expert visual assessment. Kelm et al trained a random forest ML algorithm to automatically estimate luminal cross-sectional area and detect obstructive (> 50%) stenosis, achieving a sensitivity of 95% and specificity of 67% compared with experts, at an average speed of 1.8 seconds per case. Hong et al used a CNN to automatically quantify the percentage diameter stenosis and minimal luminal area, with DL measures correlating strongly with expert manual annotations (r = 0.957 for stenosis, r = 0.984 for minimal luminal area; P < .001 for both).

CCTA-derived measures of coronary stenosis have also been integrated into ML models for outcome prediction. In 10 030 patients, Motwani et al trained a Logit. Boost algorithm using 25 clinical variables and 44 visually determined CCTA parameters of CAD extent and severity for the prediction of 5-year all-cause mortality. The resultant ML score (AUC, 0.79) outperformed traditional CCTA-based segment scores (AUC, 0.64 for both segment stenosis score and segment involvement score) and the Framingham risk score (AUC, 0.61; P < .001 for all) . Among the highest ranked variables in the ML model were the number of noncalcified segments and number of vessels with diameter stenosis less than 50%.

Coronary Plaque Characterization and Quantification

CCTA also enables assessment of plaque morphology, which previously could only be evaluated using invasive intracoronary imaging. Qualitative "high-risk plaque" features (positive remodeling, low attenuation plaque, spotty calcification, and napkin-ring sign) derived from CCTA have predictive value for acute coronary syndrome . Of these features, identification of the napkin-ring sign is most prone to interreader variability as it relies exclusively on visual assessment .Kolossváry et al sought to use CCTA-based radiomics to improve the detection of napkin-ring sign. Of 4400 radiomic features analyzed in this study, 440 (9.9%) exhibited high diagnostic accuracy (AUC > 0.80). Most of these features were textural or geometric, describing the complex spatial distribution of voxels. In another study, radiomic analysis was shown to outperform qualitative features at CCTA for the identification of vulnerable plaques determined by using intracoronary imaging. Finally, Kolossváry et al combined CCTA-based radiomic analysis with ML for the identification of histologically determined advanced atherosclerotic lesions. After using 1919 radiomic features to train eight independent ML models, a test model based on least angle regression and fitted with the 13 most predictive parameters was able to outperform visual CCTA assessment (AUC, 0.73 vs 0.65; P = .04).In a study by Motoyama et al (49), the presence of qualitative high-risk plaque at CCTA (defined by positive remodeling and/or low attenuation plaque) was an independent predictor of future acute coronary syndrome. Importantly, however, the cumulative number of events was similar among patients with and without high-risk plaques; this was primarily attributed to the diffuse nature of coronary atherosclerosis. In more recent studies, CCTA-based quantification of plaque volume and burden in the entire coronary tree using software applications has demonstrated independent prognostic value . In a landmark post hoc analysis of the multicenter Scottish COmputed Tomography of the HEART (SCOT-HEART) trial with 5-year follow-up, Williams et al showed that patients with a high >4%) low-attenuation noncalcified plaque burden were five times more likely to develop myocardial infarction than patients with a low (≤4%) plaque burden, independent of risk factors, stenosis severity, or CAC score.

CCTA-derived quantitative plaque measures have been incorporated into ML models to enhance outcome prediction. In a lesion-level analysis of a matched cohort of patients with and without acute coronary syndrome, Al'Aref et al input qualitative and quantitative plaque features measured by conventional methods into an XGBoost algorithm for the prediction of culprit lesions associated with acute coronary syndrome. The ML model provided superior performance (AUC, 0.77) compared with quantitative plaque features or qualitative high-risk plaque features alone.

Lesion-specific ischemia by invasive fractional flow reserve, which has a well-established association with adverse cardiac events , has been used as the outcome for training AI algorithms. Dey et al combined conventional quantitative plaque and vessel-based metrics in an ML model that provided superior prediction for lesion-specific ischemia (AUC, 0.84) compared with stenosis severity (AUC, 0.76) or pretest probability of CAD (AUC, 0.63). The burdens of noncalcified plaque and low-attenuation noncalcified plaque provided the highest ML information gain Noninvasive fractional flow reserve measurement derived from CCTA can also be performed with the assistance of DL techniques that identify lumen boundaries and thus enable assessment of computational fluid dynamics. In a real-world study, this method showed a LogitBoost-based model incorporating baseline clinical variables as well as qualitative and quantitative plaque parameters to have greater discriminatory value in identifying patients with rapid plaque progression compared with ML models with clinical variables or qualitative plaque features alone, and also compared with traditional risk scores. Quantitative plaque parameters provided the highest information gain for ML, followed by qualitative plaque parameters and clinical variables.

Detecting Coronary Inflammation

Beyond coronary assessment, CCTA imaging of pericoronary adipose tissue (PCAT) enables detection of coronary inflammation and several AI techniques have recently been applied to PCAT quantification. Oikonomou et al

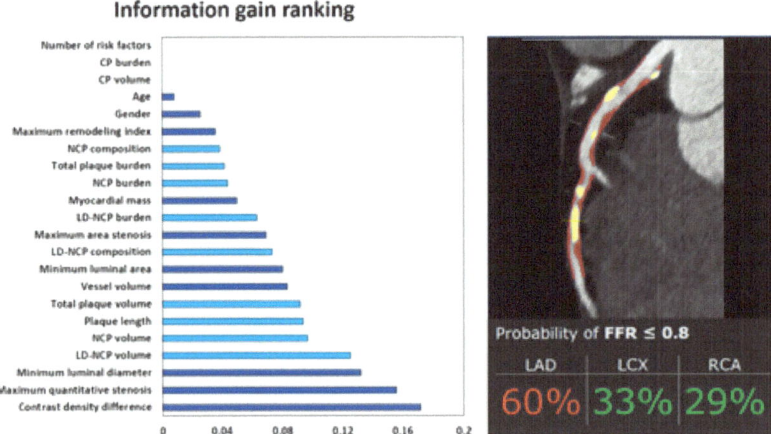

Fig.7.6 Machine learning (ML) prediction of lesion-specific ischemia. The left panel shows information gain ranking of variables in a coronary CT angiography (CCTA)–based ML model used to predict lesion-specific ischemia by invasive fractional flow reserve. Quantitative plaque measures are shown in light blue, and other CCTA and clinical variables are shown in dark blue. The right panel is a case example of the ML prediction applied to a symptomatic patient undergoing CCTA, with noncalcified plaque (NCP) and calcified plaque (CP) shown in red and yellow overlay, respectively. Invasive fractional flow reserve (FFR) of the left anterior descending artery (LAD) was positive (0.73). LCX = left circumflex artery, LD-NCP = low-density noncalcified plaque, RCA = right coronary artery. (Reprinted, with permission)

(AUC, 0.94) outperformed conventional CCTA stenosis assessment (AUC, 0.83) and PET (AUC, 0.87; P < .01 for both) for the detection of per-vessel ischemia when compared with invasive angiography as the reference standard .An ML framework has also demonstrated promising results in predicting the risk of rapid plaque progression. In patients undergoing serial CCTA over a median interval of 3.3 years, Han et al input radiomic features extracted from PCAT into a random forest ML model to develop a patient-level "fat radiomic profile." When tested in 1575 participants from the SCOT-HEART trial, this metric had incremental value for MACE prediction beyond traditional CCTA-based risk stratification (AUC, 0.88 vs 0.75; P < .001).In a prospective case-control study, Lin et al (56) examined 1103 radiomic features of PCAT in patients with and without acute myocardial infarction. Using XGBoost, an ML model integrating clinical data, the average CT attenuation of PCAT, and PCAT radiomic features (AUC, 0.87) outperformed a model with clinical data and PCAT attenuation (AUC, 0.77; P = .001) and clinical data alone (AUC, 0.87 vs 0.76; P < .001) in identifying patients with myocardial infarction . Textural features of PCAT provided the greatest variable importance in the radiomics-based ML model . Together, these studies show how combining advanced CCTA-based quantification of PCAT with ML can identify new imaging biomarkers of the so-called vulnerable patient.

4.Nuclear Cardiology

Early studies of AI in nuclear cardiology used quantitative and functional parameters from SPECT myocardial perfusion imaging (MPI) for the prediction of obstructive CAD at invasive angiography.Arsanjani et al combined imaging measures (including stress total perfusion deficit and inducible ischemic and ejection fraction changes) with clinical data and stress electrocardiogram changes using LogitBoost. The integrated ML model provided superior accuracy for detecting obstructive CAD compared with not only total perfusion deficit alone or visual analysis, but also with an ML model without clinical data. Recently, Betancur et al used 1638 MPI scans from REgistry of Fast Myocardial Perfusion Imaging with NExt generation SPECT (REFINE SPECT) for training of a DL algorithm to directly analyze polar map images and detect obstructive CAD . This model outperformed standard total perfusion deficit assessment (AUC, 0.80 vs 0.78; P < .01), with a computation time of less than 0.5 second per patient.MPI data have also been input into ML models for outcome prediction. In another REFINE SPECT substudy, Hu et al used LogitBoost to combine measures of regional perfusion deficits with stress test and clinical variables to predict early revascularization. The per-vessel and per-patient prediction by ML was higher than that of standard quantitative analysis using total perfusion deficit or expert visual analysis. In a subsequent report, Hu et al used clinical and stress perfusion parameters from all 20 414 patients from the REFINE SPECT registry to develop an ML model for automatic rest scan cancellation based on prognostic safety. An XGBoost algorithm was trained on the data to predict MACE, and the resultant ML score was used to select patients for simulated cancellation of their rest scans. This resulted in lower annualized MACE rates compared with rest scan cancellation by conventional clinical criteria. For example, the algorithm could potentially cancel

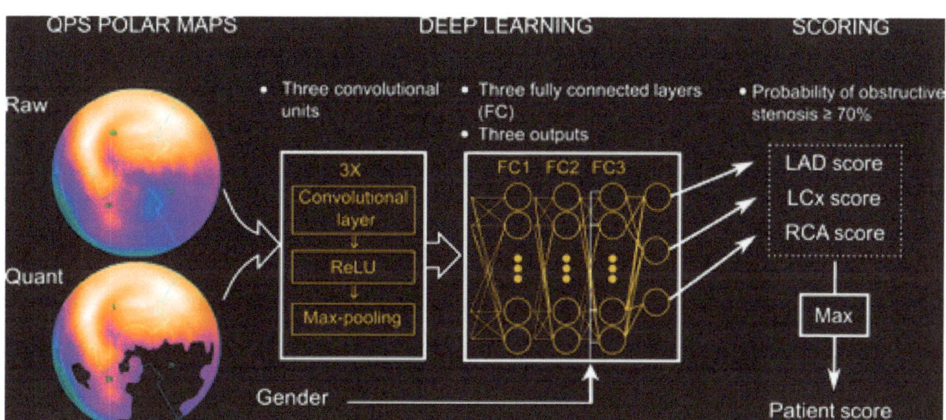

Fig.7.7 Deep learning prediction of obstructive coronary artery disease (CAD) from myocardial perfusion imaging. SPECT polar map images are directly connected to the convolutional neural network, and patterns of perfusion defects are identified by feature extraction (left). These image features then pass through three fully connected layers (FC) in a deep learning process (center), which predicts the probability of obstructive CAD in each vascular territory (right). LAD = left anterior descending artery, LCx = left circumflex artery, Max = maximum probability of obstructive CAD, QPS = quantitative perfusion SPECT, ReLU = rectified linear unit (linear function mapping input to output values), RCA = right coronary artery. (Reprinted, with permission)

60% of the rest scans, and in these patients the annual MACE risk would be 1.4%; the same cancellation rate based on visual scoring would result in an annual 2.1% MACE rate. These findings lend support to the clinical adoption of such an ML approach, which could reduce radiation exposure and health care costs while ensuring prognostic safety.

Betancur et al applied a LogitBoost algorithm for the prediction of 3-year MACE risk in 2619 patients undergoing clinically indicated exercise or pharmacologic MPI. They showed a comprehensive ML model integrating imaging, stress test, and clinical variables to outperform expert visual interpretation, automated measures of total perfusion deficit, or ML with only imaging variables (AUC, 0.81 vs 0.73, 0.71, and 0.65, respectively; $P < .01$ for all). Further, the combined ML model provided a 26% ($P < .001$) risk reclassification for MACE compared with visual analysis. Different ML algorithms using MPI and clinical data have been tested in parallel against traditional statistical methods for the prediction of cardiac death. In an analysis by Haro Alonso et al , a support vector machine model with 49 features had the highest accuracy compared with a baseline logistic regression model with 122 features (AUC, 0.83 vs 0.76; $P < .0001$). A least absolute shrinkage and selection operator approach minimized the number of predictive features to six, while providing slightly better accuracy than logistic regression (AUC, 0.77; $P = .045$). These findings highlight the role of ML in selecting the most important predictive variables, enabling the relevance of risk factors to be readily appreciated within the time constraints of clinical practice.Automated cardiovascular risk assessment can also be performed using a hybrid imaging approach. In patients undergoing 82Rb PET/CT, Išgum et al applied an ML method of automated CAC scoring to low-dose CT attenuation correction images, which are routinely acquired after the PET studies. There was excellent agreement between automated CT attenuation correction scoring and the reference standard of dedicated CAC scoring CT with manual quantification ($\kappa = 0.79–0.82$). Hence, this AI approach is not only highly feasible but may enable clinical cardiovascular risk assessment using the CT attenuation correction component of PET/CT MPI without the need for any additional protocols or radiation exposure.

Challenges to AI Implementation

Although the described AI applications hold great promise for cardiovascular risk stratification, there are several barriers to their clinical implementation. First, the accuracy of ML models will always be limited by the availability and quality of data used for training. Hence, ML algorithms may not perform as well in areas of cardiovascular imaging that do not generate large data sets, such as with rare diseases, uncommon presentations of common diseases, or historic archived images. Further, standardization of image acquisition protocols and formats is required before data from different institutions can be input into a standard AI model. Second, running AI algorithms to handle vast data sets can be computationally expensive, thereby limiting their widespread availability. However, advances in increasingly affordable hardware (eg, graphics processing units) and software (eg, cloud-based computing services) solutions will facilitate the integration and storage of imaging big data. Finally, AI algorithms trained and tested at a single institution may not be generalizable to different cohorts. Thus, all models will require external validation across multiple centers and imaging vendors before their widespread clinical adoption. Moreover, as patient characteristics, disease patterns, and image acquisition and reconstruction techniques change over time, AI models may benefit from continuous updating using large and dynamic data sets.

Summary

Noninvasive cardiovascular imaging is data-rich and primed for AI-powered solutions. AI can be used to quantify cardiovascular risk by two main methods: (a) through the direct application of DL algorithms to image data for automated quantification of prognostic biomarkers; or (b) through integration of conventional or AI-based imaging metrics with tabular data in ML models for individualized outcome prediction. For all the potential applications, however, high-quality data and model validation on unseen data sets are key to success. real-time prognostication and guide personalized therapy.

Bibliography And Acknowledgement

- Agatston AS, Janowitz WR, Hildner FJ, Zusmer NR, Viamonte M Jr, Detrano R. Quantification of coronary artery calcium using ultrafast computed tomography. J Am Coll Cardiol 1990;15(4):827–832
- Al'Aref SJ, Maliakal G, Singh G, et al.. Machine learning of clinical variables and coronary artery calcium scoring for the prediction of obstructive coronary artery disease on coronary computed tomography angiography: analysis from the CONFIRM registry. Eur Heart J 2020;41(3):359–367
- Al'Aref SJ, Singh G, Choi JW, et al.. A Boosted Ensemble Algorithm for Determination of Plaque Stability in High-Risk Patients on Coronary CTA. JACC Cardiovasc Imaging 2020;13(10):2162–2173
- Antonopoulos AS, Sanna F, Sabharwal N, et al.. Detecting human coronary inflammation by imaging perivascular fat. Sci Transl Med 2017;9(398):eaal2658.
- Arbab-Zadeh A, Hoe J. Quantification of coronary arterial stenoses by multidetector CT angiography in comparison with conventional angiography methods, caveats, and implications. JACC Cardiovasc Imaging 2011;4(2):191–202.
- Arsanjani R, Xu Y, Dey D, et al.. Improved accuracy of myocardial perfusion SPECT for detection of coronary artery disease by machine learning in a large population. J Nucl Cardiol 2013;20(4):553–562.
- Betancur J, Commandeur F, Motlagh M, et al.. Deep Learning for Prediction of Obstructive Disease From Fast Myocardial Perfusion SPECT: A Multicenter Study. JACC Cardiovasc Imaging 2018;11(11):1654–1663.
- Betancur J, Otaki Y, Motwani M, et al.. Prognostic Value of Combined Clinical and Myocardial Perfusion Imaging Data Using Machine Learning. JACC Cardiovasc Imaging 2018;11(7):1000–1009.
- Budoff MJ, Diamond GA, Raggi P, et al.. Continuous probabilistic prediction of angiographically significant coronary artery disease using electron beam tomography. Circulation 2002;105(15):1791–1796.
- Budoff MJ, Shaw LJ, Liu ST, et al.. Long-term prognosis associated with coronary calcification: observations from a registry of 25,253 patients. J Am Coll Cardiol 2007;49(18):1860–1870
- Callister TQ, Cooil B, Raya SP, Lippolis NJ, Russo DJ, Raggi P. Coronary artery disease: improved reproducibility of calcium scoring with an electron-beam CT volumetric method. Radiology 1998;208(3):807–814.
- Chang HJ, Lin FY, Lee SE, et al.. Coronary Atherosclerotic Precursors of Acute Coronary Syndromes. J Am Coll Cardiol 2018;71(22):2511–2522.
- Commandeur F, Goeller M, Razipour A, et al.. Fully Automated CT Quantification of Epicardial Adipose Tissue by Deep Learning: A Multicenter Study. Radiol Artif Intell 2019;1(6):e190045
- Commandeur F, Slomka PJ, Goeller M, et al.. Machine learning to predict the long-term risk of myocardial infarction and cardiac death based on clinical risk, coronary calcium, and epicardial adipose tissue: a prospective study. Cardiovasc Res 2020;116(14):2216–2225.
- De Mauro A, Greco M, Grimaldi M. A formal definition of Big Data based on its essential features. Library Rev 2016;65(3):122–135.
- Deo RC. Machine Learning in Medicine. Circulation 2015;132(20):1920–1930.
- Dey D, Gaur S, Ovrehus KA, et al.. Integrated prediction of lesion-specific ischaemia from quantitative coronary CT angiography using machine learning: a multicentre study. Eur Radiol 2018;28(6):2655–2664
- Dey D, Slomka PJ, Leeson P, et al.. Artificial Intelligence in Cardiovascular Imaging: JACC State-of-the-Art Review. J Am Coll Cardiol 2019;73(11):1317–1335.
- Dey D, Wong ND, Tamarappoo B, et al.. Computer-aided non-contrast CT-based quantification of pericardial and thoracic fat and their associations with coronary calcium and Metabolic Syndrome. Atherosclerosis 2010;209(1):136–141.
- Driessen RS, Danad I, Stuijfzand WJ, et al.. Comparison of Coronary Computed Tomography Angiography, Fractional Flow Reserve, and Perfusion Imaging for Ischemia Diagnosis. J Am Coll Cardiol 2019;73(2):161–173
- Eisenberg E, McElhinney PA, Commandeur F, et al.. Deep Learning-Based Quantification of Epicardial Adipose Tissue Volume and Attenuation Predicts Major Adverse Cardiovascular Events in Asymptomatic Subjects. Circ Cardiovasc Imaging 2020;13(2):e009829.
- Erbel R, Möhlenkamp S, Moebus S, et al.. Coronary risk stratification, discrimination, and reclassification improvement based on quantification of subclinical coronary atherosclerosis: the Heinz Nixdorf Recall study. J Am Coll Cardiol 2010;56(17):1397–1406.
- Esteva A, Robicquet A, Ramsundar B, et al.. A guide to deep learning in healthcare. Nat Med 2019;25(1):24–29.
- Friedman J, Hastie T, Tibshirani R. Additive logistic regression: a statistical view of boosting (with discussion and a rejoinder by the authors). Ann Stat 2000;28:337–407
- Gernaat SAM, van Velzen SGM, Koh V, et al.. Automatic quantification of calcifications in the coronary arteries and thoracic aorta on radiotherapy planning CT scans of Western and Asian breast cancer patients. Radiother Oncol 2018;127(3):487–492.
- Gorter PM, de Vos AM, van der Graaf Y, et al.. Relation of epicardial and pericoronary fat to coronary atherosclerosis and coronary artery calcium in patients undergoing coronary angiography. Am J Cardiol 2008;102(4):380–385.
- Han D, Kolli KK, Al'Aref SJ, et al.. Machine Learning Framework to Identify Individuals at Risk of Rapid Progression of Coronary Atherosclerosis: From the PARADIGM Registry. J Am Heart Assoc 2020;9(5):e013958
- Haro Alonso D, Wernick MN, Yang Y, Germano G, Berman DS, Slomka P. Prediction of cardiac death after adenosine myocardial perfusion SPECT based on machine learning. J Nucl Cardiol 2019;26(5):1746–1754
- Hong Y, Commandeur F, Cadet S, et al.. Deep learning-based stenosis quantification from coronary CT Angiography. Proc SPIE Int Soc Opt Eng 2019;10949:109492I
- Hu LH, Betancur J, Sharir T, et al.. Machine learning predicts per-vessel early coronary revascularization after fast myocardial perfusion SPECT: results from multicentre REFINE SPECT registry. Eur Heart J Cardiovasc Imaging 2020;21(5):549–559.

- Hu LH, Miller RJH, Sharir T, et al.. Prognostically safe stress-only single-photon emission computed tomography myocardial perfusion imaging guided by machine learning: report from REFINE SPECT. Eur Heart J Cardiovasc Imaging doi:10.1093/ehjci/jeaa134. Published online June 12, 2020. Accessed November 21, 2020 .
- Išgum I, de Vos BD, Wolterink JM, et al.. Automatic determination of cardiovascular risk by CT attenuation correction maps in Rb-82 PET/CT. J Nucl Cardiol 2018;25(6):2133–2142 [Published correction appears in J Nucl Cardiol 2018;25(6):2143.].
- Johnson NP, Tóth GG, Lai D, et al.. Prognostic value of fractional flow reserve: linking physiologic severity to clinical outcomes. J Am Coll Cardiol 2014;64(16):1641–1654.
- Kang D, Dey D, Slomka PJ, et al.. Structured learning algorithm for detection of nonobstructive and obstructive coronary plaque lesions from computed tomography angiography. J Med Imaging (Bellingham) 2015;2(1):014003.
- Kelm BM, Mittal S, Zheng Y, et al.. Detection, grading and classification of coronary stenoses in computed tomography angiography. Med Image Comput Comput Assist Interv 2011;14(Pt 3):25–32
- Kolossváry M, Karády J, Kikuchi Y, et al.. Radiomics versus Visual and Histogram-based Assessment to Identify Atheromatous Lesions at Coronary CT Angiography: An ex Vivo Study. Radiology 2019;293(1):89–96.
- Kolossváry M, Karády J, Szilveszter B, et al.. Radiomic Features Are Superior to Conventional Quantitative Computed Tomographic Metrics to Identify Coronary Plaques With Napkin-Ring Sign. Circ Cardiovasc Imaging 2017;10(12):e006843
- Kolossváry M, Kellermayer M, Merkely B, Maurovich-Horvat P. Cardiac Computed Tomography Radiomics: A Comprehensive Review on Radiomic Techniques. J Thorac Imaging 2018;33(1):26–34
- Kolossváry M, Park J, Bang JI, et al.. Identification of invasive and radionuclide imaging markers of coronary plaque vulnerability using radiomic analysis of coronary computed tomography angiography. Eur Heart J Cardiovasc Imaging 2019;20(11):1250–1258.
- Krittanawong C, Zhang H, Wang Z, Aydar M, Kitai T. Artificial Intelligence in Precision Cardiovascular Medicine. J Am Coll Cardiol 2017;69(21):2657–2664.
- Lessmann N, van Ginneken B, Zreik M, et al.. Automatic Calcium Scoring in Low-Dose Chest CT Using Deep Neural Networks With Dilated Convolutions. IEEE Trans Med Imaging 2018;37(2):615–625.
- Lin A, Dey D, Wong DTL, Nerlekar N. Perivascular Adipose Tissue and Coronary Atherosclerosis: from Biology to Imaging Phenotyping. Curr Atheroscler Rep 2019;21(12):47
- Lin A, Kolossváry M, Išgum I, Maurovich-Horvat P, Slomka PJ, Dey D. Artificial intelligence: improving the efficiency of cardiovascular imaging. Expert Rev Med Devices 2020;17(6):565–577
- Lin A, Kolossváry M, Yuvaraj J, et al.. Myocardial Infarction Associates With a Distinct Pericoronary Adipose Tissue Radiomic Phenotype: A Prospective Case-Control Study. JACC Cardiovasc Imaging 2020;13(11):2371–2383.
- Maurovich-Horvat P, Hoffmann U, Vorpahl M, Nakano M, Virmani R, Alkadhi H. The napkin-ring sign: CT signature of high-risk coronary plaques? JACC Cardiovasc Imaging 2010;3(4):440–444
- Min JK, Dunning A, Lin FY, et al.. Age- and sex-related differences in all-cause mortality risk based on coronary computed tomography angiography findings: results from the International Multicenter CONFIRM (Coronary CT Angiography Evaluation for Clinical Outcomes: An International Multicenter Registry) of 23,854 patients without known coronary artery disease. J Am Coll Cardiol 2011;58(8):849–860
- Motoyama S, Ito H, Sarai M, et al.. Plaque Characterization by Coronary Computed Tomography Angiography and the Likelihood of Acute Coronary Events in Mid-Term Follow-Up. J Am Coll Cardiol 2015;66(4):337–346.
- Motoyama S, Sarai M, Harigaya H, et al.. Computed tomographic angiography characteristics of atherosclerotic plaques subsequently resulting in acute coronary syndrome. J Am Coll Cardiol 2009;54(1):49–57.
- Motwani M, Dey D, Berman DS, et al.. Machine learning for prediction of all-cause mortality in patients with suspected coronary artery disease: a 5-year multicentre prospective registry analysis. Eur Heart J 2017;38(7):500–507
- Nakanishi R, Slomka P, Rios R, et al.. Machine Learning Adds to Clinical and CAC Assessments in Predicting 10-Year CHD and CVD Deaths. JACC Cardiovasc Imaging doi:10.1016/j.jcmg.2020.08.024. Published online October 28, 2020. Accessed November 21, 2020.
- Oikonomou EK, Williams MC, Kotanidis CP, et al.. A novel machine learning-derived radiotranscriptomic signature of perivascular fat improves cardiac risk prediction using coronary CT angiography. Eur Heart J 2019;40(43):3529–3543
- Otsuka K, Fukuda S, Tanaka A, et al.. Napkin-ring sign on coronary CT angiography for the prediction of acute coronary syndrome. JACC Cardiovasc Imaging 2013;6(4):448–457.
- Takx RAP, de Jong PA, Leiner T, et al.. Automated coronary artery calcification scoring in non-gated chest CT: agreement and reliability. PLoS One 2014;9(3):e91239.
- van Velzen SGM, Lessmann N, Velthuis BK, et al.. Deep Learning for Automatic Calcium Scoring in CT: Validation Using Multiple Cardiac CT and Chest CT Protocols. Radiology 2020;295(1):66–79.
- Williams MC, Kwiecinski J, Doris M, et al.. Low-Attenuation Noncalcified Plaque on Coronary Computed Tomography Angiography Predicts Myocardial Infarction: Results From the Multicenter SCOT-HEART Trial (Scottish Computed Tomography of the HEART). Circulation 2020;141(18):1452–1462.
- Wolterink JM, Leiner T, Takx RAP, Viergever MA, Isgum I. Automatic Coronary Calcium Scoring in Non-Contrast-Enhanced ECG-Triggered Cardiac CT With Ambiguity Detection. IEEE Trans Med Imaging 2015;34(9):1867–1878.
- Yeboah J, McClelland RL, Polonsky TS, et al.. Comparison of novel risk markers for improvement in cardiovascular risk assessment in intermediate-risk individuals. JAMA 2012;308(8):788–795

Current and Future Applications of Artificial Intelligence in Coronary Artery Disease

CHAPTER

Clinically significant atherosclerosis of the coronary arteries, known as coronary artery disease (CAD), is an endemic condition that is associated with significant morbidity and mortality. For instance, CAD is reported to have affected 20.1 million American adults between 2015 and 2018 .Current societal guidelines emphasize the importance of early detection and risk stratification in the appropriate age and risk groups, with the goal of implementation of goal-directed medical therapies that can alter the natural trajectory of CAD to a less morbid course. Traditional population-derived primary and secondary prevention cardiovascular risk assessment tools (e.g., Framingham risk score, ASCVD, TIMI score, GRACE score, etc.) have historically relied on patient-level data that are easily retrievable and practical to utilize in the clinical setting. Despite their importance, such tools are inherently limited by design due to relying on regression models that make many mathematical assumptions that often do not hold in a real-world setting, such as collinearity between variables and homogeneity of effects. The complex nature and multifactorial pathology of CAD make such regression-based tools less generalizable across different populations.

Recently, the digitization of health records has improved access to large repositories of clinical and imaging datasets for clinical care and research purposes. This is coupled with advances in diagnostic tools that are available for the detection and quantification of CAD. To that end, recent studies have highlighted the usefulness of these tools in enhancing risk assessment and decision making through incorporation of different yet complementary findings from these imaging modalities (e.g., quantitative and qualitative plaque features on computed tomographic imaging of the coronary circulation coupled with functional and physiologic findings on stress-test imaging). In addition, there has been an increasing interest in using the plethora of data in electronic health records and genomic data for better risk assessment .Such tools are being integrated in practice as complementary methods to traditional tools.Yet, despite the ever-increasing amounts of data, risk-prediction methods have been historically limited by what was possible with traditional statistical tools. The concept of Artificial Intelligence (AI) was introduced to mankind as early as the 1950s, with its employment in medical sciences commencing in the 1970s . AI has gained momentum recently, fueled by an improvement in computational power, accumulation of data, and cloud processing. With the attempt to transfer a significant portion of human intelligence to machines, there has been a concerted effort aimed at harnessing the power of AI for biomedical applications in the past two decades Machine learning (ML) is a subfield of AI that involves the creation of algorithms that analyze large datasets without prior assumptions and learn rules and patterns between variables to make predictions and classifications

On the other hand, deep learning (DL) is a subset of ML geared towards image analysis and utilizes more intricate algorithms known as neural networks with multiple deep, hidden layers. Specifically, while ML usually relies on structured data with handcrafted features often in tabular form, DL algorithms can input both structured and raw, unstructured data (e.g., images, video, and text) and extract their own features.

ML algorithms can incorporate a larger number of variables from different modalities, including both patient-level clinical parameters as well as two- and three-dimensional imaging data that take into account the multidimensional nonlinear interactions between variables

Implementing such techniques in healthcare mainly aims to improve the accuracy of risk prediction and customize clinical decisions to each individual, which is the overarching theme in the goal of achieving precision medicine. In this paper, we summarize the recent advances in ML and current attempts at improving predictive analytics with relevance to CAD. We also elucidate on the role of AI in genetics, the incremental role of AI in improving post-procedure risk prediction and long-term mortality. Lastly, we discuss the limitations and potential near-future applications of AI within cardiovascular medicine.

1. Integration of Genetics and AI in Cardiovascular Diseases

Over the last two decades, the emergence of technologies able to measure biological processes at a large scale have resulted in an enormous influx of data. For instance, the completion of the Human Genome Project has paved the way to design single-nucleotide polymorphism (SNP) and mRNA microarrays, which can broadly test for millions of genetic variants in a simple point-of-care test. This has paved the way for the emergence of modern data-driven sciences such as genomics and other "omics" .Genome-wide association studies (GWASs) operate by simultaneous comparison of millions of SNPs between diseased individuals and disease-free controls to detect a statistically significant association between an SNP locus and a particular condition. Erdmann et al. reported that up until the year 2018, GWASs have successfully identified 163 distinct genetic loci for SNPs that are associated with CAD. The risk for expressing a complex trait like CAD can be represented by a mathematical model that assumes a normal distribution of a binary outcome (i.e., CAD or no CAD) and captures the aggregate influence of multiple genetic variants that are predisposed to disease. Such a model is referred to as a polygenic risk score (PRS). PRSs were proposed early on to improve risk stratification in CAD risk models, especially when combined with traditional cardiovascular risk factors. However, the complex genetic architecture along with the multifactorial nature of CAD have been major challenges in CAD risk prediction. For instance, Kathiresan et al. built a genetic risk score to predict major adverse cardiovascular events based on nine different dyslipidemia-related SNPs previously identified in GWASs. Adding the genetic score to a Cox proportional hazard model along with traditional risk factors did not improve predictive accuracy as measured by the C statistic model; however, there was a significant improvement in the net reclassification index, which accounts for correct movement of categories (assigning high-risk for patients who developed the disease, and low-risk for those who were disease-free. Brautbar et al. also suggested a genetic risk score to predict coronary heart disease based on SNPs. Adding the genetic risk score to traditional risk factors in a Cox proportional hazard model only modestly improved the area under the curve (AUC) for prediction of coronary heart disease from 0.742 to 0.749 ($\Delta = 0.007$; 95% CI, 0.004–0.013). ML and particularly DL algorithms are inherently designed to extract patterns and associations from large-scale data, including clinical and genomic data. Given the complexity and multifaceted nature of cardiovascular diseases in general, and CAD in particular, an approach that integrates all these factors into a risk-stratification model would be expected to better predict incident events than existent models

Multiple studies have emphasized the role of ML in identifying genetic variants and expression patterns associated with CAD from mRNA arrays using differential expression analysis and protein–protein interaction networks . For example, Zhang et al. used ML to perform differential expression analysis on mRNA profiles from CAD patients and healthy controls to identify a set of differentially expressed genes between the two groups, then built a network representation of functional protein–protein interaction. The top 20 genes in the network were identified using a maximal clique centrality (MCC) algorithm. Finally, to test the performance, a logistic regression model was built using the top five predictor genes to classify individuals into the presence or absence of CAD. The model achieved an AUC of 0.9295 and 0.8674 in the training and internal validation sets respectively .

Dogan et al. built an ensemble model of eight random-forest (RF) classifiers to predict the risk of symptomatic CAD using genetic and epigenetic variables along with clinical risk factors. The model was trained on a cohort derived from the Framingham heart study (n = 1545) and utilized variables derived from genome-wide array chips to extract epigenetic (DNA methylation loci) and genetic (SNP) profiles. The initial number of available variables were 876,014 SNP and DNA methylation (CpG) loci, which required multiple reduction steps, ending up with 4 CpG and 2 SNP predictors fed into the model along with age and gender. The model predicted symptomatic CAD with an accuracy, sensitivity, and specificity of 0.78, 0.75, and 0.80, respectively, in the internal validation cohort (n = 142). For comparison, a similar ensemble model was built using clinical risk factors only as predictor variables and had an accuracy, sensitivity, and specificity of 0.65, 0.42, and 0.89, respectively . Pattarabanjird et al. tested multiple ML models to predict anatomical CAD severity (extent of diameter stenosis) in a binary fashion using clinical variables along with SNP loci. Quantitative coronary angiography and the Gensini score, which is a summation score that quantifies the severity of CAD by accounting for the segment-based most severe stenosis and the location of the stenosis within the coronary arteries, were used to assess model performance. The best-performing model (Sequential Neural Network; training set n = 325 and internal validation set n = 82) accurately classified CAD severity with AUC of 0.84 in the validation set . Similarly, Naushad et al. trained ML models to predict the presence of CAD and the percentage of coronary diameter stenosis using clinical and genetic variables. The best-performing model (an ensemble model; training set n = 648) accurately predicted CAD using 11 variables (clinical and genetic variants) with an AUC of 0.96 in the training set. The model also predicted the percentage of diameter stenosis with a correlation of 82.5% with the actual stenosis assessed using the gold-standard invasive angiography. However, these models were not internally nor externally validated

Finally, the coronary artery calcium (CAC) score, calculated using the Agatston method on noncontrast ECG-gated cardiac computed tomography, is an established strong predictor of major adverse cardiovascular events in asymptomatic individuals. Genomic studies have previously focused on identifying genetic loci linked to CAC . Oguz et al. suggested the use of ML algorithms to predict advanced CAC from SNP arrays and clinical variables. They identified a set of SNPs that ranked the highest in predictive importance and correlated with advanced CAC scores, defined as the 89th–99th percentile CAC scores in the derivation and replication cohorts, and trained different RF models to predict advanced CAC scores using clinical and genetic variables. Adding SNPs to clinical variables significantly improved AUC from 0.61 ± 0.02 to 0.83 ± 0.01; ($p < 0.001$) [26] for prediction of advanced CAC scores.

2. Risk Prediction Models and Imaging Modalities for Estimating Pretest Probability of CAD

Traditionally, stratifying patients presenting with stable chest pain using pretest probability (PTP) estimates of CAD has been commonly used to help with decision-making regarding downstream testing and the choice of an appropriate diagnostic modality. Historically, the Diamond–Forrester model—developed using age, sex, and chest pain characteristics—was used as a clinician's risk stratification tool in predicting the PTP of CAD . However, numerous studies showed its limitation in overestimating PTP by approximately threefold, especially in women This led to the development of the updated Diamond–Forrester model (UDF) and the CAD consortium score.These scores, incorporating demographic and clinical risk factors, have been proven to be better at predicting the risk of CAD.Therefore, improving the ability to predict CAD using more accurate risk-assessment modeling is imperative, given the potential to reduce downstream testing and associated costs. Using clinical and demographic features, ML models have been employed to estimate the PTP of CAD..In a recent multicenter cross-sectional study, a deep neural network algorithm based on the facial profile of individuals was able to achieve a higher performance than traditional risk scores in predicting PTP of CAD (AUC for the ML model 0.730 vs. 0.623 for Diamond –Forrester and 0.652 for the CAD consortium, p

, $p < 0.001$) . Though the study is limited by the lack of external validity and low specificity (54%), such approaches can potentially lead to a paradigm change in CAD management by facilitating earlier detection and initiation of primary prevention using readily available parameters, such as an individual's facial profile.When available, a CAC score has been shown to add to the PTP of CAD, with a CAC score of zero identifying low-risk patients who might not need additional testing . ML models, combining clinical and imaging parameters, have been shown to have higher predictive power than traditional risk scores when predicting the PTP of obstructive CAD . Al'Aref et al. included 25 clinical and demographic features to devise a ML model which, when combined with the Agatston CAC score, fared better than the ML model or CAD consortium score alone or in combination with the CAC score (AUC 0.881 for ML + CAC as compared to 0.866, 0.773, and 0.734 for the CAD consortium + CAC, ML model, and CAD consortium respectively, $p < 0.05$) . As expected, CAC, age, and gender were the highest-ranked features in the model

Various ML algorithms based on stress imaging, particularly single-photon emission computed tomography (SPECT), have been devised to facilitate the prediction of CAD. These models combined the clinical and demographic characteristics with the quantitative variables, as evaluated via SPECT to better predict CAD compared with the visual interpretation or quantitative variables alone

Cardiac phase-space analysis is a novel noninvasive diagnostic platform that combines advanced disciplines of mathematics and physics with ML . Thoracic orthogonal voltage gradient (OVG) signals from a patient are evaluated by cardiac phase-space analysis to quantify physiological and mathematical features associated with CAD. The analysis is performed at the point of care without the need for a change in physiologic status or radiation. Initial multicenter results suggest that resting cardiac phase-space analysis may have comparable diagnostic utility to functional tests currently used to assess CAD Finally, the assessment of regional wall motion abnormalities (RWMAs) on echocardiography has been associated with the presence of obstructive CAD, and as such can be useful in helping clinicians with downstream decision-making. Recently, a deep-learning model developed by Kusunose et al. achieved performance similar to that of experienced cardiologists in the assessment of RWMAs on echocardiography (AUC of 0.99 vs. 0.98, $p = 0.15$) . Other than the assessment of obstructive CAD, machine learning has found its wide applicability in echocardiography to predict ventricular capacities, abnormal valvular function, as well as cardiac hemodynamics.

3. Artificial Intelligence in Management of CAD in the Emergency Department

Chest pain is a common emergency department presentation, and distinguishing cardiac from noncardiac pain causes is crucial for optimal management. Modalities such as electrocardiography (ECG) serve as a quick way to recognize patterns associated with unstable CAD, and in particular acute coronary syndromes (ACSs). Deep neural networks have shown a consistent performance in image recognition, and models have hence been devised to identify patterns related to CAD and myocardial infarction (MI) .By reducing interobserver variability and providing accurate results efficiently, this approach holds the promise of improving workflow across healthcare systems, while helping patients in areas of limited medical infrastructure and specialized care.

Cardiac biomarkers, such as high-sensitivity troponin, have been well-validated as markers of myocardial ischemia and damage. High-sensitivity troponin I (hs-cTnI) assay forms the core of the 'rule in and rule out' clinical decision pathway as per ESC 2020 chest pain guidelines and 2021 ACC/AHA chest pain guidelines . For instance, a very low hs-cTnI at hospital admission or a negative one-hour delta troponin (in the background of a low hs-cTnI value at admission) has a high negative predictive value (>99%) for ACS . On the other hand, a high admission hs-cTnI value or a significant increase in values in an hour portends a high positive-predictive value (70–75%), warranting additional downstream testing

Using the strategy mentioned above, approximately one-third of the patients fall in the 'indeterminate' zone. Diagnosis and management of this group is challenging, necessitating an approach based on clinical history, pre-existing risk factors, serial hs-cTnI trends, and further imaging. A recent ML model based on three clinical (age, sex, and prior percutaneous coronary intervention) as well as levels of three biomarkers (hs-cTnI, KIM-1, and adiponectin) demonstrated excellence in predicting obstructive CAD in the validation cohort (AUC 0.86 for prediction of >50% diameter stenosis). Notably, the model performed remarkably well in patients in the 'indeterminate' zone, with AUC of 0.88 and a positive predictive value of 93%, hence identifying patients who will benefit from further testing. The 2021 American College of Cardiology/American Heart Association (ACC/AHA) chest pain guidelines advocate for the use of coronary CT angiography (CCTA) in intermediate-risk patients presenting with acute chest pain who either have no known history or a history of nonobstructive CAD (defined ascoronary artery disease with less than 50% diameter stenosis). Given the ability of CCTA toaccurately define coronary anatomy and extent/distribution of atherosclerotic plaque, it has been consistently shownnoninvasive imaging modality for patient selection, particularly for those who might require further invasive evaluation. However, interpretation of CCTA scans requires expertise and is time-intensive. Therefore, automatic interpretation of CCTA, which can lead to a significant reduction in the processing times, is highly desirable. ML algorithms have recently been developed, achieving a 70–75% reduction in reading time compared to that required for human interpretation (2.3 min for AI vs. 7.6–9.6 min for human readers). Though the model described performed slightly lower than highly experienced readers in interpreting CCTA (AUC 0.93 vs. 0.90 for human vs. AI, $p < 0.05$), when combined with low-experience human readers, it augmented the reader's

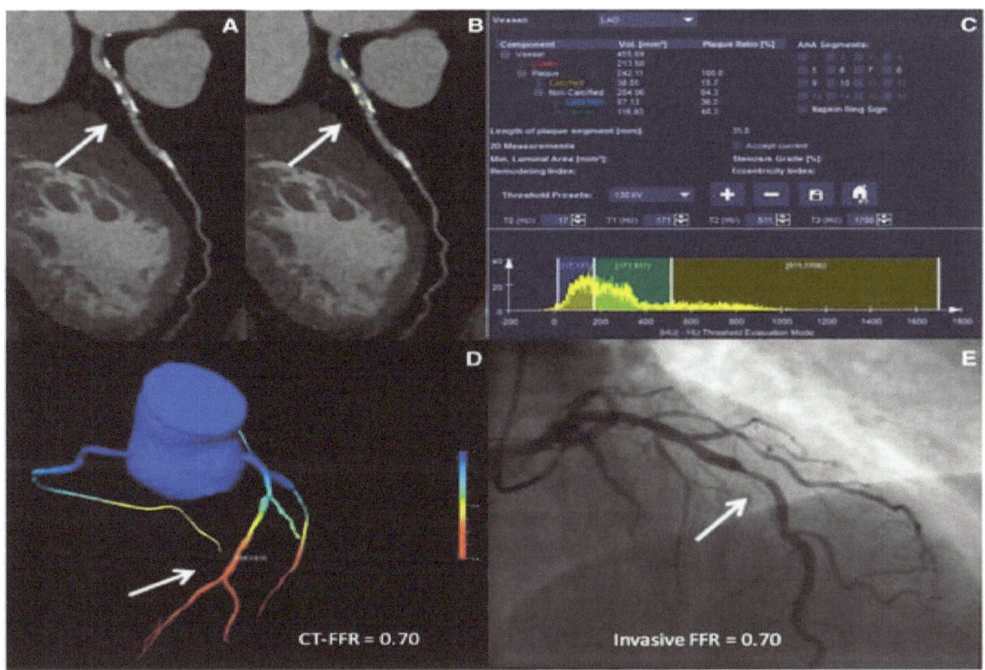

Fig.8.1 ML-based fractional flow reserve from cardiac CT (CT-FFRML). Machine-learning-based coronary plaque analysis quantifies atherosclerotic plaque into calcified and noncalcified components (A,B). This is further integrated with other quantitative parameters (C) and transformed into 3-D images of the vessels to give CT-FFRML (D), which has been shown to have a good correlation with invasive fractional flow reserve (FFR—E). Adapted with permission from Von Knebel Doeberitz et al.

ability to correctly reclassify obstructive CAD (per-vessel net reclassification index (NRI) 0.07, $p < 0.001$) . In addition, ML has been applied for various segmentation and classification tasks on cardiac CT imaging, from automatic segmentation of calcified and noncalcified plaque to automated calculation of the Agatston CAC score, and finally quantification of cardiac structures on CT imaging Therefore, the application of ML could provide reliable results in real time, while bridging the dearth of experts in low-resource settings.

Stress testing, which provides an estimate of myocardial perfusion and viability, has been recommended as an alternative to CCTA in intermediate-risk chest pain patients. Myocardial perfusion imaging, particularly SPECT, has been employed to recognize patients who might need an invasive evaluation, with a diagnostic sensitivity of 75–88% and specificity of 60–79% .SPECT can be evaluated qualitatively in terms of size, severity, location, and reversibility of perfusion defect, and quantitatively, in terms of total perfusion deficit (TPD), summed stress score (SSS), summed rest score (SRS), as well as stress and rest volumes . Automatically generated polar maps (representing radiotracer distribution in a two-dimensional plane) after three-dimensional segmentation of the left ventricle (LV) have been used as raw data for quantitative analysis. After the LV polar map is divided into 17 segments, each of the segments is graded on a scale of 0–4 based on the severity of ischemia.

The scores are then summated to generate SSS and SRS. Polar maps also provide information about the overall extent and magnitude of ischemia, in terms of TPD . These objective variables extracted from the quantitative analysis offer an increased degree of reproducibility and can be incorporated into risk scores to predict mortality.The diagnostic accuracy of qualitative and quantitative approaches is comparable, as has been shown in numerous studies . A deep convolutional neural network-based model derived from polar maps had a superior performance compared to TPD in predicting obstructive coronary artery disease (the AUC for ML were 0.80 and 0.76 vs. 0.78 and 0.73 for TPD on a per-patient and per-vessel basis respectively, $p < 0.01$). In addition to diagnosis, models to predict early revascularization (<90 days from SPECT) have been developed and have demonstrated better performance than individual SPECT variables on a per-patient and a per-vessel level

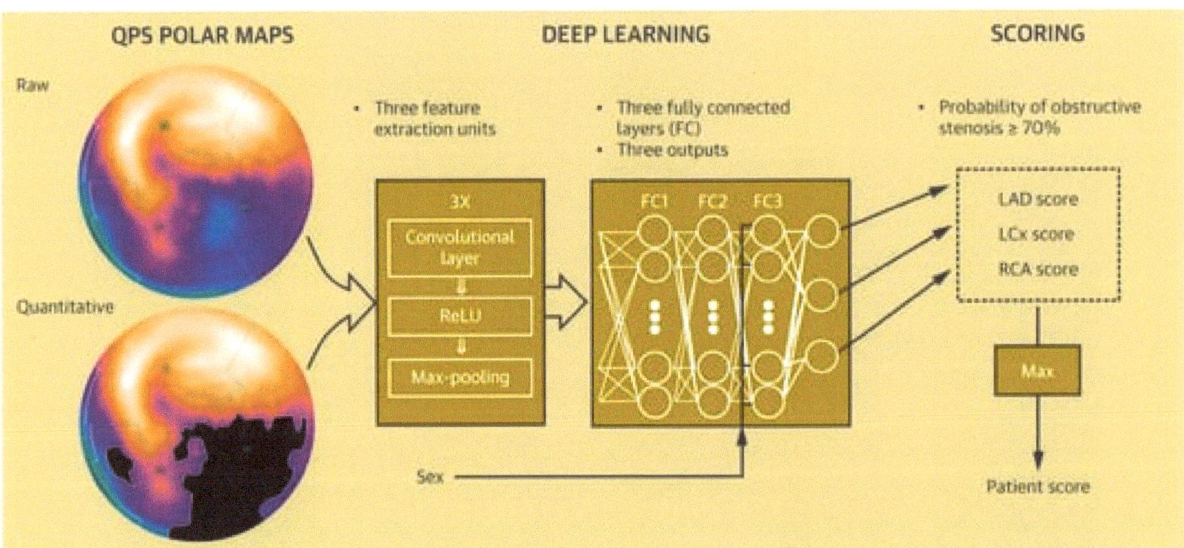

Fig.8.2 Deep-learning model to predict obstructive CAD from polar maps. Raw polar maps and extent polar maps (maps with abnormal pixels representing ischemia blackened out) are fed into deep neural networks, with the extracted data used to calculate scores for individual vessels to predict the probability of CAD. Adapted with permission from Betancur et al. Elsevier.

4. Artificial Intelligence to Predict Functionally Obstructive CAD and Lesion-Specific Ischemia as a Gatekeeper to the Catheterization Laboratory

One of the inherent limitations of CCTA is its limited ability to predict the functional significance of coronary stenosis. To overcome this shortcoming, CT-derived fractional flow reserve (FFRCT) was developed based on the critical concept of computational fluid dynamics (CFD), with numerous trials demonstrating its strong correlation with invasive fractional flow reserve (FFR) as determined by invasive coronary angiography (ICA) . Rabbat et al. demonstrated that FFRCT added to CCTA safely deferred ICA in patients with CAD of indeterminate hemodynamic significance. In addition, a high proportion of those who underwent ICA were revascularized . These studies and others led to FFRCT being incorporated in the 2021 ACC/AHA chest pain guidelines in intermediate-risk patients to detect lesion-specific ischemia in proximal or middle segments of the coronary arteries and determined to have atherosclerotic plaque with 40% to 90% diameter stenosis.Despite its excellent correlation, the off-site computation of FFRCT hampers its use in real time, owing to the need for longer processing times To overcome this limitation and to allow for quick computation of a value for the functional significance of a particular lesion, novel ML approaches based on artery lumen segmentation. left ventricular myocardial segmentation and artery centerline tracking have been proposed.

A .ML-Based CT-FFR Estimation and Diagnostic Accuracy

Based on the concept of artery lumen segmentation, the ML-based FFR estimation (CT-FFRML) has generated significant interest in the past few years. The CT-FFRML model was trained on 12,000 synthetically generated coronary geometric datasets and used deep neural networks, allowing for automatic computation of FFR in real-time [93]. Coenen et al. performed a multicenter, prospective study to evaluate the diagnostic performance of CT-FFRML to predict lesion-specific ischemia, comparing it with traditional CCTA parameters, with invasive FFR being the gold standard . They demonstrated an excellent correlation between CT-FFRML and FFRCT (r = 0.997) and a superior performance of CT-FFRML over traditional CCTA in predicting lesion-specific ischemia (AUC: 0.84 vs. 0.69, $p < 0.001$ on a per-vessel level). Since then, multiple retrospective studies have been performed to evaluate the diagnostic accuracy of CT-FFRML, validated against the gold-standard invasive FFR. They have further demonstrated superior diagnostic performance of CT-FFRML over CTA stenosis severity and quantitative atherosclerotic plaque features derived from CCTA. To further highlight the incremental diagnostic value of CT-FFRML over anatomic plaque features derived from CCTA in vessels with intermediate stenosis, several other studies have been performed [99,102,103,106]. Tang et al. evaluated the diagnostic value of CT-FFRML in predicting lesion-specific ischemia [103]. Based on a study sample of 122 vessels in 101 patients, CT-FFRML performed better than anatomic CCTA parameters (AUC 0.96 for CT-FFRML vs. 0.63 for CCTA on a per-vessel basis $p < 0.05$).

B. Impact of Calcification Burden on the Performance of CT-FFRML

The impact of coronary calcification on the diagnostic performance of CCTA has been well-established, with more extensive calcification limiting the ability of CCTA to evaluate for the presence of obstructive CAD]. Multiple indices have been devised to compute a CAC score, with the Agatston score, calcium volume, calcification remodeling index (CRI), and segmental arc calcification method being common examples . The Agatston Score (AS) is the most widely validated approach, which summates the calcium score (function of peak density and area of the lesion) of the individual lesions across all coronary artery segments . CRI provides a lesion-specific calcium estimate and is calculated as a ratio of the cross-sectional luminal area of the most severely calcified site to the proximal luminal area. The segmental arc calcification method estimates lesion-specific calcium burden by measuring the greatest circumferential extent of coronary calcium, grading as nil (noncalcified), mild (0–90°), moderate (90–180°), and severe

(>180°) calcification. Recent studies have evaluated the performance of CT-FFRML with varying calcification burden as assessed by the parameters mentioned above. Tesche et al. did a retrospective analysis using 482 vessels in 314 patients to evaluate the impact of calcifications on the performance of CT-FFRML [104]. They showed a statistically significant decrease in discriminatory power of CT-FFRML, measured in terms of AUC with increasing Agatston scores (AUC for CT-FFRML 0.85 and 0.81 in low–intermediate Agatston score (1–400) and high Agatston score (>400) ranges respectively, p = 0.04). Di Jiang et al. [98] evaluated the impact of calcification arc and CRI on the performance of CT-FFRML. No statistically significant difference was found in the discriminatory power of CT-FFRML with increasing calcification burden. In the proportion of patients where the Agatston score was available, there was no difference in the diagnostic performance of CT-FFRML across severity of calcification. The difference from Tesche et al. can be explained by a lower mean Agatston score (288 vs. 492 and 138 vs. 187 at a per-patient and per-vessel level, respectively) and smaller sample size (n = 150) for whom the Agatston score was available, resulting in low power to detect a difference.Furthermore, Koo et al. [99] carried out a similar study and found no impact of increasing Agatston score on the performance of CT-FFRML. Interestingly, a sizeable proportion of the sample had higher coronary calcification (mean Agatston score of 311 on a per-vessel basis). More research in this area is needed in order to further validate the diagnostic performance of CT-FFRML across varying degrees of coronary calcification.

C. CT-FFRML in Predicting Revascularization Events

CT-FFRML has been shown to be a better predictor than plaque features derived from CCTA for the determination of the presence of lesion-specific ischemia, but whether CT-FFRML influences the eventual treatment plan and outcomes (as guided by ICA-FFR) remains an active area of investigation [115,116,117,118]. Qiao et al. demonstrated the added benefit of CT-FFRML compared to relying on an anatomy-based strategy in patients with stable chest pain (reduction rate of ICA by 54.5% and 4.4% fewer revascularizations). Additionally, this study demonstrated that adding CT-FFRML to CCTA can decrease the rate of unnecessary ICA by 35.2% (thereby increasing the proportion of revascularizations when ICA is undertaken), truly acting as a gatekeeper to ICA. Furthermore, lower CT-FFRML was associated with higher major adverse cardiovascular event (MACE) risk when compared to diameter stenosis on CCTA (HR, 6.84 vs. 1.47) or ICA (HR, 6.84 vs. 1.84). Liu et al. found a similar rate of MACE (2.9%) after revascularization based on either combining CCTA stenosis ≥ 50% and CT-FFRML ≤ 0.8 or ICA stenosis ≥ 75% in a 2-year follow-up . This study further highlighted the use of CT-FFRML as a gatekeeper to ICA with a positive impact on lower healthcare costs.

CT-FFRML comes with its own set of shortcomings. The diagnostic performance of the CT-FFRML model is lower, with the invasive FFR closely approaching the diagnostic threshold of 0.8 . Traditional statistical and DL approaches have shown that stenosis severity; plaque characteristics, such as low-density, noncalcified plaque; and remodeling index are independent predictors of lesion-specific ischemia that are not related to CT-FFRML.An integrated DL approach in the future that combines clinical features, anatomical plaque characteristics, vessel features, and functional assessment could potentially overcome this limitation.

5. Artificial Intelligence in the Field of Intracoronary Imaging

During ICA, intravascular ultrasound (IVUS) and optical coherence tomography (OCT) have been widely adopted for coronary luminal imaging, and some of the main applications involve assessment of plaque burden and optimization of stent placement . IVUS uses ultrasound waves to generate cross-sectional images of coronary vessels with axial and lateral resolution ranging from 70–200 microns and 200–400 microns, respectively The penetration depth of IVUS is 10 mm, which allows for a complete cross-sectional analysis of the coronary vessel walls . IVUS can help describe plaque characteristics, with high-risk plaques (plaques with large necrotic cores) appearing as areas of echo-attenuation . On the other hand, calcifications in the IVUS frame indicate a calcified plaque, with heavily calcified plaque increasing the risk of stent underexpansion during percutaneous coronary intervention (PCI) .Virtual histology IVUS (VH-IVUS) is another technique derived from radiofrequency data from IVUS, allowing for in vivo assessment of plaque composition . By characterizing plaque features and vessel dimensions, IVUS has found its pre-procedural role in the quantitative and qualitative assessment of atherosclerotic plaque as well as interventional planning, ranging from vessel dimension assessment and evaluation of stent placement. Post-procedurally, IVUS can be employed to visualize stent expansion, identify stent edge dissection, stent mal-apposition, and confirm the presence of in-stent thrombosis in the right clinical context. Given the benefits, IVUS has been shown to optimize stent implantation and improve outcomes, including revascularization, MACE, and mortality when used routinely in the cardiac catheterization laboratory .

On the other hand, OCT works on the principle of near-infrared light waves, generating cross-sectional images with a much higher axial and lateral resolution of 10 microns and 20–40 microns, respectively This allows for a detailed view of the lumen–plaque interface, providing accurate dimensions of the luminal area and better plaque characterization. The vulnerability of a plaque is a function of the thickness of its fibrous cap, the size of the necrotic core, and the presence of macrophages. A thin, fibrous cap; sizeable necrotic core; and increased macrophages increase the risk of plaque rupture and subsequent ACS . Given the high resolution provided by OCT, it is considered a gold-standard invasive imaging modality for detecting thin-cap fibroatheroma (TCFA), which, pathologically, is a precursor of vulnerable plaque and clinically proven to be an independent predictor of MACE . A significant drawback of OCT is its inherent low penetration depth (1–2 mm), which makes IVUS a better modality for a full-thickness analysis of vessel wall.

Though fascinating, IVUS and OCT have a low adoption rate in the US, being employed only at tertiary-care centers owing to cost, need for additional procedural time, and the associated technical complexities . By using deep-learning algorithms to optimize the workflow associated with image acquisition and interpretation, ML has the potential to reduce procedural costs and time required, which are the two major hindrances to the widespread use of IVUS and OCT.

A. Artificial Intelligence to Optimize Peri-Intervention Workflow

To predict OCT-derived TCFA on IVUS images, Bae et al. created a ML model, enrolling 517 patients who underwent ICA . A total of 40,908 IVUS-OCT co-registered sections in 517 coronary arteries were divided into training and testing sets in a ratio of 4:1. An artificial-neural-network-based model using 17 features achieved the highest performance with a sensitivity and specificity of 85 ± 4% and 79 ± 6%, respectively, and good discriminatory power (AUC of 0.80 ± 0.08). Larger plaque burden, minimal diameter, decreased lumen area, and increased lumen eccentricity were seen to be strongly associated with OCT-derived TCFAs. Min et al. utilized a deep learning algorithm (densely connected convolutional neural network) on 35,678 OCT frames to automatically detect TCFAs from OCT images . After the frames were interpreted for the presence/absence of TCFA, data was fed into the algorithm to devise a deep-learning model. By achieving high sensitivity and specificity of 88.7 ± 3.4% and 91.8 ± 2.0% on the test data, such deep-learning models can significantly reduce processing times and allow for easy interpretation when it comes to identifying a vulnerable high-risk plaque.As mentioned earlier, IVUS can help characterize high-risk plaques, which appear as areas of attenuation on IVUS frames due to the presence of a large necrotic core. Identifying such lesions becomes imperative to reduce the incidence of complications such as periprocedural MI. To accurately classify plaque characteristics and to facilitate detection of high-risk lesions, Cho et al. described a deep-learning algorithm to accurately differentiate IVUS segments as attenuated or calcified, or plaque without attenuation or calcification. A total 598 vessels in 598 patients were evaluated, and a DL model with five-fold cross-validation was developed.

The deep-learning model closely correlated with the expert read, and correlation coefficients for calcification, attenuation, and no attenuation or calcification were 0.79, 0.74, and 0.99, respectively.Stent underexpansion is a frequently encountered entity that has been associated with an increased risk of in-stent restenosis. Studies have demonstrated the postprocedural minimum stent area (MSA) and IVUS-measured stent length to be independent predictors for in-stent restenosis Min et al. devised a deep-learning model to predict stent underexpansion based on pre-PCI IVUS frames . They evaluated 618 coronary lesions from 618 patients undergoing pre- and postprocedural IVUS and divided them into training and testing sets in to predict stent underexpansion. The stent areas and volumes predicted via the CNN correlated well with poststenting IVUS (r for stent area and volume 0.832 and 0.958, respectively). The most important features predicting stent underexpansion were luminal area, external elastic membrane (EEM) area (both at the reference and the target), and plaque area of the region of interest.

To predict OCT-derived TCFA on IVUS images, Bae et al. created a ML model, enrolling 517 patients who underwent ICA . A total of 40,908 IVUS-OCT co-registered sections in 517 coronary arteries were divided into training and testing sets in a ratioa 5:1 ratio. A convolutional neural network (CNN)model was used to predict

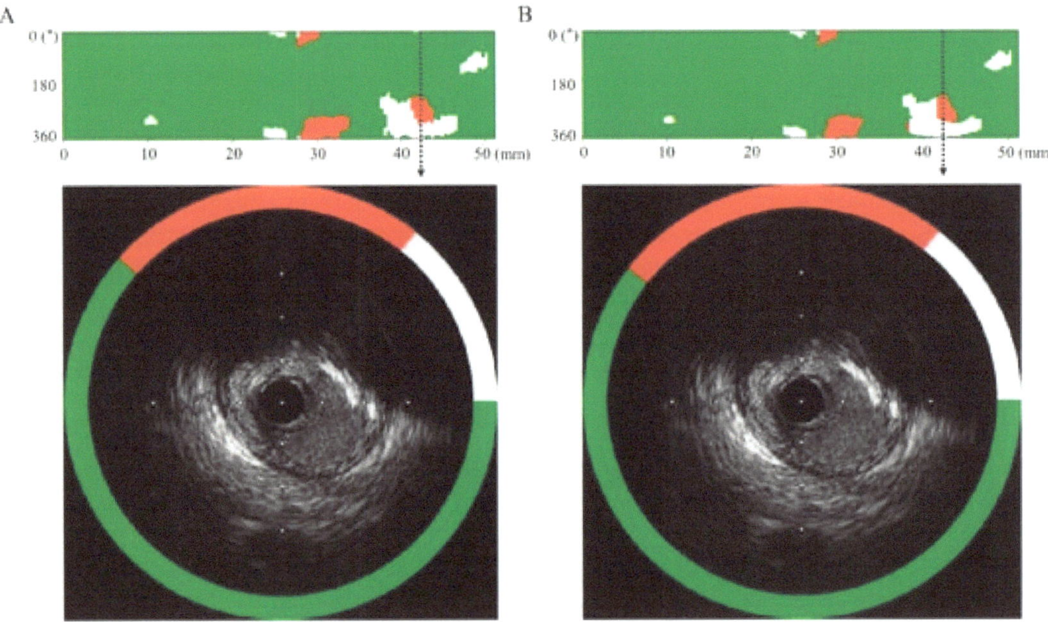

FFig.8.3 ML(A) vs. human (B) interpretations for plaque characterization for IVUS images. The upper panel shows representation of plaque features along the long axis of the vessel (x-axis represents the distance from ROI (region of interest) and y-axis represents the angular position (0–360°) of the plaque. The lower panel shows the plaque characterization on a cross-sectional view of the IVUS frame. Attenuation, calcification, and regions without attenuation or calcification are represented by red, white, and green respectively. Adapted with permission from Cho et al.

stent area. Features extracted from the CNN a 5:1 ratio. A convolutional neural network (CNN)model was used to predict the poststenting stent area. Features extracted from the CNN were combined with additional image-derived features via a boosted ensemble algorithm, which yielded sensitivity and specificity of 68% and 98%, respectively, and an AUC of 0.95 the poststenting of 4:1. An artificial-neural-network-based model using 17 features achieved the highest performance with a sensitivity and specificity of 85 ± 4% and 79 ± 6%, respectively, and good discriminatory power (AUC of 0.80 ± 0.08). Larger plaque burden, minimal diameter, decreased lumen area, and increased lumen eccentricity were seen to be strongly associated with OCT-derived TCFAs. Min et al. utilized a deep learning algorithm (densely connected convolutional neural network) on 35,678 OCT frames to automatically detect TCFAs from OCT images .After the frames were interpreted for the presence/absence of TCFA, data was fed into the algorithm to devise a deep-learning model. By achieving high sensitivity and specificity of 88.7 ± 3.4% and 91.8 ± 2.0% on the test data, such deep-learning models can significantly reduce processing times and allow for easy interpretation when it comes to identifying a vulnerable high-risk plaque

As mentioned earlier, IVUS can help characterize high-risk plaques, which appear as areas of attenuation on IVUS frames due to the presence of a large necrotic core. Identifying such lesions becomes imperative to reduce the incidence of complications such as periprocedural MI. To accurately classify plaque characteristics and to facilitate detection of high-risk lesions, Cho et al. described a deep-learning algorithm to accurately differentiate IVUS segments as attenuated or calcified, or plaque without attenuation or calcification.

A total 598 vessels in 598 patients were evaluated, and a DL model with five-fold cross-validation was developed. The deep-learning model closely correlated with the expert read, and correlation coefficients for calcification, attenuation, and no attenuation or calcification were 0.79, 0.74, and 0.99, respectively The most important features predicting stent underexpansion were luminal area, external elastic membrane (EEM) area (both at the reference and the target), and plaque area of the region of interest.

B.Applications of Artificial Intelligence in Intra and Post-Intervention Workflow

Optimal stent expansion is vital to successful outcomes, with stent underexpansion predisposing to stent restenosis and a greater stent expansion exposing the procedure to a risk of stent edge dissection .IVUS, by allowing direct visualization of vessel architecture, can help in the earlier identification and management of these complications. Nishi et al. developed a ML model to compute the luminal area and the vessel area accurately, as well as the stent area, which exhibited an excellent correlation between ML-derived and expert-derived dimensions while dramatically reducing the time required for segmentation of IVUS images (37 s) compared with expert analysis Virtual histology IVUS (VH-IVUS) is a well-studied intracoronary imaging modality used for in vivo visualization of high-risk plaques . Zhang et al. devised a deep-learning model to predict the location of high-risk plaques in nonculprit vessels in patients who underwent IVUS at baseline and after one year . Though large-scale validation is required, the model predicted the occurrence of TCFAs, plaque burden >70%, and minimal luminal area ≤4 mm2 reasonably well at a one-year follow-up on a per-lesion level.

C.Artificial Intelligence-Based Post-Procedure Risk Prediction Models

In addition to early detection and the institution of guideline-directed therapy in the appropriate risk strata, accurate prediction of unheralded adverse events forms the cornerstone for managing CAD. Identifying the high-risk target population can potentially provide a window for aggressive risk factor modulation, thereby reducing mortality and contributing towards better health at a population level. Multiple risk-prediction models have been developed to predict in-hospital mortality and the long-term risk of MACE in high-risk cohorts PCI is a relatively safe procedure, with a reported overall in-hospital mortality rate of 1–2% . The risk of complications increases with increasing patient morbidity, with an incidence of technical difficulties and periprocedural complications 2.2 times higher than in the average population . The Mayo clinic risk score (MCRS) and New York State risk score (NYSRS) were developed to predict in-hospital and 30-day mortality in patients undergoing PCI. Both scores performed equivalently well, showing an excellent discriminative ability to identify patients at a higher risk for in-hospital and 30-day mortality . They employed regression-based models, assuming a linear interplay between patient variables and mortality outcomes. ML models have been recently developed to potentially uncover complex and nonlinear relationships between multiple factors, hence improving diagnostic accuracy over current models.

Zack et al. evaluated 11,709 patients to train two RF regression models—one using 52 demographic and clinical parameters to predict in-hospital mortality and the second model also incorporating 358 discharge variables in addition to the 52 admission parameters to predict 180-day cardiovascular mortality and 30-day heart failure rehospitalization.They compared the model performances against logistic regression models trained using the same variables. No significant difference was found between the RF model and logistic regression in predicting in-hospital mortality (AUC 0.923 vs. 0.925, $p = 0.84$). The ML model performed significantly better than the logistic regression model for prediction of 30-day heart failure hospitalizations (AUC 0.899 vs. 0.846, $p = 0.003$) and 180-day cardiovascular death (AUC 0.881 vs. 0.812, $p = 0.02$).Al'Aref et al. [163] developed a supervised machine learning approach to predict in-hospital mortality among patients undergoing PCI. Utilizing 479,804 patients from the New York state registry, they utilized 49 clinical, angiographic, and periprocedural event characteristics to create a ML model via adaptive boosting. It performed better than the logistic regression model (AUC 0.927 for ML vs. 0.908 for logistic regression, $p < 0.01$). Age and ejection fraction emerged as the most important variables predicting mortality.

Periprocedural bleeding is one of the most common complications of PCI and has been linked to adverse in-hospital outcomes. Current risk scores such as the NCDR bleeding risk-prediction model and the simplified NCDR bleeding-risk score have performed modestly well in identifying patients at a high risk of periprocedural bleeding . To improve the performance of the existing risk model, an ML-based model was developed on 3,316,465 patients enrolled in the CathPCI registry. In addition to the 31 variables used in the existing model, 28 new variables were incorporated to devise an integrated model via the gradient-boosting approach. The blended model using ML had a higher discriminatory power than the existing model (C statistic 0.82 vs. 0.78, $p < 0.05$) and improved the positive predictive value to 26.6%, compared with 21.5% for the existent model.

One of the primary challenges faced in the PCI era is in-stent restenosis, which is linked to neointimal proliferation due to vascular wall damage [168]. The incidence of ISR has been estimated to be 20–40% for bare metallic stents and 10–15% for drug-eluting stents .Smaller vessel size, increasing stent length, complex lesion morphology, diabetes mellitus, and prior bypass surgery are risk factors for stent restenosis . These factors have been incorporated with other variables to devise risk models such as PRESTO 1, PRESTO 2, and EVENT scores to provide an estimated risk of ISR . These models have a modest discriminatory power in predicting ISR, leaving room for improvement. A big-data approach incorporated 68 variables relating to clinical, demographic, and angiographic characteristics to devise a risk prediction model for ISR.The ML model, when applied post-PCI, achieved a higher discriminatory power (AUC for the precision recall curve was 0.45 vs. 0.31, 0.27, and 0.18 for PRESTO-1, PRESTO-2, and EVENT, respectively, $p < 0.05$) to predict ISR at 12 months. Interestingly, post-PCI TIMI flow was one of the prominent predictors of ISR, alongside diabetes mellitus and the presence of ≥2 vessel CAD. Though the model requires external validation, given the small sample size of the population ($n = 263$), the study yet again underscores the merit of ML in identifying crucial parameters from a vast dataset to predict outcomes

D.Artificial Intelligence-Based Long-Term Mortality and MACE Prediction Models

Prognostic modeling via ML has been validated with the use of electronic health records (EHRs) integrated with clinical scores and imaging modalities to predict MACE . Utilizing the array of data available in EMR and identifying patterns based on clinical course, ML models have been used to create a personalized treatment algorithm (ML4CAD) for every patient, based on risk factors,past medical history, time present in the EMR system, and medications. The illustrated model makes clinical decisions for patients based on these factors and suggests a decision with an aim to increase prescription effectiveness, evaluated in the terms of time from initial diagnosis to the first potential adverse event (time to adverse event, TAE). The model had superior performance when compared to standard of care, increasing the time to adverse event (TAE) from 4.56 to 5.66 years (24.3% increase), hence furthering the idea of precision medicine .

Imaging findings, such as CAC score quantified from cardiac computed tomography, are an independent risk factor adding to the traditional clinical risk factors in predicting long-term risk of cardiovascular events Noncontrast CT imaging, other than providing information on the CAC score, provides valuable measures such as epicardial adipose tissue (EAT) volume, and EAT attenuation, all of which have been shown to provide additional information regarding the long-term risk of cardiovascular disease Extracting these pieces of data can be tedious and labor-intensive, and automated techniques can result in more standardized evaluations in a more time-efficient manner.

Multiple ML techniques have been proposed to automatically evaluate CAC score from dedicated cardiac and non-EKG gated chest CT scans ML techniques incorporating CAC score and other imaging parameters have been shown to be a better predictor than the traditional risk scores employed for cardiovascular disease risk stratification. An ensemble-boosting model developed by Nakanishi et al. incorporating a total of 77 clinical and imaging variables had a superior discriminatory power for predicting coronary heart disease deaths than imaging and clinical data alone (AUC for ML model: 0.845 compared to 0.821 and 0.781 for clinical data and CAC respectively, $p < 0.001$)

Apart from CAC scoring and traditional CT metrics, the role of EAT volume and attenuation in the prediction of future cardiovascular risk has been an active area of research. Deep-learning approaches to automatically compute EAT volume and EAT attenuation from CT have been developed,significantly reducing generation time from 15 min to 2 s . Eisenberg et al. demonstrated an independent association between deep-learning-derived EAT volume and attenuation with the risk of future MACE, defined as myocardial infarction, late (>180 days) revascularization, and cardiac death (HR:1.35, $p < 0.01$ and 0.83, $p = 0.01$, demonstrating a direct correlation with EAT volume and an inverse correlation with EAT attenuation respectively) . Subsequently, these parameters have been combined with other physiologic and radiology variables to develop new deep-learning approaches, which have further been shown tohave a higher predictive value than the traditional risk scores.Apart from its role in CAD diagnosis, CCTA has been shown to have an incremental prognostic value in terms of short- and long-term risk prediction. Results from the CONFIRM registry validated two CCTA parameters, namely the number of proximal segments with stenosis > 50% and the number of proximal segments with mixed or calcified plaque as important prognostic markers above the predictive value of the Framingham risk score (FRS)

A multitude of ML approaches have been described, combining imaging parameters with clinical and demographic parameters for better prognostication of cardiovascular outcomes Including 10,030 patients with suspected CAD from the CONFIRM registry, Motwani et al. utilized a boosting ensemble algorithm using 25 clinical and 44 CCTA parameters . The ML algorithm performed better in predicting 5-year all-cause mortality than CCTA segment stenosis score or FRS (AUC 0.79 for ML vs. 0.664 for segment stenosis score and 0.61 for FRS, respectively, $p < 0.001$). More recently, models incorporating high-risk plaque features with the traditional imaging and clinical parameters have performed better than either of the parameters in isolation Although anatomical CT scores and plaque features provide useful diagnostic and prognostic data, the complex interplay of factors at the molecular level, in addition to patient-level characteristics leading to specific phenotypic manifestations in terms of plaque burden and features, is not well-elucidated and remains an area of active research. In particular, elucidating important factors that "drive" the process of atherosclerotic plaque formation and progression is not only vital from a therapeutic perspective, but it can also improve risk-assessment strategies. Recent studies have demonstrated that coronary artery inflammation inhibits lipid accumulation in the perivascular adipose tissue [200]. This results in a higher attenuation of the affected perivascular area, identified on CCTA as the fat attenuation index (FAI). FAI has been shown to be a sensitive marker of coronary inflammation, with higher FAI values (≥−70.1 HU) independently predicting cardiovascular mortality A posthoc analysis of the CRISP-CT study showed an incremental value of adding FAI to high-risk plaque characteristics, pointing towards a more significant role of these precursor lesions in predicting patient outcomes. A more recent ML approach created a pericoronary fat 'radiomic' profile (FRP), identifying radiomic variables predicting tissue inflammation, fibrosis, and vascularity on CCTA . The incorporation of FRP significantly improved the MACE predictive ability of the traditional model (AUC for traditional + FRP 0.88 vs. 0.754 for the traditional model, $p < 0.001$). Using a cut-off of 0.63, individuals in the high FRP group were at a higher risk of MACE (HR = 10.84, $p < 0.001$). Importantly, Kaplan–Meir analysis showed an additional value of FRP over high-risk plaque (HRP) characteristics in predicting long-term survival (HR for the FRP-/HRP+ subgroup 5.97, p = 0.03 compared to 43.33 for the FRP+/HRP+ subgroup). Such 'radiotranscriptomic' approaches incorporating molecular biology and radiology and evaluating their interaction via artificial intelligence can help uncover deeper relationships between metabolic pathways and clinical outcomes, helping to better understand the pathophysiology and elements involved in the clinical progression of cardiovascular disease.With significant developments occurring in the last decade in terms of data processing and analytics, AI can provide new and sophisticated tools that could help us to better understand disease processes, which ultimately should translate into better patient care and outcomes . Nevertheless, AI comes with its own set of limitations. ML models lack interpretability and suffer from the 'black box' problem . ML models based on neural networks and ensemble methods are inherently complex and are derived from complicated mathematical algorithms. 'Explainable (interpretable) machine learning', whereby simple approximations of the model are devised to make it more understandable, is being developed to overcome the black box problem.

Another limitation of ML encountered at the model-development phase is sampling bias and lack of external validation [207,208]. ML learning models usually derive their weights from large datasets. Datasets, particularly those derived from EHRs, might be skewed and not representative of the entire population, leading to significant sampling bias and limited generalizability. A few models have tried to address this problem by stratifying the datasets at the model-development phase to ensure not to lose representation of any subgroup and preserve the model's generalizability. Nevertheless, randomized controlled trials are needed to potentially overcome this bias and establish the model performance against the standard clinical parameters. In addition, imputation methods such as MICE have been used to address the missing data issue Furthermore, the creation of bigger datasets by pooling data from multiple hospital systems has led to a lack of standardization of datasets, potentially compromising the quality of analysis. Datasets might internally differ from each other because of the different mechanisms used to generate them. For instance, one dataset might define the presence of diabetes mellitus through ICD-10 codes, while another dataset might define it using glycemic indices, such as the hemoglobin A1c. On a similar theme, ML models developed by using imaging modalities deserve a special mention. For instance, differences can exist at the level of image scanning (different scanner characteristics and vendors), image quality (radiation dose, motion artifacts), and image processing (reconstruction filters, post-processing) which can potentially lead to significant variability and differences of the assimilated data. A prerequisite to the development of any ML model is the centralization of data, which is tedious given the different image processing algorithms employed at various institutions. This lack of standardization needs to be addressed before AI can be fully integrated into clinical practice.

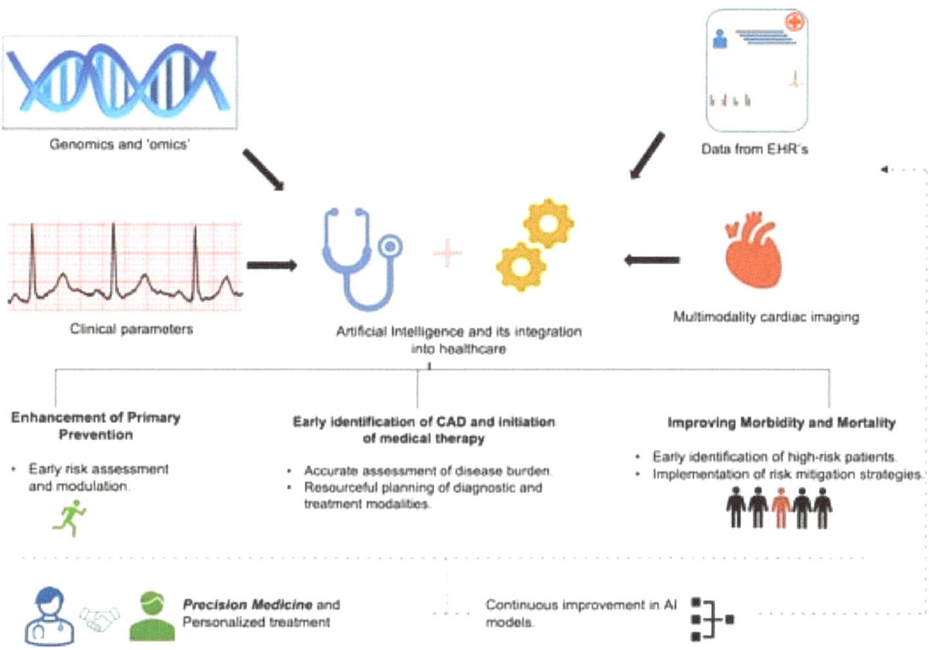

Fig.8.4 Current applicability and future directions for AI in coronary artery disease.

Overfitting is another concern encountered during ML model development, which occurs when the algorithm learns the data 'too well' and interprets the signal noise as concepts . This usually happens with smaller datasets and can lead to a lack of external validity, despite high performance in the training and internal validation datasets. A definite solution is k-fold cross-validation, whereby data is randomly divided into an arbitrary k number of partitions. The model is trained using k − 1 number of data subsets and tested on the remaining subset. This process is repeated k total number of times, using different combinations of training and testing datasets to select the best model hyper-parameters to yield the final model. This can potentially reduce noise and lead to better generalizability of the model in the overall population.Apart from the problems encountered at the model development and training phase, there are a few noteworthy practical limitations to the implementation of ML within healthcare workflows. Firstly, unauthorized data access is an issue, as handling such large amounts of data also poses a risk of leaking sensitive patient information, thereby violating patient confidentiality and privacy Furthermore, comparisons between various machine-learning methods are difficult, given the different combinations of model parameters and different population characteristics used for in model development. Hence, it becomes difficult for physicians to compare and choose one model over the other. Prospective future trials, comparing these models on the same dataset, are needed to select the best algorithm fit for integration into routine clinical decision-making. Proper integration of AI can only be achieved once these models are embedded within EHRs. However, the full implementation and assimilation of developed AI models into EHRs can be a complex issue, as it depends on organizational resources and patient-privacy policies. Furthermore, available algorithms may be limited to off-the-shelf ML models, rather than more intricate and complex neural networks, which is easier to implement in a real clinical setting. Yet, a data-driven approach utilizing advanced analytic techniques can help clinicians and patients to make informed decisions, improve care, and optimize workflow efficiency.

Bibliography And Acknowledgement

- Acharya, U.R.; Fujita, H.; Sudarshan, V.K.; Oh, S.L.; Adam, M.; Koh, J.E.W.; Tan, J.H.; Ghista, D.N.; Martis, R.J.; Chua, C.K.; et al. Automated detection and localization of myocardial infarction using electrocardiogram: A comparative study of different leads. Knowl.-Based Syst. 2016, 99, 146–156
- Agatston, A.S.; Janowitz, W.R.; Hildner, F.J.; Zusmer, N.R.; Viamonte, M., Jr.; Detrano, R. Quantification of coronary artery calcium using ultrafast computed tomography. J. Am. Coll. Cardiol. 1990, 15, 827–832.
- Al'Aref, S.J.; Singh, G.; van Rosendael, A.R.; Kolli, K.K.; Ma, X.; Maliakal, G.; Pandey, M.; Lee, B.C.; Wang, J.; Xu, Z.; et al. Determinants of In-Hospital Mortality after Percutaneous Coronary Intervention: A Machine Learning Approach. J. Am. Heart Assoc. 2019, 8, e011160
- Ali, Z.A.; Karimi Galougahi, K.; Maehara, A.; Shlofmitz, R.A.; Ben-Yehuda, O.; Mintz, G.S.; Stone, G.W. Intracoronary Optical Coherence Tomography 2018: Current Status and Future Directions. JACC Cardiovasc. Interv. 2017, 10, 2473–2487
- Aragam, K.G.; Natarajan, P. Polygenic Scores to Assess Atherosclerotic Cardiovascular Disease Risk: Clinical Perspectives and Basic Implications. Circ. Res. 2020, 126, 1159–1177.
- Arbab-Zadeh, A.; Miller, J.M.; Rochitte, C.E.; Dewey, M.; Niinuma, H.; Gottlieb, I.; Paul, N.; Clouse, M.E.; Shapiro, E.P.; Hoe, J.; et al. Diagnostic accuracy of computed tomography coronary angiography according to pre-test probability of coronary artery disease and severity of coronary arterial calcification. The CORE-64 (Coronary Artery Evaluation Using 64-Row Multidetector Computed Tomography Angiography) International Multicenter Study. J. Am. Coll. Cardiol. 2012, 59, 379–387
- Arjmand Shabestari, A. Coronary artery calcium score: A review. Iran Red. Crescent. Med. J. 2013, 15, e16616.
- Arnett, D.K.; Blumenthal, R.S.; Albert, M.A.; Buroker, A.B.; Goldberger, Z.D.; Hahn, E.J.; Himmelfarb, C.D.; Khera, A.; Lloyd-Jones, D.; McEvoy, J.W.; et al. 2019 ACC/AHA Guideline on the Primary Prevention of Cardiovascular Disease: A Report of the American College of Cardiology/American Heart Association Task Force on Clinical Practice Guidelines. Circulation 2019, 140
- Arsanjani, R.; Dey, D.; Khachatryan, T.; Shalev, A.; Hayes, S.W.; Fish, M.; Nakanishi, R.; Germano, G.; Berman, D.S.; Slomka, P. Prediction of revascularization after myocardial perfusion SPECT by machine learning in a large population. J. Nucl. Cardiol. 2015, 22, 877–884.
- Arsanjani, R.; Xu, Y.; Dey, D.; Fish, M.; Dorbala, S.; Hayes, S.; Berman, D.; Germano, G.; Slomka, P. Improved accuracy of myocardial perfusion SPECT for the detection of coronary artery disease using a support vector machine algorithm. J. Nucl. Med. 2013, 54, 549–555.
- Arsanjani, R.; Xu, Y.; Dey, D.; Vahistha, V.; Shalev, A.; Nakanishi, R.; Hayes, S.; Fish, M.; Berman, D.; Germano, G.; et al. Improved accuracy of myocardial perfusion SPECT for detection of coronary artery disease by machine learning in a large population. J. Nucl. Cardiol. 2013, 20, 553–562
- Baskaran, L.; Maliakal, G.; Al'Aref, S.J.; Singh, G.; Xu, Z.; Michalak, K.; Dolan, K.; Gianni, U.; van Rosendael, A.; van den Hoogen, I.; et al. Identification and Quantification of Cardiovascular Structures From CCTA: An End-to-End, Rapid, Pixel-Wise, Deep-Learning Method. JACC Cardiovasc. Imaging 2020, 13, 1163–1171.
- Baskaran, L.; Ying, X.; Xu, Z.; Al'Aref, S.J.; Lee, B.C.; Lee, S.E.; Danad, I.; Park, H.B.; Bathina, R.; Baggiano, A.; et al. Machine learning insight into the role of imaging and clinical variables for the prediction of obstructive coronary artery disease and revascularization: An exploratory analysis of the CONSERVE study. PLoS ONE 2020, 15, e0233791
- Betancur, J.; Commandeur, F.; Motlagh, M.; Sharir, T.; Einstein, A.J.; Bokhari, S.; Fish, M.B.; Ruddy, T.D.; Kaufmann, P.; Sinusas, A.J.; et al. Deep Learning for Prediction of Obstructive Disease From Fast Myocardial Perfusion SPECT: A Multicenter Study. JACC Cardiovasc. Imaging 2018, 11, 1654–1663.
- Betancur, J.; Hu, L.H.; Commandeur, F.; Sharir, T.; Einstein, A.J.; Fish, M.B.; Ruddy, T.D.; Kaufmann, P.A.; Sinusas, A.J.; Miller, E.J.; et al. Deep Learning Analysis of Upright-Supine High-Efficiency SPECT Myocardial Perfusion Imaging for Prediction of Obstructive Coronary Artery Disease: A Multicenter Study. J. Nucl. Med. 2019, 60, 664–670
- Biagini, E.; Shaw, L.J.; Poldermans, D.; Schinkel, A.F.; Rizzello, V.; Elhendy, A.; Rapezzi, C.; Bax, J.J. Accuracy of non-invasive techniques for diagnosis of coronary artery disease and prediction of cardiac events in patients with left bundle branch block: A meta-analysis. Eur. J. Nucl. Med. Mol. Imaging 2006, 33, 1442–1451.
- Bittencourt, M.S.; Hulten, E.; Polonsky, T.S.; Hoffman, U.; Nasir, K.; Abbara, S.; Di Carli, M.; Blankstein, R. European Society of Cardiology-Recommended Coronary Artery Disease Consortium Pretest Probability Scores More Accurately Predict Obstructive Coronary Disease and Cardiovascular Events Than the Diamond and Forrester Score: The Partners Registry. Circulation 2016, 134, 201–211.
- Boeddinghaus, J.; Nestelberger, T.; Twerenbold, R.; Neumann, J.T.; Lindahl, B.; Giannitsis, E.; Sörensen, N.A.; Badertscher, P.; Jann, J.E.; Wussler, D.; et al. Impact of age on the performance of the ESC 0/1h-algorithms for early diagnosis of myocardial infarction. Eur. Heart J. 2018, 39, 3780–3794
- Brautbar, A.; Pompeii, L.A.; Dehghan, A.; Ngwa, J.S.; Nambi, V.; Virani, S.S.; Rivadeneira, F.; Uitterlinden, A.G.; Hofman, A.; Witteman, J.C.; et al. A genetic risk score based on direct associations with coronary heart disease improves coronary heart disease risk prediction in the Atherosclerosis Risk in Communities (ARIC), but not in the Rotterdam and Framingham Offspring, Studies. Atherosclerosis 2012, 223, 421–426.
- Brown, A.J.; Teng, Z.; Calvert, P.A.; Rajani, N.K.; Hennessy, O.; Nerlekar, N.; Obaid, D.R.; Costopoulos, C.; Huang, Y.; Hoole, S.P.; et al. Plaque Structural Stress Estimations Improve Prediction of Future Major Adverse Cardiovascular Events After Intracoronary Imaging. Circ. Cardiovasc. Imaging 2016, 9,
- Cabitza, F.; Rasoini, R.; Gensini, G.F. Unintended Consequences of Machine Learning in Medicine. JAMA 2017, 318, 517–518.
- Cassese, S.; Byrne, R.A.; Tada, T.; Pinieck, S.; Joner, M.; Ibrahim, T.; King, L.A.; Fusaro, M.; Laugwitz, K.L.; Kastrati, A. Incidence and predictors of restenosis after coronary stenting in 10 004 patients with surveillance angiography. Heart 2014, 100, 153–159.

- Chao, H.; Shan, H.; Homayounieh, F.; Singh, R.; Khera, R.D.; Guo, H.; Su, T.; Wang, G.; Kalra, M.K.; Yan, P. Deep learning predicts cardiovascular disease risks from lung cancer screening low dose computed tomography. Nat. Commun. 2021, 12, 2963.
- Chen, C.-C.; Chen, C.-C.; Hsieh, I.C.; Liu, Y.-C.; Liu, C.-Y.; Chan, T.; Wen, M.-S.; Wan, Y.-L. The effect of calcium score on the diagnostic accuracy of coronary computed tomography angiography. Int. J. Cardiovasc. Imaging 2011, 27, 37–42
- Cheng, J.M.; Garcia-Garcia, H.M.; de Boer, S.P.; Kardys, I.; Heo, J.H.; Akkerhuis, K.M.; Oemrawsingh, R.M.; van Domburg, R.T.; Ligthart, J.; Witberg, K.T.; et al. In vivo detection of high-risk coronary plaques by radiofrequency intravascular ultrasound and cardiovascular outcome: Results of the ATHEROREMO-IVUS study. Eur. Heart J. 2014, 35, 639–647. .
- Cho, H.; Kang, S.J.; Min, H.S.; Lee, J.G.; Kim, W.J.; Kang, S.H.; Kang, D.Y.; Lee, P.H.; Ahn, J.M.; Park, D.W.; et al. Intravascular ultrasound-based deep learning for plaque characterization in coronary artery disease. Atherosclerosis 2021, 324, 69–75.
- Chowdhary, S.; Ivanov, J.; Mackie, K.; Seidelin, P.H.; Dzavík, V. The Toronto score for in-hospital mortality after percutaneous coronary interventions. Am. Heart J. 2009, 157, 156–163.
- Collet, J.P.; Thiele, H.; Barbato, E.; Barthelemy, O.; Bauersachs, J.; Bhatt, D.L.; Dendale, P.; Dorobantu, M.; Edvardsen, T.; Folliguet, T.; et al. 2020 ESC Guidelines for the management of acute coronary syndromes in patients presenting without persistent ST-segment elevation. Eur. Heart J. 2021, 42, 1289–1367.
- Commandeur, F.; Slomka, P.J.; Goeller, M.; Chen, X.; Cadet, S.; Razipour, A.; McElhinney, P.; Gransar, H.; Cantu, S.; Miller, R.J.H.; et al. Machine learning to predict the long-term risk of myocardial infarction and cardiac death based on clinical risk, coronary calcium, and epicardial adipose tissue: A prospective study. Cardiovasc. Res. 2020, 116, 2216–2225
- Cook, C.M.; Petraco, R.; Shun-Shin, M.J.; Ahmad, Y.; Nijjer, S.; Al-Lamee, R.; Kikuta, Y.; Shiono, Y.; Mayet, J.; Francis, D.P.; et al. Diagnostic Accuracy of Computed Tomography–Derived Fractional Flow Reserve: A Systematic Review. JAMA Cardiol. 2017, 2, 803–810
- Detrano, R.; Guerci, A.D.; Carr, J.J.; Bild, D.E.; Burke, G.; Folsom, A.R.; Liu, K.; Shea, S.; Szklo, M.; Bluemke, D.A.; et al. Coronary Calcium as a Predictor of Coronary Events in Four Racial or Ethnic Groups. N. Engl. J. Med. 2008, 358, 1336–1345
- Dey, D.; Slomka, P.J.; Leeson, P.; Comaniciu, D.; Shrestha, S.; Sengupta, P.P.; Marwick, T.H. Artificial Intelligence in Cardiovascular Imaging: JACC State-of-the-Art Review. J. Am. Coll. Cardiol. 2019, 73, 1317–1335.
- Di Jiang, M.; Zhang, X.L.; Liu, H.; Tang, C.X.; Li, J.H.; Wang, Y.N.; Xu, P.P.; Zhou, C.S.; Zhou, F.; Lu, M.J.; et al. The effect of coronary calcification on diagnostic performance of machine learning-based CT-FFR: A Chinese multicenter study. Eur. Radiol. 2021, 31, 1482–1493.
- Dogan, M.V.; Grumbach, I.M.; Michaelson, J.J.; Philibert, R.A. Integrated genetic and epigenetic prediction of coronary heart disease in the Framingham Heart Study. PLoS ONE 2018, 13,
- Druey, S.; Wildi, K.; Twerenbold, R.; Jaeger, C.; Reichlin, T.; Haaf, P.; Gimenez, M.R.; Puelacher, C.; Wagener, M.; Radosavac, M. Early rule-out and rule-in of myocardial infarction using sensitive cardiac Troponin I. Int. J. Cardiol. 2015, 195, 163–170.
- Eisenberg, E.; McElhinney, P.A.; Commandeur, F.; Chen, X.; Cadet, S.; Goeller, M.; Razipour, A.; Gransar, H.; Cantu, S.; Miller, R.J.H.; et al. Deep Learning-Based Quantification of Epicardial Adipose Tissue Volume and Attenuation Predicts Major Adverse Cardiovascular Events in Asymptomatic Subjects. Circ. Cardiovasc. Imaging 2020, 13,
- Eraslan, G.; Avsec, Ž.; Gagneur, J.; Theis, F.J. Deep learning: New computational modelling techniques for genomics. Nat. Rev. Genet. 2019, 20, 389–403.
- Erdmann, J.; Kessler, T.; Munoz Venegas, L.; Schunkert, H. A decade of genome-wide association studies for coronary artery disease: The challenges ahead. Cardiovasc. Res. 2018, 114, 1241–1257. [
- Fanaroff, A.C.; Zakroysky, P.; Dai, D.; Wojdyla, D.; Sherwood, M.W.; Roe, M.T.; Wang, T.Y.; Peterson, E.D.; Gurm, H.S.; Cohen, M.G.; et al. Outcomes of PCI in Relation to Procedural Characteristics and Operator Volumes in the United States. J. Am. Coll. Cardiol. 2017, 69, 2913–2924.
- Farhadian, M.; Dehdar Karsidani, S.; Mozayanimonfared, A.; Mahjub, H. Risk factors associated with major adverse cardiac and cerebrovascular events following percutaneous coronary intervention: A 10-year follow-up comparing random survival forest and Cox proportional-hazards model. BMC Cardiovasc. Disord. 2021, 21, 38.
- Ferguson, J.F.; Matthews, G.J.; Townsend, R.R.; Raj, D.S.; Kanetsky, P.A.; Budoff, M.; Fischer, M.J.; Rosas, S.E.; Kanthety, R.; Rahman, M.; et al. Candidate gene association study of coronary artery calcification in chronic kidney disease: Findings from the CRIC study (Chronic Renal Insufficiency Cohort). J. Am. Coll. Cardiol. 2013, 62, 789–798.
- Foldyna, B.; Udelson, J.E.; Karády, J.; Banerji, D.; Lu, M.T.; Mayrhofer, T.; Bittner, D.O.; Meyersohn, N.M.; Emami, H.; Genders, T.S.S.; et al. Pretest probability for patients with suspected obstructive coronary artery disease: Re-evaluating Diamond-Forrester for the contemporary era and clinical implications: Insights from the PROMISE trial. Eur. Heart J. Cardiovasc. Imaging 2019, 20, 574–581.
- Fujii, K.; Carlier, S.G.; Mintz, G.S.; Yang, Y.M.; Moussa, I.; Weisz, G.; Dangas, G.; Mehran, R.; Lansky, A.J.; Kreps, E.M.; et al. Stent underexpansion and residual reference segment stenosis are related to stent thrombosis after sirolimus-eluting stent implantation: An intravascular ultrasound study. J. Am. Coll. Cardiol. 2005, 45, 995–998.
- Gaur, S.; Ovrehus, K.A.; Dey, D.; Leipsic, J.; Botker, H.E.; Jensen, J.M.; Narula, J.; Ahmadi, A.; Achenbach, S.; Ko, B.S.; et al. Coronary plaque quantification and fractional flow reserve by coronary computed tomography angiography identify ischaemia-causing lesions. Eur. Heart J. 2016, 37, 1220–1227
- Genders, T.S.; Steyerberg, E.W.; Alkadhi, H.; Leschka, S.; Desbiolles, L.; Nieman, K.; Galema, T.W.; Meijboom, W.B.; Mollet, N.R.; de Feyter, P.J.; et al. A clinical prediction rule for the diagnosis of coronary artery disease: Validation, updating, and extension. Eur. Heart J. 2011, 32, 1316–1330

- Gimenez, M.R.; Twerenbold, R.; Jaeger, C.; Schindler, C.; Puelacher, C.; Wildi, K.; Reichlin, T.; Haaf, P.; Merk, S.; Honegger, U. One-hour rule-in and rule-out of acute myocardial infarction using high-sensitivity cardiac troponin I. Am. J. Med. 2015, 128, 861–870.
- Guner, L.A.; Karabacak, N.I.; Akdemir, O.U.; Karagoz, P.S.; Kocaman, S.A.; Cengel, A.; Unlu, M. An open-source framework of neural networks for diagnosis of coronary artery disease from myocardial perfusion SPECT. J. Nucl. Cardiol. 2010, 17, 405–413
- Hachamovitch, R.; Hayes, S.W.; Friedman, J.D.; Cohen, I.; Berman, D.S. A prognostic score for prediction of cardiac mortality risk after adenosine stress myocardial perfusion scintigraphy. J. Am. Coll. Cardiol. 2005, 45, 722–729.
- Hadamitzky, M.; Achenbach, S.; Al-Mallah, M.; Berman, D.; Budoff, M.; Cademartiri, F.; Callister, T.; Chang, H.J.; Cheng, V.; Chinnaiyan, K.; et al. Optimized prognostic score for coronary computed tomographic angiography: Results from the CONFIRM registry (COronary CT Angiography Evaluation For Clinical Outcomes: An InteRnational Multicenter Registry). J. Am. Coll. Cardiol. 2013, 62, 468–476.
- Han, C.; Shi, L. ML–ResNet: A novel network to detect and locate myocardial infarction using 12 leads ECG. Comput. Methods Programs Biomed. 2020, 185, 105138.
- Han, D.; Kolli, K.K.; Gransar, H.; Lee, J.H.; Choi, S.Y.; Chun, E.J.; Han, H.W.; Park, S.H.; Sung, J.; Jung, H.O.; et al. Machine learning based risk prediction model for asymptomatic individuals who underwent coronary artery calcium score: Comparison with traditional risk prediction approaches. J. Cardiovasc. Comput. Tomogr. 2020, 14, 168–176
- Han, D.; Lee, J.H.; Rizvi, A.; Gransar, H.; Baskaran, L.; Schulman-Marcus, J.; Hartaigh, B.ó.; Lin, F.Y.; Min, J.K. Incremental role of resting myocardial computed tomography perfusion for predicting physiologically significant coronary artery disease: A machine learning approach. J. Nucl. Cardiol. 2018, 25, 223–233.
- Hannan, E.L.; Farrell, L.S.; Walford, G.; Jacobs, A.K.; Berger, P.B.; Holmes, D.R., Jr.; Stamato, N.J.; Sharma, S.; King, S.B., 3rd. The New York State risk score for predicting in-hospital/30-day mortality following percutaneous coronary intervention. JACC Cardiovasc. Interv. 2013, 6, 614–622
- Holder, L.; Lewis, S.; Abrames, E.; Wolin, E.A. Review of SPECT myocardial perfusion imaging. J. Am. Osteopath. Coll. Radiol. 2016, 5, 5–13.
- Hong, M.K.; Mintz, G.S.; Lee, C.W.; Park, D.W.; Choi, B.R.; Park, K.H.; Kim, Y.H.; Cheong, S.S.; Song, J.K.; Kim, J.J.; et al. Intravascular ultrasound predictors of angiographic restenosis after sirolimus-eluting stent implantation. Eur. Heart J. 2006, 27, 1305–1310
- Hoshino, M.; Zhang, J.; Sugiyama, T.; Yang, S.; Kanaji, Y.; Hamaya, R.; Yamaguchi, M.; Hada, M.; Misawa, T.; Usui, E.; et al. Prognostic value of pericoronary inflammation and unsupervised machine-learning-defined phenotypic clustering of CT angiographic findings. Int. J. Cardiol. 2021, 333, 226–232
- Hu, L.H.; Betancur, J.; Sharir, T.; Einstein, A.J.; Bokhari, S.; Fish, M.B.; Ruddy, T.D.; Kaufmann, P.A.; Sinusas, A.J.; Miller, E.J.; et al. Machine learning predicts per-vessel early coronary revascularization after fast myocardial perfusion SPECT: Results from multicentre REFINE SPECT registry. Eur. Heart J. Cardiovasc. Imaging 2020, 21, 549–559.
- Huang, M.-S.; Wang, C.-S.; Chiang, J.-H.; Liu, P.-Y.; Tsai, W.-C. Automated Recognition of Regional Wall Motion Abnormalities Through Deep Neural Network Interpretation of Transthoracic Echocardiography. Circulation 2020, 142, 1510–1520.
- Hwang, I.-C.; Park, H.E.; Choi, S.-Y. Epicardial Adipose Tissue Contributes to the Development of Non-Calcified Coronary Plaque: A 5-Year Computed Tomography Follow-up Study. J. Atheroscler. Thromb. 2017, 24, 262–274.
- Itu, L.; Rapaka, S.; Passerini, T.; Georgescu, B.; Schwemmer, C.; Schoebinger, M.; Flohr, T.; Sharma, P.; Comaniciu, D. A machine-learning approach for computation of fractional flow reserve from coronary computed tomography. J. Appl. Physiol. 2016, 121, 42–52.
- Iverson, A.; Stanberry, L.I.; Tajti, P.; Garberich, R.; Antos, A.; Burke, M.N.; Chavez, I.; Gössl, M.; Henry, T.D.; Lips, D.; et al. Prevalence, Trends, and Outcomes of Higher-Risk Percutaneous Coronary Interventions Among Patients without Acute Coronary Syndromes. Cardiovasc. Revasc. Med. 2019, 20, 289–292.
- Jaarsma, C.; Leiner, T.; Bekkers Sebastiaan, C.; Crijns Harry, J.; Wildberger Joachim, E.; Nagel, E.; Nelemans Patricia, J.; Schalla, S. Diagnostic Performance of Noninvasive Myocardial Perfusion Imaging Using Single-Photon Emission Computed Tomography, Cardiac Magnetic Resonance, and Positron Emission Tomography Imaging for the Detection of Obstructive Coronary Artery Disease. J. Am. Coll. Cardiol. 2012, 59, 1719–1728. [
- Johnson, K.M.; Dowe, D.A. Prognostic Implications of Coronary CT Angiography: 12-Year Follow-Up of 6892 Patients. AJR Am. J. Roentgenol. 2020, 215, 818–827.
- Johnson, K.M.; Johnson, H.E.; Zhao, Y.; Dowe, D.A.; Staib, L.H. Scoring of Coronary Artery Disease Characteristics on Coronary CT Angiograms by Using Machine Learning. Radiology 2019, 292, 354–362.
- Johnson, K.W.; Torres Soto, J.; Glicksberg, B.S.; Shameer, K.; Miotto, R.; Ali, M.; Ashley, E.; Dudley, J.T. Artificial Intelligence in Cardiology. J. Am. Coll. Cardiol. 2018, 71, 2668–2679.
- Kathiresan, S.; Melander, O.; Anevski, D.; Guiducci, C.; Burtt, N.P.; Roos, C.; Hirschhorn, J.N.; Berglund, G.; Hedblad, B.; Groop, L.; et al. Polymorphisms associated with cholesterol and risk of cardiovascular events. N. Engl. J. Med. 2008, 358, 1240–1249.
- Kawasaki, T.; Kidoh, M.; Kido, T.; Sueta, D.; Fujimoto, S.; Kumamaru, K.K.; Uetani, T.; Tanabe, Y.; Ueda, T.; Sakabe, D.; et al. Evaluation of Significant Coronary Artery Disease Based on CT Fractional Flow Reserve and Plaque Characteristics Using Random Forest Analysis in Machine Learning. Acad. Radiol. 2020, 27, 1700–1708.
- Keller, T.; Zeller, T.; Ojeda, F.; Tzikas, S.; Lillpopp, L.; Sinning, C.; Wild, P.; Genth-Zotz, S.; Warnholtz, A.; Giannitsis, E. Serial changes in highly sensitive troponin I assay and early diagnosis of myocardial infarction. JAMA 2011, 306, 2684–2693.
- Kinnaird, T.D.; Stabile, E.; Mintz, G.S.; Lee, C.W.; Canos, D.A.; Gevorkian, N.; Pinnow, E.E.; Kent, K.M.; Pichard, A.D.; Satler, L.F.; et al. Incidence, predictors, and prognostic implications of bleeding and blood transfusion following percutaneous coronary interventions. Am. J. Cardiol. 2003, 92, 930–935

- Lee, J.-G.; Kim, H.; Kang, H.; Koo, H.J.; Kang, J.-W.; Kim, Y.-H.; Yang, D.H. Fully Automatic Coronary Calcium Score Software Empowered by Artificial Intelligence Technology: Validation Study Using Three CT Cohorts. Korean J. Radiol. 2021, 22, 1764–1776.
- Li, D.; Xiong, G.; Zeng, H.; Zhou, Q.; Jiang, J.; Guo, X. Machine learning-aided risk stratification system for the prediction of coronary artery disease. Int. J. Cardiol. 2021, 326, 30–34.
- Lih, O.S.; Jahmunah, V.; San, T.R.; Ciaccio, E.J.; Yamakawa, T.; Tanabe, M.; Kobayashi, M.; Faust, O.; Acharya, U.R. Comprehensive electrocardiographic diagnosis based on deep learning. Artif. Intell. Med. 2020, 103, 101789
- Lin, S.; Li, Z.; Fu, B.; Chen, S.; Li, X.; Wang, Y.; Wang, X.; Lv, B.; Xu, B.; Song, X.; et al. Feasibility of using deep learning to detect coronary artery disease based on facial photo. Eur. Heart J. 2020, 41, 4400–4411
- Liu, C.Y.; Tang, C.X.; Zhang, X.L.; Chen, S.; Xie, Y.; Zhang, X.Y.; Qiao, H.Y.; Zhou, C.S.; Xu, P.P.; Lu, M.J.; et al. Deep learning powered coronary CT angiography for detecting obstructive coronary artery disease: The effect of reader experience, calcification and image quality. Eur. J. Radiol. 2021, 142, 109835.
- Mahajan, N.; Polavaram, L.; Vankayala, H.; Ference, B.; Wang, Y.; Ager, J.; Kovach, J.; Afonso, L. Diagnostic accuracy of myocardial perfusion imaging and stress echocardiography for the diagnosis of left main and triple vessel coronary artery disease: A comparative meta-analysis. Heart 2010, 96, 956–966
- Malik, A.H.; Yandrapalli, S.; Aronow, W.S.; Panza, J.A.; Cooper, H.A. Intravascular ultrasound-guided stent implantation reduces cardiovascular mortality—Updated meta-analysis of randomized controlled trials. Int. J. Cardiol. 2020, 299, 100–105.
- Muscogiuri, G.; Chiesa, M.; Trotta, M.; Gatti, M.; Palmisano, V.; Dell'Aversana, S.; Baessato, F.; Cavaliere, A.; Cicala, G.; Loffreno, A.; et al. Performance of a deep learning algorithm for the evaluation of CAD-RADS classification with CCTA. Atherosclerosis 2020, 294, 25–32.
- Nair, A.; Kuban, B.D.; Tuzcu, E.M.; Schoenhagen, P.; Nissen, S.E.; Vince, D.G. Coronary Plaque Classification With Intravascular Ultrasound Radiofrequency Data Analysis. Circulation 2002, 106, 2200–2206.
- Nakanishi, R.; Rajani, R.; Cheng, V.Y.; Gransar, H.; Nakazato, R.; Shmilovich, H.; Otaki, Y.; Hayes, S.W.; Thomson, L.E.; Friedman, J.D.; et al. Increase in epicardial fat volume is associated with greater coronary artery calcification progression in subjects at intermediate risk by coronary calcium score: A serial study using non-contrast cardiac CT. Atherosclerosis 2011, 218, 363–368.
- Nous, F.M.A.; Budde, R.P.J.; Lubbers, M.M.; Yamasaki, Y.; Kardys, I.; Bruning, T.A.; Akkerhuis, J.M.; Kofflard, M.J.M.; Kietselaer, B.; Galema, T.W.; et al. Impact of machine-learning CT-derived fractional flow reserve for the diagnosis and management of coronary artery disease in the randomized CRESCENT trials. Eur. Radiol. 2020, 30, 3692–3701
- O'Connor, G.T.; Malenka, D.J.; Quinton, H.; Robb, J.F.; Kellett, M.A., Jr.; Shubrooks, S.; Bradley, W.A.; Hearne, M.J.; Watkins, M.W.; Wennberg, D.E.; et al. Multivariate prediction of in-hospital mortality after percutaneous coronary interventions in 1994-1996. Northern New England Cardiovascular Disease Study Group. J. Am. Coll. Cardiol. 1999, 34, 681–691.
- Patel, V.L.; Shortliffe, E.H.; Stefanelli, M.; Szolovits, P.; Berthold, M.R.; Bellazzi, R.; Abu-Hanna, A. The coming of age of artificial intelligence in medicine. Artif. Intell. Med. 2009, 46, 5–17.
- Qiao, H.Y.; Tang, C.X.; Schoepf, U.J.; Tesche, C.; Bayer, R.R., 2nd; Giovagnoli, D.A.; Todd Hudson, H., Jr.; Zhou, C.S.; Yan, J.; Lu, M.J.; et al. Impact of machine learning-based coronary computed tomography angiography fractional flow reserve on treatment decisions and clinical outcomes in patients with suspected coronary artery disease. Eur. Radiol. 2020, 30, 5841–5851.
- Rabbat, M.; Leipsic, J.; Bax, J.; Kauh, B.; Verma, R.; Doukas, D.; Allen, S.; Pontone, G.; Wilber, D.; Mathew, V.; et al. Fractional Flow Reserve Derived from Coronary Computed Tomography Angiography Safely Defers Invasive Coronary Angiography in Patients with Stable Coronary Artery Disease. J. Clin. Med. 2020, 9, 604
- Ranka, S.; Reddy, M.; Noheria, A. Artificial intelligence in cardiovascular medicine. Curr. Opin. Cardiol. 2021, 36, 26–35
- Sandstedt, M.; Henriksson, L.; Janzon, M.; Nyberg, G.; Engvall, J.; De Geer, J.; Alfredsson, J.; Persson, A. Evaluation of an AI-based, automatic coronary artery calcium scoring software. Eur. Radiol. 2020, 30, 1671–1678.
- Tang, C.X.; Wang, Y.N.; Zhou, F.; Schoepf, U.J.; Assen, M.V.; Stroud, R.E.; Li, J.H.; Zhang, X.L.; Lu, M.J.; Zhou, C.S.; et al. Diagnostic performance of fractional flow reserve derived from coronary CT angiography for detection of lesion-specific ischemia: A multi-center study and meta-analysis. Eur. J. Radiol. 2019, 116, 90–97
- Tat, E.; Bhatt, D.L.; Rabbat, M.G. Addressing bias: Artificial intelligence in cardiovascular medicine. Lancet Digit Health 2020, 2,
- van Rosendael, A.R.; Maliakal, G.; Kolli, K.K.; Beecy, A.; Al'Aref, S.J.; Dwivedi, A.; Singh, G.; Panday, M.; Kumar, A.; Ma, X.; et al. Maximization of the usage of coronary CTA derived plaque information using a machine learning based algorithm to improve risk stratification; insights from the CONFIRM registry. J. Cardiovasc. Comput. Tomogr. 2018, 12, 204–209
- Vokinger, K.N.; Feuerriegel, S.; Kesselheim, A.S. Mitigating bias in machine learning for medicine. Commun. Med. 2021, 1, 25.
  Wu, C.; Hannan, E.L.; Walford, G.; Ambrose, J.A.; Holmes, D.R., Jr.; King, S.B., 3rd; Clark, L.T.; Katz, S.; Sharma, S.; Jones, R.H. A risk score to predict in-hospital mortality for percutaneous coronary interventions. J. Am. Coll. Cardiol. 2006, 47, 654–660.
- Xie, Z.; Dong, N.; Sun, R.; Liu, X.; Gu, X.; Sun, Y.; Du, H.; Dai, J.; Liu, Y.; Hou, J.; et al. Relation between baseline plaque features and subsequent coronary artery remodeling determined by optical coherence tomography and intravascular ultrasound. Oncotarget 2017, 8, 4234–4244.
- Yeri, A.; Shah, R.V. Comparison of Computational Fluid Dynamics and Machine Learning-Based Fractional Flow Reserve in Coronary Artery Disease. Circ. Cardiovasc. Imaging 2018, 11,
- Zreik, M.; van Hamersvelt, R.W.; Khalili, N.; Wolterink, J.M.; Voskuil, M.; Viergever, M.A.; Leiner, T.; Isgum, I. Deep Learning Analysis of Coronary Arteries in Cardiac CT Angiography for Detection of Patients Requiring Invasive Coronary Angiography. IEEE Trans. Med. Imaging 2020, 39, 1545–1557.

Machine Learning and Artificial Intelligence to Improve Peripheral Artery Disease Management

CHAPTER

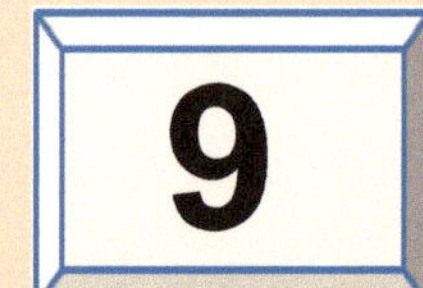

Peripheral artery disease is an atherosclerotic disorder which, when present, portends poor patient outcomes. Low diagnosis rates perpetuate poor management, leading to limb loss and excess rates of cardiovascular morbidity and death. Machine learning algorithms and artificially intelligent systems have shown great promise in application to many areas in health care, such as accurately detecting disease, predicting patient outcomes, and automating image interpretation. Although the application of these technologies to peripheral artery disease are in their infancy, their promises are tremendous. In this review, we provide an introduction to important concepts in the fields of machine learning and artificial intelligence, detail the current state of how these technologies have been applied to peripheral artery disease, and discuss potential areas for future care enhancement with advanced analytics.

The first Circulation Research Compendium on Peripheral Artery Disease (PAD) was assembled in 2015, powerfully noting that many with PAD are dying of neglect. Despite being a major atherosclerotic disease with a global prevalence of >200 million,2 physicians often fail to diagnose PAD, due in part to conflicting screening recommendations, low patient and provider awareness, and the high prevalence of asymptomatic or atypical symptoms. Even once recognized by clinicians, rates of initiation of evidence-based therapies lag that of other atherosclerotic diseases, such as coronary artery disease.

The large amount of undiagnosed PAD cases is unfortunate because preventive therapies, such as statins and antithrombotic agents, can save both life and limb. Recent years have seen a major investment in identifying effective treatments for PAD, including several randomized clinical trials of both medical and revascularization approaches. At the same time, health care is at major crossroads—with the generation of massive amounts of data from sources such as electronic health records (EHRs), medical imaging, wearables, and large-scale genetic sequencing. The high volume of data provide opportunities to revolutionize how care for vascular patients is delivered.

Since the publication of the original Compendium, multiple medical specialties have sought to leverage "Big Data" and advanced analytics, but the real-world integration of artificially intelligent systems and medicine remains in its infancy. When applied to PAD, advanced analytics promise to identify latent disease, refine disease and risk phenotyping, and aid treatment choices with consideration of the full breadth of demographic, biological, and clinical data . Artificial intelligence (AI)-based vascular imaging tools will also provide support for diagnostic, prognostic, and intraoperative settings. Given that PAD care is often fragmented across different locations and specialties, AI can also aid with integrating care data points, thereby promoting the holistic, interdisciplinary care that is critical to optimizing management and outcomes.

This chapter reviews contributions of AI and machine learning (ML) to PAD care and explores what integration of AI and PAD care can mean for patients, internists, surgeons, and the multidisciplinary care team as a whole. In some instances, we draw from developments in other vascular diseases such as carotid and aortic aneurysm disease, highlighting the need to develop AI for PAD specifically to help rescue patients from dying of neglect.

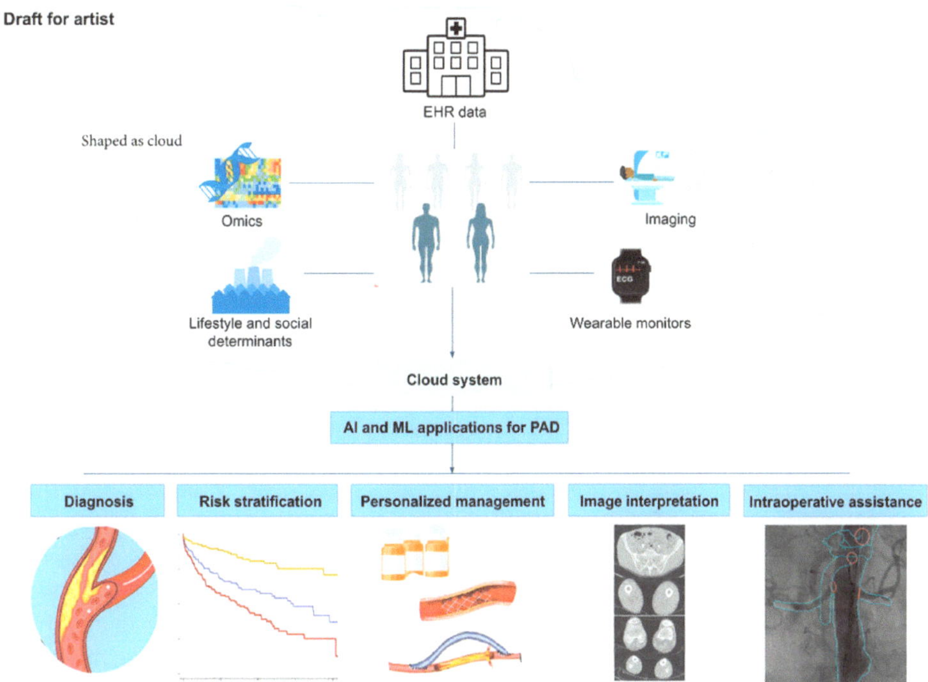

Fig.9.1 Applications of AI and ML across the spectrum of peripheral artery disease care, spanning diagnosis, risk stratification, management, and intraoperative guidance.AI, artificial intelligence. EHR, electronic health record. ML, machine learning. PAD, peripheral artery disease. (Illustration credit: Ben Smith)

What we know about AI and ML?

AI can be defined as the use of computer algorithms to automate a specific task with the goal of mimicking human thought processes and learning. For example, digital assistants such as Apple's Siri and Amazon's Alexa are powered by a range of AI technologies that enable each system to understand, parse, and respond to speech in a manner similar to a human's response. These digital assistants also "learn" over time to improve the accuracy of their responses. And while AI encompasses task automation, AI is powered by computational algorithms, broadly known as ML algorithms, which enable this automation.There are many types of ML algorithms that are broadly classified by the way in which each algorithm "learns". Learning, as it applies to ML algorithms, involves applying a mathematical formula or series of formulas to data such that relationships between features (or variables) can be summarized mathematically. The final result of this application is a model that represents the mathematical summary. This model can then be applied to new data to estimate expected values (eg, predict laboratory values or yes/no patient outcomes).

When algorithms are provided data where the outcome or class (disease, nondiseased) are labeled this is considered supervised learning—supervised because the ground truth is known and provided to the algorithm. In unsupervised learning, there is no ground truth label and the algorithm finds structure within the data. we summarize different ML algorithms based on the type of learning methods employed. Key terms for interpreting ML model development are listed

Vascular Disease Diagnosis

Disease Detection Using Supervised Learning Approaches

ML models can enable automated disease detection. One of the first studies to demonstrate the utility of using ML to identify undiagnosed PAD was published in 2016 (Online Dataset I).26 Data were derived from a clinical trial of patients presenting for elective coronary angiography. Of all patients included in the study, 17% had PAD and 68% of these patients were undiagnosed at study enrollment, confirming that PAD is underrecognized.

Integrating disparate data variables spanning sociodemographics, medical history, genetic, and coronary angiography findings, our group developed a classification model that was trained in a hypothesis-free fashion to identify cases of patients with PAD who were previously undiagnosed. The most accurate PAD prediction model was based on a random forest algorithm . Supervised Learning). The final model included over 120 baseline characteristics and achieved an area under the receiver operating curve (AUC) of 0.84 for PAD classification, notably outperforming classifications made on the basis of traditional linear models using the same data (AUC=0.60). Additionally, the ML model achieved a sensitivity of 76% compared with 57% from a traditional linear model. Such improvements in sensitivity can significantly improve detection of undiagnosed patients with PAD.Other efforts to apply ML algorithms have attempted to predict angiographically significant or advanced disease based on proteomics and functional metrics, respectively. In a study using data from patients referred for diagnostic coronary or peripheral angiography, a least absolute selection and shrinkage operator regression model combined >50 clinical variables and 109 biomarkers to predict obstructive PAD, defined as >50% stenosis in at least 1 peripheral vessel. The final model incorporated hypertension and 6 biomarkers and had an AUC of 0.85 for obstructive PAD. Authors concluded that the tool may be used as a gatekeeper for invasive angiography and predict need for revascularization. Another study sought to identify patients at risk of critical limb ischemia in a cohort with critical limb ischemia (cases) and no PAD (controls) (defined as toe-brachial index <0.7 and >0.7, respectively). Authors developed an ML model using data on demographics, 6-minute walk test distance, symptom scores derived from vascular quality of life questionnaire, and calf circumference. Their random forest and generalized linear algorithms resulted in similar AUCs of 0.69 and 0.68 for identifying cases of critical limb ischemia, respectively.

Disease Detection Using Natural Language Processing

Because of the large amount of text data in the EHR, natural language processing (NLP) methods have been analyzed as a tool to identify cases of PAD. For example Afzal et al applied a rule-based NLP Natural Language Processing) to notes retrieved from the Mayo clinical data warehouse with the goal of automating detection of prevalent PAD. First, in analyzing 300 364 notes from a community-based cohort, the NLP model was built using PAD-related concepts and keywords (eg, "lower extremity, occlusive disease") to ascertain PAD status (defined as Ankle Brachial Index ≤0.9 or >1.4). Authors optimized the NLP model by reviewing and sequentially excluding select note types that led to the most false positives to maximize accuracy. Compared with a disease detection model based on International Classification of Diseases and Current Procedural Terminology codes, the NLP model was more accurate (92% versus 82%), had a higher PPV (93% versus 74%), and greater specificity (93% versus 64%) for identifying true PAD cases.29 Similarly, to identify severity of PAD, Afzal et al30 refined their NLP models and established the superiority of using NLP algorithms to classify patients with critical limb ischemia relative to billing codes (F1 Scores: NLP 90% versus billing code 76%, P<0.001)

Recently, Weissler et al31 also leveraged NLP methodology to query Duke University Medical Center's EHR system to identify patients with PAD. In comparison to Afzal et al, rather than using rule-based algorithms applied to predefined note types or sections, Weissler and colleagues trained an embedding-based NLP algorithm using notes from all clinical encounters and evaluated model performance on a broader PAD cohort adjudicated by imaging reports, surgical/ intervention documentation, and ABIs. Clinical notes were analyzed using an algorithm known as hierarchical Label-Embedding Attention Model that considered the frequency of individuals words, their learned representations, and the aggregate implication of numerous notes from each patient. Word embeddings were aggregated from all notes for a given patient and served as input to a neural network that generated a classification probability for PAD status. The NLP model applied to free-text outperformed a PAD classification strategy based on structured billing and procedure codes, with an AUC of 0.888 versus 0.801 (P<0.0001), respectively

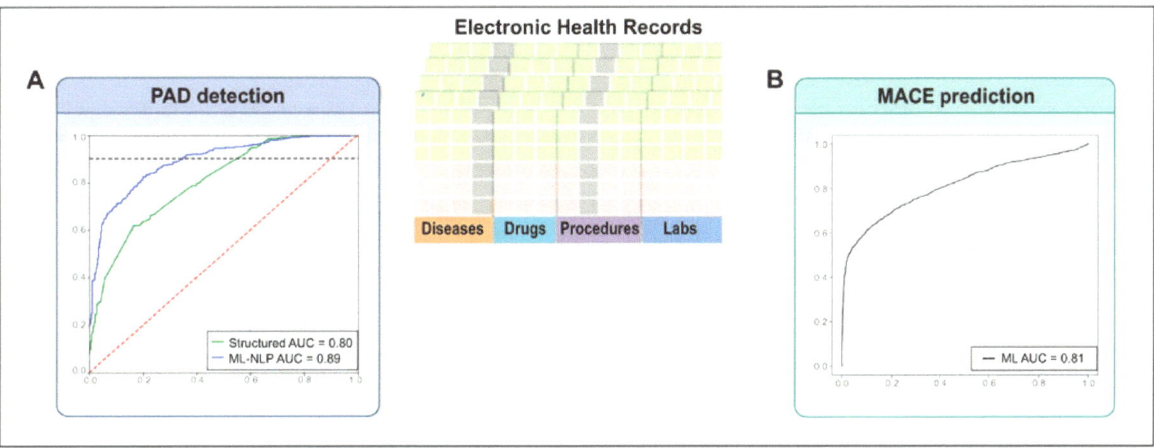

Fig.9.2 **When applied to the EHR, machine learning models reliably identify PAD and predict future cardiovascular events**. A, ML-based natural language processing (ML-NLP) of clinical notes identifies patients with PAD more accurately than structured data based on administrative diagnosis codes. B, By incorporating structured and unstructured EHR data, ML algorithms accurately risk stratify PAD patients at high risk for major adverse cardiovascular events (MACE). AUC, area under the receiver operating curve. EHR, electronic health record. MACE, major adverse cardiovascular event. PAD, peripheral artery disease. X-axis represents 1-specificity. Y-axis represents sensitivity. A, modified from Weissler et al.31 B, modified from Ross et al.

Disease Detection Using Complementary Clinical and Genetic Data

Although not yet applied to PAD detection, investigators have sought to combine the rich data from the EHR with genetic information, paving the way for the development and deployment of personalized health applications For example, Li et al developed an ML model to combine whole-genome sequencing and EHR data to automate identification of those with abdominal aortic aneurysms (AAAs). Their ML algorithm examined the clinical relevance of > 23 million genetic variants—agnostically identified genes with disease-distinct mutational patterns—and incorporated EHR data to complement predictions from individual genomes. EHR data utilized in the model included lifestyle and physiological measurements such as fasting glucose, lipid profiles, waist-to-hip ratios, and more. Compared with a genome-only model (AUC=0.69) or an EHR-only model (AUC=0.78), integrating both data sources resulted in a significant increase in the ML model's predictive power for AAA development (AUC=0.80, $P<1\times10^{-3}$).

Efforts to combine EHR data with genetic risk assessment of other vascular disease processes such as PAD have been hampered by lack of large enough sample sizes to identify unique genetic risks. However, with the recent landmark genome-wide association study on PAD in the large-scale biobank, the Million Veteran Program,33 we now have the ability to combine genetic susceptibility with EHR data. Such data could potentially be combined to create a precision health screening platform for vascular disease. These platforms would enable health care systems to identify individuals with high pretest probability of having or developing highly morbid diseases. Targeted early diagnosis and treatment may subsequently reduce disease complications, improve patient outcomes, and decrease health care costs

Vascular Disease Phenotyping and Management

Identifying Unique Disease Subtypes With Unsupervised Clustering

PAD shares many risk factors with coronary artery disease, including hypertension, smoking, and hyperlipidemia. However, there is growing evidence that suggests PAD is a more distinct atherosclerotic disorder. For example, unlike in the coronary and carotid vasculature, the presence of unstable plaques that lead to acute events is relatively uncommon in PAD. These findings suggest that their shared risk factors may contribute differently to disease pathogenesis, in addition to having unique pathophysiologic mechanisms. Further, within the PAD population, there is broad heterogeneity in clinical profiles and outcomes To help resolve disease heterogeneity, ML approaches can be applied for deep phenotyping of PAD.

Unsupervised cluster analysis has emerged as a promising approach to discovering clinically unique phenotypes in complex diseases Unsupervised Learning Rather than being limited to a known handful of risk factors, clustering algorithms can group patients based on robust, multidimensional patient data. Unsupervised clustering holds a number of advantages: it can generate novel disease subgroups, reveal population health patterns, and generate actionable information to tailor therapies. Such approaches have been applied to identify distinct phenotypes, reveal differences in population practice patterns, and detect subgroup heterogeneity in responses to common and new therapies.A more nuanced understanding of the unique characteristics of PAD and risk factors specific to individual patients can generate insights on the remaining curious distinctions that impact PAD severity, as well as differences between PAD and other atherosclerotic disorders like coronary artery disease or cerebrovascular disease. While prior cluster analyses have relied on analysis of one type of data with complete observations, advances in unsupervised algorithms are now enabling discovery of patient phenotypes using mixed categories of data and even missing data entries.39,40 These clustering frameworks are particularly suited for the data present in the EHR and will enable us to resolve phenotypic heterogeneity and personalize PAD management.

Identifying Appropriate Medical Treatment for Vascular Disease

The current approach to medical management of PAD is largely based on a reductionist methods—where patients with largely similar symptoms and broad diagnoses are given the same treatments. However, with the growing evidence base of therapies for PAD, there are now more options to consider beyond aspirin, high-intensity statins, and smoking. Even so, the increased costs of newer treatments and their attendant risks must be considered when selecting an appropriate treatment strategy and prescribing newer agents.

ML models can assist with matching preventative efforts to patients who may most benefit from new or existing drugs, and achieve appropriate polypharmacy, which is especially prevalent in the highly comorbid PAD population. For example, Hansen et al used random forest to investigate warfarin-drug interactions with 220 drug groups from >61 000 prescriptions of patients with atrial fibrillation. ML approaches have also been developed to model polypharmacy side effects with networks of drug-protein interactions, drug-drug interactions, and protein-protein interactions. With numerous treatment guidelines for PAD and its frequent comorbid conditions, training such algorithms on patients with PAD can help develop plans that synchronize therapy and limit interactions leading to side effects. AI tools that can automate identification of PAD subgroups and integrate data such as polypharmacy interactomes and even pharmacogenetics will advance us from the conventional reductionist approach to personalized PAD care.In addition, advanced data science methods may be used to characterize long-term treatment safety in a real-world setting, including questions that are not likely to be addressed in clinical trials. For instance, in trials of cilostazol for the treatment of claudication, patients with congestive heart failure (CHF) were excluded largely based on theoretical safety concerns of a drug from a similar class. To conduct safety surveillance, Leeper and colleagues used NLP to mine clinical notes from patients with PAD and identify a subset of patients with CHF who were prescribed cilostazol. They found no adverse impact of cilostazol on cardiovascular events or mortality on patients with PAD, including in patients with CHF.

Novel Approaches to Risk Prediction

Predicting Cardiovascular Outcomes

PAD confers increased cardiovascular morbidity and mortality, including MI, stroke, and cardiovascular death.44 Unlike conventional risk models that incorporate a handful of risk factors, ML approaches have the advantage of being able to consider 100s of different risk factors and identify risk factors for which complex relationships amplify or attenuate risk.

There has been significant interest in using EHR data for risk stratification. A major challenge in this application is to coerce enough structure into EHR data with processing pipelines that are reproducible and portable across multiple health care settings (eg, institutions, geographic locations). Through an analysis of a clinical trial database, ML models have been developed to predict mortality risk in patients with PAD.26 Advancing efforts into the real-world EHR from 2 different medical institutions, our group recently built a risk stratification model that accurately identifies which patients with PAD are most likely to go on to have a major adverse cardiovascular event (MACE) before event occurrence . EHR data were coded using the Observational Medical Outcomes Partnership Common Data Model, which enables transformation of disparate date types present in the EHR into a cohesive database structure In our specific models, data included patient prescriptions, laboratory values, International Classification of Diseases and Current Procedural Terminology codes, and annotated text from clinical notes. A random forest algorithm was then applied to the EHR data from both institutions. Interestingly, clinical text was vital for optimal model performance, where removal resulted in a significant decline in model AUC. The final predictive model was able to accurately discriminate between patients with PAD at high versus low risk of MACE occurrence (AUC=0.81) and showed good calibration (Brier score=0.10

Predicting Limb Outcomes

Vascular specialists are also keenly interested in limb-related outcomes. One study by Davis et al applied a combination of regularized linear regression algorithms Supervised Learning) to predict surgical site infections after lower extremity revascularization. Combining elastic net and random forest algorithms, their model had an AUC of 0.66 for post-bypass surgical site infections and identified a number of patient and procedure risk factors, including modifiable factors such as iodine-only skin preparation.

To continue to advance applications of ML and AI for PAD, evidence supporting reliable model prediction of amputation and acute limb ischemia are needed. Major adverse limb events (MALEs) are associated with a dire prognosis for patients with PAD, including MACE, prolonged hospitalization, and downstream impairments in quality of life.Even so, there are no well-vetted ML-based MALE prognostication tools. Such developments would be welcome given the far-reaching implications of MALE on PAD outcomes and care. Considerations of what type of data to utilize for MALE prognostication are important. Data from noninvasive studies based on velocity and stenosis criteria are abundant but can be unreliable and underestimate disease severity.EHR data can be considered given its depth and breadth; however, EHR data may miss important physiological markers. More than likely, a multimodal data approach will be needed where clinical data in the EHR or elsewhere are merged with imaging data (eg, hemodynamic noninvasive studies or computed tomography) to develop the most accurate MALE prognostic tools.

Computer Vision for Image Interpretation and Diagnosis

Carotid Atherosclerosis Imaging

Computer vision is a branch of AI in which deep learning algorithms are applied to automate analysis of images and videos. Computer vision for medical image analysis has shown great promise in multiple use cases including use cases specific to vascular disease. Successes in the application of computer vision have particularly begun to shape interpretation of carotid ultrasound images identifying features that correlate with stroke risk, such as the lipid core, fibrous cap and vessel-wall volume.

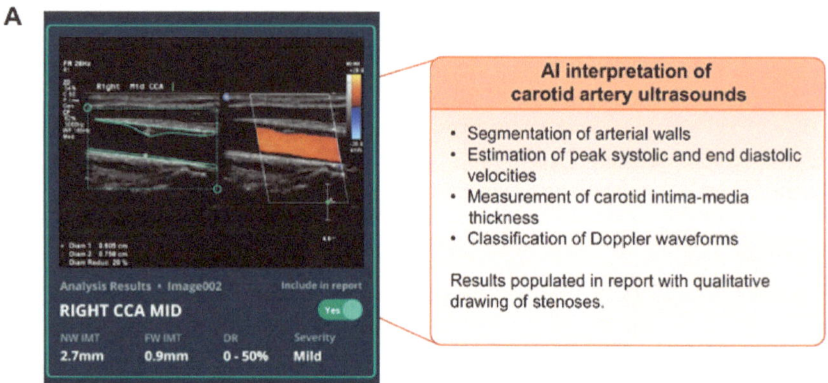

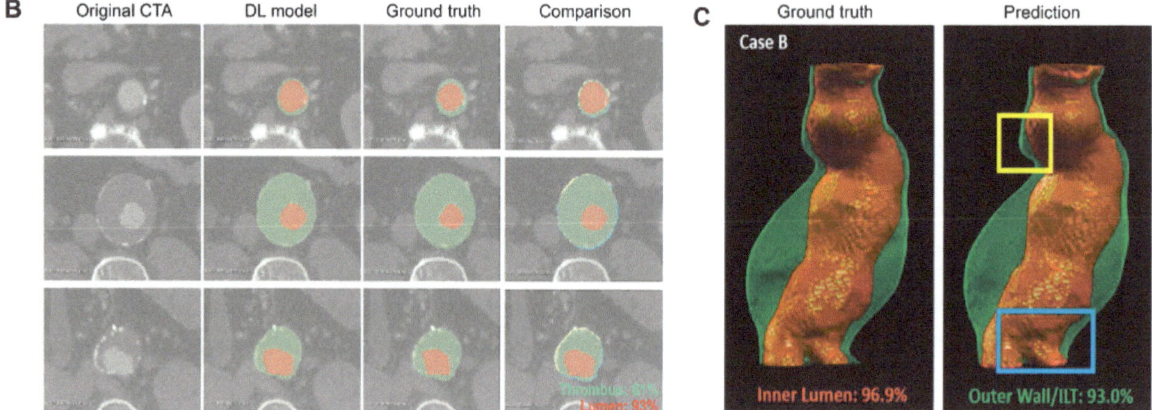

Fig.9.3 **Imaging assessment of carotid atherosclerosis and AAA disease using deep learning.**
A, AI software enables automated analysis and reporting of carotid ultrasounds. B,C, Deep learning pipelines have also been developed for fully automated volumetric analysis of AAA disease from CT images. B, Representative axial CTA slices are shown for automated segmentation of the aortic lumen (red) and thrombus (green) and the manually extracted ground truth. Key for comparison image: true positive lumen and thrombus (green and yellow, respectively), false negatives (red), false positives (blue). C, 3D U-Net output for the inner wall and outer wall/ILT (intraluminal thrombus) along with its respective ground truth. Points of discrepancy are boxed. Percentages in B-C represent the Dice coefficient. AAA, abdominal aortic aneurysm. AI, artificial intelligence. CTA, computed topography angiography. DL, deep learning. A, modified from See-Mode AVA user interface.63 B, modified from Caradu et al.68 C, modified from Chandrashekar et al.

One AI solution was developed by See-Mode AVA (See-ModeAugmented Vascular Analysis, Singapore). Their software can perform automated carotid vessel segmentation and measure intima-media thickness. The software was developed using a convolutional neural network. The model accurately estimated carotid intima-media thickness and achieved a correlation of 0.93 with experts, which was greater than the correlation between experts. See-Mode AVA's deep learning software received premarket FDA clearance in late 2020 for analysis of carotid and lower extremity ultrasounds and generation of reports including carotid intima-media thickness, velocities, and waveform type. This software is exciting as widespread adoption can lead to more timely diagnosis and easier postoperative surveillance. In addition, AI vascular ultrasound tools can assist with obtaining high-quality images, which would be especially impactful in resource-poor settings where experienced sonographers may not be available. For example, AI software can provide real-time guidance during localization and interrogation of vascular structures (Caption Health, Brisbane, CA) and automate image enhancement for optimized quality (ContextVision, Sweden).

Additional automated methods for carotid plaque characterization have been achieved using MRI data. Wu et al report a deep neural network that diagnoses carotid atherosclerosis after being trained on manually labeled vessel-wall MRI images to learn visual features separately from the lumen and outer wall areas. Their model included use of a pretrained CNN developed specifically for biomedical imaging segmentation known as U-Net. This segmentation process involves labeling specific parts of images and with this labeled data deep learning algorithms learn important features that are predictive of predefined outcomes. In Wu et al's work, performance of the trained modified U-Net CNN was evaluated in 2 test datasets and could successfully diagnose carotid atherosclerosis (AUC, 0.92–0.95).

Aortic Aneurysm Imaging

While most computer vision algorithms such as CNNs are trained on 2-dimensional images, 3-dimensional (3D) CNNs provide the opportunity to automate characterization of lesions for which additional measurements are of great importance. The clinical significance of aneurysm disease, for example, is better characterized by capturing 3-dimensional features such as volume, rather than just length and/or width. Applying a 3D CNN for post-endovascular aneurysm repair (EVAR) endoleak detection, Hahn et al demonstrate that these deep learning algorithms are able to identify multiple types of post-EVAR endoleaks with high performance (AUC=0.94). Using a 3D U-Net CNN, they also automate detection of AAA diameter and other key features such as AAA and endograft volumes. Other groups have applied U-Net CNNs for preoperative assessment of patients with AAAs, extracting aortic and thrombus volumes from computed tomography angiograms (CTAs) and noncontrast images. Application areas for automated AAA diagnosis and characterization are many, such as aiding vascular surgeons with surveillance and providing volumetric measurements that may be of greater prognostic value than diameter.Tools that can identify patients who may benefit from different endovascular repair approaches could also be helpful to vascular surgical practice.

PAD Imaging

Applications of computer vision algorithms to PAD-specific imaging are just starting to be reported and have the possibility to inform approaches to revascularization and potentially reduce the number of invasive diagnostic studies. Ara et al developed a computer vision model to automate classification of Doppler waveforms and detect aortoiliac, femoral-popliteal, and tibial trifurcation disease. Their model classified waveforms using a CNN, followed by a hierarchical neural network that integrated waveform classifications at each segment to classify normal versus diseased segments. In one model, CNN had an accuracy of 0.69, 1, and 0.86 for classifying mono-, bi-, and triphasic waveforms, respectively. In detecting disease, the hierarchical model achieved high F1 scores of 0.98 in normal arteries, 0.91 on aortoiliac disease, 0.93 on femoral-popliteal disease, and 0.85 on tibial trifurcation disease.

Another important imaging modality for PAD is CTA, where automatic peripheral vessel identification may be used for localizing and quantifying disease, defining runoff, and helping define surgical or endovascular targets . A recent study by Dai et al developed a CNN to interpret lower extremity CTAs and classify disease in above-knee and below-knee arteries. They used 17 050 axial images from 265 patients to develop a CNN that classifies above-knee artery stenosis into 5 classes (0, 1%–50%, 51%–69%, 70–99%, 100%) and below-knee artery stenosis into 3 classes (0%–50%, 51%–99%, and 100%). Using digital subtraction angiography as the reference standard, their model achieved an accuracy of >90% in the majority of stenosis classes. The lowest accuracies were 79% for 51-69% stenosis in above-knee segments and 88% for 51-99% stenosis in below-knee segments. For both above and below-knee segments, CNN classifications had similar accuracies (P=0.27 and P=0.81) and specificities (P=0.12 and P=0.97) as radiologist reads, but had significantly lower sensitivities (P<0.001 and P=0.02).

Innovative studies in MRI analysis have also been recently reported and may reduce the time and labor-intensive processing of MRI images. Zhang et al73 developed a computer vision model to accelerate mapping of calf muscle perfusion from dynamic contrast-enhanced MRIs. Their feedforward neural network was developed using 48 MRI scans, including pre- and post-exercise scans from healthy subjects and patients with PAD.The model had comparable exercise-stimulated perfusion estimates as the reference standard based on tracer kinetic analysis (correlation efficient=0.95) and generated the calf muscle perfusion maps much faster (<1 second versus 80 minutes). The Yuan group has also reported an efficient and accurate deep learning approach developed to evaluate atherosclerosis in the popliteal arteries Using knee MRI scans from an osteoarthritis cohort study, their CNN reduced vessel wall segmentation times from 4 hours to 8 minutes and performed similarly as human readers (Dice coefficient: 0.79). Following segmentation, their model was trained to quantify vessel features including mean wall thickness, maximum wall thickness, wall area, and lumen area, for which correlation coefficients were 0.73, 0.78, 0.90, and 0.99

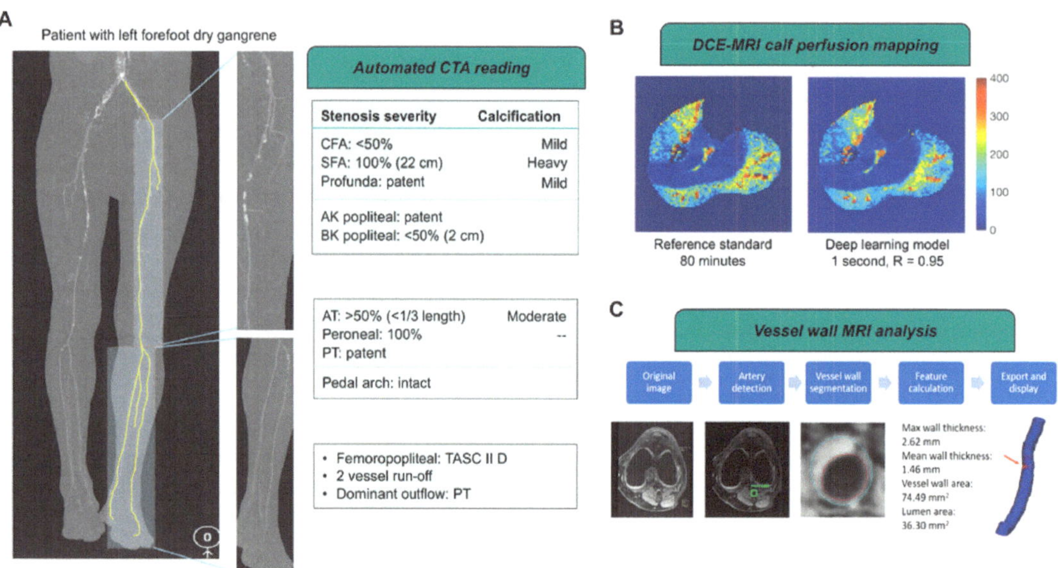

Fig.9.4 Computer vision for PAD imaging interpretation.

A, AI systems may automate interpretation of CTAs and generate reports based on TASC II classification. B,C, Computer vision algorithms may also enable more efficient processing of MRI images without compromising accuracy. Computer vision models generate accurate calf muscle perfusion maps in less than 1 second, compared to 180 minutes by standard modeling (B, modified from Zhang et al.73). Using standardized knee MRIs, fully automated pipelines for assessing atherosclerosis burden in the popliteal arteries have also been reported (C, modified from Chen et al.75). AI, artificial intelligence. AK, above knee. AT, anterior tibial. BK, below knee. CFA, common femoral artery. CTA, computed topography angiography. DCE-MRI, dynamic contrast-enhanced magnetic resonance imaging. R, correlation coefficient. PT, posterior tibial. SFA, superficial femoral artery. TASC II, Trans-Atlantic Intersociety Consensus II.

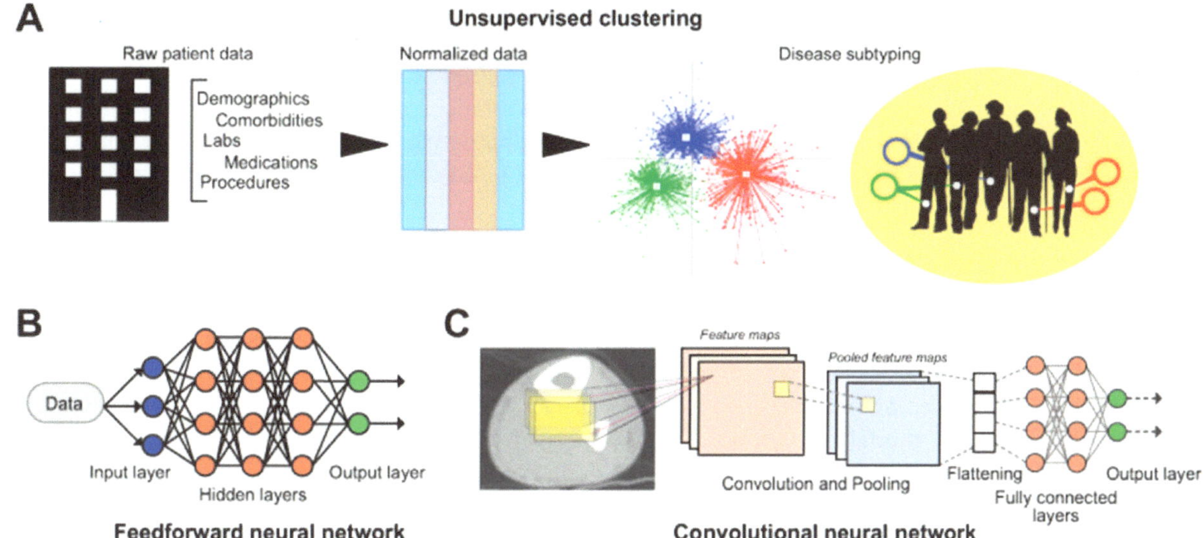

Fig.9.5. Framework for unsupervised cluster analysis and types of deep neural networks.
A, Unsupervised cluster analysis can reveal clinically relevant patterns in data in a process where raw high-dimensional data is mathematically summarized and clustered. This general framework may be used to derive unique disease subtypes from patient data elements in a clinical database or the electronic health record. B, Feedforward neural network, composed of an input layer, multiple hidden layers, and an output layer. C, Convolutional neural networks capture local image features which are down-sampled in pooling layers to retain the most valuable features. Many pooled feature maps then pass through a flatten layer to form a single linear vector, thereby enabling input to fully connected layers that perform image classification. A, modified from Ross et al.

Vascular Image-Based Prognostication

Extending from disease characterization and detection to prediction and prognosis, ML-aided image interpretation offers an opportunity to improve risk stratification. A seminal example of this is predicting the presence, progression, and development of diabetic retinopathy.78 Following demonstration of accurate diagnosis, AI software for retinal evaluation subsequently moved to prospective studies and one company received FDA approval in 2018 (IDx-DR, Iowa City, IA Beyond disease-specific screening, the developments by Google Health and multiple academic research teams exemplify the broader capabilities of deep learning models for prognostication and their ability to discover hidden associations. For example, one AI-system is able to predict sex, smoking status, systolic blood pressure, and risk of MACE based solely on retinal image analysis

Computer-Aided Prediction of Stroke

Automatically incorporating image-derived features into a vascular risk stratification tool has shown early potential in AI software developed by Suri and colleagues (Online Dataset II) Investigators developed a 3D CNN for characterization of carotid ultrasounds and detection of symptomatic or asymptomatic carotid stenosis. The network was trained and tested on ultrasounds from 150 asymptomatic patients and 196 with symptomatic disease. The 3D CNN framework was benchmarked against 2 types of deep learning models that were developed using a process known as transfer learning .Rather than training a network from scratch, transfer learning fine-tunes a CNN that is pretrained on a large dataset of natural images (eg, of scenes, animals, and plants) for medical image tasks.Compared with the two fine-tuned pretrained models, the de novo 3D CNN model better discriminated between symptomatic and asymptomatic plaques (AUC=0.79, 0.83, and 0.96, respectively). The authors note that an AI platform could be used by vascular surgeons to guide patient selection for intervention, and they highlight the need for external model validation beyond their single-center. With 100 000 carotid ultrasounds planned for public release by the UK Biobank study there is a major opportunity to train more ML models using this robust imaging and associated longitudinal data, potentially improving prediction of stroke based on earlier stage disease and uncovering new features predictive of adverse outcomes.

Computer-Aided Prediction of Aneurysm Growth and Rupture

There has also been special interest in image-derived prediction models for aneurysm growth and rupture. One group combined a deep learning and a computational model of growth and remodeling to predict AAA sac expansion. To overcome the need for a large volume of longitudinal data, investigators pretrained a deep neural network known as a deep belief network on 32 900 computer generated samples, then fine-tuned the network on longitudinal CT scans from 20 patients. At 9 months, their model produced accurate predictions of maximum AAA diameter with a root mean square error of 1.8 millimeters

Another intriguing study predicted AAA growth based on 3 automated geometric features, including maximum diameter, radius of curvature, and undulation index (a measure of surface concavity). This model predicted annual AAA growth with a root mean square error of 1.3 mm and had AUCs of 0.80 for slow growth (<2.5 mm/year) and 0.79 for fast growth (>5 mm/year). In a study using follow-up CTAs from 22 patients treated with EVAR, López-Linarez et al extracted biomechanical features to predict ongoing aneurysm evolution. CNNs were used for AAA segmentation, followed by principal components analysis of the aneurysm strain fields that were then used as input for a support vector machine algorithm. Their ML model demonstrated a good correlation between the principal components of biomechanical strain and long-term prognosis, achieving an AUC of 0.89 for post-EVAR sac expansion or rupture.

Computer Vision-Aided Prediction of MACE and MALE

In prediction of MACE, one study by Pickhardt and colleagues evaluated the prognostic value of a panel of automated biometric measures from abdominal CTs. The burden of abdominal aortic calcification was quantified using a CNN and was found to predict MACE in 9223 generally healthy asymptomatic adults, outperforming the Framingham risk score.89 In particular, all AUC values (2-, 5-, and 10-year) for abdominal aortic calcification were significantly greater than Framingham risk score and further improved when combined with other automated measures such as visceral-to-subcutaneous fat and muscle density. For example, the 5-year AUC of 3 imaging biomarkers and Framingham risk score was 0.74 versus 0.69 for MACE (P<0.05), respectively. Building off prior work quantifying the burden of popliteal atherosclerosis from knee MRIs,74 Chen et al75 recently investigated whether the fully automated vessel wall features correlate with cardiovascular risk. High cardiovascular risk was defined as individuals ≥65 years old with a history of smoking, hypertension, BMI≥25 kg/m2, and one of the following: lower extremity revascularization, stroke/TIA, MI, diabetes, current smoking, BMI≥30 kg/m2, or age ≥75 years. A number of automated vessel measures discriminated between high and low-risk groups, with the greatest discrimination achieved by the ratio of maximum/minimum vessel wall thickness (AUC=0.79) and maximum wall thickness (AUC=0.73; Online Dataset II). Given that these studies were performed on commonly obtained scans from low-risk asymptomatic individuals, their findings highlight the potential utility of ML models that harnesses the readily available information embedded in imaging for improved cardiovascular risk assessment.

Automated derivation of imaging features that specifically predict hard MALE events such as major amputation or need for peripheral reintervention would be a major advance, especially given that what we have interpreted as abnormal from standard noninvasive studies has been inconsistently shown to correlate with clinical outcomes or success. By simultaneously assessing and integrating focal and diffuse disease patterns, ML models may be trained to learn the relationship between CTA images and clinically significant restenosis that occurs with recurrent symptoms or delayed wound healing. Deep learning algorithms have indeed shown progress in predicting functionally significant coronary lesions from coronary CTA, achieving similar accuracies as invasive fractional flow reserve measurements

Optimizing Behavior and Lifestyle Modifications

There have been growing applications of AI and ML in behavioral science to study, recommend, and influence human behaviors. By developing tailored interventions, ML-based decision support systems can help prioritize lifestyle changes for patients in a personally meaningful way. Chi et al used data from the Atherosclerosis Risk in Communities study to develop an ML model that identifies lifestyle changes that maximally reduce an individual's 10-year cardiovascular risk (defined as coronary artery disease event or stroke). This model then formed the basis for a decision support "ML expert system" that made optimized lifestyle recommendations adjusting for patient preferences and limitations (eg, time, food). When comparing the original and optimized recommendations in a clinical trial simulation, the optimized recommendations resulted in a relative risk reduction of 8.6% in patients with single lifestyle changes and 9.9% in patients with multiple lifestyle changes.

AI and ML systems have also been effective in increasing adherence to anticoagulation therapy and incentivizing regular physical activity These developments were each enabled by smartphones and created opportunities for continuous monitoring, enhanced communication, and personalized feedback. Labovitz et al used an AI mobile application (AiCure, New York, NY) that uses computer vision and neural networks to visually confirm medication ingestion and provide reminders within the hour and before the end of a missed dosing window. In a randomized trial of 28 patients with recent ischemic strokes, the AI platform improved adherence to anticoagulation (100% in AI group, 50% in patients without daily monitoring), including a 67% improvement with compliance in patients taking direct oral anticoagulantsIn another study of 27 sedentary patients with type 2 diabetes, individuals received a smartphone-based pedometer, a personal plan for physical activity, and personalized reinforcement messages that encouraged adherence.Investigators used reinforcement learning (RL), a type of algorithm that learns by observing the result of an action taken . The algorithm thus gradually improves in predicting the types and frequency of feedback that effectively encourage physical activity. Compared with individuals who received identical once-weekly reminders, patients in the RL group increased physical activity levels and experienced a superior reduction in HbA1c compared with the control group, with an average improvement of 0.28%.

RL could similarly promote supervised exercise therapy for patients with PAD, which is increasingly being delivered through mobile health technologies. RL algorithms could potentially be combined with the Society for Vascular Surgery supervised exercise therapy mobile application, which began pilot study in early 2021. The app implements a provider-prescribed 12-week program of exercise and live health and wellness coaching. Combined with the engagement from mobile health technologies, RL algorithms could add an important component of adaptive messaging to better incentivize exercise and automate certain coaching elements to expand the availability of an exercise therapy coaching program to a broader patient population.

Guiding Vascular Surgical Care

Open versus endovascular revascularization is an age old question for vascular surgeons and specialists. While there have been thousands of studies published on optimal surgical strategies, many are small and underpowered. Although clinical trials offer "gold standard" evidence, costs, struggles with enrollment, patient disease heterogeneity, and potential ethical concerns of withholding surgical treatments can limit their impact on vascular surgical care. Bringing personalized guidance to aid in the choice of surgical approach based on an individual's unique data remains an ideal. Potential solutions include drawing from the large experience of previous patients and surgical outcomes to predict a patient's likely response to open and/or surgical treatments. Initiative's such as Stanford Medicine's "green button service" utilize EHRs to compile real-world evidence and support treatment decisions at the point-of-care (Atropos Health, Palo

Alto, CA) The service has helped clinicians across a variety of medical specialties, and drawing from surgical cohorts would enable use by vascular surgeons and specialists. For vascular specialists, this could add an additional dimension of data to the decision-making process by incorporating evidence based on collective real-world practices. Intraoperatively, AI companies are using advanced algorithms to improve the success of image-guided interventions. In one example, AI software is used to provide fully automated 3D overlays onto live fluoroscopic images and continuously adjust to patient movement and deformations due to wires and other devices (Cydar Medical, United Kingdom). This cloud-based AI system has been applied to standard and fenestrated EVAR and has preliminarily been shown to reduce radiation exposure and optimize operative workflow without the need for additional equipment to be installed.

Challenges and Future Considerations

Although the majority of developments around ML and AI are in their early days with regards to vascular disease, the studies highlighted in this review demonstrate that the practice of medicine and surgery for the vascular patient is on the brink of evolution.

To date, promising predictive capabilities have been harnessed primarily from retrospective data modeling. Moving forward, prospective validation in real-world settings will enable our ability to truly assess their clinical utility. It will be necessary to demonstrate meaningful end points when compared with standard-of-care to ensure that the technology developed will help move the needle forward.

For example EHR-enabled identification of latent PAD and enhanced diagnostic accuracy could be associated with greater adherence to guideline-directed therapy. Subsequent demonstration of improved clinical outcomes will be important as there are many historical examples of screening programs that led to overdiagnosis of early but benign disease and overtreatment.

Bibliography And Acknowledgement

- Aboyans V, Criqui MH, Abraham P, Allison MA, Creager MA, Diehm C, Fowkes FG, Hiatt WR, Jönsson B, Lacroix P, et al; American Heart Association Council on Peripheral Vascular Disease; Council on Epidemiology and Prevention; Council on Clinical Cardiology; Council on Cardiovascular Nursing; Council on Cardiovascular Radiology and Intervention, and Council on Cardiovascular Surgery and Anesthesia. Measurement and interpretation of the ankle-brachial index: a scientific statement from the American Heart Association.Circulation. 2012; 126:2890–2909
- Abràmoff MD, Lavin PT, Birch M, Shah N, Folk JC. Pivotal trial of an autonomous AI-based diagnostic system for detection of diabetic retinopathy in primary care offices.NPJ Digit Med. 2018; 1:39.
- Abul-Husn NS, Kenny EE. Personalized medicine and the power of electronic health records.Cell. 2019; 177:58–69.
- Afzal N, Mallipeddi VP, Sohn S, Liu H, Chaudhry R, Scott CG, Kullo IJ, Arruda-Olson AM. Natural language processing of clinical notes for identification of critical limb ischemia.Int J Med Inform. 2018; 111:83–89.
- Afzal N, Sohn S, Abram S, Scott CG, Chaudhry R, Liu H, Kullo IJ, Arruda-Olson AM. Mining peripheral arterial disease cases from narrative clinical notes using natural language processing.J Vasc Surg. 2017; 65:1753–1761.
- Agbo CC, Mahmoud QH, Eklund JM. Blockchain technology in healthcare: a systematic review.Healthcare (Basel). 2019; 7:56.
- Ahmad T, Lund LH, Rao P, Ghosh R, Warier P, Vaccaro B, Dahlstrom U, O'Connor CM, Felker GM, Desai NR. Machine learning methods improve prognostication, identify clinically distinct phenotypes, and detect heterogeneity in response to therapy in a large cohort of heart failure patients.J Am Heart Assoc. 2018; 7:
- Ahmad T, Pencina MJ, Schulte PJ, O'Brien E, Whellan DJ, Piña IL, Kitzman DW, Lee KL, O'Connor CM, Felker GM. Clinical implications of chronic heart failure phenotypes defined by cluster analysis.J Am Coll Cardiol. 2014; 64:1765–1774
- Anand SS, Caron F, Eikelboom JW, Bosch J, Dyal L, Aboyans V, Abola MT, Branch KRH, Keltai K, Bhatt DL, et al. Major adverse limb events and mortality in patients with peripheral artery disease: the COMPASS trial.J Am Coll Cardiol. 2018; 71:2306–2315
- Ara L, Luo X, Sawchuk A, Rollins D. Automate the peripheral arterial disease prediction in lower extremity arterial doppler study using machine learning and neural networks.Paper presented at: BCB '19: Proceedings of the 10th ACM International Conference on Bioinformatics; September 7-10, 2019, Niagra Falls, NY, USA
- Arcadu F, Benmansour F, Maunz A, Willis J, Haskova Z, Prunotto M. Deep learning algorithm predicts diabetic retinopathy progression in individual patients.NPJ Digit Med. 2019; 2:92.
- Arya S, Khakharia A, Binney ZO, DeMartino RR, Brewster LP, Goodney PP, Wilson PWF. Association of statin dose with amputation and survival in patients with peripheral artery disease.Circulation. 2018; 137:1435–1446

- Ata R, Gandhi N, Rasmussen H, El-Gabalawy O, Gutierrez S, Ahmad A, Suresh S, Ravi R, Rothenberg K, Aalami O. Clinical validation of smartphone-based activity tracking in peripheral artery disease patients.NPJ Digit Med. 2018; 1:66.
- Berger JS, Ladapo JA. Underuse of prevention and lifestyle counseling in patients with peripheral artery disease.J Am Coll Cardiol. 2017; 69:2293–2300.
- Bhatt DL, Peterson ED, Harrington RA, Ou FS, Cannon CP, Gibson CM, Kleiman NS, Brindis RG, Peacock WF, Brener SJ, et al; CRUSADE Investigators. Prior polyvascular disease: risk factor for adverse ischaemic outcomes in acute coronary syndromes.Eur Heart J. 2009; 30:1195–1202.
- Bora A, Balasubramanian S, Babenko B, Virmani S, Venugopalan S, Mitani A, de Oliveira Marinho G, Cuadros J, Ruamviboonsuk P, Corrado GS, et al. Predicting the risk of developing diabetic retinopathy using deep learning.Lancet Digit Health. 2021.
- Brass EP, Lewis RJ, Lipicky R, Murphy J, Hiatt WR. Risk assessment in drug development for symptomatic indications: a framework for the prospective exclusion of unacceptable cardiovascular risk.Clin Pharmacol Ther. 2006; 79:165–172.
- Caradu C, Spampinato B, Vrancianu AM, Berard X, Ducasse E. Fully automatic volume segmentation of infra-renal abdominal aortic aneurysm CT images with deep learning approaches versus physician controlled manual segmentation [published online ahead of print December 9, 2020]. J Vasc Surg
- Castelli WP. Epidemiology of coronary heart disease: the Framingham study.Am J Med. 1984; 76:4–12.
- Chandrashekar A, Handa A, Lapolla P, Shivakumar N, Ngetich E, Grau V, Lee R. Prediction of abdominal aortic aneurysm growth using geometric assessment of computerised tomography images acquired during the aneurysm surveillance period [published online ahead of print December 29, 2020 Ann Surg.
  Chandrashekar A, Handa A, Shivakumar N, Lapolla P, Uberoi R, Grau V, Lee R. A deep learning pipeline to automate high-resolution arterial segmentation with or without intravenous contrast [published online ahead of print November 23, 2020].Ann Surg
- Chen L, Canton G, Liu W, Hippe DS, Balu N, Watase H, Hatsukami TS, Waterton JC, Hwang JN, Yuan C. Fully automated and robust analysis technique for popliteal artery vessel wall evaluation (FRAPPE) using neural network models from standardized knee MRI.Magn Reson Med. 2020; 84:2147–2160.
- Chi CL, Nick Street W, Robinson JG, Crawford MA. Individualized patient-centered lifestyle recommendations: an expert system for communicating patient specific cardiovascular risk information and prioritizing lifestyle options.J Biomed Inform. 2012; 45:1164–1174.
- Coenen A, Kim YH, Kruk M, Tesche C, De Geer J, Kurata A, Lubbers ML, Daemen J, Itu L, Rapaka S, et al. Diagnostic accuracy of a machine-learning approach to coronary computed tomographic angiography-based fractional flow reserve: result from the MACHINE consortium.Circ Cardiovasc Imaging. 2018; 11:e007217.
- Connell A, Black G, Montgomery H, Martin P, Nightingale C, King D, Karthikesalingam A, Hughes C, Back T, Ayoub K, et al. Implementation of a digitally enabled care pathway (Part 2): qualitative analysis of experiences of health care professionals.J Med Internet Res. 2019; 21:
- Cooke JP, Chen Z. A compendium on peripheral arterial disease.Circ Res. 2015; 116:1505–1508.
  Criqui MH, Aboyans V. Epidemiology of peripheral artery disease.Circ Res. 2015; 116:1509–1526. doi: 10.1161/CIRCRESAHA.116.303849
- Dai L, Zhou Q, Zhou H, Zhang H, Cheng P, Ding M, Xu X, Zhang X. Deep learning-based classification of lower extremity arterial stenosis in computed tomography angiography.Eur J Radiol. 2021; 136:109528
- Davis FM, Sutzko DC, Grey SF, Mansour MA, Jain KM, Nypaver TJ, Gaborek G, Henke PK. Predictors of surgical site infection after open lower extremity revascularization.J Vasc Surg. 2017; 65:1769–1778
- Dennis BM, Stonko DP, Callcut RA, Sidwell RA, Stassen NA, Cohen MJ, Cotton BA, Guillamondegui OD. Artificial neural networks can predict trauma volume and acuity regardless of center size and geography: a multicenter study.J Trauma Acute Care Surg. 2019; 87:181–187.
- Duff S, Mafilios MS, Bhounsule P, Hasegawa JT. The burden of critical limb ischemia: a review of recent literature.Vasc Health Risk Manag. 2019; 15:187–208
- Duscha BD, Piner LW, Patel MP, Crawford LE, Jones WS, Patel MR, Kraus WE. Effects of a 12-week mHealth program on functionalcapacity and physical activity in patients with peripheralartery disease.Am J Cardiol. 2018; 122:879–884.
- Esserman LJ, Thompson IM, Reid B, Nelson P, Ransohoff DF, Welch HG, Hwang S, Berry DA, Kinzler KW, Black WC, et al. Addressing overdiagnosis and overtreatment in cancer: a prescription for change.Lancet Oncol. 2014; 15:e234–
- Esteva A, Kuprel B, Novoa RA, Ko J, Swetter SM, Blau HM, Thrun S. Dermatologist-level classification of skin cancer with deep neural networks.Nature. 2017; 542:115–118.
- Fenton JJ, Weyrich MS, Durbin S, Liu Y, Bang H, Melnikow J. Prostate-Specific Antigen-Based Screening for Prostate Cancer: A Systematic Evidence Review for the US Preventive Services Task Force. 2018; 319:1914–1931.
- Ferket BS, Spronk S, Colkesen EB, Hunink MG. Systematic review of guidelines on peripheral artery disease screening.Am J Med. 2012; 125:198–208.
- Gerhard-Herman MD, Gornik HL, Barrett C, Barshes NR, Corriere MA, Drachman DE, Fleisher LA, Fowkes FG, Hamburg NM, Kinlay S, et al. 2016 AHA/ACC guideline on the management of patients with lower extremity peripheral artery disease: executive summary: a report of the American College of Cardiology/American Heart Association Task Force on Clinical Practice Guidelines.Circulation. 2017; 135:e686
- Ghorbani A, Ouyang D, Abid A, He B, Chen JH, Harrington RA, Liang DH, Ashley EA, Zou JY. Deep learning interpretation of echocardiograms.NPJ Digit Med. 2020; 3:10.
- Gianfrancesco MA, Tamang S, Yazdany J, Schmajuk G. Potential biases in machine learning algorithms using electronic health record data.JAMA Intern Med. 2018; 178:1544–1547.
- Gombar S, Callahan A, Califf R, Harrington R, Shah NH. It is time to learn from patients like mine.NPJ Digit Med. 2019; 2:16

- Gulshan V, Peng L, Coram M, Stumpe MC, Wu D, Narayanaswamy A, Venugopalan S, Widner K, Madams T, Cuadros J, et al. Development and validation of a deep learning algorithm for detection of diabetic retinopathy in retinal fundus photographs.JAMA. 2016; 316:2402–2410.
- Hahn S, Perry M, Morris CS, Wshah S, Bertges DJ. Machine deep learning accurately detects endoleak after endovascular abdominal aortic aneurysm repair.JVS: Vascular Science. 2020; 1:5–12.
- Hannun AY, Rajpurkar P, Haghpanahi M, Tison GH, Bourn C, Turakhia MP, Ng AY. Cardiologist-level arrhythmia detection and classification in ambulatory electrocardiograms using a deep neural network.Nat Med. 2019; 25:65–69.
- Hansen PW, Clemmensen L, Sehested TS, Fosbøl EL, Torp-Pedersen C, Køber L, Gislason GH, Andersson C. Identifying drug-drug interactions by data mining: a Pilot Study of Warfarin-Associated Drug Interactions.Circ Cardiovasc Qual Outcomes. 2016; 9:621–628.
- Hess CN, Bonaca MP. Contemporary review of antithrombotic therapy in peripheral artery disease.Circ Cardiovasc Interv. 2020; 13:e009584.
- Hinton GE, Osindero S, Teh YW. A fast learning algorithm for deep belief nets.Neural Comput. 2006; 18:1527–1554
- Hippe DS, Balu N, Chen L, Canton G, Liu W, Watase H, Waterton JC, Hatsukami TS, Hwang JN, Yuan C. Confidence weighting for robust automated measurements of popliteal vessel wall magnetic resonance imaging.Circ Genom Precis Med. 2020; 13:e002870.
- Hirsch AT, Criqui MH, Treat-Jacobson D, Regensteiner JG, Creager MA, Olin JW, Krook SH, Hunninghake DB, Comerota AJ, Walsh ME, et al. Peripheral arterial disease detection, awareness, and treatment in primary care.JAMA. 2001; 286:1317–1324.
- Jiang Z, Do HN, Choi J, Lee W, Baek S. A deep learning approach to predict abdominal aortic aneurysm expansion using longitudinal data.Frontiers in Physics. 2020; 7.
  Jung K, Covington S, Sen CK, Januszyk M, Kirsner RS, Gurtner GC, Shah NH. Rapid identification of slow healing wounds.Wound Repair Regen. 2016; 24:181–188.
- Kinlay S. Outcomes for clinical studies assessing drug and revascularization therapies for claudication and critical limb ischemia in peripheral artery disease.Circulation. 2013; 127:1241–1250.
- Klarin D, Lynch J, Aragam K, Chaffin M, Assimes TL, Huang J, Lee KM, Shao Q, Huffman JE, Natarajan P, et al; VA Million Veteran Program. Genome-wide association study of peripheral artery disease in the Million Veteran Program.Nat Med. 2019; 25:1274–1279
- Kullo IJ, Leeper NJ. The genetic basis of peripheral arterial disease: current knowledge, challenges, and future directions.Circ Res. 2015; 116:1551–1560.
- Labovitz DL, Shafner L, Reyes Gil M, Virmani D, Hanina A. Using artificial intelligence to reduce the risk of nonadherence in patients on anticoagulation therapy.Stroke. 2017; 48:1416–1419.
- Leeper NJ, Bauer-Mehren A, Iyer SV, Lependu P, Olson C, Shah NH. Practice-based evidence: profiling the safety of cilostazol by text-mining of clinical notes.PLoS One. 013; 8:
  Li J, Pan C, Zhang S, Spin JM, Deng A, Leung LLK,
- Dalman RL, Tsao PS, Snyder M. Decoding the genomics of abdominal aortic aneurysm.Cell. 2018; 174:1361–1372.e10.
  Li RC, Asch SM, Shah NH. Developing a delivery science for artificial intelligence in healthcare.NPJ Digit Med. 2020; 3:107
- Littlejohns TJ, Holliday J, Gibson LM, Garratt S, Oesingmann N, Alfaro-Almagro F, Bell JD, Boultwood C, Collins R, Conroy MC, et al. The UK Biobank imaging enhancement of 100,000 participants: rationale, data collection, management and future directions.Nat Commun. 2020; 11:2624
- López-Linares K, García I, García A, Cortes C, Piella G, Macía I, Noailly J, González Ballester MA. Image-based 3D characterization of abdominal aortic aneurysm deformation after endovascular aneurysm repair.Front Bioeng Biotechnol. 2019; 7:267.
- Lyell D, Coiera E. Automation bias and verification complexity: a systematic review.J Am Med Inform Assoc. 2017; 24:423–431.
- Mandel JC, Kreda DA, Mandl KD, Kohane IS, Ramoni RB. SMART on FHIR: a standards-based, interoperable apps platform for electronic health records.J Am Med Inform Assoc. 2016; 23:899–908. doi: 10.1093/jamia/ocv189
- Maurel B, Martin-Gonzalez T, Chong D, Irwin A, Guimbretière G, Davis M, Mastracci TM. A prospective observational trial of fusion imaging in infrarenal aneurysms.J Vasc Surg. 2018; 68:1706.e1–1713.e1.
- McCarthy CP, Ibrahim NE, van Kimmenade RRJ, Gaggin HK, Simon ML, Gandhi P, Kelly N, Motiwala SR, Mukai R, Magaret CA, et al. A clinical and proteomics approach to predict the presence of obstructive peripheral arterial disease: from the Catheter Sampled Blood Archive in Cardiovascular Diseases (CASABLANCA) Study.Clin Cardiol. 2018; 41:903–909.
- McDermott MM. Lower extremity manifestations of peripheral artery disease: the pathophysiologic and functional implications of leg ischemia.Circ Res. 2015; 116:1540–1550.
- McNair D, Price WN. Health Care AI: Law, Regulation, Policy.Artificial Intelligence in Health Care: The Hope, the Hype, the Promise, the Peril. 2020.
- Menard MT, Farber A, Assmann SF, Choudhry NK, Conte MS, Creager MA, Dake MD, Jaff MR, Kaufman JA, Powell RJ, et al. Design and rationale of the best endovascular versus best surgical therapy for patients with critical limb ischemia (BEST-CLI) trial.J Am Heart Assoc. 2016; 5
- Misra S, Shishehbor MH, Takahashi EA, Aronow HD, Brewster LP, Bunte MC, Kim ESH, Lindner JR, Rich K; American Heart Association Council on Peripheral Vascular Disease; Council on Clinical Cardiology; and Council on Cardiovascular and Stroke Nursing. Perfusion assessment in critical limb ischemia: principles for understanding and the development of evidence and evaluation of devices: a scientific statement from the American Heart Association.Circulation. 2019; 140:e657–e672.
- Myers KD, Knowles JW, Staszak D, Shapiro MD, Howard W, Yadava M, Zuzick D, Williamson L, Shah NH, Banda JM, et al. Precision screening for familial hypercholesterolaemia: a machine learning study applied to electronic health encounter data.Lancet Digit Health. 2019;

- Nam JG, Park S, Hwang EJ, Lee JH, Jin KN, Lim KY, Vu TH, Sohn JH, Hwang S, Goo JM, et al. Development and validation of deep learning-based automatic detection algorithm for malignant pulmonary nodules on chest radiographs.Radiology. 2019; 290:218–228.
- Observational Health Data Sciences and Informatics. The Book of OHDSI.2019. Accessed March 18, 2021
  Ouyang D, He B, Ghorbani A, Yuan N, Ebinger J, Langlotz CP, Heidenreich PA, Harrington RA, Liang DH, Ashley EA, et al. Video-based AI for beat-to-beat assessment of cardiac function.Nature. 2020; 580:252–256.
- Patel MR, Conte MS, Cutlip DE, Dib N, Geraghty P, Gray W, Hiatt WR, Ho M, Ikeda K, Ikeno F, et al. Evaluation and treatment of patients with lower extremity peripheral artery disease: consensus definitions from Peripheral Academic Research Consortium (PARC).J Am Coll Cardiol. 2015; 65:931–941.
- Pickhardt PJ, Graffy PM, Zea R, Lee SJ, Liu J, Sandfort V, Summers RM. Automated CT biomarkers for opportunistic prediction of future cardiovascular events and mortality in an asymptomatic screening population: a retrospective cohort study.Lancet Digit Health. 2020; 2:e192–e200
- Poplin R, Varadarajan AV, Blumer K, Liu Y, McConnell MV, Corrado GS, Peng L, Webster DR. Prediction of cardiovascular risk factors from retinal fundus photographs via deep learning.Nat Biomed Eng. 2018; 2:158–164.
- Popplewell MA, Davies H, Jarrett H, Bate G, Grant M, Patel S, Mehta S, Andronis L, Roberts T, Deeks J, et al; BASIL-2 Trial Investigators. Bypass versus angio plasty in severe ischaemia of the leg - 2 (BASIL-2) trial: study protocol for a randomised controlled trial.Trials. 2016; 17:11.
- Qutrio Baloch Z, Raza SA, Pathak R, Marone L, Ali A. Machine learning confirms nonlinear relationship between severity of peripheral arterial disease, functional limitation and symptom severity.Diagnostics (Basel). 2020; 10:515.
- Rolls AE, Maurel B, Davis M, Constantinou J, Hamilton G, Mastracci TM. A comparison of accuracy of image- versus hardware-based tracking technologies in 3D fusion in aortic endografting.Eur J Vasc Endovasc Surg. 2016; 52:323–331
- Ronneberger O, Fischer P, Brox T. U-Net: Convolutional Networks for Biomedical Image Segmentation.arXiv. 2015.
  Ross EG, Jung K, Dudley JT, Li L, Leeper NJ, Shah NH. Predicting future cardiovascular events in patients with peripheral artery disease using electronic health record data.Circ Cardiovasc Qual Outcomes. 2019; 12:e004741.
- Ross EG, Shah N, Leeper N. Statin intensity or achieved LDL? practice-based evidence for the evaluation of new cholesterol treatment guidelines.PLoS One. 2016; 11
- Ross EG, Shah NH, Dalman RL, Nead KT, Cooke JP, Leeper NJ. The use of machine 26. learning for the identification of peripheral artery disease and future mortality risk.J Vasc Surg. 2016; 64:1515–1522.
- Saba L, Biswas M, Suri HS, Viskovic K, Laird JR, Cuadrado-Godia E, Nicolaides A, Khanna NN, Viswanathan V, Suri JS. Ultrasound-based carotid stenosis measurement and risk stratification in diabetic cohort: a deep learning paradigm.Cardiovasc Diagn Ther. 2019; 9:439–461.
- Sarikaya R. The Technology Behind Personal Digital Assistants: an overview of the system architecture and key components.IEEE Signal Processing Magazine. 2017; 34:67.
- Talebi S, Madani MH, Madani A, Chien A, Shen J, Mastrodicasa D, Fleischmann D, Chan FP, Mofrad MRK. Machine learning for endoleak detection after endovascular aortic repair.Sci Rep. 2020; 10:18343. doi: 10.1038/s41598-020-74936-7
- Udell M, Horn C, Zadeh R, Boyd S. Generalized low rank models.arXiv. 2014. Preprint posted online 5 May 2015
  Wanhainen A, Mani K, Golledge J. Surrogate markers of abdominal aortic aneurysm progression.Arterioscler Thromb
- Vasc Biol. 2016; 36:236–244.
  Ward A, Sarraju A, Chung S, Li J, Harrington R, Heidenreich P, Palaniappan L, Scheinker D, Rodriguez F. Machine learning and atherosclerotic cardiovascular disease risk prediction in a multi-ethnic population.NPJ Digit Med. 2020; 3:125
- Weissler EH, Zhang J, Lippmann S, Rusincovitch S, Henao R, Jones WS. Use of natural language processing to improve identification of patients with peripheral artery disease.Circ Cardiovasc Interv. 2020; 13:
- Wolterink JM, Leiner T, de Vos BD, van Hamersvelt RW, Viergever MA, Išgum I. Automatic coronary artery calcium scoring in cardiac CT angiography using paired convolutional neural networks.Med Image Anal. 2016; 34:123–136.
- Wu J, Xin J, Yang X, Sun J, Xu D, Zheng N, Yuan C. Deep morphology aided diagnosis network for segmentation of carotid artery vessel wall and diagnosis of carotid atherosclerosis on black-blood vessel wall MRI.Med Phys. 2019; 46:5544–5561.
- Yasaka K, Akai H, Abe O, Kiryu S. Deep learning with convolutional neural network for differentiation of liver masses at dynamic contrast-enhanced CT: a preliminary study.Radiology. 2018; 286:887–896.
- Yeo LL and Sharma VK. Automatic Detection and Measurement of Atherosclerotic Plaques in Carotid Ultrasound Using Deep Learning.International Stroke Conference. 2020.
- Yom-Tov E, Feraru G, Kozdoba M, Mannor S, Tennenholtz M, Hochberg I. Encouraging physical activity in patients with diabetes: intervention using a reinforcement learning system.J Med Internet Res. 2017; 19:e338.
- Zhang JL, Conlin CC, Li X, Layec G, Chang K, Kalpathy-Cramer J, Lee VS. Exercise-induced calf muscle hyperemia: rapid mapping of magnetic resonance imaging using deep learning approach.Physiol Rep. 2020; 8:e14563.
- Zhou R, Fenster A, Xia Y, Spence JD, Ding M. Deep learning-based carotid media-adventitia and lumen-intima boundary segmentation from three-dimensional ultrasound images.Med Phys. 2019; 46:3180–3193.
- Zierler RE, Jordan WD, Lal BK, Mussa F, Leers S, Fulton J, Pevec W, Hill A, Murad MH. The Society for Vascular Surgery practice guidelines on follow-up after vascular surgery arterial procedures.J Vasc Surg. 2018; 68:256–284
- Zitnik M, Agrawal M, Leskovec J. Modeling polypharmacy side effects with graph convolutional networks.Bioinformatics. 2018; 34:i457–i466
- Zreik M, Lessmann N, van Hamersvelt RW, Wolterink JM, Voskuil M, Viergever MA, Leiner T, Išgum I. Deep learning analysis of the myocardium in coronary CT angiography for identification of patients with functionally significant coronary artery stenosis.Med Image Anal. 2018; 44:72–85.

Artificial Intelligence And Automation In Valvular Heart Diseases

CHAPTER 10

Artificial intelligence (AI), which is a branch of computer science that attempts to create machines that perform tasks as though they possessed human brainpower, and this is gradually changing the landscape of the healthcare industry . Clini-cal procedures that were supposed to, and could only be performed by human experts previously can now been carried out by machines in a more accurate and efficient way. Recently, cardiologists and radiologists have cooperated with computer scientists and have developed a fully automated echocardiography interpretation system for clini-cal practice. Cardiovascular diseases affect 48% of the population (≥ 20 years old) and is the leading cause of death. Echocardiography is an effective method to monitor the state of the heart and allows early diagnosis before the onset of symptoms. However, in primary care clinics and poorer regions, there are inadequately experienced radiologists for echocardiography interpretation, let alone patient follow-up. There is group of researchers who trained AI systems using over 14,000 echocardiograms for multiple tasks including view classification and quantification of chamber volume, ejection fraction and longitudinal strain. The AI system validated its accuracy in diagnosing several cardiac diseases after testing on over 8000 cardiograms obtained from routine clinical flow . Such an AI system holds great potential for the transformation of current clinical practice models as well as the popularization of quality healthcare. The above example is only the tip of the ice-berg in the application of AI in medicine for over half a century. Since "AI" was first proposed by John MacCarthy at the Dartmouth College Conference in 1956, great efforts have been made for apply-ing AI to almost all phases of clinical practice. In 1960s, the concept of "computer-assisted diagnosis" emerged with attempts to use mathematical formalism to interpret clinical problems, although they have little practical value, it has paved the way for subsequent expert systems .In 1970s,researchers began to shift attention to studying the reasoning process of clinicians and simulate it on computer systems, which gave birth to the first generation of medical AI products, i.e. MYCIN. It attempts to diagnose infectious diseases and provide appropriate medication therapies based on over 200 rules that in the form of "if (precon-dition), then (conclusion or action)". Although MYCIN showed reliability in 63% of the cases of bacteremia .it is more like an advanced version of a textbook which has the function of automatic retrievals with little "intelligence". Moreover, the interactions between each rule should be defined by human experts which is extremely arduous with increasingly new knowledge added to the system. However, automatic interpretation of electrocar-diograms has gained great benefits from the rule--based AI system. During the same period, a new model, i.e. the probabilistic reasoning was used to simulate the process of expert decision making . Unlike the categorical mode of reasoning utilized by MYCIN, the probabilistic model assign weight to every symptom and clinical finding to indicate its possibility of occurrence for a certain disease. Based on this, new systems including the present illness program, INTERNIST, CASNET were developed. With the introduction of "artificial neural network" in 1980s, machine learning began to flourish. Machine learning endows computers with the ability to learn patterns from data and perform tasks without explicit programming It has showed great power in developing robust risk prediction models, redefining patient classes and other tasks with the popularization of electronic health records and digital imaging systems.In 2006, the introduction of deep learning by LeCun et al.

achieved unprecedented progress in im-age recognition and other domains, which brought a new renaissance to the development of AI and made automated medical imaging interpretation one of the hottest topics in AI. AI can generally be classified as either weak AI or strong AI. Strong AI is an intelligence construct that has the ability to understand and think as a human being. Weak AI is limited to a specific or narrow area, which is often designed to perform time-consuming tasks and analyze data in ways that humans sometimes cannot. In this review, a brief introduction to AI is provided and highlights its application in the clinical flow of diagnosing and treating valvular heart diseases, including heart sound auscultation, medical image analysis (echocardiography, cardiac computed tomography [CT] and cardiac magnetic resonance [CMR]), risk factor identification, mortality prediction and robotic surgery.

Fundamental concepts in AI

Machine learning

In essence, machine learning is an extension to traditional statistical methods for dealing with large data sets and variables. It enables computers to learn rules and even uncover new patterns from data through a series of algorithms. Most impor-tantly, machine learning can gradually optimize the "reasoning process" between inputs and outputs. Machine learning can be broadly classified into three classes: supervised learning, unsupervised learning and reinforcement learning.

In supervised learning, machines learn the mapping relations between input variables and labeled outcomes and are able to predict outcomes according to inputs. For example, after training with echocardiograms that are labeled with given disease categories, machines are able to assign these disease labels to new echocardiograms. Common computational approaches in supervised learning include artificial neural network (ANN), support vector machine, k-nearest neighbor, naive Bayesian model and decision tree model, among others. Unsupervised learning aims to uncover hid-den structures in unlabeled data and classify it into separate categories, which means machines are only trained with input variables and automatically find potential classification rules.For example, with unsupervised learning, machines uncovered three cardiac phenotypes in patients diagnosed with type 2 diabetes mellitus according to their echocardiograms Common computational approaches include hierarchical clustering, k-means clustering and principle component analysis. Reinforcement learning signifies that machines learn strategies which can obtain the maximum reward through interaction with the environment or outcomes. Unlike the static mode of supervised or unsupervised learning, it is a dynamic learning process. Q-learning, an example of reinforcement learning, has been utilized in clinical trials of lung cancer to find the optimal individualized therapies

Artificial neural network and deep learning

Artificial neural network is composed of multiple interconnected artificial neurons which mimic the biological brain. As mentioned above, ANN is actually a computational model. ANN learns from large amounts of data and continuously optimizes the weight of each connection between neurons. Figure 1B shows a typical ANN, which is also called multilayer perceptron, is composed of three layers: input layer, hidden layer and output layer. Each layer contains multiple neurons that are responsible for different functions. The input layer receives numerical variables from data, each value in first layer neurons combines with the weight of the connection, which is then propagated to a hidden layer where the values are integrated, while an output layer generates the final value which represents an outcome. Each neuron in the hid-den layer can also set up a threshold to determine whether the information should propagate to the next layer. Now suppose that a database that includes patient data (such as age, body mass index, laboratory results and images results) prior to cardiac surgery and operation results (alive or dead), a mortality prediction model can be built with ANN. Patient variables are input into the neurons in the first layer, the outputs are set as 1 for alive and 0 for dead. The weight of each connection and the excitation threshold of each neuron in the hidden layer are gradually optimized by learning from the data. In this way, after trained with sufficient cases,the ANN model can be accurate enough to predict surgical outcome in new patients.

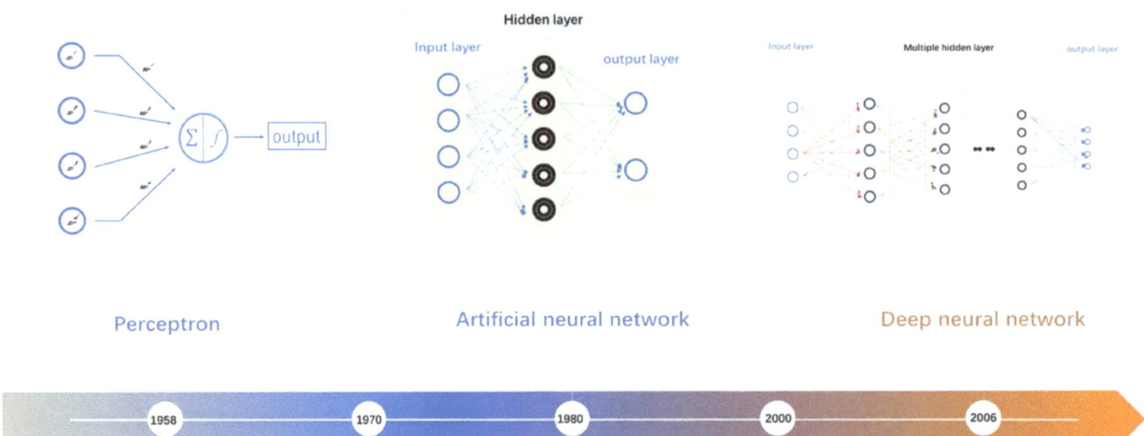

Fig. 10.1 Schematic diagram of the evolvement of artificial neural network. Perceptron, also called single layer neural network, was proposed by Rosenblatt in 1958 (A), classic artificial neural network, also known as double layer neural network or multilayer perceptron (B), deep neural network (C).

It can be imagined that, with more hidden layers, the computational results will be more ac-curate, but this meanwhile requires greater com-putational power using more training data. Thanks to the rapid development of computer processors and arrival of the era of big data, and also the in-troduction of "pre-training process", "fine-tuning technique" by Hinton et al. which decreases the training time substantially, multilayer ANN which is also known as "deep learning" becomes a reality. It now represents the most advanced AI technology. The biggest advantage of deep neural network is that it allows the computing model to automatically extract the features of the data by abstracting the data layer by layer and learning the representative and discriminant features.

Computer vision

Computer vision is a main research field in AI, which simulates the human vision with imaging systems and computers. The main tasks involved in computer vision can be divided into three levels. The basic level includes image acquiring and processing techniques such as noise filtering, image enhancement, image segmentation, patternrecognition. For middle level computer vision, computers should be able to draw conclusions and make decisions based on the information obtained from the basic level. For the top level, computersrecognition. For middle level computer vision, computers should be able to draw conclusions and make decisions based on the information obtained from the basic level. For the top level, computershave the capability to "think" and can understand images like humans do. For now, the first two levels of computer vision are mostly applied to the analy-sis of medical images and assist in diagnosis. As described below, many algorithms and commercial software have been developed for automating the analysis of medical images, which are more accu-rate and efficient compared to human endeavour.

Expert system

Expert systems are in their earliest application of AI in medicine, and will keep playing an impor-tant role in healthcare. In brief, expert systems are a computer program that simulates human experts in solving problems . It is also called a knowl-edge-based system because it contains a large amount of knowledge and experience from experts. A typical medical expert system is composed of two modules: knowledge base and control system, the latter can be further divided into a human-computerinteractive component, an explanation component, a knowledge acquisition component and an infer-ence engine. The knowledge base is composed of medical knowledge from experts, case-specific knowledge from patients and intermediate results from the reasoning process

Application of AI and automation in diagnosis of valvular heart diseases

AI-assisted "cardiac auscultation"

In spite of the diverse alternatives of imaging tools being the major diagnostic approach to valvu-lar heart diseases (VHDs), physical examination, is the cornerstone of clinical diagnosis and should be the primary screening method for VHDs. Common physical examinations for VHDs include general inspection, pulse palpation, percussion of heart boarder and heart sound auscultation, etc. Among these, auscultation plays a key role of diagnosing VHDs. Valvular heart diseases manifest as heart murmurs or/and extra heart sound before the stress of hemodynamic changes causing other signs and symptoms including dyspnea, fatigue, angina, cough and hemoptysis. While cardiac auscultation provides significant diagnostic and prognostic information for cardiac disease, it is not an easy skill to master, especially when innocent murmurs are confronted. Although experienced clinicians have reached an accuracy over 90% in identifying innocent murmurs from pathologic murmurs, less-experienced residents and primary care physicians perform less than satisfactorily . In addition, auscultation is a highly subjective process which may cause bias when evaluating the intensity, location and shape of murmurs. For over a cen-tury, tools for cardiac auscultation is a mechanical stethoscope, however, it can neither store nor play back sounds . Thanks to the inventionThanks to the invention of electronic (digital) stethoscope, the forgoing problems have been well solved, more than that, it provides clinicians with a handy way of "see-ing" the heart sound through phonocardiogram. AI-assisted cardiac auscultation in practice refers to the auto-interpretation of phonocardiogram, which belongs to the domain of signal processing. Key steps involved in heart sound analysis could be summarized as segmentation, feature extraction and classification . Each step is fulfilled through a multitude of algorithms with the ultimate goal of precisely identifying the pathological events underlying heart sounds.

Heart sounds segmentation.

Segmentation aims to locate the fundamental elements includ-ing the first heart sound (S1), systolic period, the second heart sound (S2) and diastolic period in each cardiac cycle. Training machines to think like human so as to solve problems is to mimic the thinking process of human brain to a certain extent. When interpreting heart sounds, A human expert would firstly locate the two fundamental heart sounds then discriminate S1 from S2 by its pitch, intensity and duration, finally the systolic and diastolic regions are determined, as is the process with computational analysis, but in a more logical and mathematical way. In the early exploration of heart sound seg-mentation, electrocardiograph or/and carotid pulse was/were obtained concurrently with phonocar-diogram.Transformation equation g(n) was used to compute the smooth energy curve of electrocardiograph signal, then the peaks in g(n) was determined as the beginning of S1 and the systolic period, the dicrotic notch of carotid pulse curve was recognized as the beginning of S2 . This approach apparently is impractical in routine clinical work. Envelop-based (or amplitude threshold-based) segmentation algorithm was first introduced by Liang et al. to locate S1 and S2. Envelop of a signal signifies the smooth curves outlining its upper or lower extremes The envelop of the original heart sound waveform was first extracted using specific transformation equations, then a threshold value was selected to filter noise and low intensity signals, the peaks exceed the threshold value were recognized as the S1 and S2, S1 was differentiated form S2 based on an as-sumption that the systolic period was shorter than the diastolic period.A well-fitted extraction equation would allow only two peaks to exceed the threshold when interpreting the normal heart sound, therefore identification accuracy depends largely on an envelope extraction equation.Di-verse methods are used to calculate the envelopewere created including normalized

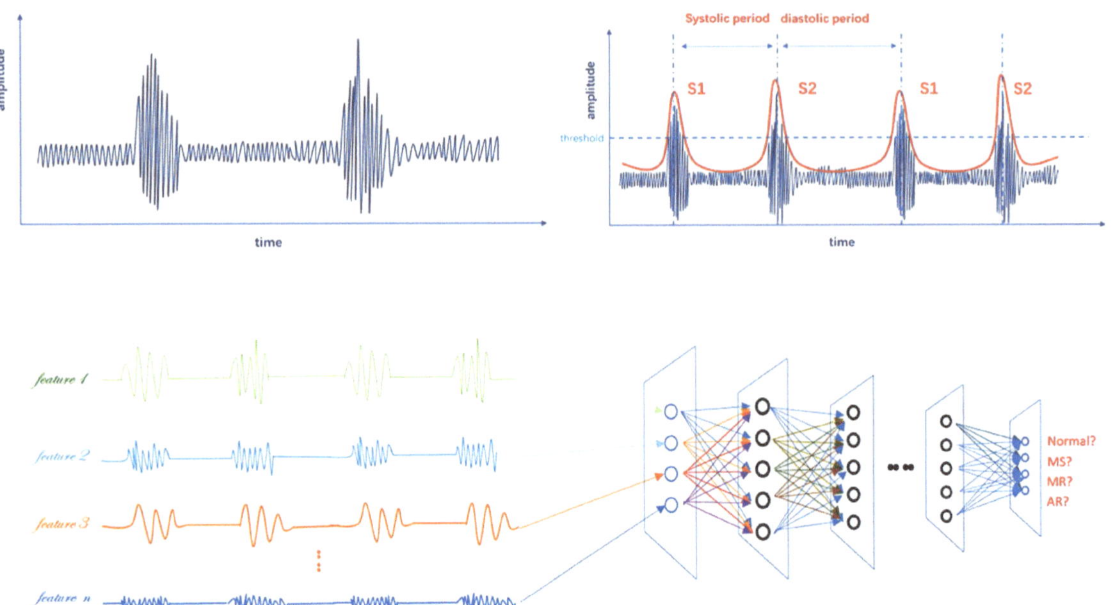

Fig.10.2 Process of artificial intelligence-assisted auscultation. A normal phonocardiogram (A), heart sound segmen-tation (B), feature extraction (C), heart sound classification by deep neural network (D).

Shan-non energy , single-DOF analytical model , wavelet decomposition method [24], Viola integral approach and others. However, the envelope-based segmentation method often leads to problems like weak peaks or extra peaks which reduce accuracy of the results. The application of machine learning algorithms to heart sound segmentation based on features substantially improves the segmentation results (see feature extraction below). Hidden Markov Model (HMM) is the most widely used in the task .To train the HMM, adequate samples pre-labeled with the accurate location of S1, S2, systolic and diastolic period are required at the output end; sequences of feature vectors extracted from original phonocardiogram or transformed envelope are used as the observation end of HMM. Recently, utilization of deep learning achieves even higher precision compared to other classification methods in heart sound segmentation

Feature extraction and feature selection.

This step aims to select and extract discriminative features either for more precise segmentation of heart sound or for following the disease clas-sification step. Feature means the characteristic of an object by which the human brain recognizes and distinguishes it automatically. The concept of feature is similar to "variable" in regression analy-sis. Features that can be recognized by machines tend to be presented in the form of numbers or symbols. A human expert draws physiological or pathological information from heart sound through features including heart rate, heart rhythm, timing and shape of the murmur, pitch of the heart sound, and extra heart sound among others. As for phono-cardiogram, the features are based on time-domain, frequency-domain, and time-frequency complex do-main.Time-domain features include intervals (interval of S1 and S2, systolic intervals, diastolic intervals, the ratio of each component to the cardiac cycle etc.) and amplitude (mean absolute amplitude of S1 and S2 interval). Frequency-domain features refer to the power spectrum of each heart sound component across frequency bands. Theoreti-cally the more input of features into machine train-ing, the better the classification performance it will achieve. In practice, with the number of training samples being set, the classification performance will drop off when the number of feature inputs exceeds a certain value. In order to exclude the redundant features and improve the classification efficiency, feature selection is often required

Classification and detection of VHDs.

This step aims to classify the phonocardiograms into cardiac disease categories using suitable classi-fiers. Classifier in machine learning refers to the algorithm that learns to assign labels to testing data from training data. This learning process can be supervised or unsupervised. Briefly speaking, supervised learning assigns given labels to data while unsupervised learning seeks labels that could be assigned to data. In the present case, labels are given disease categories like mitral stenosis, mitral regurgitation, aortic stenosis, etc. therefore, supervised learning algorithms/ classifiers are uti-lized. The common classifiers used in heart sound classification include a support vector machine , neural networks , HMM , etc. After a careful combination of algorithms used in segmentation, feature extraction and classification, previous studies showed promising and inspiring results in detecting VHDs from phonocardiograms. For instance, an intelligent diagnostic system developed by Sun could discriminate aortic regurgitation, mitral regurgitation, pulmo-nary stenosis with accuracy of 98.9%, 98.4% and 98.7%, respectively. Thompson et al. utilized a murmur detection algorithm developed by CSD labs to distinguish no murmurs and innocent mur-murs from pathologic murmurs. 3180 phonocar-diograms recorded at five different chest location from 603 cases were tested, the algorithm had good sensitivity, specificity and accuracy in detecting a pathologic murmur, which are 93%, 81% and 88%, respectively. The algorithm showed the highest ac-curacy (90%) using recordings from the left upper and lower sternal boarder. However, it was unable to analyze the recordings with precision which had a high heart rate and low signal quality

AI-assisted interpretation of echocardiography

Although heart sounds auscultation is con-venient, cost-effective and a quick way to diagnose VHDs, it only provides qualitative diagnostic information. To further confirm the diagnosis of VHDs as well as to assess the etiology, severity, ventricular responses and prognosis, imaging tools including echocardiography, CMR, multi-slice CT (MSCT) or even cardiac catheterization are indispensable

Echocardiography is the "heart" of cardiology.
It is the preferred method of diagnosing and guid-ing the treatment of VHDs as well as other cardiac diseases. However, echocardiographic examination is a time-consuming process which usually takes hours from inspection, analysis to formal report which make it impractical in emergency settings. Moreover, typical echocardiographic examination produces large amounts of data including images from multiple views and up to 70 videos which would cause cognitive overload and be prone to error. In addition, due to the characteristic of multiple views in examination, the problems of intra-observer and inter-observer variability inevi-tably arise. The application of AI and automation in echocardiography would a allow consistent, quick and accurate measurement which promises a more accurate diagnosis and improved patient care.

Image segmentation-valve leaflet detection and tracking.

Segmentation and recognition of anatomical structures from original medical images are preprocessing steps for subsequent quantitative analysis and diagnosis. Morphologi-cal characteristics and motion pattern of the heart valves are key information to diagnose VHDs and to assist surgical valve repair or percutaneous intervention. While many studies have sought the approaches to segment heart chambers and detect endocardial boarder which were reviewed by Noble and Boukerroui , relatively few studies of the segmentation of heart valves and annulus have been published. The reasons for difficulty in segmenting and tracking the heart valves in echocardiographic sequences can be summarized as follows: poor image quality due to low frame rate, speckle noise and artifact which may resultin missing boundaries; (2) lack of features to dis-criminate heart valve from adjacent myocardium for those structures have similar intensity and texture; (3) fast and irregular valve motion making it hard to establish correspondence between frames. Re-ported approaches for valve segmentation including active contour models , thin tissue detector combined with graph cut outlier detection method , J-spline method multi-atlas joint label fusion , trajectory spectrum learning algorithm and neural network

Active contour models (ACM) is the first and most widely used segmentation algorithm for the heart valve. The segmentation process is based on ACM and is initiated by manual placement of contour close to the target, which means it is not fully automated. Zhou et al. formulated the problems of valve detection and tracking as outliner detection in the low-rank representation based on different motion patterns between leaflets and the heart wall, which is fully automated requiring no user interaction. Recently, there is a growing trend of applying machine learning to valve seg-mentation. This approach shifts the manual input to a training phase which makes segmentation fully automated .Ionasec et al. utilized spec-trum learning algorithm and boundary detectors to locate and refine mitral leaflets based on anatomical landmarks in four-dimensional (4D) transesopha-geal echocardiograms and CT which allows precise morphological and functional quantification, and a large amount of data as well as high computational power were required to train the model. Recently, a novel UNet architecture based on a convolutional neural network was utilized by Costa et al. to segment mitral valves in PLAX and A4C views. The biggest strength of UNet architecture is that it does not require a large training dataset to produce accurate results.

Automated quantitative analysis.

Precise and reliable quantitative analysis of stenosis and regurgitation is crucial to severity assessment, prognosis prediction and to evaluate whether sur-gery or intervention is needed. Proximal isoveloc-ity surface area (PISA) method is widely used in measuring mitral valve orifice area and calculating the regurgitant volume.Conventional PISA method of two-dimensional echocardiography is based on the assumption that the shape of the proximal flow convergence region is hemispheric, which is not quite true . The development of three-dimensional (3D) color Doppler echocar-diography enables direct measurement of PISA without assumptions, thereby reducing errors . However, it is not indicated for routine clinical use because it is a time-consuming procedure, thus in desperate need of an automated algorithm. Grady et al. proposed the first automated PISA measurement system based on a random walker algorithm. The system was initiated by the manual input of two points (one at the valve annulus and one at the coaptation site), followed by automated segmentation of valve annulus and the isovelocity region. The segmentation results were then used to generate 3D meshes for computing PISA. In vitro experiments validated its accuracy in measuring PISA, effective regurgitant surface area (EROA) and regurgitant volume. Further in vivo experi-ments showed that measurement of EROA on pa-tients with magnetic resonance (MR) by automated algorithm was significantly correlated with manual measurement of vena contracta . Cobey et al. proposed another novel automated method based on Halcon H Develop Machine Vision. 3D images of PISA were first sliced into 2 mm-thick sequential cuts, the algorithm traced the boundary of each slice and the arc lengths between each slice from which the 3D surface area was generated and computed. Another method of quantitatively assessing MR is to use regurgitant fraction which is calculated from mitral inflow and stroke volume . Wang et al. proposed a novel automated system for estimating mitral inflow and aortic out-flow. The system first detected the left ventricular wall, mitral annulus and left ventricular outflow tract using marginal space learning and placed the measurement plane. The 3D motions of these structures were tracked through a whole cardiac circle to construct and adjust the measurement plane, then the volume of mitral inflow and left ventricular outflow was computed by aggregating color flow values in the 3D space In addition to these pioneering studies, several commercial software have been developed including Mitral Valve Quantification (Philips Medical Imaging, Andover, MA) eSie Valve (Siemens Healthcare, Mountain View, CA, USA) Mitral Valve Navigator (Philips Medical Systems).Auto Valve Analysis (Siemens; California, USA) , eSie PISA Volume Analysis (Siemens Medi-cal Solutions USA, Inc., Mountain View, CA) which aim to automate the quantitative analysis of 3D echocardiography.

These approaches can reduce the measurement time substantially and provide more accurate and reproducible results. The aforementioned automated algorithms and commercial software have validated their reliability in quantitatively measuring aortic and mitral valve apparatus parameters and regurgitation volume

AI-assisted interpretation of cardiac CT images

Computed tomography is not employed as the preferred diagnostic method of VHD. It generally serves as a complementary role when echocardi-ography is insufficient or inclusive. Nevertheless, cardiac CT has prominent advantages in the evalu-ation of valve calcification and annulus geometry. It is the golden standard for annulus sizing and an indispensable tool in preoperative planning of transcatheter aortic valve replacement (TAVR). Reliable measurement of aortic valve annulus size, aortic root dimension and the height of coronary ostia are crucial for appropriate transcatheter valve prosthesis selection and intraprocedural valve po-sitioning which may improve success rate and re-duce postoperative complications. In recent years, advances in 3D image techniques have enabled reconstruction of patient-specific models of aortic valve apparatus. Several automated algorithms and commercial software for aortic valve segmentation and quantification have been developed for pre-operative planning of transcathether aortic valve implantation (TAVI).

Patient-specific 3D modeling of aortic valve.

Ionasec et al. proposed the first dy-namic patient-specific aortic valve model from 4D CT images. A generic physiological model which can represent aortic valve and its pathological variations was constructed first, patient-specific parameters of the model were estimated from volu-metric sequences by trajectory spectrum learning, marginal space learning and discriminative learn-ing. Their study was further improved with shape forest to constrain the classical statistical shape model Waechter et al. extracted the aortic valve geometry from CT images using model-based segmentation and applies pattern search method to detect the coronary ostia. The whole heart geom-etry (including heart chambers and great vessels) was first roughly modeled, a generic aortic mesh model was established and boundary detector were trained by annotated images aiming to build more detailed models of the aortic valve and root, the coronary ostia was then detected on the surface of the aortic root. Segmentation results allowed a series of clinical measurements including the di-ameters of annulus and the distance between ostia and aortic valve, etc. Considering that VHDs often involve multivalvular lesion which require joint as-sessment, Grbic et al. proposed an integrated model for quantification of all heart valves from 4D CT images based on marginal space learning and multi-linear shape models. Another study of Grbic et al. [69] extracted both the volumetric model of the aortic valve and calcification, which is closely correlated with postoperative regurgitation

Landmarks detection and quantitative measurement.

A number of parameters should be measured with precision for surgical planning before TAVI. These include annulus diameter, an-nulus area, angulation of annulus plane and the distance from annulus to coronary ostia to name a few. The annulus diameter is crucial for selection of the appropriate valve prosthesis. Size mismatching may either cause post-operative perivalvular regurgita-tion or annulus rupture. A short distance between aortic annulus and coronary ostia indicates elevated risk of coronary obstruction after valve deployment. Annulus plane angulation determines the position of an X-ray tube C-arm during operations to achieve an optimal view of valve delivery. Accurate segmentation of the aorta, aortic valve apparatus and detection of anatomic land-marks (coronary ostium, aortic commissures and aortic hinges) is the prerequisite for reliable meas-urement of the above parameters. Zheng et al. proposed a robust hierarchical approach by first segmenting the global aorta using marginal space learning from which the position of the anatomical landmarks can be roughly inferred, followed by us-ing specific landmark detectors to refine each land-mark.Elattar et al.used thresholding and connected component analysis to detect the region of interest, from which aortic root was extracted using 3D normalized cut.

Two coronary ostia and three valve hinge points were then detected on the surface of aortic root by intensity projection map and Gaussian curvature map. Lalys et al. used a hybrid approach which integrated thresholding, model-based method, statistical-based method and a 3D contour model in the procedure, however, a user-specific point is needed to define the vol-ume of interest. Recently, colonial walk algorithm, which is a machine learning method, was utilized by Al et al. to automatically localize the land-marks. Several commercial software including three mensio valves (3mensio Medical Imaging BV, the Netherlands) Syngo (Siemens Healthcare, Erlangen, Germany) , Intelli-Space Portal (Philips Medical Systems, Cleveland, OH) , have been available for routine clini-cal use. Together with the aforementioned al-gorithms, these pioneering techniques showed reliable aortic annulus measurements A comparative study between 3 mensio, Intelli- Space Portal (version 7.0), IntelliSpace Portal (version 9.0) and manual measurement concerning annulus parameters, time-cost and reproducibility was performed [81]. Results showed that Intelli-Space Portal (version 9.0) allowed the fastest and most reproducible measurements, parameters derived from either method can be used inter-changeably in prosthesis sizing. Moreover, Samim et al. performed a prospective cohort study to compare angiography and MSCT (using 3mensio) in predicting the annulus plane and choosing the C-arm position . The study included 35 patients in an angiography cohort and 36 patients in an MDCT cohort. The utilization of MDCT was associated with a significant reduction of prosthesis implanting time, radiation exposure and contrast delivery. A reduction of postoperative complications and 30-day mortality was observed in patients in the MDCT cohort.

AI-assisted interpretation of CMR

Cardiac magnetic resonance is the second-line technique in the assessment of VHDs. A standard CMR scan takes about an hour followed by tedi-ous image processing which is both time and labor consuming. However, it is the golden standard in the assessment of cardiac morphology, volume and function due to its high spatial resolution [82]. MR cine imaging and phase-contrast velocity imaging are gaining increasing importance in studying val-vular function.

Particularly, CMR have advantages over other imaging tools in the quantification of regurgitation when the regurgitant jet is highly eccentric.

Automated cardiac chamber segmentation and cardiac volume measurement have been widely studied in MR images as reviewed by Bernard et al. [83] and Petitjean et al. [84]. Several large CMR image datasets (Sunnybrook, STACOM, MICCAI RV and kaggle), which are free to access, have been released in the last decade in conjunction with international challenges to automatically segment left ventricle, right ventricle, end-diastolic volume and end-systolic volume Commercial software such as SuiteHEART® (Neosoft, Pewaukee, Wisconsin, USA) which allows automated quantification of biventricular volumes and function is now available . The regurgitant volume and fraction in isolated aortic or mitral regurgitation can be calculated from left ventricle and right ventricle stroke volume , however, to date, the aforementioned automated methods have not applied in quantification of valve regurgitation. AI-assisted CMR which allows automated diagnosis of VHDs is underexplored. However, several pioneering studies have achieved many valuable results. Fries et al. developed a novel supervised deep learning model for aortic valve malformation classification using unlabeled MR images. 570 patients were classified as bicuspid aortic valve from a cohort of 9230 patients from the UK biobank. These individuals showed a significant lower major adverse cardiac event-free survival rate compared to individuals with a normal aortic valve.

Risk factor identification and in-hospital mortality prediction of cardiac surgery

Preoperative assessment of surgical risk is an important procedure in cardiac surgery which guides the selection of surgery, intervention or nonsurgical treatment. Great progress has been made in risk factor identification and mortality pre-diction. Risk score models including EuroSCORE, STS score and ACEF scores have been widely used . The linear regression model is the most widely used in analyzing a correlation between risk variables and cardiac adverse events. However, there is a growing trend of utilizing machine learn-ing methods in developing prediction models which outperform traditional scoring systems.

Nilsson et al. were among the first to use an ANN model to identify risk factors and predict mortality in cardiac surgery. 72 risk factors were evaluated from 18,362 patients, 34 of the factors were identified as relevant to mortality. Receiver operating characteristic (ROC) area of the ANN model for mortality prediction was significantly larger than logistic EuroSCORE model (0.81 vs. 0.79). For isolated valve surgery (with or without coronary artery bypass grafting), the ROC area of the ANN model was 0.76 vs. 0.72 of the logistic models. Celi et al. achieved an even larger ROC area using ANN, Bayesian network and lo-gistic regression (0.941, 0.931, 0.854) compared to EuroSCORE (0.648). Allyn et al. utilized a novel ensemble machine learning method which integrates the results from four isolated machine learning algorithms to predict cardiac surgery mortality. 6250 patients were enrolled in the study, Chi-square filtering was utilized to extract relevant variables. Results showed that the ensemble ma-chine learning model had a significantly stronger discriminatory power for operative mortality than EuroSCORE II (ROC area: 0.795 vs. 0.737). Recently, Hernandez-Suarez firstly applied four machine learning algorithms in mortality predic-tion after TAVI 10,883 patients were enrolled in the study. Logistic regression, ANN, Naïve bayes and random forest which are the four top supervised learning algorithms all showed good discriminative performance. The best prediction model obtained by logistic algorithm (ROC area: 0.92) have close discriminative power with state-of-the-art National Inpatient Sample TAVR score model.

Moreover, ANN and machine learning algo-rithm have been applied in other fields such as pre-diction of length of stay in intensive care unit after cardiac surgery , post-operative complications , both short-term and long-term mortality after heart transplantation . However, the downside of current studies is that few studies have been dedicated to isolated cardiac surgery procedures

Intelligent cardiac operating room: Towards autonomous robotic surgery

which is partially due to a lack of sufficient samples to feed machine training. The introduction of minimally invasive strate-gies and a surgical robot in cardiac surgery prom-ises quicker recovery and less postoperative complications and mortality. While having many superiorities over human hands such as tremor resistance and scalable motion, current robotic systems are merely teleoperated devices under human control which entirely possess no autonomy. Since automation has gained great success in other robotic fields which have increased safety, accuracy and efficiency, it is reasonable to assume that the same benefit will be gained by developing autonomous surgical robots. To achieve the level of fully "autonomous", the surgical robot should possess the ability to "see", "think" and "act". "see" refers to perception of the surgical field and itself through sensors. "think" is the process of receiving information and calculating the future status that it needs to achieve in the following "act" . Recently, European research council launch the Autonomous Robotic Surgery (ARS) project aiming to developing a unified framework for the autonomous execution of robotic tasks . Main research objectives include establish-ment of global action model by analyzing current robotic surgical data, patient specific intervention models, design of controllers, perception of overall surgical situations, and assessment of the surgical robot capability.

Though at an experimental stage, the feasi-bility of autonomous robots performing simple surgical tasks like suture and knot typing have been demonstrated. Penesar et al. developed a novel Smart Tissue Autonomous Robot (STAR) which was able to perform linear continuous suture, it successfully completed in-vivo end-to-end anastomosis of porcine small intestine with few suturing mistakes, no complications were observed in 7 day follow-up. Although the STAR system realized autonomous suture, the step of knot typing remained manual. In the context of endoscopic surgery or robot-assisted surgery,the task of knot typing is cumbersome which re-quires manipulation of many subtle movements in a confined space

Through training a recurrent neural network on 3D loop trajectories generated by human surgeon, the Endoscopic Partial-Auton-omous Robot (EndoPAR) was able to accurately perform the winding portion of a knot-tying task [99]. To date however, robots are unable to fully perform autonomous knot tying.

Transcatheter therapy has been accepted as an alternative to traditional cardiac valvular surgery especially in patients with high surgical risk in recent years. Catheters are inserted either from peripheral vessel or the cardiac apex to deploy valve prothesis or occlusion device. In either case, the catheters need to be precisely navigated to the intervention site which is a very challenging task in a beating heart. Inspired by wall following, which is used by thigmotactic animals to locate and navi-gate themselves in low-visibility environments, Fagogenis et al. developed an autonomous intracardiac catheter navigation system. With hybrid imaging and touch sensor installed on the catheter tip, which can provide clear images of what it has touched and identify it as blood, valve or myocardium. The catheter created continuous low-force contact with the surrounding tissue and followed the cardiac wall to achieve autonomous navigation. With the navigation system, authors designed a robotic catheter, inserted from the cardiac apex, which can autonomously navigate to the aortic valve and deploy an occlusion device into the leak site on a porcine model. The in-vivo animal experiments demonstrate that an autono-mous robot catheter was non-inferior to human experts

Conclusions

Artificial intelligence is changing the land-scape of healthcare. The inclusion of AI and automated algorithms in medical image analysis are very promising for they require less measure-ment time and meanwhile provide more accurate and reproducible results, which make them ideal helpers in a busy clinical flow. Machine learning methods can make full use of patient data and build more powerful prediction models of cardiac surgery compared to traditional statistical ap-proaches. Moreover, the autonomous surgical robot, although in its infancy, holds great promise for improved safety and efficiency in cardiac surgery and intervention.

Bibliography And Acknowledgement

- Al WA, Jung HoY, Yun IID, et al. Automatic aortic valve land-mark localization in coronary CT angiography using colonial walk. PLoS One. 2018; 13(7):
- Allyn J, Allou N, Augustin P, et al. A Comparison of a Machine Learning Model with EuroSCORE II in Predicting Mortality after Elective Cardiac Surgery: A Decision Curve Analysis. PLoS One. 2017; 12(1
- Backhaus SJ, Staab W, Steinmetz M, et al. Fully automated quan-tification of biventricular volumes and function in cardiovascular magnetic resonance: applicability to clinical routine settings. J Cardiovasc Magn Reson. 2019; 21(1): 24, Baeßler B, Mauri V, Bunck AC, et al. Software-automated multi-detector computed tomography-based prosthesis-sizing in tran-scatheter aortic valve replacement: Inter-vendor comparison and relation to patient outcome. Int J Cardiol. 2018; 272: 267–272,
- Beam AL, Kohane IS. Big data and machine learning in health care. JAMA. 2018; 319(13): 1317–1318, doi: 10.1001/jama.2017.18391, indexed in Pubmed: 29532063.
- Benjamin EJ, Muntner P, Alonso A, et al. Heart Disease and Stroke Statistics — 2019 Update: A Report From the American Heart Association. Vol. 139, Circulation. 2019.
- Bernard O, Cervenansky F, Lalande A, et al. Deep learning tech-niques for automatic MRI cardiac multi-structures segmentation and diagnosis: is the problem solved? IEEE Trans Med Imag-ing. 2018; 37(11): 2514–2525
- Calleja A, Thavendiranathan P, Ionasec RI, et al. Automated quantitative 3-dimensional modeling of the aortic valve and root by 3-dimensional transesophageal echocardiography in normals, aortic regurgitation, and aortic stenosis: comparison to computed tomography in normals and clinical implications. Circ Cardio-vasc Imaging. 2013; 6(1): 99–108,
- Celi LA, Galvin S, Davidzon G, et al. A database-driven deci-sion support system: customized mortality prediction. J Pers Med. 2012; 2(4): 138–148, doi: 10.3390/jpm2040138, indexed in Pubmed: 23766893.
- Chen C. Computer vision in medical imaging. Vol. 2. World Scientific. 2014.
- Chen TE, Yang SI, Ho LT, et al. S1 and S2 Heart Sound Rec-ognition Using Deep Neural Networks. IEEE Trans Biomed Eng. 2017; 64(2): 372–380,
- Choi J, Hong GR, Kim M, et al. Automatic quantification of aortic regurgitation using 3D full volume color doppler echocardiogra-phy: a validation study with cardiac magnetic resonance imaging. Int J Cardiovasc Imaging. 2015; 31(7): 1379–1389
- Cobey FC, McInnis JA, Gelfand BJ, et al. A method for automat-ing 3-dimensional proximal isovelocity surface area measure-ment. J Cardiothorac Vasc Anesth. 2012; 26(3): 507–511,
- Costa E, Martins N, Sultan MS, et al. Mitral valve leaflets segmentation in echocardiography using convolutional neural networks. 6th IEEE Port Meet Bioeng ENBENG 2019 Proc. 2019: 1–4.
- de Agustin JA, Viliani D, Vieira C, et al. Proximal isovelocity sur-face area by single-beat three-dimensional color Doppler

- de Agustin JA, Viliani D, Vieira C, et al. Proximal isovelocity sur-face area by single-beat three-dimensional color Doppler echo-cardiography applied for tricuspid regurgitation quantification. J Am Soc Echocardiogr. 2013; 26(9): 1063–1072
- Delgado V, Ng ACT, Schuijf JD, et al. Automated assessment of the aortic root dimensions with multidetector row com-puted tomography. Ann Thorac Surg. 2011; 91(3): 716–723, doi: 10.1016/j.athoracsur.2010.09.060, indexed in Pubmed: 21352985.
- Dwivedi AK, Imtiaz SA, Rodriguez-Villegas E. Algorithms for au-tomatic analysis and classification of heart sounds-A systematic review. IEEE Access. 2019; 7(c): 8316–45.
- Elattar M, Wiegerinck E, van Kesteren F, et al. Automatic aortic root landmark detection in CTA images for preprocedural plan-ning of transcatheter aortic valve implantation. Int J Cardiovasc Imaging. 2016; 32(3): 501–511,
- Elattar MA, Wiegerinck EM, Planken RN, et al. Automatic seg-mentation of the aortic root in CT angiography of candidate pa-tients for transcatheter aortic valve implantation. Med Biol Eng Comput. 2014; 52(7): 611–618,
- Ernande L, Audureau E, Jellis CL, et al. Clinical implications of echocardiographic phenotypes of patients with diabetes mel-litus. J Am Coll Cardiol. 2017; 70(14): 1704–1716,
- Fagogenis G, Mencattelli M, Machaidze Z, et al. Autonomous Ro-botic Intracardiac Catheter Navigation Using Haptic Vision. Sci Robot. 2019; 4(29),
- Fahad HM, Ghani Khan MU, Saba T, et al. Microscopic abnormal-ity classification of cardiac murmurs using ANFIS and HMM. Mi-crosc Res Tech. 2018; 81(5): 449–457,
- Falk V, Baumgartner H, Bax JJ, et al. ESC/EACTS Guidelines for the management of valvular heart disease. Eur J Cardio-thoracic Surg. 2017; 52: 616–664.
- Fries JA, Varma P, Chen VS, et al. Weakly supervised classifica-tion of rare aortic valve malformations using unlabeled cardiac MRI sequences. bioRxiv. 2018; 2019: 1–25, doi: 10.1038/s41467-019-11012-3.
- Garcia-Ruiz A, Gagner M, Miller JH, et al. Manual vs robotically assisted laparoscopic surgery in the performance of basic ma-nipulation and suturing tasks. Arch Surg. 1998; 133(9): 957–961,
- Gill D, Gavrieli N, Intrator N. Detection and identification of heart sounds using homomorphic envelogram and self-organiz-ing probabilistic model. Comput Cardiol. 2005; 32: 957–60.
- Grady L, Datta S, Kutter O, et al. Regurgitation Quantification Using 3D PISA in Volume Echocardiograhy. In: Fichtinger G, editors. pMedical Image Comuting and Comuter-AssisteInter-vention -- MICCAI 2011. Berlin, Heidelberg: Sringer Berlin Heidelberg. 2011: 512–519.
- Grbic S, Ionasec R, Mansi T, et al. Advanced intervention plan-ning for Transcatheter Aortic Valve Implantations (TAVI) from CT using volumetric models. Proc Int Symp Biomed Imaging. 2013: 1424–1427.
- Grbic S, Ionasec R, Vitanovski D, et al. Complete valvular heart apparatus model from 4D cardiac CT. Med Image Anal. 2012; 16(5): 1003–1014.
- Grespan L, Fiorini P, Colucci G. Looking Ahead: The Future of Robotic Surgery. In: The Route to Patient Safety in Robotic Sur-gery [Internet]. Cham: Springer International Publishing. 2019: 157–162,
- Guez D, Boroumand G, Ruggiero NJ, et al. Automated and Manual Measurements of the Aortic Annulus with ECG-Gated Cardiac CT Angiography Prior to Transcatheter Aortic Valve Replacement: Comparison with 3D-Transesophageal Echocar-diography. Acad Radiol. 2017; 24(5): 587–593
- Hernandez-Suarez DF, Kim Y, Villablanca P, et al. Machine Learning Prediction Models for In-Hospital Mortality After Transcatheter Aortic Valve Replacement. JACC Cardiovasc In-terv. 2019; 12(14): 1328–1338,
- Hinton GE, Osindero S, Teh YW. A fast learning algorithm for deep belief nets. Neural Comput. 2006; 18(7): 1527–1554,
- Ionasec RI, Georgescu B, Gassner E, et al. Dynamic Model-Driven Quantitative and Visual Evaluation of the Aortic Valve from 4D CT. In: Metaxas D, editors. Medical Image Comuting and Comuter-Assisted Intervention. MICCAI 2008. Berlin, Hei-delberg: Sringer Berlin Heidelberg. 2008: 686–694.
- Ionasec RI, Voigt I, Georgescu B, et al. Patient-specific modeling and quantification of the aortic and mitral valves from 4-D cardiac CT and TEE. IEEE Trans Med Imaging. 2010; 29(9): 1636–1651,
- Iwata A, Ishii N, Suzumura N, et al. Algorithm for detecting the first and the second heart sounds by spectral tracking. Med Biol Eng Comput. 1980; 18(1): 19–26,
- Jiang Z, Choi SA. cardiac sound characteristic waveform method for in-home heart disorder monitoring with electric stethoscope. Expert Syst Appl. 2006; 31(2): 286–98.
- Kagiyama N, Toki M, Hara M, et al. Efficacy and Accuracy of Novel Automated Mitral Valve Quantification: Three-Dimensional Transesophageal Echocardiographic Study. Echocardiography. 2016; 33(5): 756–763,
- Khalid S, Khalil T, Nasreen SA. survey of feature selection and feature extraction techniques in machine learning. Proc 2014 Sci Inf Conf SAI. 2014; 2014: 372–378.
- Koos R, Mahnken AH, Dohmen G, et al. Association of aortic valve calcification severity with the degree of aortic regurgitation after transcatheter aortic valve implantation. Int J Cardiol. 2011; 150(2): 142–145.
- Kumar D, Carvalho P, Antunes M, et al. Heart murmur clas-sification with feature selection. Conf Proc IEEE Eng Med Biol Soc. 2010; 2010: 4566–4569,
- Kwak C. Kwon O-W. Cardiac disorder classification by heart sound signals using murmur likelihood and hidden Markov model state likelihood. IET Signal Process. 2012; 6(4): 326.
- LaFaro RJ, Pothula S, Kubal KP, et al. Neural Network Predic-tion of ICU Length of Stay Following Cardiac Surgery Based on Pre-Incision Variables. PLoS One. 2015; 10(12):
- Lalys F, Esneault S, Castro M, et al. Automatic aortic root seg-mentation and anatomical landmarks detection for TAVI pro-edure planning. Minim Invasive Ther Allied Technol. 2019; 28(3): 157–164,

- Lehner RJ, Rangayyan RM. A three-channel microcomputer system for segmentation and characterization of the phonocar-diogram. IEEE Trans Biomed Eng. 1987; 34(6): 485–489,
- Liang H, Lukkarinen S, Hartimo I. Heart sound segmentation algorithm based on heart sound envelogram. 1997; 24: 105–108.
- Liu X, Cheung Y, Ming Y, et al. Automatic mitral valve leaflet tracking in Echocardiography via constrained outlier pursuit and region-scalable active contours. Neurocomputing. 2014; 144: 47–57
- Martin S, Daanen V, Troccaz J, et al. Tracking of the mitral valve leaflet in echocardiography images. 3rd IEEE Int Symp Biomed Imaging Nano to Macro. 2006; 2006: 181–184.
- Mayer H, Gomez F, Wierstra D, et al. system for robotic heart surgery that learns to tie knots using recurrent neural networks. Adv Robot. 2008; 13(14): 1521–1537.
- Mediratta A, Addetia K, Medvedofsky D, et al. 3D echocardio-graphic analysis of aortic annulus for transcatheter aortic valve replacement using novel aortic valve quantification software: Comparison with computed tomography. Echocardiography. 2017; 34(5): 690–699
- Mikić I, Krucinski S, Thomas JD. Segmentation and tracking in echocardiographic sequences: active contours guided by optical flow estimates. IEEE Trans Med Imaging. 1998; 17(2): 274–284,
- Moustris GP, Hiridis SC, Deliparaschos KM, et al. Evolution of autonomous and semi-autonomous robotic surgical systems: a review of the literature. Int J Med Robot. 2011; 7(4): 375–392,
- Nashef SAM, Roques F, Sharples LD, et al. EuroSCORE II. Eur J Cardiothorac Surg. 2012; 41(4): 734–44; discussion 744, doi: 10.1093/ejcts/ezs043, indexed in Pubmed: 22378855.
- Nilsson J, Ohlsson M, Höglund P, et al. The International Heart Transplant Survival Algorithm (IHTSA): a new model to improve organ sharing and survival. PLoS One. 2015; 10(3):
- Nilsson J, Ohlsson M, Thulin L, et al. Risk factor identification and mortality prediction in cardiac surgery using artificial neural networks. J Thorac Cardiovasc Surg. 2006; 132(1): 12–19, doi: 10.1016/j.jtcvs.2005.12.055, indexed in Pubmed: 16798296.
- Noble JA, Boukerroui D. Ultrasound image segmentation: a survey. IEEE Trans Med Imaging. 2006; 25(8): 987–1010
Olmez T, Zumray D. Classification of heart sounds using an arti-ficial neural network. Pattern Recognit Lett. 2003; 24: 617–629.
- Panesar S, Cagle Y, Chander D, et al. Artificial Intelligence and the Future of Surgical Robotics. Ann Surg. 2019; 270(2): 223– 226
- Pennell DJ Cardiovascular magnetic resonance Circulation. 2010; 121(5): 692–705.
- Petitjean C, Dacher JN. A review of segmentation methods in short axis cardiac MR images. Med Image Anal. 2011; 15(2): 169–184, doi: 10.1016/j.media.2010.12.004, indexed in Pubmed: 21216179.
- Potes C, Parvaneh S, Rahman A, et al. Ensemble of feature-based and deep learning-based classifiers for detection of abnormal heart sounds. Comput Cardiol. 2016; 43: 621–624.
- Pouch AM, Wang H, Takabe M, et al. Fully automatic segmenta-tion of the mitral leaflets in 3D transesophageal echocardio-graphic images using multi-atlas joint label fusion and deform-able medial modeling. Med Image Anal. 2014; 18(1): 118–129,
- Puppe F. Systematic introduction to expert systems: Knowledge representations and problem-solving methods. Springer Science & Business Media. 2012.
- Safara F, Doraisamy S, Azman A, et al. Multi-level basis selection of wavelet packet decomposition tree for heart sound classifica-tion. Comput Biol Med. 2013; 43(10): 1407–1414,
- Samim M, Stella PR, Agostoni P, et al. Automated 3D analysis of pre-procedural MDCT to predict annulus plane angulation and C-arm positioning: benefit on procedural outcome in patients re-ferred for TAVR. JACC Cardiovasc Imaging. 2013; 6(2): 238–248
- Schmidt SE, Holst-Hansen C, Graff C, et al. Segmentation of heart sound recordings by a duration-dependent hidden Markov model. Physiol Meas. 2010; 31(4): 513–529, doi: 10.1088/0967-3334/31/4/004, indexed in Pubmed: 20208091.
- Schneider RJ, Perrin DP, Vasilyev NV, et al. Mitral annulus segmentation from 3D ultrasound using graph cuts. IEEE Trans Med Imaging. 2010; 29(9): 1676–1687,
- Schwartz WB, Patil RS, Szolovits P. Artificial intelligence in medicine. Where do we stand? N Engl J Med. 1987; 316(11): 685–688
- Shang Y, Yang X, Zhu L, et al. Region competition based ac-tive contour for medical object extraction. Comput Med Im-aging Graph. 2008; 32(2): 109–117,
- Shortliffe EHA. rule-based comuter rogram for advising hysi-cians regarding antimicrobial theray selection. In: Proceedings of the Annual ACM Conference. ACM. 1974; 739.
- Siefert AW, Icenogle DA, Rabbah JPM, et al. Accuracy of a mitral valve segmentation method using J-splines for real-time 3D echocardiography data. Ann Biomed Eng. 2013; 41(6): 1258–1268,
- Springer DB, Tarassenko L, Clifford GD. Logistic Regression-HSMM-Based Heart Sound Segmentation. IEEE Trans Biomed Eng. 2016; 63(4): 822–832,
- Sultan MS, Martins N, Costa E, et al. Virtual M-Mode for Echo-cardiography: A New Approach for the Segmentation of the An-terior Mitral Leaflet. IEEE J Biomed Health Inform. 2019; 23(1): 305–313
- Sun S, Jiang Z, Wang H, et al. Automatic moment segmentation and peak detection analysis of heart sound pattern via short-time modified Hilbert transform. Comput Methods Programs Biomed. 2014; 114(3): 219–230,
- Sun S. An innovative intelligent system based on automatic diagnostic feature extraction for diagnosing heart diseases. Knowledge-Based Syst. 2015; 75: 224–238, doi: 10.1016/j.kno-sys.2014.12.001.
- Swee JKY, Grbić S. Advanced transcatheter aortic valve implan-tation (TAVI) planning from CT with ShapeForest. Lect Notes Comput Sci. (including Subser Lect Notes Artif Intell Lect Notes Bioinformatics). 2014; 8674 LNCS(Part 2): 17–24.
- Szolovits P, Pauker SG. Categorical and probabilistic reason-ing in medical diagnosis. Artif Intell [Internet]. 1978 Aug 1; 11(1–2):115–44.

- Tavel ME. Cardiac auscultation. A glorious past -- but does it have a future? Circulation. 1996; 93(6): 1250–1253,
- Thavendiranathan P, Liu S, Datta S, et al. Quantification of chron-ic functional mitral regurgitation by automated 3-dimensional peak and integrated proximal isovelocity surface area and stroke volume techniques using real-time 3-dimensional volume color doppler echocardiography: In vitro and clini. Circ Cardiovasc Imaging. 2013; 6(1): 125–133.
- Thavendiranathan P, Phelan D, Thomas JD, et al. Quantitative assessment of mitral regurgitation: validation of new methods. J Am Coll Cardiol. 2012; 60(16): 1470–1483, Thompson WR, Reinisch AJ, Unterberger MJ, et al. Artificial intelligence-assisted auscultation of heart murmurs: validation by virtual clinical trial. Pediatr Cardiol. 2019; 40(3): 623–629,
- Thottakkara P, Ozrazgat-Baslanti T, Hupf BB, et al. Application of Machine Learning Techniques to High-Dimensional Clinical Data to Forecast Postoperative Complications. PLoS One. 2016; 11(5
- Ton J. Cleophas AHZ. Machine Learning in Medicine. 2013;1920–30. LeCun Y, Bengio Y, Hinton G. Deep learning. Nature. 2015; 521(7553): 436–444
- Topol EJ. High-performance medicine: the convergence of human and artificial intelligence. Nat Med. 2019; 25(1): 44–56, doi: 10.1038/s41591-018-0300-7, indexed in Pubmed: 30617339.
- Uğuz H. A biomedical system based on artificial neural network and principal component analysis for diagnosis of the heart valve diseases. J Med Syst. 2012; 36(1): 61–72 Waechter I, Kneser R, Korosoglou G, et al. Patient Secific Mod-els for Planning and Guidance of Minimally Invasive Aortic Valve Imlantation. In: Jiang T, Navab N, Pluim JPW, Viergever MA, edi-tors. Medical Image Comuting and Comuter-Assisted Interven-tion -- MICCAI 2010. Sringer Berlin Heidelberg. 2010: 526–533.
- Wang Y, Georgescu B, Datta S, et al. Automatic cardiac flow quantification on 3D volume color Doppler data. Proc - Int Symp Biomed Imaging. 2011; C(Lv): 1688–1691.
- Watanabe Y, Morice MC, Bouvier E, et al. Automated 3-dimensional aortic annular assessment by multidetector computed tomography in transcatheter aortic valve implantation. JACC Cardiovasc Interv. 2013; 6(9): 955–964,
- Zhang J, Gajjala S, Agrawal P, et al. Fully automated echocar-diogram interpretation in clinical practice. Circulation. 2018; 138(16): 1623–1635,
- Zhang W, Guo X, Yuan Z, et al. Heart sound classification and recognition based on eemd and correlation dimension. J Mech Med Biol. 2014; 14(04): 1450046.
- Zhang W, Han J, Deng S. Heart sound classification based on scaled spectrogram and tensor decomposition. Expert Syst Appl. 2017; 84: 220–231.
- Zhao Y, Zeng D, Socinski MA, et al. Reinforcement learning strat-egies for clinical trials in nonsmall cell lung cancer. Biometrics. 2011; 67(4): 1422–1433,
- Zheng Y, John M, Liao R, et al. Automatic aorta segmentation and valve landmark detection in C-arm CT for transcatheter aortic valve implantation. IEEE Trans Med Imaging. 2012; 31(12): 2307–2321.
- Zhou X, Yang C, Yu W. Automatic mitral leaflet tracking in echo-cardiography by outlier detection in the low-rank representation. Proc IEEE Comput Soc Conf Comput Vis Pattern Recognit. 2012: 972–979.

Artificial Intelligence In The Diagnosis And Management Of Cardiac Arrhythmias

As artificial intelligence (AI) has entered the medical field in recent years, machine learning (ML) approaches have made progress in assisting healthcare professionals in optimizing personalized treat-ment in a given situation, in particular in electrocardiography and image interpretation. Artificial intelligence methodologies are increasingly being adopted into all aspects of patient care and are paving the way to minimally invasive or non-invasive treatment modalities. This article offers a state-of-the-art overview on milestones achieved, but also on future integration of this information into diagnostic and therapeutic measures, and its likely impact on all aspects of arrhyth-mia care. Integration of all individual information in combination with AI solutions is likely to revolutionize electrophysiology (EP) interven-tions in the near future

Cardiac electrical signal analysis using artificial intelligence methodologies

Human intelligence is characterized by the capability of learning, reasoning, analysing, and decision-making. When machines mimic the use of these capabilities, it can be termed AI. Although the concept and the term AI have been used for over six decades.its usage has skyrocketed over the last decade. Whilst ML is the most commonly used term for AI, it only denotes one of the methodologies of AI Most of the AI applications in EP are based on the analysis of signals that represent cardiac electrical activity, with the signal varying with the type of sensor and underlying technology. Two of the most com-monly used signals are electrocardiogram (ECG) and photo plethys-mography (PPG). Photo plethysmography is more contemporary and has been used in some of the wearable devices including watches, wrist bands, and smartphones. Fundamental AI processes employed in analysing data obtained from these devices are essentially similar Following data collection, data are pre-processed, feature engin-eering carried out, and followed by classification by one of the ML methodologies.The ML methodology is first trained using the 'training data' with appropriate labels. The second stage involves ML methodology assessment using a 'validation data set' and fine tuning the algorithm. Following these two steps, the ML algo-rithm would then be ready to be used with a third 'test set'. Performance of the algorithm is expressed using values such as sensi-tivity, specificity, accuracy, receiver operating curve (ROC), and area under ROC (AUC).

Arrhythmia detection using artificial intelligence

Since digitalization of ECG, AI methods have been employed in com-puterized interpretation of ECGs. Whilst ML methods revealed high sensitivity and specificity for detecting normal sinus rhythm, their abilities were lower than expert cardiologists for the identification of cardiac arrhythmias.5 One of the main deterrents have been the pres-ence of noise, small or varying P waves resulting in over diagnosis of atrial fibrillation (AF), paced rhythms, poor-quality ECGs, tremor, and previously untrained rhythms. With better ML algorithms, noise reduction techniques and advanced feature extraction, selection and reduction methods [including use of the unsupervised deep neural network (DNN)], computerized interpretation of ECGs has clearly improved arrhythmia detection achieving an accuracy close to 95% Hannun et al.8 developed an end to end deep learning (DL) ap-proach for ECG analysis by using a DNN for identifying 12 rhythm abnormalities by using 91 232 single-lead ECGs. When validated against independent data reported by a committee of certified cardiologists, their algorithm was shown to be superior to an average car-diologist in identifying these rhythm abnormalities (ROC 0.97 vs. 0.78). With the development of unsupervised DNN algorithms, more interest has been generated amongst researchers for identifying hid-den diseased state signatures in a 12-lead ECG. So far, it has been shown to be feasible to detect hyperkalaemia, heart failure,hypoglycaemia, and even changes in emotional states using 12-lead ECG. Attia et al. at Mayo Clinic Rochester assessed the feasibility of identifying previous episodes of or impending AF using an AI-enabled 12-lead ECG in normal sinus rhythm. They used 0.65 million ECGs to train, validate, and test the AI algorithm in a 7:1:2 ratio and found that AI-enabled ECG recorded during normal sinus rhythm performed well as a screening test to identify AF with an accuracy of 79.4% and this improved to 83.4% when it was a first ECG following an episode of AF. Additional multiple ECGs improved the model accuracy lead-ing to the hypothesis that structural changes that may precede AF including myocyte hypertrophy, fibrosis, or chamber dilatation may result in subtle multifaceted changes in ECG that may otherwise be unrecognized by the human eye but are detectable by a DNN. This observation has important clinical implications with potential point-of-care identification of individuals at the risk of AF and for the em-bolic stroke of undetermined source.Deep neural network has also been used to predict hypertrophic cardiomyopathy (HCM), age and sex, and plasma dofetilide concentration from ECG.

Advancements in sensor technology, telecommunications (increased availability of wireless, Wi-Fi, Bluetooth and smartphone technologies), availability of web-based data storage, and AI-aided analysis have seen rapid growth of handheld and wearable cardiac monitoring systems. Whilst several handheld devices are available, the AliveCor Heart Monitor, an ECG-based system, has been studied extensively for AF detection in symptomatic patients. In most of these studies, AliveCor Heart Monitor achieved well over 90% sensitivity and speci-ficity for AF detection both in outpatient and hospital settings. In a comparison with traditional transtelephonic monitor, AliveCor Heart Monitor achieved 100% sensitivity and 97% specificity for AF and atrial flutter detection. Similar results were seen with the use of PPG-based systems coupled with AI-aided analysis. In the WATCH AF trial, Do¨rr et al. studied the efficacy of a smartphone PPG-based algorithm in AF detection. The PPG algorithm achieved a sensitivity of 93.7%, a specificity of 98.2%, and an accuracy of 96.1%to detect AF.

In a recent community-based trial on the utility of a smartwatch in AF detection (Apple Heart Study), smartwatch in conjunction with a pulse notification algorithm showed promising results in 0.41 million participants with no prior history of AF. The smartwatch application collected single 1-min tachograms every 2 h. If a smartwatch-based ir-regular pulse notification algorithm identified possible AF, the partici-pant was notified to have further simultaneous 7-day monitoring using an ECG patch. The smartwatch-based algorithm had a positive predictive value of 0.84 (95% confidence interval 0.76–0.92) for iden-tifying AF during the simultaneous monitoring period. Similar results were shown in yet another population-based AF screening study using a PPG algorithm in conjunction with smart devices.Chen et al.studied AF detection using a smart wristband equipped with both ECG and PPG sensors, comparing ECG and PPG individually as well as in combination. They demonstrated higher ac-curacy of 97.5% for AF detection with the combination against 94.7%and 93.2% with ECG and PPG, respectively. Wasserlauf et al. compared smartwatch detection of AF using a DL algorithm (episodes lasting >_1 h) with an insertable loop record-er. They analysed 348 h of simultaneously recorded data. The smartwatch algorithm achieved 97.5% and 97.7% for episode sensitiv-ity and duration sensitivity, respectively.

Artificial intelligence-enabled monitoring systems are affordable and reliable, can be used for continuous ambulatory monitoring, and will facilitate the detection of vulnerable groups.32 A step closer to the holy grail of early AF detection within the community in other-wise

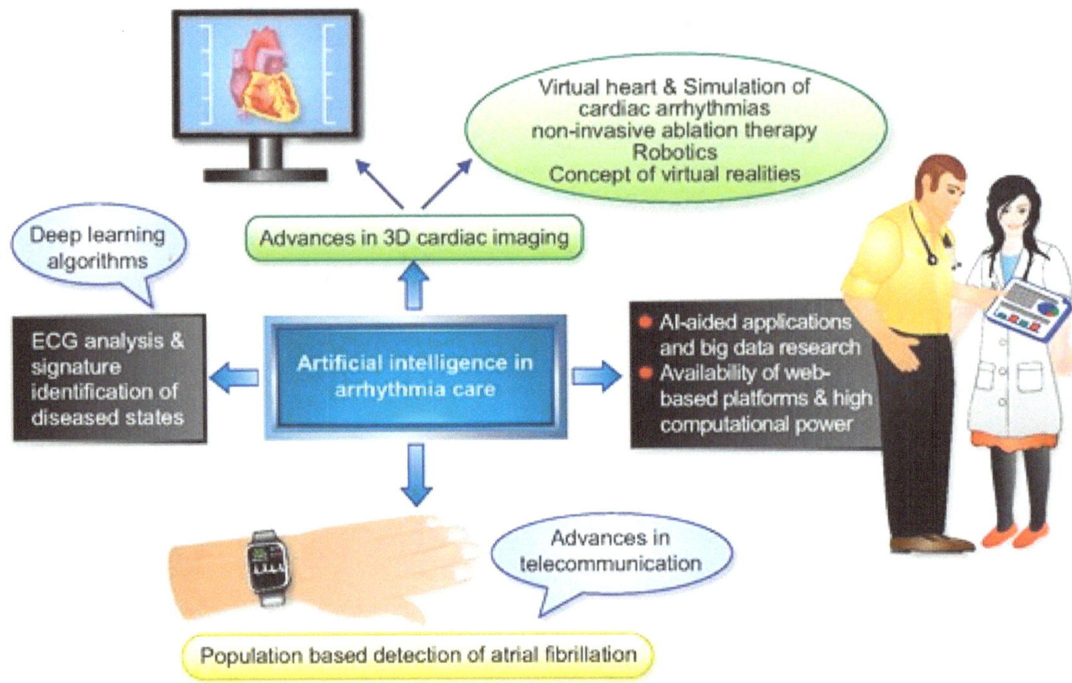

Fig. 11.1 Graphical Abstract Artificial intelligence-enhanced arrhythmia care.

asymptomatic patients may in fact initiate a paradigm shift in ar-rhythmia detection.

Artificial intelligence and cardiac devices

Most of the pacemaker and defibrillator functions use rule-based algorithms. Rate response feature in a pacemaker, which incorpo-rates the ability of the device to vary the pacing rate based on an input from a biosensor; tachycardia detection and deliverance of an appro-priate therapy by an implantable defibrillator, are some of the illustra-tions of the rule-based decision-making. A rule-based algorithm is referred to as a simplest form of AI but it differs from ML in its inabil-ity to learn. In rule-based algorithms, rules are laid down by humans based on the domain expertise, whereas ML methodologies learn ac-tively from the training data and create their own rules for decision-making, which may not be transparent in some instances.Machine learning algorithms are finding their use with cardiac devices both in arrhythmia detection and prediction of future events. Machine learning methods have been employed in automated external defibrillators in the development of shock advicealgorithms. Recently, Nguyen et al. developed an algorithm for the detection of shockable and non-shockable rhythms using ML. They used both boosting classifier and convolutional neural network as a feature extractor with a sensitivity and specificity of 95.21% and 99.31%, respectively. This shock advice algorithm was a considerable improvement over existing algorithms and in keeping with the stand-ards set by the American Heart Association guidelines. More re-cently, a DL technique was introduced to identify any cardiac device model from a chest radiograph.Machine learning methods have been used to improve cardiac resynchronization therapy (CRT) outcomes prediction, paving the way for better patient selection. In a proof of concept, single centre study, ML algorithm in conjunction with natural language proc-essing was applied to electronic health records. This model suc-cessfully identified subgroups of patients who were unlikely to benefit from CRT. An ML algorithm using naive Bayes classifier using patient variables including age, sex, QRS duration and morphology, left ventricular ejection fraction and end-diastolic diameter, New York Heart Association functional class, presence of AF, and epicar-dial left ventricular lead was superior to existing guidelines in predict-ing event-free survival post-CRT.

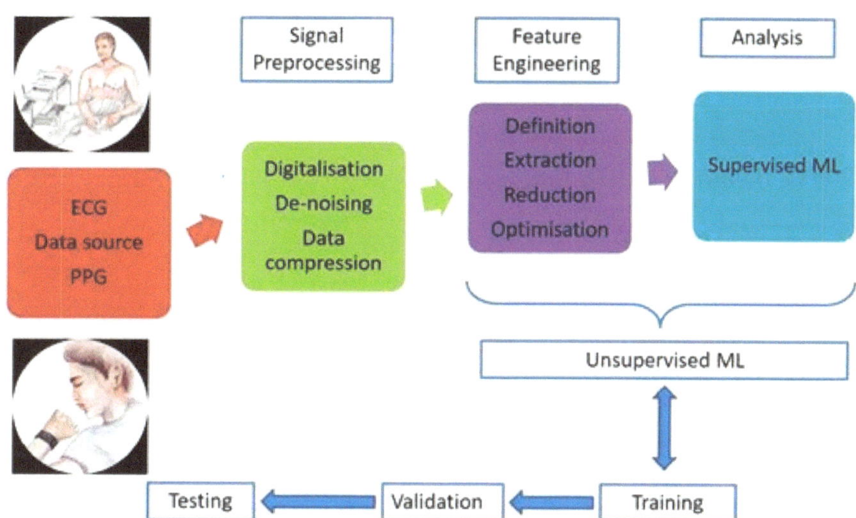

Fig 11.2 Schematic representation of steps involved in cardiac impulse analysis from the data acquisition to analysis by machine learning algorithm. ECG, electrocardiogram; ML, machine learning; PPG, photo plethysmography.

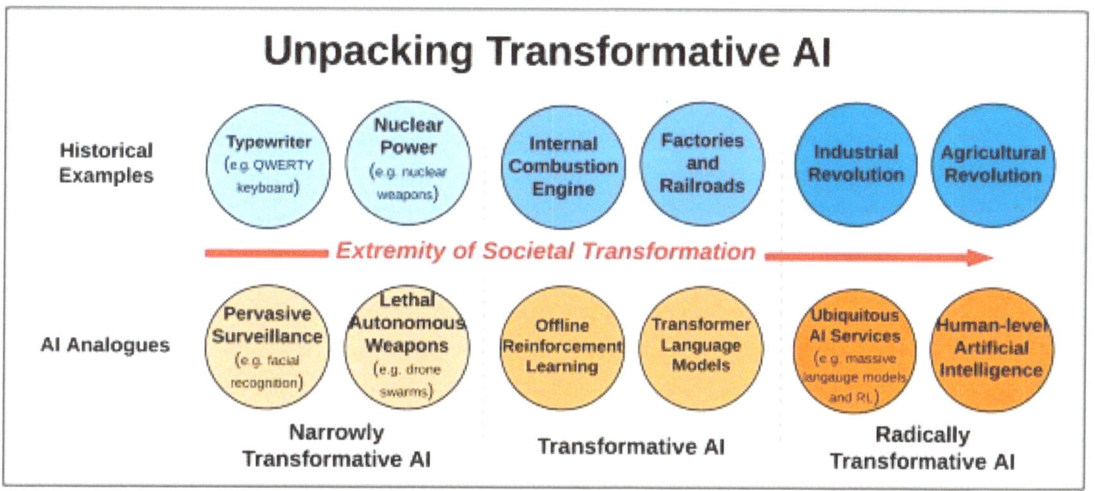

Fig.11.3 Our proposed levels of transformative AI and analogous AI technologies compared with historical examples of transformative GPTs

Machine learning algorithms including random forests and convo-luted neural networks, when applied to the AF signature burden obtained using continuous remote monitoring data in patients with cardiac implantable electronic devices, were superior in predicting stroke compared to the widely used CHA2DS2-VASc score. An en-semble method using ML model in conjunction with CHA2DS2-VASc score had better sensitivity and specificity when compared to using CHA2DS2-VASc score alone and improved AUC from 0.52 to 0.63.

Multimodal integrative approach to predict sites of arrhythmia origins and role of machine learning

Non-invasive characterization of arrhythmia prior to attempting abla-tive therapy is gaining favour amongst electrophysiologists. This ap-proach aids in focused targeting of the cardiac region of interest. One of the important contributors to this being ML aided advances in car-diac 3D imaging.Application of DL methods including convolutional neural net-work has improved the speed of acquisition, time efficiency, recon-struction quality of images,and accuracy of cardiac magnetic resonance (CMR) segmentation. Machine learning techniques have been applied to improve myocardial tissue characterization and texture analysis and define the heterogeneous nature of the scarred myocardium in late gadolinium enhancement (LGE) CMR images in patients post-myocardial infarction.

Automated CMR analysis using a convolutional neural network al-gorithm was shown to be similar in precision to human analysis for measuring left ventricular ejection fraction and left ventricular mass but was 186 times faster.

In a proof of concept study, Fahmy et al. used U-Net deep convo-luted networks with 150 operational layers to quantify scar volumes in patients with HCM. A strong correlation was observed between the manually and automatically segmented scar volumes.

Cardiac magnetic resonance-defined scar regions have gained con-siderable importance and form the basis of some of the ablation strat-egies including scar homogenization and scar de-channelling in ventricular tachycardia (VT) ablation. These advancements have also paved the way for the concept of targeting fibrotic substrate that can perpetuate rotors, in addition to pulmonary vein isolation in patients with persistent AF.

Advances of ML-aided imaging have set the stage for the devel-opment of several novel concepts in EP including non-invasive local-ization of arrhythmia foci with high precision, personalized virtual heart modelling including simulation of cardiac arrhythmias and con-cept of non-invasive ablation.

In parallel with developments in cardiac imaging, further advance-ments have been made in ECG acquisition with the development of body surface mapping (using up to 252 electrodes instead of standard 12 leads). Electrocardiography imaging systems that integrate body surface mapping with non-contrast computed tomography (CT) that simultaneously records electrode location and geometry of cardiac surface can localize focal activation of atrial or ventricular ectopy on the 3D reconstruction of the patient's heart using an inverse solution approach.

The Amycard 01C (EP Solutions SA, Yverdon-les-Bains, Switzerland) and ECVUE (CardioInsight Technologies Inc., Cleveland, OH, USA) systems are now commercially available and are able to locate atrial and ventricular arrhythmias. As they provide a simultaneous, quasi global view of the entire atrial or ventricular ac-tivation, these systems allow to visualize even AF. Using this technique, focal trigger and rotor sites are identified, which is impossible using the conventional sequential mapping techniques .

View into ventricular onset (VIVO, Catheter Precision) is a next-generation non-invasive mapping system that combines knowledge of the exact location of the surface 12-lead ECG stickers with careful-ly reconstructed cardiac anatomy from either CMR or CT imaging (Figure 4, right). With the VIVO platform, prediction of the focus of premature ventricular electrical activity and VT focus is correct in 85% and 88% of patients, respectively.

Using a multimodal integrative approach, feasibility of combining body surface mapping, cardiac gated multidetector CT, and/or delayed contrast-enhanced magnetic resonance (MR) imaging on a common platform This approach was useful in understanding complex accessory pathway previously resistant to ablation and to identify rotor trajectories in patients with AF

Software (Automatic Detection of Arrhythmic Substrate, ADAS-VT, Galgo Medical SL, Barcelona, Spain), which processes LGE CMR images offline to characterize 3D scar architecture to be merged with electro anatomical mapping (EAM) during the ablation proced-ure, has been shown to facilitate the ablation procedure.

With the development of methods for non-invasive localization of arrhythmia focus, several groups have reported on their experience of using radiation therapy in patients with mostly ischaemic ventricu-lar arrhythmia. Robinson et al. reported successful utilization of radiotherapy in a cohort of patients with treatment-refractory epi-sodes of VT or cardiomyopathy related to premature ventricular contractions. They identified scar regions using ECG imaging, cardiac anatomical imaging and delivered Focused stereotactic body radiation therapy (SBRT) with marked reduction in arrhythmia burden, reduced

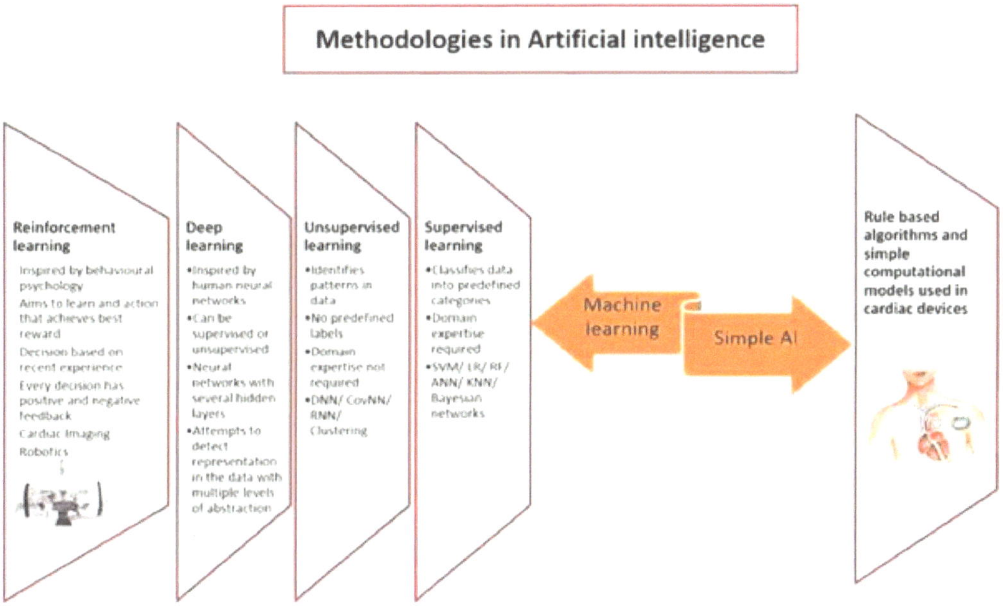

Methodologies in Artificial intelligence

Reinforcement learning
Inspired by behavioural psychology
Aims to learn and action that achieves best reward
Decision based on recent experience
Every decision has positive and negative feedback
Cardiac Imaging
Robotics

Deep learning
- Inspired by human neural networks
- Can be supervised or unsupervised
- Neural networks with several hidden layers
- Attempts to detect representation in the data with multiple levels of abstraction

Unsupervised learning
- Identifies patterns in data
- No predefined labels
- Domain expertise not required
- DNN/ CovNN/ RNN/ Clustering

Supervised learning
- Classifies data into predefined categories
- Domain expertise required
- SVM/ LR/ RF/ ANN/ KNN/ Bayesian networks

Machine learning

Simple AI

Rule based algorithms and simple computational models used in cardiac devices

Fig. 11.4 Artificial intelligence methodologies with their individual characteristics. AI, artificial intelligence; ANN, artificial neural network; CovNN, convolutional neural network; DNN, deep neural network; KNN, K-nearest neighbours; LR, logistic regression; RF, random forest; RNN, recurrent neural network; SVM, support vector machine.

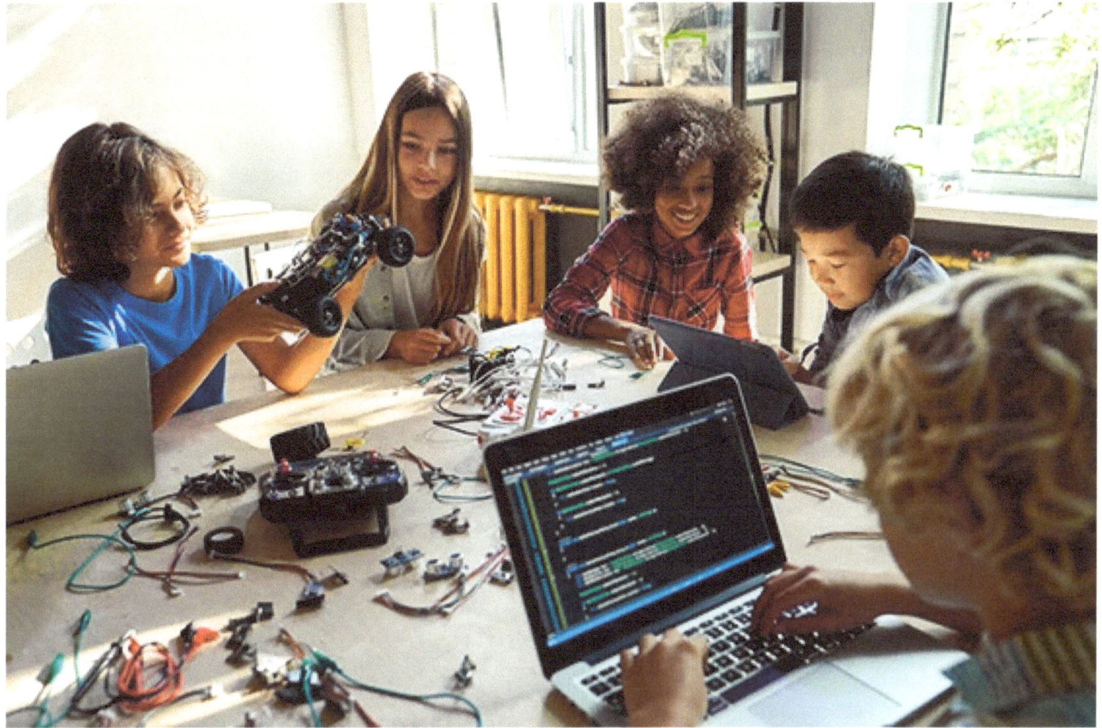

Fig. 11.5 Generative AI opens new horizons and challenges for education. But we urgently need to take action to ensure that new AI technologies are integrated into education on our terms. It is our duty to prioritize safety, inclusion, diversity, transparency and quality — as stated in the UNESCO Recommendation on the Ethics of Artificial Intelligence adopted unanimously by our Member States.Stefania Giannini UNESCO Assistant Director-General for Education

use of anti-arrhythmic medication and improved quality of life following therapy. Overall survival was 89% and 72% at the end of 6 and 12 months, respectively.

In addition, first-in-man treatment of paroxysmal AF using SBRT in two patients has been reported with the demonstration of safety and efficacy of delivering SBRT lesion set in the left atrium confirmed by presence of fibrosis. Results from these initial pilot studies and case reports are encouraging. However, more robust data are required from larger clinical trials with longer follow-up to show long-term safety of these techniques, which are of great interest but still under evaluation.

Personalized virtual heart modelling—a new paradigm

Considerable advances in cellular modelling technology have paved the way for the development of a computerized human cardiac myo-cyte.68 Virtual ventricular myocytes, with predefined electrophysio-logical properties, and predictable functional changes in response to surroundings including ion channel changes and myocardial ischaemia have been developed.

Trayanova et al. envisaged the creation of a computerized but per-sonalized virtual heart mode. Contrast-enhanced MR images of the patient's heart were used to create near identical geometrical models of the cardiac chambers and were populated with virtual car-diac myocytes with physiological properties pertaining to the cells from a designated location. Previously validated rule-based algo-rithms were applied for fibre orientation to compute heart models. These computed virtual hearts were electrophysiological twins to the patient's heart on which various stimulation protocols could be applied to induce ventricular arrhythmias of different morphologies and identify critical isthmus zones for these arrhythmias.As a proof of concept, this study of virtual heart modelling was used for non-invasive risk assessment of sudden cardiac death in a high-risk population undergoing cardioverter defibrillator implant-ation. The virtual heart arrhythmia risk predictor approach (VARP) was evaluated retrospectively in a cohort of 41 patients executing simulations to evaluate patient specific VT inducibility and found to be superior to other predictors including left ventricular ejection fraction. Predictive capability of this novel targeted approach needs further evaluation in larger studies.

Yet another proof of concept study evaluated the use of virtual heart modelling in patients undergoing VT ablation. Virtual hearts were modelled from patients' contrast-enhanced MR images and VT induction carried out as in the VARP study. Once VT induction was carried out, the optimal ablation strategy was performed virtually. This technique was termed virtual heart arrhythmia ablation targeting (VAAT). When compared retrospectively in 21 patients undergoing VT ablation, it was found to correspond well with real ablation lesions. The VAAT strategy was further tested prospectively in 5 patients undergoing VT ablation in two different centres. VAAT lesions were merged with an EAM system and an ablation was carried out at these sites without further prior mapping. The clinical outcomes for these patients were encouraging with no further VT episodes post-ablation.

Virtual hearts and machine learning in atrial fibrillation

Machine learning methodologies in conjunction with atrial computa-tional models were used to define re-entrant driver locations in AF.80 Segmented LGE CMR scans were used to identify atrial fibrosis in 21 patients with persistent AF. Fibrotic and non-fibrotic regions were identified and were assigned with region-specific tissue properties. Atrial fibrillation was induced using multisite atrial pacing in these vir-tual atrial models. Phase mapping with an unsupervised density-based spatial cluster algorithm was used to define re-entrant driver loca-tions. Over 80% of re-entrant driver locations matched to the fibrosis border zones.The first-in-human clinical study of virtual heart models to guide ablation in patients with persistent AF used personalized atrial geo-metric models created using segmented LGE MR scans done prior to the procedure.81 Rapid pacing was carried out from 40 uniformly dis-tributed bi-atrial sites. The model response was analysed to deter-mine the optimal ablation lesion set to eliminate all possible persistent re-entrant drivers identified using above mentioned ML

Table 11.1 Overview of feature engineering processes employed during development of machine learning methods

Feature engineering		
Definition	**Extraction**	**Optimization**
• Most informative and non-redundant characteristics of data signals • Represented in a numerical form and together form a feature vector • Data represented as features is computationally processed by ML algorithms	• In supervised ML methods feature extraction is done by experts in the domain • In unsupervised and DL methodologies feature engineering is done by the algorithm itself • Features used for cardiac signal analysis—time intervals, morphological amplitudes, areas or distances	• Selection of appropriate features is crucial for the success of ML methodology • Algorithms used for relevant feature identification—particle swarm optimization, etc. • Algorithms used for dimensionality reduction—principal component analysis and linear discriminant analysis

DL, deep learning; ML, machine learning.

Table 11.2 Commonly used machine learning classification algorithms

Algorithm	Learning method	Description	Utility in EP ML
Support vector machine	• Most commonly used supervised learning method	• Used to classify complex non-linear data • Creates 'hyperplane' that non-linearly separates the two classes in a feature space • Good classification and generalization properties	• Arrhythmia classification using heart rate variability • VF detection algorithm in automated external defibrillators
Random Forest	• Supervised learning method	• Ensemble learning methods that combine multiple decision trees (algorithms) • Decision trees arranged in a hierarchical manner • Final prediction derived by calculating the mean or mode of the individual DT's decision	• Classification of ECG beats • CRT outcomes prediction
Bayesian networks	• Supervised learning method	• Graphical structures to represent knowledge about an uncertain domain • Represent variables and their probabilistic relationships • HMM—one of the frequently used examples of BNs	• Classification of ECG beats • CRT outcomes prediction
Neural networks	• Can be supervised or unsupervised learning method	• Computational model mimicking biological neural networks • Data is propagated in a hierarchical manner via nodes in each layer • Input/target pairs are used during model training	• Classifying large amounts of data • Classification of ECG beats
Convolutional neural networks	• Can be supervised or unsupervised learning method	• Evolved form of deep neural networks (multiple hidden layers between input and output) • Convolution layers produce a spatially dependent feature for the subsequent layer • Most widely used DL	• For deciphering diseased state footprints in 12-lead ECG • Cardiac imaging

BN, bayesian networks; CRT, cardiac resynchronization therapy; DL, deep learning; ECG, electrocardiogram; EP, electrophysiology; HMM, Hidden Markov Models; ML, machine learning; VF, ventricular fibrillation.

Table 11.3 Diagnostic accuracy of artificial intelligence-aided devices in identifying atrial fibrillation

Study	Device and AI algorithm	Signal analysed	AF detection
The iREAD Study William *et al.*[17]	Algorithm using smartphone (Kardia Mobile Cardiac Monitor) and handheld cardiac rhythm recorder vs. physician-interpreted ECG	ECG	96.6% sensitivity and 94.1% specificity for AF detection
HUAWEI Heart Study Guo *et al.*[18]	Wristband/wristwatch-based irregular pulse notification algorithm	PPG	Positive predictive value of PPG signals being 91.6% (95% CI 91.5–91.8%)
Apple Heart Study Perez *et al.*[19]	Smartwatch-based irregular pulse notification algorithm vs. subsequent monitoring with ECG patch	Initial PPG followed by simultaneous PPG and ECG	Smartwatch-based algorithm had a positive predictive value of 0.84 (95% CI 0.76–0.92) for observing AF during the simultaneous monitoring period
Chen *et al.*[20]	Smart wristband device enabled by AF-identifying AI algorithm vs. wristband ECG reviewed by physicians	PPG and ECG	Sensitivity, specificity, and accuracy were 88.00%, 96.41%, and 93.27%, respectively, for PPG and 87.33%, 99.20%, and 94.76% for ECG
Wasserlauf *et al.*[21]	Apple Watch with KardiaBand (enabled by convoluted neural network algorithm) vs. insertable cardiac monitor	ECG	97.5% and 97.7% for episode sensitivity and duration sensitivity, respectively
WATCH AF trial Dörr *et al.*[22]	Smartwatch-based algorithm vs. cardiologists' diagnosis by electrocardiography	PPG	Sensitivity of 93.7% (95% CI 89.8–96.4%), specificity of 98.2% (95% CI 95.8–99.4%), and 96.1% accuracy (95% CI 94.0–97.5%)

AF, atrial fibrillation; AI, artificial intelligence; CI, confidence interval; ECG, electrocardiogram; PPG, photo plethysmography.

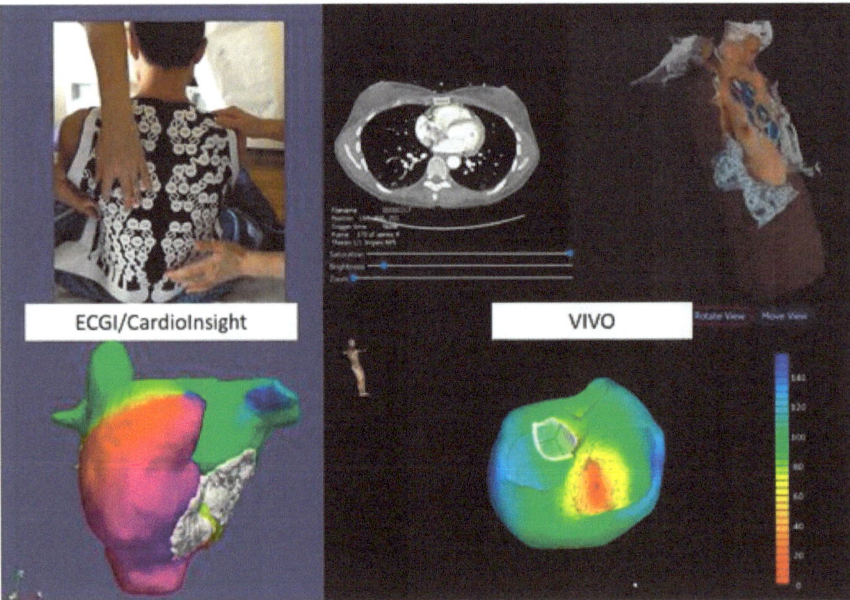

Fig.11.6 Left panel: Example of non-invasive simultaneous mapping of atrial fibrillation of both the right and left atrium using the electrocardiogram imaging technology. Several mechanisms occur in various areas of the atria simultaneously and thereby maintain atrial fibrillation. Right panel: Example of non-invasive simultaneous mapping of ventricular ectopy using the view into ventricular onset technology.

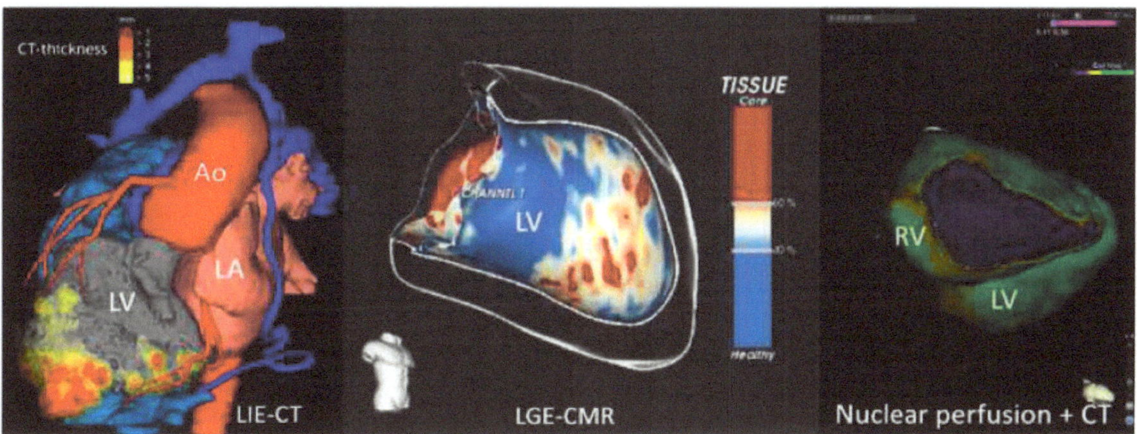

Fig.11.7 Left panel: 3D image information from computed tomography and myocardial thickness in a patient with coronary artery disease and ap-ical scar after myocardial infarction. Middle panel: Image information of late gadolinium enhancement from cardiac magnetic resonance imaging of the left ventricle with identification of the potentially arrhythmogenic channels within the scar responsible for ventricular re-entrant tachycardia. Right panel: Example of perfusion information from functional nuclear imaging superimposed on a contrast computed tomography scan in a patient with arrhythmogenic right ventricular disease. Ao, aorta; CMR, cardiac magnetic resonance; LA, left atrium; LGE, late gadolinium enhancement; LV, left ventricle; RV, right ventricle.

methodologies) sustaining AF and other atrial arrhythmias; the opti-mal ablation lesion set created using this approach was called OPTIMA: OPtimal Target Identification via Modelling of Arrhythmogenesis was then loaded onto the EAM mapping system and the ablation was carried out without prior mapping. This was a proof of concept feasibility study and was not designed to evaluate procedure outcomes. In fact, outcomes reported from 10 patients were encouraging with no further recurrence of persistent AF.

In a study combining ML and personalized computational model-ling, an ML algorithm was shown to predict AF recurrence post-pulmonary vein isolation in patients with paroxysmal AF. In this proof of concept study, features were derived from patient's pre-pulmonary vein isolation LGE MR images and also from the results of AF simulations carried out on their personalized computational model. Random forests were used for unbiased feature selection, and ten-fold nested cross-validation was used to train, validate, and test quadratic discriminant analysis ML classifier. Most predictive features were used as input to this classifier. This ML algorithm predicted post-pulmonary vein isolation AF recurrence with an average valid-ation sensitivity and specificity of 82% and 89%, respectively, and a validation AUC of 0.82.

Intracardiac data and machine learning applications in atrial fibrillation

Large quantities of intracardiac data are recorded during EP procedures. Recent advances in ML methodologies have encouraged researchers to apply these techniques to the intracardiac electro-grams and EAM data with a view to define extra pulmonary ablation sites in AF. Schilling et al. showed the feasibility of classifying complex frac-tionated atrial electrograms in an objective way using fuzzy decision tree algorithm retrospectively on intracardiac electrograms. Atrial electrograms were classified into four subgroups ranging from non-fractionated with high frequency to continuous activity achieving a correct rate of 81 ± 3%. Electrograms with continuous activity were detected correctly 100% of the time.

In a proof of concept study, McGillivray et al. developed random forest supervised ML algorithm to locate re-entrant circuits driving AF using indirect feature measurements, derived from electrograms in a simulated model. The model correctly identified 95.4% of drivers in the simulation model.

In a recent study, Alhusseini et al.85 developed an ML algorithm to classify intracardiac electrical patterns during AF. They used a convo-luted neural network DL approach to analyse EAM data obtained from bi-atrial sites using basket catheters. Spatial maps of activation were created to identify the presence of rotational activation fea-tures. Algorithm compared well with a team of experts with an ac-curacy of 97.3% when the experts were in unanimous agreement and 85.1% in more difficult instances. Convoluted neural network accur-acy in the test set was similar for locations containing termination sites (95.6%) or otherwise (94.2%). With ML-guided ablation strategies becoming a possibility for the near future, electrophysiologists would need real-time access to inte-grated data from different sources including EAM and 3D cardiac imaging. Availability of this information with the ability to manipulate the data for better visualization whilst still operating in a sterile field would enhance operator dexterity and procedural efficacy during complex ablations. Holographic visualization of real-time catheter position, cardiac geometry, EAM, and ablation data in an EP lab has been shown to be feasible. Systems to provide augmented reality solutions in EP labs are currently being developed for future use87 and would certainly aid in better and efficient work flow.

Robotics in electrophysiology and potential role of machine learning

To deliver catheter ablation safely to a high degree of precision reducing the impact of operator variability in level of training and technical skill, robotic ablation can be seen as a valuable tool to help improve access to the same level of accuracy in a reproducible fashion.In the field of EP, robotic navigation was introduced 20 years ago. The two concepts proposed were either a mechanical sheath system guiding a conventional ablation catheter via computer-enhanced technique (Hansen & Amigo) or a magnetic platform (Stereotaxis).

A more recent contender is another mechanical system, which uses acoustic energy for both imaging and lesion deployment (Vytronus). 3D reconstruction using ultrasound imaging is performed automatically and the robotic system months deploys acoustic energy com-pletely automatically along an operator designed ablation line. First-in-human experience was reported in a cohort of 52 patients with paroxysmal AF undergoing pulmonary vein isolation using low inten-sity collimated ultrasound (LICU). Acute pulmonary vein isolation was achieved in 77.3% and 94.2% of patients using LICU only and LICU with enhanced software, respectively, with continued freedom from atrial arrhythmia recurrence at 12 months

A vast body of evidence has been published for the magnetic navi-gation system (Niobe, Stereotaxis), which in combination with 3D EAM systems (CARTO or ACUTUS) plus 3D image integration, can be applied to all arrhythmias.

Feasibility of using an ML algorithm to guide automated electro-anatomical voltage mapping was previously demonstrated using re-mote magnetic navigation system. The ML algorithm used learning from demonstration framework utilizing prior knowledge from ex-pert mapping procedures and Gaussian process model-based active learning.

Non-invasive ML-aided identification of the ablation targets using 3D imaging and personalized heart modelling followed by robotic ab-lation of these pre-defined locations appears to be an exciting pro-spect for the future. This approach, if successful, could limit the number of catheters to a minimum and could be both more time and cost-efficient.

Is artificial intelligence bridging the gaps in arrhythmia care?

Recent research into AI-enabled ECG has rekindled interest into ob-servational-based research. Artificial intelligence-enabled ECG has been shown to identify patients with persistent AF, left ventricular systolic dysfunction, and HCM and the list is likely to grow in time with emerging evidence from ongoing research. This ubiquitous car-diac investigation has a potential to be a powerful screening tool at point of care, an innovation that may have a significant impact on community-based diagnosis of latent cardiac conditions, even more so in the under privileged parts of the world. In an acute setting, AI-enabled ECG may aid in the rapid identifica-tion of life threatening electrolyte imbalance and patients at imminent risk of cardiac arrest who may need more intensive moni-toring. Severe restrictions imposed by the recent COVID-19 pan-demic resulted in some of the AI-enabled technologies such as QT interval monitoring using AI-enabled mobile devices, approved by regulatory authorities to see the light of the day in clinical practice.

Advancements in sensor technology and wireless communications with ability to link devices over internet of things have made continu-ous heart rhythm monitoring feasible, albeit resulting in an exponen-tial increase in data to be analysed. Review of such data by a skilled personnel is nearly impossible due to time and resource constraints. Artificial intelligence solutions can effectively analyse these data in a time and a resource efficient manner. Artificial intelligence-assisted near real-time analysis of data from wearable devices has prompted the contemplation of newer research into novel treatment strategies such as pill in the pocket anticoagulation following an epi-sode of AF.Machine learning algorithms have shown their utility to further personalized patient care by improving existing guidelines, which aid in clinical decision-making regarding anticoagulation in the at-risk population and patient selection for cardiac device therapy. Superiority of ML methodologies over traditional rule-based algo-rithms in handling big data may facilitate data analysis from multiple data sources to identify the impending risk of life threatening arrhyth-mia or heart failure episodes in a timely manner.

Artificial intelligence-enabled technological advancements are aid-ing in arrhythmia focus identification prior to EP procedures. In time, AI-enabled ECG may better contribute to accurate localization of ac-cessory pathway or arrhythmia focus. There is a vast potential for the application of ML methodologies to intracardiac data including EAM, for better characterization of an arrhythmia to aid in selection of the ideal ablation strategy.

Limitations and challenges

Machine learning methodologies are not error free, best example being overfitting, a phenomenon resulting from a disproportionate number of features in comparison to the amount of data in the training set.As a result of overfitting, the ML algorithm performs very well on the training set whilst performing poorly on the test set with poor generalizability. It has to be appreciated that traditional statistic-al methods may be superior in analysing lesser amount of data whilst ML offers the ability to handle high computational power to classify large amounts of data efficiently.

Some of the ML methodologies are opaque, and as a consequence, it may not possible to verify how an algorithm arrives at its conclu-sions. This current lack of transparency in methodology, often referred to as black box nature of ML can affect clinicians' confi-dence when applying ML-based technologies in active clinical deci-sion-making. Defining regulatory guidelines for these self-learning, non-transparent yet accurate ML methods can be challenging.

Artificial intelligence is a data science, and hence, the importance of the quality of the data used to train and validate ML algorithms can-not be overstated. There is a greater need for collaboration and data sharing between research centres to collate large quantities of robust healthy data to improve the generalizability of ML methodolo-gies. This highlights yet another challenge relating to data security and privacy. More transparency about how data are shared and stricteradherence to data management laws is essential in research involving ML methodologies.

Increasing use of ML algorithms in clinical decision-making101 is likely to challenge the concept of personal responsibility and a physi-cians fiduciary relationship towards patients, necessitating regula-tory guidelines to clarify the distribution of liability in the event of mishaps involving AI-aided technologies. Cardiologists in the near term are likely to be keen on AI-aided rather than AI-dictated clinical decision-making for patient management.

Abstract

The field of cardiac electrophysiology (EP) had adopted simple artificial intelligence (AI) methodologies for decades. Recent renewed interest in deep learning techniques has opened new frontiers in electrocardiography analysis including signature identification of diseased states. Artificial intelligence advances coupled with simultaneous rapid growth in computational power, sensor technology, and availability of web-based platforms have seen the rapid growth of AI-aided applications and big data research. Changing lifestyles with an expansion of the concept of internet of things and advancements in telecommunication technology have opened doors to population-based detec-tion of atrial fibrillation in ways, which were previously unimaginable. Artificial intelligence-aided advances in 3D cardiac imaging heralded the concept of virtual hearts and the simulation of cardiac arrhythmias. Robotics, completely non-invasive ablation therapy, and the con-cept of extended realities show promise to revolutionize the future of EP.

In this review, we discuss the impact of AI and recent techno-logical advances in all aspects of arrhythmia care.

Conclusion

Artificial intelligence has considerable impact on all aspects of patient management in the field of cardiac EP from the identification of ar-rhythmia to therapy (invasively and non-invasively). Simple AI techni-ques have been established in the form of computerized interpretation of electrocardiography and rule-based algorithms for cardiac devices. Recent advances with the use of DL techniques are paving the way for newer research in arrhythmia detection and arrhythmogenic focus identification. The most recent AI-aided advancements in cardiac imaging invigorated the attempts to develop better non-invasive mapping techniques to guide targeted ablation therapies (invasive and non-invasive). This is a new paradigm shift and promises personalized 'state of the art' precision care for patients with complex cardiac arrhythmias. The combination of advanced communication and imaging technologies have helped the rapid adoption of AI techniques and big data research as evidenced by the exponential growth of literature on AI-aided research. It may well be that we are in the midst of an AI-led profound change in patient care.

Bibliography And Acknowledgement

- Acharya UR, Oh SL, Hagiwara Y, Tan JH, Adam M, Gertych A, Tan R. A deep convolutional neural network model to classify heartbeats. Comput Biol Med 2017;89:389–396.
- Al'Aref SJ, Anchouche K, Singh G, Slomka PJ, Kolli KK, Kumar A, Pandey M, Maliakal G, van Rosendael AR, Beecy AN, Berman DS, Leipsic J, Nieman K, Andreini D, Pontone G, Schoepf UJ, Shaw LJ, Chang HJ, Narula J, Bax JJ, Guan Y, Min JK. Clinical applications of machine learning in cardiovascular disease and its relevance to cardiacimaging.EurHeartJ2019;40:1975–1986.
- Al-Ahmad A, Grossman JD, Wang PJ. Early experience with a computerized ro-botically controlled catheter system. J Interv Card Electrophysiol 2005;12:199–202.
- Alhusseini MI, Abuzaid F, Rogers AJ, Zaman JAB, Baykaner T, Clopton P, Bailis P, Zaharia M, Wang PJ, Rappel WJ, Narayan S. Machine learning to classify intra-cardiac electrical patterns during atrial fibrillation: machine learning of atrial fib-rillation. Circ Arrhythm Electrophysiol 2020;13:e008160.
- Al-Khatib SM, Stevenson WG, Ackerman MJ, Bryant WJ, Callans DJ, Curtis AB, Deal BJ, Dickfeld T, Field ME, Fonarow GC, Gillis AM, Granger CB, Hammill SC, Hlatky MA, Joglar JA, Kay GN, Matlock DD, Myerburg RJ, Page R. 2017 AHA/ACC/HRS Guideline for management of patients with ventricular arrhythmias and the prevention of sudden cardiac death: a report of the American College of Cardiology/American Heart Association Task Force on Clinical Practice Guidelines and the Heart Rhythm Society. JAmCollCardiol2018;72
- Alonso-Atienza F, Morgado E, Ferna´ndez-Martı´nez L, Garcı´a-Alberola A, Rojo-lvarez JL. Detection of life-threatening arrhythmias using feature selection and support vector machines. IEEE Trans Biomed Eng 2014;61:832–840.
- Arevalo HJ, Vadakkumpadan F, Guallar E, Jebb A, Malamas P, Wu KC, Trayanova N. Arrhythmia risk stratification of patients after myocardial infarc-tion using personalized heart models. Nat Commun 2016;7:11437.
- Aronis KN, Ali R, Trayanova N. The role of personalized atrial modeling in understanding atrial fibrillation mechanisms and improving treatment. Int J Cardiol 2019;287:139–147.
- Aronis KN, Ali RL, Liang JA, Zhou S, Trayanova N. Understanding AF mecha-nisms through computational modelling and simulations. Arrhythm Electrophysiol Rev 2019;8:210–219.
- Attia ZI, Friedman PA, Noseworthy PA, Lopez-Jimenez F, Ladewig DJ, Satam G, Pellikka PA, Munger TM, Asirvatham SJ, Scott CG, Carter RE, Kapa S. Age and sex estimation using artificial intelligence from standard 12-lead ECGs. Circ Arrhythmia Electrophysiol 2019;12:

- Attia ZI, Kapa S, Lopez-Jimenez F, McKie PM, Ladewig DJ, Satam G, Pellikka PA, Enriquez-Sarano M, Noseworthy PA, Munger TM, Asirvatham SJ, Scott CG, Carter RE, Friedman PA. Screening for cardiac contractile dysfunction using an artificial intelligence-enabled electrocardiogram. Nat Med 2019;25:70–74.
- Attia ZI, Noseworthy PA, Lopez-Jimenez F, Asirvatham SJ, Deshmukh AJ, Gersh BJ, Carter RE, Yao X, Rabinstein AA, Erickson BJ, Kapa S, Friedman P. An artifi-cial intelligence-enabled ECG algorithm for the identification of patients with atrial fibrillation during sinus rhythm: a retrospective analysis of outcome pre-diction. Lancet 2019;394:861–867.
- Attia ZI, Sugrue A, Asirvatham SJ, Ackerman MJ, Kapa S, Friedman PA, Noseworthy P. Noninvasive assessment of dofetilide plasma concentration using a deep learning (neural network) analysis of the surface electrocardio-gram: a proof ofconceptstudy.PLoSOne2018;13:e0201059.
- Avendi MR, Kheradvar A, Jafarkhani H. A combined deep-learning and deformable-model approach to fully automatic segmentation of the left ven-tricle in cardiac MRI. Med Image Anal2016;30:108–119.
- Bertagnolli L, Torri F, Paetsch I, Jahnke C, Hindricks G, Arya A, Dinov B. Cardiac magnetic resonance imaging for coregistration during ablation of ische-mic ventricular tachycardia for identification of the critical isthmus. HeartRhythmCaseRep2018;4:70–72.
- Bhaskaran A, Downar E, Chauhan VS, Lindsay P, Nair K, Ha A, Hope A, Nanthakumar K. Electroanatomical mapping–guided stereotactic radiotherapy for right ventricular tachycardia storm. HeartRhythm Case Rep 2019;5:590–592.
- Bhuva AN, Bai W, Lau C, Davies RH, Ye Y, Bulluck H, McAlindon E, Culotta V, Swoboda PP, Captur G, Treibel TA, Augusto JB, Knott KD, Seraphim A, Cole GD, Petersen SE, Edwards NC, Greenwood JP, Bucciarelli-Ducci C, Hughes AD, Rueckert D, Moon JC, Manisty C. A multicenter, scan-rescan, human and machine learning CMR study to test generalizability and precision in imaging biomarker analysis. CircCardiovascImaging2019;12:
- Boyle PM, Zghaib T, Zahid S, Ali RL, Deng D, Franceschi WH, Hakim JB, Murphy MJ, Prakosa A, Zimmerman SL, Ashikaga H, Marine JE, Kolandaivelu A, Nazarian S, Spragg DD, Calkins H, Trayanova N. Computationally guided personalized tar-geted ablation of persistent atrial fibrillation. NatBiomedEng2019;3:870–879.
- Chen E, Jiang J, Su R, Gao M, Zhu S, Zhou J, Huo Y. A new smart wristband equipped with an artificial intelligence algorithm to detect atrial fibrillation. Heart Rhythm 2020;17:847–853.
- Cheniti G, Puyo S, Martin CA, Frontera A, Vlachos K, Takigawa M, Bourier F, Kitamura T, Lam A, Dumas-Pommier C, Pillois X, Pambrun T, Duchateau J, Klotz N, Denis A, Derval N, Cochet H, Sacher F, Dubois R, Jais P, Hocini M, Haissaguerre M. Noninvasive mapping and electrocardiographic imaging in atrial and ventricular arrhythmias (CardioInsight). Card Electrophysiol Clin 2019;11: 459–471.
- Cochet H, Dubois R, Sacher F, Derval N, Sermesant M, Hocini M, Montaudon M, Haı¨ssaguerre M, Laurent F, Jaı¨s P. Cardiac arrhythmias: multimodal assess-ment integrating body surface ECG mapping into cardiac imaging. Radiology 2014;271:239–247.
- Cuculich PS, Schill MR, Kashani R, Mutic S, Lang A, Cooper D, Faddis M, Gleva M, Noheria A, Smith TW, Hallahan D, Rudy Y, Robinson CG. Noninvasive car-diac radiation for ablation of ventricular tachycardia. N Engl J Med 2017;377: 2325–2336.
- Desteghe L, Raymaekers Z, Lutin M, Vijgen J, Dilling-Boer D, Koopman P, Schurmans J, Vanduynhoven P, Dendale P, Heidbuchel H. Performance of hand-held electrocardiogram devices to detect atrial fibrillation in a cardiology and geriatric ward setting. Europace 2017;19:29–39.
- Dissanayake T, Rajapaksha Y, Ragel R, Nawinne I. An ensemble learning ap-proach for electrocardiogram sensor based human emotion recognition. Sensors 2019;19:4995.
- Do¨rr M, Nohturfft V, Brasier N, Bosshard E, Djurdjevic A, Gross S, Raichle CJ, Rhinisperger M, Sto¨ckli R, Eckstein J. The WATCH AF trial: SmartWATCHes for detection of atrial fibrillation. JACC Clin Electrophysiol 2019;5:199–208.
- Ernst S, Babu-Narayan SV, Keegan J, Horduna I, Lyne J, Till J, Kilner PJ, Pennell D, Rigby ML, Gatzoulis MA. Remote-controlled magnetic navigation and abla-tion with 3D image integration as an alternative approach in patients with intra-atrial baffle anatomy. Circ Arrhythmia Electrophysiol 2012;5:131–139.
- Ernst S, Ouyang F, Linder C, Hertting K, Stahl F, Chun J, Hachiya H, Ba¨nsch D, Antz M, Kuck KH. Initial experience with remote catheter ablation using a novel magnetic navigation system: magnetic remote catheter ablation. Circulation 2004; 109:1472–1475.
- Faddis MN, Blume W, Finney J, Hall A, Rauch J, Sell J, Bae KT, Talcott M, Lindsay B. Novel, magnetically guided catheter for endocardial mapping and radiofrequency catheter ablation. Circulation2002;106:2980–2985.
- Fahmy AS, El-Rewaidy H, Nezafat M, Nakamori S, Nezafat R. Automated ana-lysis of cardiovascular magnetic resonance myocardial native T1 mapping images using fully convolutional neural networks. J Cardiovasc Magn Reson 2019;21:7.
- Fahmy AS, Neisius U, Chan RH, Rowin EJ, Manning WJ, Maron MS, Nezafat R. Three-dimensional deep convolutional neural networks for automated myocar-dial scar quantification in hypertrophic cardiomyopathy: a multicenter multi-vendor study. Radiology 2020;294:52–60.
- Fahmy AS, Rausch J, Neisius U, Chan RH, Maron MS, Appelbaum E, Menze B, Nezafat R. Automated cardiac MR scar quantification in hypertrophic cardiomy-opathy using deep convolutional neural networks. JACC Cardiovasc Imaging2018;11:1917–1918.
- Fan YY, Li YG, Li J, Cheng WK, Shan ZL, Wang YT, Guo Y. Diagnostic performance of a smart device with photoplethysmography technology for atrial fibrillation detec-tion: pilot study (Pre-mAFA II Registry). JMIR Mhealth Uhealth 2019;7:e11437.

- Feeny AK, Rickard J, Patel D, Toro S, Trulock KM, Park CJ, LaBarbera MA, Varma N, Niebauer MJ, Sinha S, Gorodeski EZ, Grimm RA, Ji X, Barnard J, Madabhushi A, Spragg DD, Chung M. Machine learning prediction of response to cardiac resynchronization therapy: improvement versus current guidelines. Circ Arrhythm Electrophysiol 2019;12:e00731625.
- Feng Y, Guo Z, Dong Z, Zhou XY, Kwok KW, Ernst S, Lee SL. An efficient car-diac mapping strategy for radiofrequency catheter ablation with active learning. Int J Comput Assist Radiol Surg 2017;12:1199–1207.
- Figuera C, Irusta U, Morgado E, Aramendi E, Ayala U, Wik L, Kramer-Johansen J, Eftestøl T, Alonso-Atienza F. Machine learning techniques for the detection of shockable rhythms in automated external defibrillators. PLoS One 2016;11:e0159654.
- Galloway CD, Valys AV, Shreibati JB, Treiman DL, Petterson FL, Gundotra VP, Albert DE, Attia ZI, Carter RE, Asirvatham SJ, Ackerman MJ, Noseworthy PA, Dillon JJ, Friedman P. Development and validation of a deep-learning model to screen for hyperkalemia from the electrocardiogram. JAMA Cardiol 2019;4: 428–436.
- Goldenthal IL, Sciacca RR, Riga T, Bakken S, Baumeister M, Biviano AB, Dizon JM, Wang D, Wang KC, Whang W, Hickey KT, Garan H. Recurrent atrial fibril-lation/flutter detection after ablation or cardioversion using the AliveCor KardiaMobile device: iHEART results. Cardiovasc Electrophysiol 2019;30: 2220–2228.
- Goldstein BA, Navar AM, Carter RE. Moving beyond regression techniques in cardiovascular risk prediction: applying machine learning to address analytic challenges. Eur Heart J 2017;38:1805–1814.
- Grosan C, Abraham A. Intelligent systems. In: Rule-Based Expert Systems. ISRL. Vol. 17. Berlin, Heidelberg: Springer-Verlag; 2011. p.149–187.
- Guo Y, Wang H, Zhang H, Liu T, Liang Z, Xia Y, Yan L, Xing Y, Shi H, Li S, Liu Y, Liu F, Feng M, Chen Y, Lip GYH; MAFA II Investigators. Mobile photoplethys-mographic technology to detect atrial fibrillation. J Am Coll Cardiol 2019;74: 2365–2375.
- Han L, Askari M, Altman RB, Schmitt SK, Fan J, Bentley JP, Narayan SM, Turakhia MP. Atrial fibrillation burden signature and near-term prediction of stroke: a machine learning analysis. Circ Cardiovasc Qual Outcomes 2019;12: e005595.
- Hannun AY, Rajpurkar P, Haghpanahi M, Tison GH, Bourn C, Turakhia MP, Ng AY. Cardiologist-level arrhythmia detection and classification in ambulatory electrocardiograms using a deep neural network. Nat Med 2019;25:65–69.
- Himmelreich JCL, Karregat EPM, Lucassen WAM, van Weert HCPM, de Groot JR, Handoko ML, Nijveldt R, Harskamp R. Diagnostic accuracy of a smartphone-operated, single-lead electrocardiography device for detection of rhythm and conduction abnormalities in primary care. Ann Fam Med 2019;17: 403–411
- Howard JP, Fisher L, Shun-Shin MJ, Keene D, Arnold AD, Ahmad Y, Cook CM, Moon JC, Manisty CH, Whinnett ZI, Cole GD, Rueckert D, Francis DP. Cardiac rhythm device identification using neural networks. JACC Clin Electrophysiol 2019; 5:576–586.
- Hu SY, Santus E, Forsyth AW, Malhotra D, Haimson J, Chatterjee NA, Kramer DB, Barzilay R, Tulsky JA, Lindvall C. Can machine learning improve patient se-lection for cardiac resynchronization therapy? PLoS One 2019;14:
- Kalscheur MM, Kipp RT, Tattersall MC, Mei C, Buhr KA, DeMets DL, Field ME, Eckhardt LL, Page C. Machine learning algorithm predicts cardiac resynchroniza-tion therapy outcomes: lessons from the COMPANION trial. Circ Arrhythm Electrophysiol 2018;11
- Kim EJ, Davogustto G, Stevenson WG, John RM. Non-invasive cardiac radiation for ablation of ventricular tachycardia: A new therapeutic paradigm in electro-physiology. Arrhythmia Electrophysiol Rev 2018;7:8–10. Ko
- W-Y, Siontis KC, Attia ZI, Carter RE, Kapa S, Ommen SR, Demuth SJ, Ackerman MJ, Gersh BJ, Arruda-Olson AM, Friedman PA, Noseworthy P. Detection of hyper-trophic cardiomyopathy using a convolutional neural network-enabled electro-cardiogram. J Am Coll Cardiol 2020;75:722–733.
- Koivuma¨ki JT, Korhonen T, Tavi P. Impact of sarcoplasmic reticulum calcium re-lease on calcium dynamics and action potential morphology in human atrial myocytes: a computational study. PLoS Comput Biol 2011;7:e1001067.
- Kotu LP, Engan K, Skretting K, Ma˚løy F, Ørn S, Woie L, Eftestøl T. Probability mapping of scarred myocardium using texture and intensity features in CMR images. Biomed Eng Online 2013;12:91.
- Krittanawong C, Johnson KW, Rosenson RS, Wang Z, Aydar M, Baber U, Min JK, Tang WHW, Halperin JL, Narayan SM. Deep learning for cardiovascular medicine: a practical primer. Eur Heart J 2019;40:2058–2073.
- Krittanawong C, Rogers AJ, Johnson KW, Wang Z, Turakhia MP, Halperin JL, Narayan SM. Integration of novel monitoring devices with machine learning tech-nology for scalable cardiovascular management. Nat Rev Cardiol 2021;18:75–91.
- Lascano EC, Said M, Vittone L, Mattiazzi A, Mundi~na-Weilenmann C, Negroni J. Role of CaMKII in post acidosis arrhythmias: a simulation study using a human myocyte model. J Mol Cell Cardiol 2013;60:172–183.
- Lau JK, Lowres N, Neubeck L, Brieger DB, Sy RW, Galloway CD, Albert DE, Freedman S. iPhone ECG application for community screening to detect silent atrial fibrillation: a novel technology to prevent stroke. Int J Cardiol 2013;165:193–194.
- Leiner T, Rueckert D, Suinesiaputra A, Baeßler B, Nezafat R, I sgum I, Young AA. Machine learning in cardiovascular magnetic resonance: basic concepts and applications. J Cardiovasc Magn Reson 2019;21:61.
- Li Q, Rajagopalan C, Clifford G. Ventricular fibrillation and tachycardia classifica-tion using a machine learning approach. IEEE Trans Biomed Eng 2014;61: 1607–1613.
- Li Y, Bisera J, Weil MH, Member S, Tang W. An algorithm used for ventricular fibrillation detection without interrupting chest compression. IEEE Trans Biomed Eng 2012;59:78–86.
- Loo BW, Soltys SG, Wang L, Lo A, Fahimian BP, Iagaru A, Norton L, Shan X, Gardner E, Fogarty T, Maguire P, Al-Ahmad A, Zei P. Stereotactic ablative radiotherapy for the treatment of refractory cardiac ventricular arrhythmia. Circ Arrhythmia Electrophysiol 2015;8:748–750.

- Lowres N, Neubeck L, Salkeld G, Krass I, McLachlan AJ, Redfern J, Bennett AA, Briffa T, Bauman A, Martinez C, Wallenhorst C, Lau JK, Brieger DB, Sy RW, Freedman S. Feasibility and cost-effectiveness of stroke prevention through community screening for atrial fibrillation using iPhone ECG in pharmacies. The SEARCH-AF study. Thromb Haemost 2014;111:1167–1176.
- Luo CH, Rudy Y. A model of the ventricular cardiac action potential. Depolarization, repolarization, and their interaction. Circ Res 1991;68:1501–1526.
- Marques E, Filho DS, Fernandes FDA, Lacerda C, Soares DA, Seixas L, Augusto A, Sarmet MD, Gismondi RA, Mesquita ET, Mesquita CT. Artificial intelligence in cardiology: concepts, tools and challenges—"the horse is the one who runs, you must be the jockey". Arq Bras Cardiol 2020;114:718–725.
- Martin-Isla C, Campello VM, Izquierdo C, Raisi-Estabragh Z, Baeßler B, Petersen SE, Lekadir K. Image-based cardiac diagnosis with machine learning: a review. Front Cardiovasc Med 2020;7:1.
- McGillivray MF, Cheng W, Peters NS, Christensen K. Machine learning methods for locating re-entrant drivers from electrograms in a model of atrial fibrillation. R Soc Open Sci 2018;5:172434.
Misra S, van Dam P, Chrispin J, Assis F, Keramati A,
- Kolandaivelu A, Berger R, Tandri H. Initial validation of a novel ECGI system for localization of premature ventricular contractions and ventricular tachycardia in structurally normal and abnormal hearts. J Electrocardiol 2018;51:801–808.
- Moore J. The Dartmouth College Artificial Intelligence Conference: the next fifty years. AI Mag 2006;27:87–91.
- Motwani M, Dey D, Berman DS, Germano G, Achenbach S, Al-Mallah MH, Andreini D, Budoff MJ, Cademartiri F, Callister TQ, Chang HJ, Chinnaiyan K, Chow BJ, Cury RC, Delago A, Gomez M, Gransar H, Hadamitzky M, Hausleiter J, Hindoyan N, Feuchtner G, Kaufmann PA, Kim YJ, Leipsic J, Lin FY, Maffei E, Marques H, Pontone G, Raff G, Rubinshtein R, Shaw LJ, Stehli J, Villines TC, Dunning A, Min JK, Slomka PJ. Machine learning for prediction of all-cause mor-tality in patients with suspected coronary artery disease: a 5-year multicentre prospective registry analysis. Eur Heart J 2017;38:500–507.
- Nguyen MT, Nguyen BV, Kim K. Deep feature learning for sudden cardiac ar-rest detection in automated external defibrillators. Sci Rep 2018;8:17196.
- Niederer SA, Lumens J, Trayanova N. Computational models in cardiology. Nat Rev Cardiol 2019;16:100–111.
- Nygren A, Fiset C, Firek L, Clark JW, Lindblad DS, Clark RB, Giles WR. Mathematical model of an adult human atrial cell: the role of Kþ currents in repolarization. Circ Res 1998;82:63–81.
- O'Hara T, Vira´g L, Varro´ A, Rudy Y. Simulation of the undiseased human car-diac ventricular action potential: model formulation and experimental valid-ation. PLoS Comput Biol 2011;7:e1002061.
- Perez MV, Mahaffey KW, Hedlin H, Rumsfeld JS, Garcia A, Ferris T, Balasubramanian V, Russo AM, Rajmane A, Cheung L, Hung G, Lee J, Kowey P, Talati N, Nag D, Gummidipundi SE, Beatty A, Hills MT, Desai S, Granger
- CB, Desai M, Turakhia M; Apple Heart Study Investigators. Large-scale assessment of a smartwatch to identify atrial fibrillation. N Engl J Med 2019;381:1909–1917.
Petersen SE, Abdulkareem M, Leiner T. Artificial intelligence will transform car-diac imaging—opportunities and challenges. Front Cardiovasc Med 2019;6:133.
- Porumb M, Stranges S, Pescape` A, Pecchia L. Precision medicine and artificial in-telligence: a pilot study on deep learning for hypoglycemic events detection based on ECG. Sci Rep 2020;10:170.
- Prakosa A, Arevalo HJ, Deng D, Boyle PM, Nikolov PP, Ashikaga H, Blauer JJE, Ghafoori E, Park CJ, Blake RC 3rd, Han FT, MacLeod RS, Halperin HR, Callans DJ, Ranjan R, Chrispin J, Nazarian S, Trayanova N. Personalized virtual-heart technology for guiding the ablation of infarct-related ventricular tachycardia. Nat Biomed Eng 2018;2:732–740.
- Qian PC, Azpiri JR, Assad J, Gonzales Aceves EN, Cardona Ibarra CE, de la Pena C, Hinojosa M, Wong D, Fogarty T, Maguire P, Jack A, Gardner EA, Zei PC. Noninvasive stereotactic radioablation for the treatment of atrial fibrilla-tion: first-in-man experience. J Arrhythmia 2020;36:67–74.
- Qin C, Schlemper J, Caballero J, Price AN, Hajnal JV, Rueckert D. Convolutional recurrent neural networks for dynamic MR image reconstruc-tion. IEEE Trans Med Imaging 2019;38:280–290.
- Reddy VY, Neuzil P, Malchano ZJ, Vijaykumar R, Cury R, Abbara S, Weichet J, McPherson CD, Ruskin JN. View-synchronized robotic image-guided therapy for atrial fibrillation ablation: experimental validation and clinical feasibility. Circulation 2007;115:2705–2714.
- Reed MJ, Grubb NR, Lang CC, O'Brien R, Simpson K, Padarenga M, Grant A, Tuck S, Keating L, Coffey F, Jones L, Harris T, Lloyd G, Gagg J, Smith JE, Coats T.Multi-centre randomised controlled trial of a smartphone-based event re-corder alongside standard care versus standard care for patients presenting to the emergency department with palpitations and pre-syncope: the IPED (Investigation of Palpitations in the ED) study. EClinicalMedicine 2019;8:37–46.
- Robinson CG, Samson PP, Moore KMS, Hugo GD, Knutson N, Mutic S, Goddu SM, Lang A, Cooper DH, Faddis M, Noheria A, Smith TW, Woodard PK, Gropler RJ, Hallahan DE, Rudy Y, Cuculich PS. Phase I/II trial of electrophysiology-guided noninvasive cardiac radioablation for ventricular tachycardia. Circulation 2019;139:313–321.
- Sana F, Isselbacher EM, Singh JP, Heist EK, Pathik B, Armoundas A. Wearable devices for ambulatory cardiac monitoring: JACC state-of-the-art review. JAm Coll Cardiol 2020;75:1582–1592.
- Saucerman JJ, Healy SN, Belik ME, Puglisi JL, McCulloch A. Proarrhythmic con-sequences of a KCNQ1 AKAP-binding domain mutation: computational models of whole cells and heterogeneous tissue. Circ Res 2004;95:1216–1224.
- Scara` A, Sciarra L, De Ruvo E, Borrelli A, Grieco D, Palama` Z, Golia P, De Luca L, Rebecchi M, Calo` L. Safety and feasibility of atrial fibrillation ablation using AmigoRV system versus manual approach: a pilot study. Indian Pacing Electrophysiol J 2018;18:61–67.
- Schilling C, Keller M, Scherr D, Oesterlein T, Haı¨ssaguerre M, Schmitt C, Do¨ssel O, Luik A. Fuzzy decision tree to classify complex fractionated atrial electrograms. Biomed Tech

2015;60:245–255.

- Schla¨pfer J, Wellens HJ. Computer-interpreted electrocardiograms benefits and limitations. J Am Coll Cardiol 2017;70:1183–1192.
- Schlemper J, Caballero J, Hajnal JV, Price AN, Rueckert D. A deep cascade of convolutional neural networks for dynamic MR image reconstruction. IEEE Trans Med Imaging 2018;37:491–503.
- Scholz EP, Seidensaal K, Naumann P, Andre´ F, Katus HA, Debus J. Risen from the dead: cardiac stereotactic ablative radiotherapy as last rescue in a patient with refractory ventricular fibrillation storm. HeartRhythm Case Rep 2019;5: 329–332.
- Shade JK, Ali RL, Basile D, Popescu D, Akhtar T, Marine JE, Spragg DD, Calkins H, Trayanova N. Pre-procedure application of machine learning and mechanistic simulations predicts likelihood of paroxysmal atrial fibrillation recurrence fol-lowing pulmonary vein isolation. Circ Arrhythm Electrophysiol 2020;13:e008213.
- Silva JNA, Southworth M, Raptis C, Silva J. Emerging applications of virtual real-ity in cardiovascular medicine. JACC Basic Transl Sci 2018;3:420–430.
- Southworth MK, Silva JR, Silva JNA. Use of extended realities in cardiology. Trends Cardiovasc Med 2020;30:143–148.
- Stavrakis S, Stoner JA, Kardokus J, Garabelli PJ, Po SS, Lazzara R. Intermittent vs. Continuous Anticoagulation theRapy in patiEnts with Atrial Fibrillation (iCARE-AF): a randomized pilot study. J Interv Card Electrophysiol 2017;48:51–60.
- Tarakji KG, Wazni OM, Callahan T, Kanj M, Hakim AH, Wolski K, Wilkoff BL, Saliba W, Lindsay B. Using a novel wireless system for monitoring patients after the atrial fibrillation ablation procedure: the iTransmit study. Heart Rhythm 2015;12:554–559.
- Tison GH, Sanchez JM, Ballinger B, Singh A, Olgin JE, Pletcher MJ, Vittinghoff E, Lee ES, Fan SM, Gladstone RA, Mikell C, Sohoni N, Hsieh J, Marcus G. Passive detection of atrial fibrillation using a commercially available smart watch.JAMA Cardiol 2018;3:409–416.
- Tokodi M, Schwertner WR, Kova´cs A, T}ose´r Z, Staub L, Sa´rka´ny A, Lakatos BK, Behon A, Boros AM, Perge P, Kutyifa V, Sze´plaki G, Gelle´r L, Merkely B, Kosztin A. Machine learning-based mortality prediction of patients undergoing cardiac resynchronization therapy: the SEMMELWEIS-CRT score. Eur Heart J 2020;41:1747–1756.
- Trayanova NA. How personalized heart modeling can help treatment of lethal arrhythmias: a focus on ventricular tachycardia ablation strategies in post-infarction patients. Wiley Interdiscip Rev Syst Biol Med 2020;12:e147
- Tsyganov A, Wissner E, Metzner A, Mironovich S, Chaykovskaya M, Kalinin V, Chmelevsky M, Lemes C, Kuck K. Mapping of ventricular arrhythmias using a novel noninvasive epicardial and endocardial electrophysiology system. J Electrocardiol 2018;51:92–98.
- Turagam MK, Petru J, Neuzil P, Kakita K, Kralovec S, Harari D, Phillips P, Piazza D, Whang W, Dukkipati SR, Reddy V. Automated noncontact ultrasound imag-ing and ablation system for the treatment of atrial fibrillation: outcomes of the first-in-human VALUE trial. Circ Arrhythm Electrophysiol 2020;13:e007917
- Turing A. Computing machinery and intelligence. Mind 1950;LIX:433–460.
- Wasserlauf J, You C, Patel R, Valys A, Albert D, Passman R. Smartwatch per-formance for the detection and quantification of atrial fibrillation. Circ Arrhythmia Electrophysiol 2019;12:e006834.
- William AD, Kanbour M, Callahan T, Bhargava M, Varma N, Rickard J, Saliba W, Wolski K, Hussein A, Lindsay BD, Wazni OM, Tarakji KG. Assessing the accur-acy of an automated atrial fibrillation detection algorithm using smartphone technology: the iREAD study. Heart Rhythm 2018;15:1561–1565.
- Zahid S, Cochet H, Boyle PM, Schwarz EL, Whyte KN, Vigmond EJ, Dubois R, Hocini M, Haı¨ssaguerre M, Jaı¨s P, Trayanova N. Patient-derived models link re-entrant driver localization in atrial fibrillation to fibrosis spatial pattern. Cardiovasc Res 2016;110:443–454.

Advances and Future Directions in Cardiac Pacemakers

CHAPTER 12

Several strategies have been developed and are emerging to enhance device therapy. Pump efficiency is addressed with multisite left ventricle pacing and, potentially, His-Purkinje recruitment. Hardware reduction and simplification include leadless pacemakers (single component and multicomponent), and future advances may eliminate the need for batteries, which deplete over time.

Cardiac Resynchronization

Although cardiac pacing had been used historically to effectively treat bradycardia (delayed or absent activation of the entire ventricle), cardiac resynchronization therapy (CRT) introduced the concept of pacing to treat a delayed segment of the ventricle. When segments of the left ventricle (LV) contract with marked delay (most commonly of the free wall due to left bundle branch block [LBBB]), they fail to meaningfully contribute to stroke volume and cardiac output. This is termed dyssynchrony . Cardiac resynchronization improves ventricular function by pacing to improve electrical (and consequently mechanical) coordination and thus pump efficiency. It is accomplished by near simultaneous pacing of the right ventricle (RV) and LV, most commonly using an epicardial lead in the coronary sinus to restore interventricular and intraventricular synchrony. This, in turn, improves LV contractility, stroke volume, and ejection fraction (EF). CRT has been shown to reverse adverse cellular remodeling, improve ventricular function, lower levels of HF biomarkers (e.g., B-type natriuretic peptide), reduce HF hospitalization, and lower mortality However, CRT is not uniformly effective, and careful patient selection, lead positioning, and device programming are necessary to maximize its benefits. Here, we provide an overview of best practices to optimize CRT and future directions.

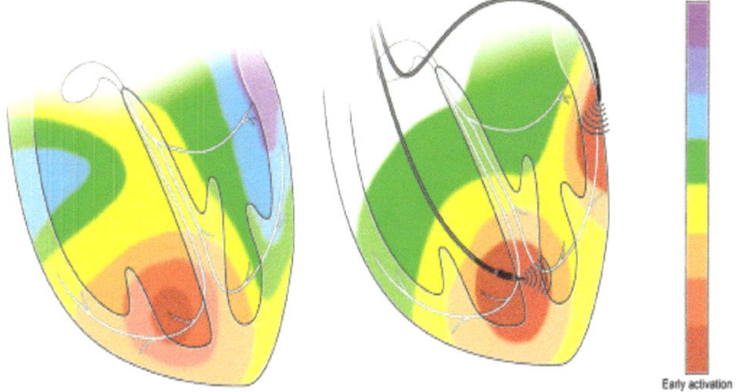

Fig. 12.1. CRT for the Treatment of Heart Failure

Left bundle branch block causes delayed electrical and mechanical activation of the LV, which in turn results in atrioventricular, interventricular, and intraventricular dyssynchrony, consequently reducing LV pump function. This results in adverse LV remodeling over time. CRT, by pacing the right and left ventricles near-simultaneously, aims to correct mechanical dyssynchrony, improve LV function, and over time, cause reverse remodeling. CRT = cardiac resynchronization therapy; LV = left ventricle/ventricular

Optimizing CRT to maximize clinical response and ventricular remodeling

The CRT response refers to the modification of the natural history of HF progression (Figure 2). Defining CRT response is complex, and numerous endpoints have been used, including New York Heart Association (NYHA) functional class and echocardiographic changes. The success of cardiac resynchronization is dependent on: 1) selection of appropriate patients; 2) maximal LV resynchronization to correct the delayed activation imposed by a conduction abnormality (i.e., pacing the correct location); and 3) continuous delivery of biventricular (BiV) pacing with every cardiac cycle to deliver the maximal "dose" of therapy. Response to CRT is determined by a host of parameters, including patient symptoms, objective measurements of functional capacity, and cardiac function. Those who demonstrate improvement in these parameters are termed responders, with super-responders referring to a subgroup with near normalization of LV function. Patients who demonstrate stabilization of LV function without experiencing the progressive decline that is expected with heart failure are termed nonprogressors. A small proportion of patients may experience a rapid decline in LV function following CRT (negative responders).

Patient selection

The selection of patients who are most likely to benefit from CRT relies heavily on the severity of HF symptoms and on electrocardiographic criteria indicative of ventricular dyssynchrony. A summary of the results of selected large, randomized, clinical trials of CRT stratified by key patient characteristics .

A

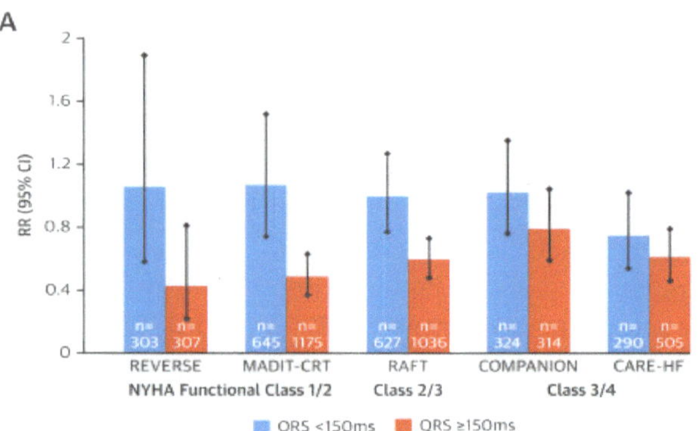

B

LVEF ≤35%, QRS Duration ≥120 ms and Sinus Rhythm

QRS morphology	QRS duration (ms)	NYHA functional class	Level of recommendation
LBBB	≥150	II, III, ambulatory IV	Class I
	120-149	II, III, ambulatory IV	Class IIa
	≥150	I + LVEF ≤30% + ischemic heart disease	Class IIb
Non-LBBB	≥150	III, ambulatory IV	Class IIa
	120-149	III, ambulatory IV	Class IIb
	≥150	II	Class IIb
	120-149	I, II	Class III (no CRT)
Significant (>40%) ventricular pacing	Any QRS	I, II, III, ambulatory IV	Class IIa

Fig.12.2 Effect of CRT in Randomized Clinical Trials and Indications for CRT for Patients in Sinus Rhythm

A) Effect of CRT on composite clinical outcomes in large randomized clinical trials. The effect of CRT on composite clinical outcomes in selected large randomized trials is stratified by patient(characteristics, including NYHA functional class and QRS duration. Patients with severely prolonged QRS duration (>150 ms) were more likely to have improved outcomes compared with those with QRS duration <150 ms. The New York Heart Association (NYHA) functional class was less predictive of clinical improvement. Adapted from Sipahi et al. (B) Indications for CRT for patients in sinus rhythm: guidelines from the American Heart Association/American College of Cardiology. Severity of heart failure symptoms, ejection fraction, cardiac rhythm, QRS morphology, and QRS duration are considered when selecting patients for

CRT. CARE-HF = Cardiac Resynchronization-Heart Failure; CI = confidence interval; COMPANION = Comparison of Medical Therapy, Pacing, and Defibrillation in Heart Failure; LBBB = left bundle branch block; LVEF = left ventricular ejection fraction; MADIT-CRT = Multicenter Automatic Defibrillator Implantation Trial–Cardiac Resynchronization Therapy; NYHA = New York Heart Association; RAFT = Resynchronization-Defibrillation for Ambulatory Heart Failure Trial; REVERSE = Resynchronization Reverses Remodeling in Systolic Left Ventricular Dysfunction; RR = relative risk.

Electrocardiographic criteria

A wide QRS complex is a marker of electrical dyssynchrony and, in the presence of an LBBB pattern, is the most powerful predictor of CRT response. All of the randomized controlled trials (RCTs) that have shown improvement in HF symptoms and survival using patients enrolled in CRT with a minimal QRS duration of 120 to 150 ms The wider the QRS complex, the greater the likelihood of response. There is interplay between the type of bundle branch block and the QRS duration, likely because a sufficiently wide right bundle branch block (RBBB) (>150 ms) reflects delay in both bundles, so that delay of the LV lateral wall activation is present, and CRT is thus effective. However, the presence of bifascicular block (RBBB with left anterior fascicular block) was not predictive of CRT response in the MADIT-CRT (Multicenter Automatic Defibrillator Implantation Trial With Cardiac Resynchronization Therapy) . Current guidelines require the presence of LBBB the QRS complex is relatively narrow (120 to 149 ms) for a Class I indication for CRT . CRT is not indicated when the QRS complex is <120 ms, as it may potentially cause harm . Women are more likely to benefit from CRT than men, particularly when the QRS duration is <150 ms (10). When patients with depressed ventricular function and a pacemaker manifest an LBBB that is caused by frequent RV pacing, upgrading to a CRT system often improves ventricular function.

An intrinsic LBBB or a mechanical dyssynchrony induced by a high percentage of RV apical pacing are the main substrates for resynchronization. In a meta-analysis of RCTs, the benefit of CRT was limited to those patients with LBBB .Patients with RBBB and a nonspecific intraventricular conduction delay with a QRS complex >150 ms may still be considered for CRT, although the strength of the indication is smaller and the likelihood of nonresponse is greater. Certain subgroups of patients with non-LBBB QRS morphologies, such as those with echocardiographic dyssynchrony, may have better outcomes after CRT .

Severity of HF

Initial RCTs predominantly enrolled patients with EF ≤35% and NYHA functional class III or ambulatory class IV (no hospital admissions within 1 month) HF.Subsequent trials included patients with EF ≤30% to 40% and asymptomatic or mild HF (NYHA functional classes I and II) However, the majority of trial participants had symptomatic HF (NYHA functional class II to IV); hence, the evidence supporting CRT for these patients is much stronger (6). Clinical scenarios that warrant special consideration are discussed later.

Atrial fibrillation

Experience in randomized trials of CRT in patients with atrial fibrillation (AF) and with symptomatic HF, QRS complex ≥120 ms, and no other indication for pacing is limited. The MUSTIC (Multisite Stimulation in Cardiomyopathies) trial reported improvement in functional status in patients with both sinus rhythm and AF. A meta-analysis of observational studies reported a greater mortality risk and a higher rate of CRT

Current guidelines recommend CRT implantation in patients with AF, HF, LVEF ≤35%, and QRS complex ≥120 ms . However, it is critical to control the ventricular response in AF to provide >99% BiV pacing .

CRT in patients who require pacing for bradycardia

RV apical pacing induces electrical and mechanical dyssynchrony, and has been associated with an increased risk of HF, particularly when pacing is frequent (>40%) and LV systolic function is depressed . In patients with atrioventricular (AV) block who require pacing, EF ≤50%, and NYHA functional class I to III HF, BiV pacing (with a defibrillator, if indicated) reduces the combined endpoint of mortality, intravenous therapy for HF, or reduction in LV end-systolic volume compared with RV-only pacing. BiV pacing can reasonably be considered in patients who are anticipated to require a high percentage of ventricular pacing and have EF ≤50% with mild HF symptoms .

Measurement of mechanical dyssynchrony for patient selection

Only patients with a QRS complex ≥120 ms were enrolled in initial CRT studies. Because many patients with EF <35% and symptomatic HF have a narrow QRS complex, to identify potential resynchronization candidates, several studies used echocardiography to identify mechanical dyssynchrony by assessing the time difference between activation of the LV septum and lateral wall with M-mode, tissue Doppler, speckle tracking, or other modalities. Three multicenter trials failed to show substantial improvement in CRT response with dyssynchrony assessment by these means, and 1 found increased mortality in patients with a QRS complex <130 ms and echocardiographic dyssynchrony . Whether these study findings reflect limitations of the specific echocardiographic assessments used or whether the strategy of using a mechanical measurement to select an electrical therapy is doomed to failure is unclear. At present, there is no role for routine echocardiographic assessment of dyssynchrony in patient selection for CRT.

Lead position;-Positioning of the LV lead at the site of latest activation to maximize resynchronization seems intuitive. The effect of the location of the LV lead for assessing CRT response has been extensively studied. Broadly, 3 metrics have been used to characterize the LV lead position to determine its effect on CRT response: anatomic LV lead position, LV local electrogram timing, and mechanical delay or scar assessment at the LV lead site.

Anatomic LV lead position

The ideal site for LV pacing is the subject of debate. However, it is clear that the closer the LV and RV electrodes are placed, the lower the potential for resynchronization. As a general rule of thumb, maximizing the distance between the RV and LV electrodes in the horizontal plane in the lateral view (or left anterior oblique [LAO] view) is associated with a better CRT response. Apical positions are unattractive, in part because they necessarily result in less separation between the RV and LV leads, and in part due to potentially nonphysiological ventricular activation. This is supported by a randomized clinical trial showing worse outcomes with apical pacing sites. Posterior and lateral positions are generally preferred. However, compelling differences in outcomes with different lead positions in large studies have been inconsistently found, perhaps due to the presence of a large target region in patients with LBBB or due to patient-specific variations in the ideal site of pacing.

LV local electrogram timing

The site of latest electrical activation can be identified using the timing of the local LV electrogram recorded during lead implantation. As an LV lead is moved within a coronary sinus tributary, the greater the time interval between the start of the surface QRS complex and the local electrogram (the QLV interval), the larger the local delay. Longer QLV intervals result in a more favorable acute hemodynamic response to CRT, long-term reverse LV remodeling, and improved quality of life . A QLV interval >50% of the QRS width was associated with fewer HF hospitalizations and death in 1 small study . Larger studies are examining the feasibility of testing multiple coronary vein tributaries.Although data regarding the feasibility of consistent lead implantation at the site of latest activation and the long-term clinical outcome using the QLV interval are lacking, this approach appears promising.

Mechanical delay or scar assessment to identify the LV lead site

In contrast to the inability of imaging-based indexes of delayed activation to select patients for CRT (see earlier discussion), these techniques appear promising when used to select attractive LV pacing sites. Optimal LV pacing sites are those with the latest mechanical activation, and undesirable sites are those with scarring, which may limit the amount of LV myocardium captured by the pacing pulse. Use of echocardiographic speckle tracking and tissue Doppler imaging improved CRT response in small studies.With speckle tracking, the ultrasound backscatter "fingerprint" is used to track the motion of specific myocardial segments. The randomized controlled TARGET (Targeted Left Ventricular Lead Placement to Guide Cardiac Resynchronization Therapy) study found a reduction in death and HF hospitalization in patients with LV lead placement at the site of latest activation identified using speckle tracking.The STARTER (Speckle Tracking Assisted Resynchronization Therapy for Electrode Region) RCT reported that patients with QRS width 120 to 149 ms and non-LBBB morphology, a group at high risk of nonresponse, were most likely to benefit from echocardiography-guided lead placement. Cardiac magnetic resonance imaging may be useful as well; BiV pacing from sites of late gadolinium enhancement (e.g., scar) increases mortality. The concept of avoiding scar for lead placement was further supported by the TARGET trial, in which echocardiogram speckle tracking was used to avoid lead implantation at sites of scarring

Computational models

Computational models of electromechanical cardiac function have shown promise in improving patient selection, lead localization, and device optimization for optimal CRT, and are the subject of ongoing research.

Multisite pacing

Because dyssynchrony is the underlying substrate for CRT, it has been proposed that pacing from more than 1 LV site may improve resynchronization and outcomes. Multisite pacing using 2 or more LV leads and multipoint pacing using 1 LV multipolar lead have shown promise in improving CRT response. The use of 2 epicardial coronary venous leads compared with 1 improves acute hemodynamic response, EF, LV end-systolic volume, and symptoms of HF in small, randomized trials .The implantation of 2 LV leads has been shown to be feasible and safe in the short term, but has a high long-term failure rate due to the inability to chronically capture using a Y adaptor to pace simultaneously from 2 leads, and due to rapid battery depletion. Studies of the effectiveness of multilead, multisite pacing have had mixed results. Multipoint pacing through a single quadripolar lead has emerged as a feasible and safe option for providing CRT. Quadripolar leads offer the advantage of multiple programmable pacing vectors, hence minimizing the chance of lead abandonment due to a high pacing threshold or phrenic nerve capture. In a national database of quadripolar lead implantation, the risk of lead deactivation and replacement was lower with quadripolar than with bipolar leads.In addition, emerging evidence from small cohorts shows hemodynamic advantages to multipoint pacing using a quadripolar lead, with acute improvement in LV systolic function .The ability to choose a pacing vector with the best hemodynamic response and the ability to capture a large region of LV myocardium by pacing from widely spaced electrodes are potential explanations for the observed improvement. In a nationwide study of over 18,000 recipients of a quadripolar lead, mortality was noted to be lower compared with patients receiving CRT with a bipolar lead. Ongoing RCTs are comparing the efficacy of quadripolar versus bipolar leads.

Endocardial LV pacing

Although all CRT has been delivered via epicardial electrodes, epicardial LV pacing introduces multiple mechanisms of nonresponse, including unsuitable coronary venous anatomy, lead dislodgement, phrenic nerve capture, and nonphysiological epicardial-to-endocardial activation. Endocardial LV pacing may allow for pacing from any noninfarcted LV site; it results in a narrower QRS complex and improved acute hemodynamic function compared with epicardial pacing (36). Endocardial pacing may be preferred due to greater flexibility in selecting the site of lead implantation, absence of phrenic nerve stimulation, and more physiological LV activation. Endocardial LV pacing using conventional pacing leads placed transapically, or through the interatrial or interventricular septum, has been described in small case series.Despite the attractive resynchronization potential, this technique is marred by a prohibitive risk of systemic thromboembolism and mitral valve regurgitation. Leadless LV electrodes under development have shown promise in reducing these complications (as discussed later).

Post-implantation management

CRT nonresponse, the absence of improvement in LV systolic function and HF symptoms, is present in 30% of recipients.Early recognition of nonresponse and its causes permits interventions to improve outcomes. A multidisciplinary approach to CRT optimization has been shown to identify a cause in 74% of nonresponders, leading to changes in device settings or therapy. Common causes for nonresponse include suboptimal lead position, lack of baseline dyssynchrony, LV lead malfunction, inadequate device settings, loss of BiV pacing, and arrhythmias . Successful CRT requires ongoing assessment of the efficacy of BiV pacing following implantation. Follow-up visits assess:

(1) HF symptoms;

(2) LV lead capture threshold

(3) percentage BiV pacing

(4) device settings; and

(5) presence of arrhythmias. When appropriate, further investigation may include an electrocardiogram (ECG), echocardiogram, oxygen consumption treadmill test, 6-min walk, and Holter monitor. CRT response is improved by ensuring:

- Effective LV capture
- A high percentage of BiV pacing and, uncommonly,
- Optimization of AV and VV intervals; or
- LV lead repositioning.

Assessing LV capture: importance of the 12-lead ECG

Poor LV lead performance due to dislodgement, high capture thresholds, phrenic nerve capture, or structural lead dysfunction may affect CRT. A 12-lead ECG facilitates assessment of LV lead performance and its contribution to overall ventricular activation. The QRS morphology during LV and BiV pacing is determined by lead position, capture latency, and the presence of anodal capture. Fig. shows the correlation between radiographic lead position and 12-lead QRS morphology during BiV pacing. Capture of the LV free wall is associated with a dominant R-wave in V1 and a QS complex in lead I, which indicate a wave front propagating away from the LV toward the RV. The absence of these features can indicate: 1) loss of LV capture; 2) LV lead dislodgement; 3) LV capture latency or conduction delay, resulting in the majority of the LV being activated by an RV lead-initiated wave front; 4) fusion between CRT and intrinsic complexes; or 5) anodal capture.

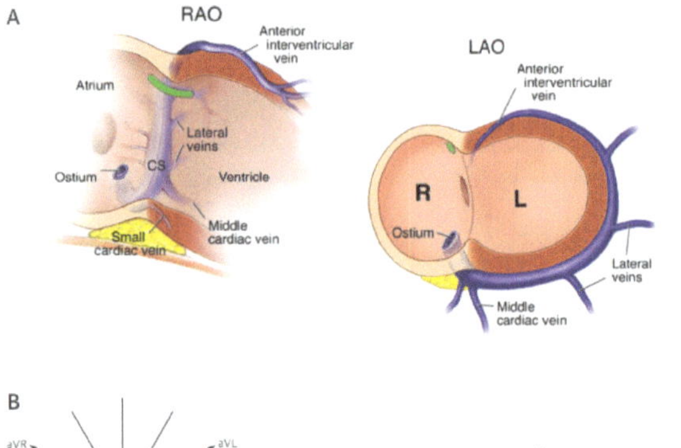

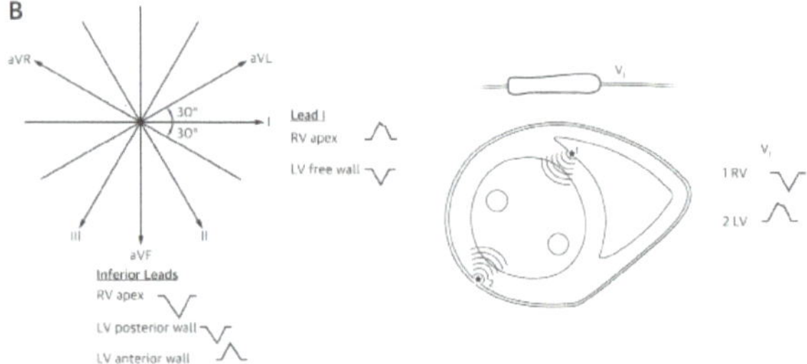

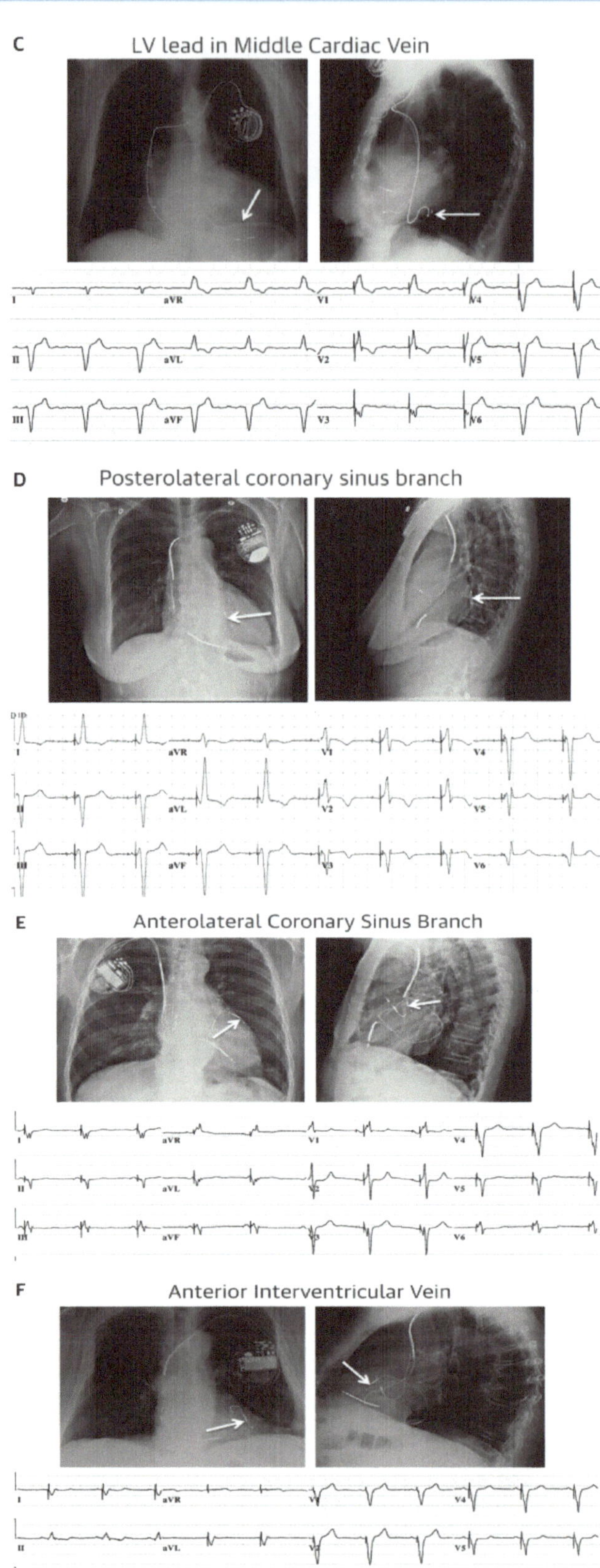

Fig.12.3 Radiographic Lead Position of Coronary Venous Lead and Paced QRS Morphology: Electroanatomic Correlation

(A) Anatomy of the coronary veins in the LAO and RAO views. Tributaries of the CS are best assessed using angiography in the LAO and RAO views during lead placement. The LAO view helps distinguish between lead placement in the lateral wall (preferred) and the septum. The RAO view helps assess whether the lead is anterior versus posterior and basal (preferred) versus apical. *(continued to next page ist column.)*

(B) Correlation between paced QRS morphology and CS lead position. The QRS morphology during coronary venous pacing can be used to confirm capture and assess satisfactory lead positioning and the contribution of LV activation to the overall biventricular paced morphology. Electrocardiographic vectors in the limb leads and the precordial leads as they correlate with coronary venous tributaries are presented here. Pacing from the lateral LV wall results in a predominantly negative vector in leads I and aVL. The inferior limb leads II, III, and aVF distinguish anterior from posterior LV pacing, with a predominantly positive vector resulting from pacing anteriorly and a negative vector resulting from posterior pacing. Precordial lead V1 is placed anteriorly and rightward on the chest. Hence, pacing the LV, the posteriorly placed ventricle, results in a predominantly positive vector (i.e., right bundle branch morphology). The exception is pacing the anterior interventricular vein, which will produce a negative vector in V1 (i.e., left bundle branch morphology). (C to F) Twelve-lead ECG and chest x-ray in the posteroanterior and lateral views showing correlation between lead position and paced QRS morphology in the (C) anterior interventricular vein, (D) anterolateral vein, (E) posterolateral vein, and (F) middle cardiac vein. Arrows in C to F point to the tip of the coronary sinus lead. CS = coronary sinus; LAO = left anterior oblique; RAO = right anterior oblique.

The LV lead capture threshold is tested independently (RV lead output programmed off) with a real-time ECG to record the paced QRS morphology and to identify loss of capture. Conceptually, if an LV lead is placed in a zone of slow electrical conduction, during synchronous BiV pacing, very little LV myocardium is stimulated by the wave front initiated by the LV electrode, and little resynchronization is present. Pre-exciting the tissue at the LV electrode (by pacing the LV ahead of the RV, also known as LV offset) to give the slowly propagating wave front a "head start" results in its greater contribution to LV activation . Serial ECGs performed with varying VV intervals can be used to identify the LV offset interval that produces a dominant R-wave in V1 and QS complex in lead I.In an observational study, increasing R-wave amplitudes in V1 and a change in axis from left to right with CRT was associated with favorable LV remodeling (41). Although there are no systematic studies of the value of ECG optimization, this is a widely available, inexpensive, and simple tool that the authors frequently use.

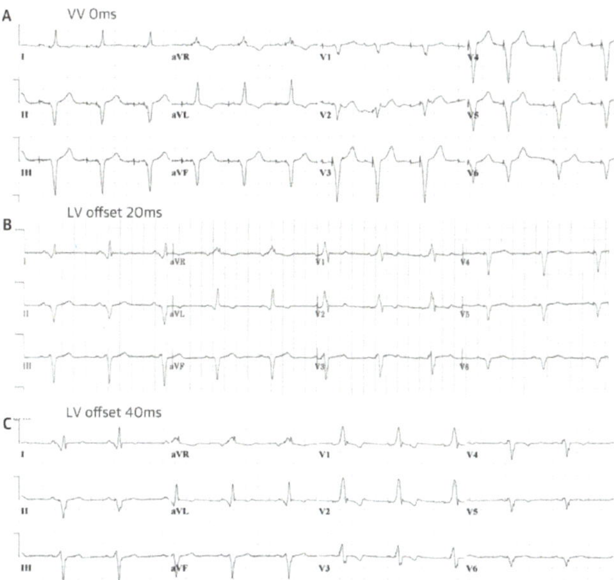

Fig.12.4 Optimization of the VV Interval Using Electrocardiography A) Simultaneous pacing of the LV and RV (LV offset 0 ms) results in a negative vector in lead V1 and an R-wave in lead I due to activation of the majority of the LV by pacing from the RV. Serial electrocardiograms are obtained with increasing pre-excitation of the LV lead in (B) (LV offset 20 ms) and (C) (LV offset 40 ms). When the LV is paced prior to the RV, the QRS morphology reflects progressively greater contribution from LV pacing with resultant positive vector in V1 and negative vector in lead I.

Anodal stimulation is an often under-recognized cause for a lack of CRT response . During pacing, electrons exit the cathode and return via the anode, with capture desired at the cathode. CRT devices allow multiple programmable pacing configurations. If pacing occurs between an LV electrode (cathode) and RV ring electrode (anode), and myocardial stimulation occurs only at the RV anode, effective CRT is not delivered. Anodal-only capture is corrected by adjusting the pacing output or configuration.

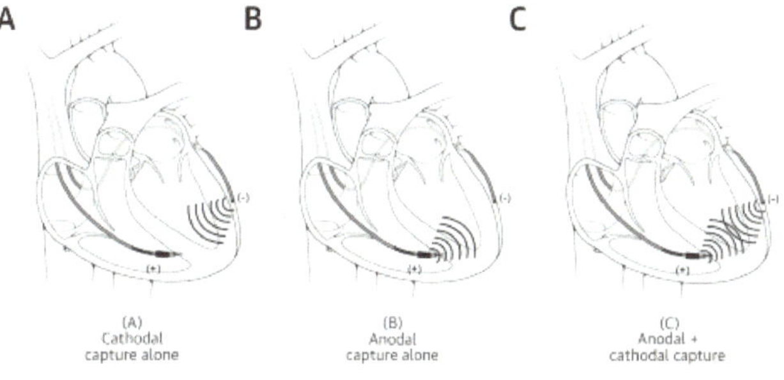

Fig. continued to next page

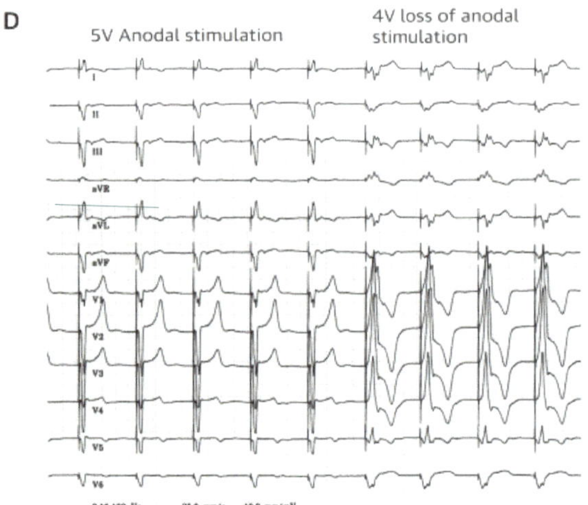

Fig. 12.5. Anodal Stimulation in a BiV Device Anodal stimulation may occur when LV pacing is configured with the LV electrode as cathode and the RV ring or coil (in a defibrillator) as anode. (A) Capture typically occurs at the LV electrode only (cathodal-only capture) producing LV paced morphology. (B) If capture occurs at the anode alone, the QRS morphology resembles RV pacing and leads to loss of resynchronization. Anodal stimulation is more likely to occur at high pacing output. (C) Capture at both the cathode and anode may rarely occur, resulting in a narrow QRS complex with maintenance of cardiac resynchronization. (D) Electrocardiogram during pacing from the LV tip electrode (cathode) to the RV coil (anode) with reducing pacing output. (Left) Pacing at output of 5 V produces a QRS complex resembling RV pacing consistent with anodal only stimulation. (Right) As the pacing output is reduced to 4 V, there is a change in QRS to LV pacing morphology. This represents loss of anodal stimulation with capture at the cathode as the pacing output is reduced.

Percentage BiV pacing: ensuring continuous CRT

The percentage of QRS complexes that are resynchronized (i.e., the CRT "dose") correlates with HF outcome and mortality. Hayes et al. reported optimal improvement in survival with

>98.4% BiV pacing; a goal of >95% is commonly used. In a large national registry, 40% and 11% of patients had <98% and <90% BiV pacing, respectively . Among patients with <98% pacing, atrial arrhythmias, premature ventricular contractions (PVCs), and inappropriately programmed AV intervals account for 30%, 17%, and 35% of pacing loss, respectively Device interrogation provides the percentage of BiV pacing, as well as clues to the reason for its loss. CRT devices have the capability to provide "trigger" pacing from the LV lead in response to a sensed event on the RV lead. This leads to fusion or pseudofusion between the intrinsic beat and LV pacing. Triggered LV pacing does not afford the same hemodynamic benefits of "true" BiV pacing, and hence should be minimized. Although some device manufacturers provide data regarding frequency of triggered LV pacing, Holter monitoring may be required to detect fused QRS morphologies in others. Frequent PVCs interfere with CRT and may independently worsen HF due to dyssynchrony. Treatment with beta-blockers or membrane-active antiarrhythmic drugs, and in select patients, catheter ablation of PVCs may improve CRT response .

Intrinsically conducted AF results in fusion and pseudofusion between LV pacing and native conduction, leading to loss of BiV pacing. Ablation of the AV node restores BiV pacing and improves CRT response (46). Routine AV node ablation in CRT recipients with permanent AF is controversial, as the benefits of response are weighed against the risks associated with pacemaker dependency. Hence, in patients with permanent AF, an initial strategy of pharmacological rate control with rapid escalation to AV node ablation if >99% BiV pacing is not achieved is reasonable. The role of antiarrhythmic drug therapy and catheter ablation to restore sinus rhythm in paroxysmal AF in improving CRT response needs further investigation.

Optimizing device programming: programming AV and VV intervals

A number of studies have optimized device AV and VV intervals to determine whether CRT response may be improved. ECG-based, echocardiographic, and intracardiac electrogram-based AV and VV interval optimization have all been tested. Although in selected cases such a strategy is used, trials of routine optimization using echocardiography and device-based AA and VV interval optimization have been universally disappointing. Optimization is not routinely performed.

Para-Hisian pacing

As noted earlier, chronic RV apical pacing is associated with an increased risk of death, HF hospitalization, and persistent AF. BiV pacing is superior to RV pacing in patients with reduced EF. However, procedural complexity, complications, increased lead burden, CRT nonresponse, and long-term costs of device replacement have led to interest in selective pacing of the proximal conduction system to mimic the natural activation of the ventricles (Figure 8). His-bundle capture enables rapid activation of the ventricles by engaging the highly branching Purkinje network. On the ECG, selective capture of the His bundle results in a QRS complex similar to normal conduction .There is an isoelectric interval from the pacing stimulus to the QRS complex that is often equal to the HV interval. The restoration of a narrow QRS complex by His pacing represents an intact His-Purkinje system or the capability of overcoming impaired conduction within the His-Purkinje system by pacing . Para-Hisian pacing can be achieved using a small-caliber pacing lead (Select Secure Model 3830, Medtronic, Minneapolis, Minnesota) delivered through specially designed sheaths (C 315 HIS) to map the AV septal region . Unipolar pacing aids selective capture of myocardial tissue at the lead tip, and is successful in 84% of patients. In patients with a wide complex, unstable escape rhythms, and diffuse infra-Hisian disease, it may not be feasible to map and place a pacing lead that results in a narrow QRS complex. Select Secure leads placed in the ventricle have a cumulative survival probability of 97.2% at 78 months, although data on long-term performance is lacking. Reliable selection of patients who are likely to have recruitment of the left-sided conduction system is challenging. His bundle pacing in patients with AV block results in higher rates of His-Purkinje system recruitment when the block is at the AV nodal level (93% to 98%) compared with when it is at the infranodal level (52% to 76%). With His-bundle pacing, sensed R waves are often smaller than with pacing at other sites due to the paucity of ventricular myocardium near the membranous septum. The pacing thresholds are often higher when compared with traditional sites, resulting in shorter battery life. There are limited data regarding extraction of leads placed on the membranous septum. Technical aspects of His-bundle pacing are discussed elsewhere. Although promising as a superior alternative to RV apical pacing, larger studies involving longer follow-up are required before widespread adoption.

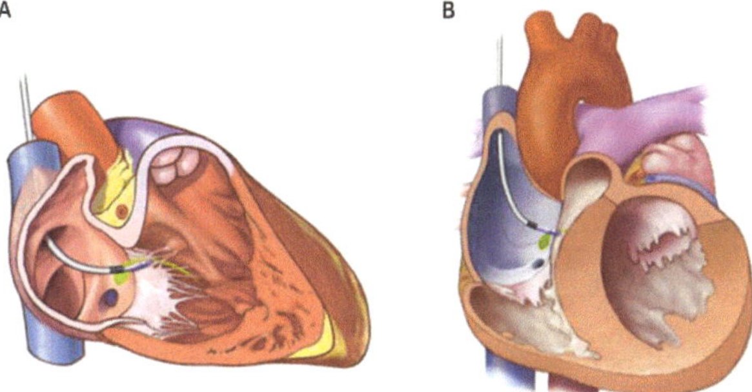

Fig.12.6 His Bundle Pacing (A) Right anterior oblique and (B) left anterior oblique views of the heart showing placement of the lead on the proximal conduction system.

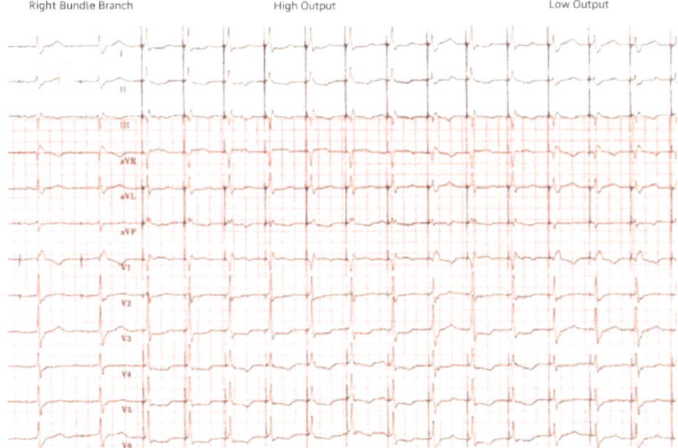

Fig.12.7 ECG Demonstrating Effects of His Bundle Pacing (Left) Atrial pacing is seen with native RBBB configuration. When high output pacing (VVI mode) is performed (middle), the QRS normalizes in duration representing recruitment of the right and left ventricular conduction system. (Right) When the output is reduced, RBBB morphology is reproducible with loss of the recruitment of the left-sided conduction system. ECG = electrocardiogram; RBBB = right bundle branch block.

Remote Monitoring of Pacemakers and Diagnostics

Worldwide, seven million people live with a cardiovascular implantable electronic device to treat bradycardias, tachyarrhythmias, or HF and require effective monitoring for long-term care. RM and remote interrogation (RI) refer to acquisition of system or patient information from a cardiovascular implantable electronic device and transmitting it to a clinic distant from the patient to enhance care. When properly implemented, they can substantially reduce clinic burden and care delay, and can improve patient outcomes. Specifically, RI is routine and scheduled, requires coordination between the patient and clinic, and mirrors an office checkup; RM is automatic data transmission that typically requires no action by the patient that is triggered by clinical and device function alerts

Remote Monitoring technology (RM)

Transtelephonic monitoring

unction can be deduced. Due to the complexity for patients and clinic, and the marked superiority of RI and RM, new pacemakers do not use TTM, although many patients with legacy devices continue to use it.

Transtelephonic monitoring (TTM) has been in use since approximately 1970, and requires a patient to make contact with skin electrodes (such as bracelets) that record a single-lead ECG and transmit it through an analog phone to the clinic. By observing the ECG and pacemaker magnet behavior, device status and battery f

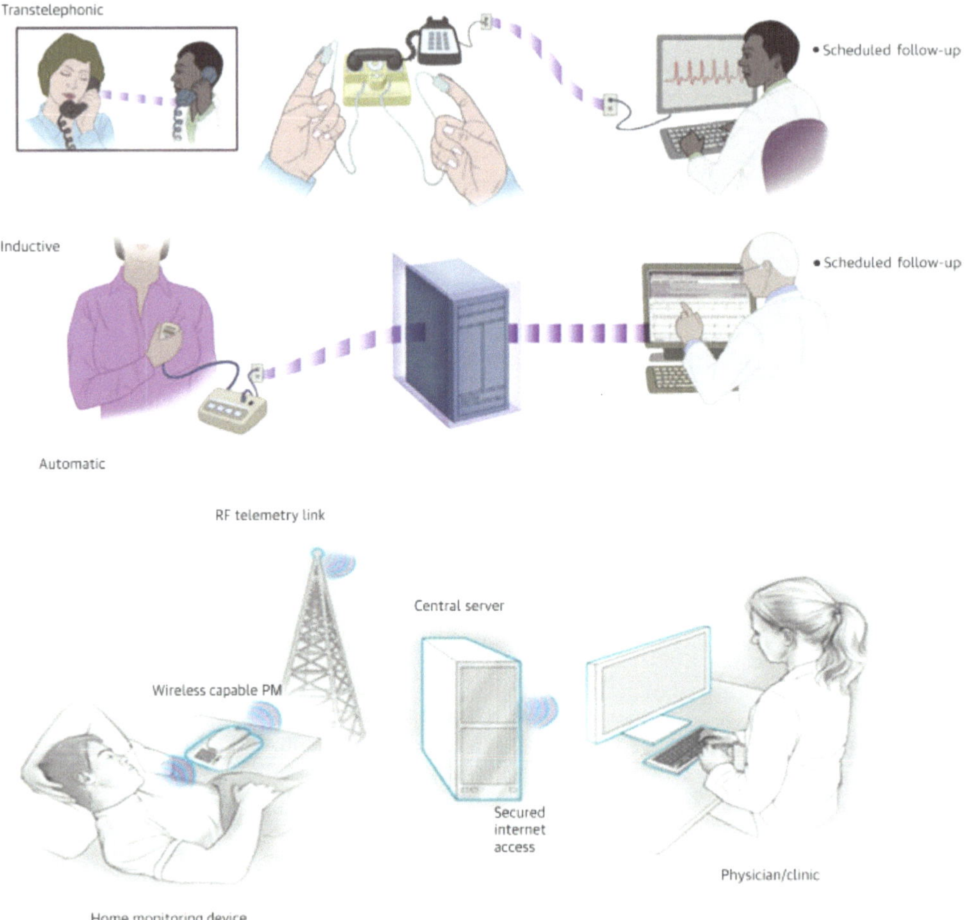

Fig.12.8 **Evolution of Techniques for Monitoring of Pacemakers:** Transtelephonic, Inductive, and Remote Wandless Monitoring Although transtelephonic and inductive monitoring provide intermittent monitoring, radiofrequency wandless monitoring can provide device- and patient-related information more continuously. Modified from Slotwiner et al. (75). PM = pacemaker; RF = radiofrequency.

Inductive transmission

RI typically uses inductive transmission. A patient holds a transmitter's inductive wand over the pacemaker to perform a full interrogation. The transmitter, in turn, connects via a landline or cellular connection to a server, which delivers a full device interrogation to the clinic that is often identical to the report created by an in-office visit. This includes: 1) battery status; 2) lead integrity; 3) lead sensing and pacing (threshold) function; 4) activity sensor statistics; 5) pacing frequency; and 6) stored arrhythmic events.

Radiofrequency RM

A wandless transmitter with radiofrequency capabilities automatically connects to the implanted pacemaker, with no action required on the patient's part, as long as he or she is within range. Typically, the transmitter is placed on or near a nightstand to enable daily communication in the event of alerts (e.g., device or rhythm abnormalities). Episodically, full transmissions that include all of the information available with RI are performed. Patients also can manually force a transmission by pushing a button on the transmitter.

In contrast to RI and TTM, RM checks patient and device status on a daily basis (as opposed to every 3 months), is fully automatic, and can verify transmissions and generate alerts when they are absent. Evidence suggests that this form of monitoring detects abnormalities sooner and may improve survival; new pacemakers either include this capability or will do so in the near future

Monitoring of device and lead function

RM effectively detects system malfunction with less delay than clinic visits with TTM (51). In a randomized study comparing RM versus in-person clinic visits augmented by TTM, the remote arm had a shorter mean time to first diagnosis of clinically actionable events (5.7 months vs. 7.7 months). Events included significant pacing threshold increases or loss of capture, changes in lead impedance, and generator battery depletion to replacement indicators.Furthermore, a randomized trial of long-term RM versus in-clinic follow-up of pacemaker recipients showed that the RM group had a similar rate of death and hospitalization for device-related or cardiovascular adverse events, demonstrating its safety

Detection of supraventricular arrhythmia and stroke prevention

Detection of asymptomatic AF using RM permits timely therapy, including the introduction of anticoagulation therapy to prevent stroke in at-risk individuals . Remotely monitored patients are also less likely to be hospitalized for atrial arrhythmias. In patients without clinical AF, subclinical atrial arrhythmias lasting 6 min or longer are associated with a significantly increased risk of ischemic stroke or embolism . Ongoing trials will determine the effect of therapy for these brief, asymptomatic events. Unrelated to stroke, atrial tachyarrhythmia detection permits medical therapy and rate control interventions, potentially accounting for the reduction in inappropriate shocks with RM and improving HF.

Detection of ventricular tachyarrhythmia

The benefit of detection of ventricular arrhythmia by RM has been demonstrated in multiple implantable cardioverter-defibrillator (ICD) studies and registries; its role in patients with pacemakers is less clear. A meta-analysis comparing RM to in-clinic visits demonstrated a nonsignificant trend toward reduced cardiovascular mortality, a similar overall shock rate, a significantly reduced inappropriate shock rate, and shorter time to the detection of atrial and ventricular arrhythmias with RM.

RM and survival

RM permits analytics on large patient numbers. In the ALTITUDE registry and Merlin network, the use of RM was associated with a lower mortality in recipients of pacemakers, ICDs, and CRT .The improved survival may have resulted from early recognition and management of arrhythmia and HF. However, a meta-analysis of RM trials found no difference in survival compared with in-office visits (indicating safety), with a potential survival benefit limited to systems using daily transmission verification (radiofrequency systems)

Heart Failure Monitoring

Current ICDs and CRT devices can monitor for HF using thoracic impedance as a surrogate for pulmonary congestion. This is sometimes used in combination with other parameters, such as heart rate variability, patient activity level, rapid ventricular rate during AF, and low CRT pacing, to detect possible worsening of HF. Although these programs can provide early warning of worsening HF, their use has not been shown to improve HF clinical outcomes and survival

Leadless Pacing

Cardiac pacemakers are extremely effective for treating symptomatic bradycardia. However, the same system paradigm has been in use for the past 50 years, namely, an implanted extravascular pulse generator connected to a lead that traverses the vasculature to make contact with the endocardium. Although reliable and effective, complications are almost universally caused by the lead, which is a polyurethane- or silicone-encapsulated conductor that is subject to repetitive mechanical motion with each cardiac cycle and with shoulder girdle motion, exposing its constituent materials to mechanical stress and fracture (Figure 12) (59). Because pulse generator pockets are extravascular, they may serve as a nidus for bacterial growth by providing a surface for bacterial biofilm elaboration; the lead then serves as a conduit for bacterial entry to the blood pool. Moreover, leads are inherently thrombogenic, eliciting fibrotic reactions that make removal technically challenging, with a risk of venous perforation, valve disruption, hemothorax, and death. Lead thrombogenicity also introduces a risk of stroke in the setting of venosystemic shunts. Last, by crossing the tricuspid valve, a lead can impinge on leaflet motion, promote clinically significant tricuspid regurgitation, and impair the response to cardiac resynchronization Given the effectiveness of pacemakers and the host of potential lead-related complications, a leadless pacemaker was developed.

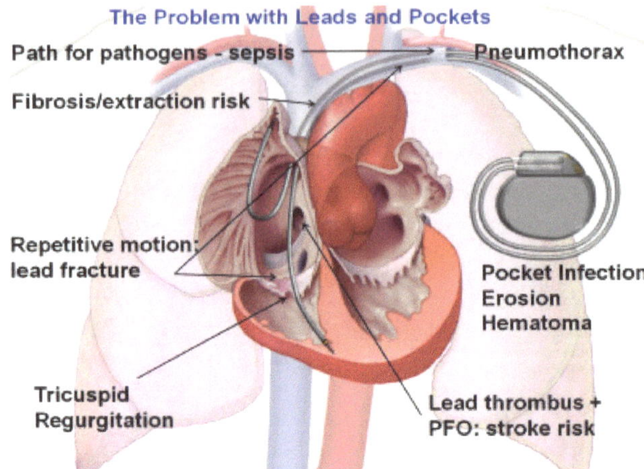

Fig. 12.9 Mechanisms of Complications in Pacemaker with Extravascular Pockets and Transvenous Leads Limitations of traditional transvenous pacemakers include increased risk of infection, thromboembolism, and lead failure, among others. PFO = patent foramen ovale

Leadless pacemakers have been developed using 2 distinct strategies: single-component and multicomponent systems. With single-component systems, the entire pacemaker (battery, electronics, stimulating electrodes, and sensors) is compressed into a small capsule that is delivered into the heart using a deflectable sheath. Advantages of this strategy include greater energy efficiency,system simplicity, and ease of implantation. Limitations, however, include retrieval of intracardiac systems years later after battery depletion, and uncertain thrombus and infection risk. With a multicomponent system, a small "seed" is placed within a cardiac chamber to act as an energy transducer. A second, extrathoracic component beams energy (ultrasound or radio waves) to the seed, and the seed then converts the energy to a pacing pulse.

Single-component leadless pacing

In single-component leadless pacemakers, the pulse generator and sensing and pacing electrodes are all entirely self-contained in a capsule designed for intraventricular placement, eliminating the need for pockets and leads. There are currently 2 devices that have been widely tested in humans:

the Nanostim leadless cardiac pacemaker (LCP) (St. Jude Medical, St. Paul, Minnesota), and the MICRA transcatheter pacing system (TPS) (Medtronic), both of which can deliver single-chamber rate-responsive ventricular pacing .The systems are placed via an 18- (LCP) or 24-F (TPS) sheath inserted in a femoral vein, and are delivered to the RV apical septum (Figure 14). The systems differ with regard to fixation mechanism. The LCP uses an active fixation helix, with rotation of the entire device via a delivery catheter handle control knob at the time of implantation, whereas the TPS has integrated electrically inert nitinol tines that are used solely for fixation. In the initial trial experience for both systems, successful implantation occurred in over 95% of cases, with major complications in 4% to 6.5% of cases, perforation or effusion in 1.5% to 1.6% of cases, and adequate pacing measures at 6 months in 90% to 98.3%. The TPS is physically smaller than the LCP (0.8 cm3 vs. 1.0 cm3), but has a larger diameter (24-F vs. 18-F introducer sheath) and a smaller battery, with shorter anticipated longevity at nominal settings (9.6 years vs. 14.7 years) . The TPS uses autocapture technology to algorithmically use the lower energy pacing pulses to extend longevity, and uses radiofrequency telemetry, which may permit daily alerts and passive follow-up for true RM. The LCP uses conductive telemetry, which saves battery charge, but requires placement of patches on the skin for pacemaker communication. Direct comparisons between systems have not been performed.

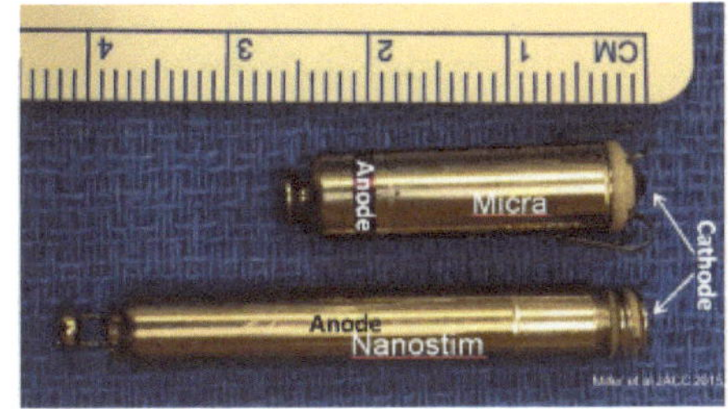

Device	Size	Means of Fixation	Patients	Successful Implantation	Major Complications	Perforation or Effusion	Device Dislodgement	Adequate Pacing Measures at 6 Mo
	cm^3		no.	%	%	%	%	%
Nanostim	1.0	Helical wire screw	526	95.8	6.5	1.5	1.1	90.0
Micra	0.8	Tines	725	99.2	4.0	1.6	0	98.3

Fig.12.10 Single-Component Leadless Pacemakers
The MICRA (Medtronic, Minneapolis, Minnesota) and Nanostim (St. Jude Medical, St. Paul, Minnesota) leadless pacemakers are compared.Reprinted with permission from Miller et al. and Link et al.

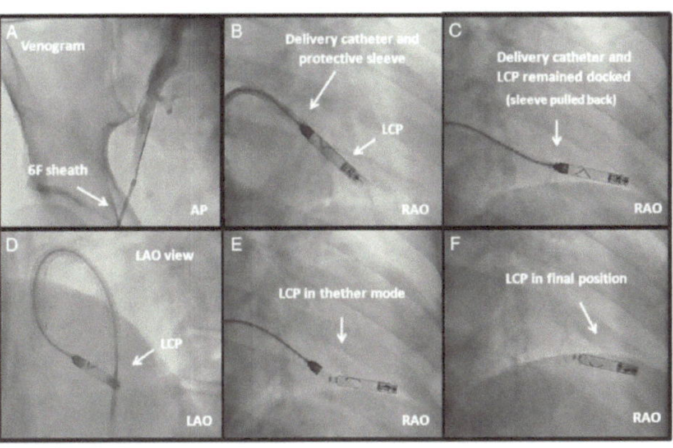

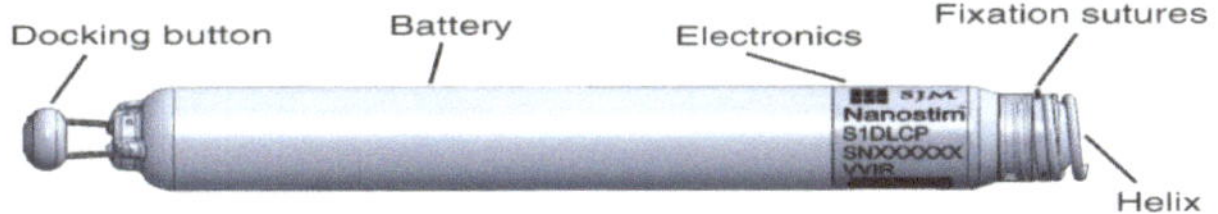

Fig 12.11 Leadless Pacemaker Implantation
Leadless cardiac pacemaker implantation steps. (A) A venogram may optionally be performed; (B) The LCP is positioned into the RV by deflecting the catheter and placed 0.5–1 cm from the RV apex; (C and D) Protective cover is pulled back to expose the flexible part of the catheter; (E) The pacemaker is undocked from the delivery catheter while a tethered connection is maintained. In case the position is suboptimal, the LCP can be reengaged, unscrewed, and repositioned. (F) The LCP is released by rotating the release knob of the catheter.

Ideal management of leadless pacemakers after battery depletion is not known. Little data exists regarding removal of chronically implanted systems. Both available pacemakers have a posterior docking button designed to facilitate late device retrieval.In the TPS experience, 7 of 9 attempts at percutaneous retrieval were successful, including all attempts within 6 months of implantation . Specifically designed removal tools have been developed for the LCP. Fourteen of 15 removal attempts were successful in a recent report; 4 of 4 acute removals (<6 weeks) and 10 of 11 chronic removals (implant duration 88 to 1,188 days). The 1 failed removal was because of inaccessibility of the proximal hub due to its position under the tricuspid valve. Given that leadless pacemakers are one-fiftieth the volume of the typical RV, device deactivation and insertion of a replacement may be a viable strategy for battery depletion for those patients who outlive their pacemaker's battery.Both leadless pacemaker systems have been compared with cohorts of transvenous pacemaker recipients, although direct, prospective randomized comparisons are lacking bloodstream

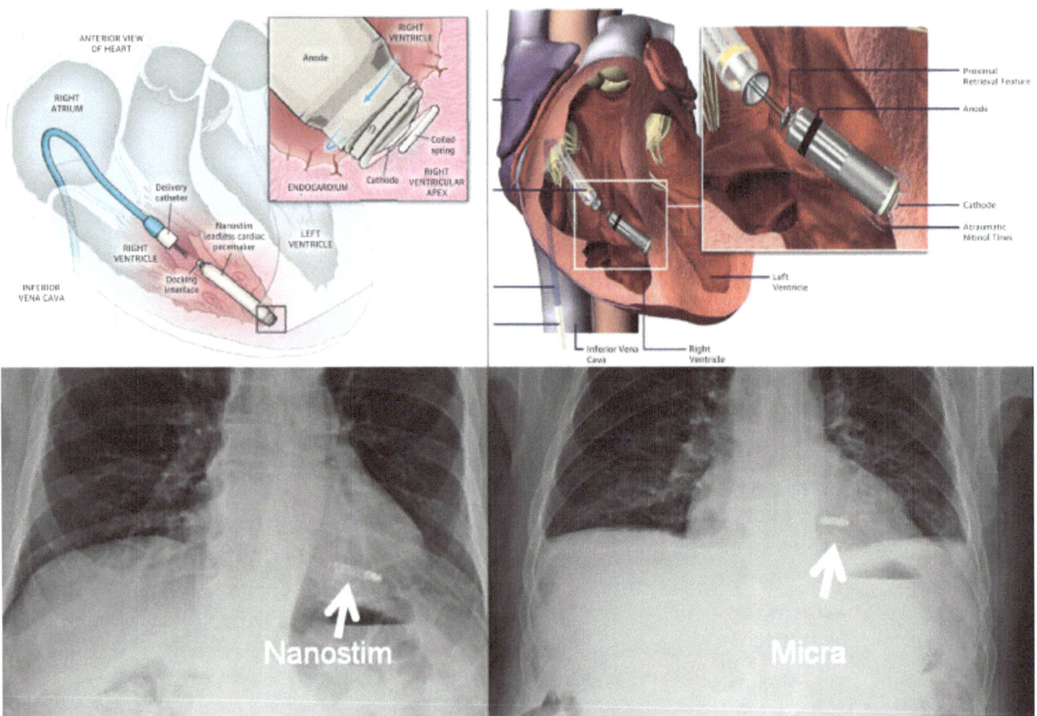

Fig.12.12 Leadless Pacemaker Fixation Mechanism and Radiographic Appearance (Left) Nanostim active fixation leadless pacemaker. (Right) Micra passive fixation transcatheter pacing system. Top panels adapted from Reddy et al. (62) and Reynolds et al.

In these analyses, the leadless pacemaker was associated with fewer short- and intermediate-term complications. This was driven largely by reductions in or the absence of lead complications, infections, and pocket complications. Across all leadless devices, infections appear rare, perhaps due to the lack of an extravascular pocket with direct connection to the bloodstream

The major limitation of current-generation leadless pacemakers is their ability to only perform single-chamber ventricular pacing. Thus, for most patients with sinus node dysfunction, or sinus rhythm and AV block, dual-chamber transvenous devices are preferred. Similarly, patients in need of cardiac resynchronization are not candidates for single-component leadless pacemakers. Patients with inferior vena cava filters and mechanical tricuspid valves are not candidates. Although chronic device embolization has not been reported, it remains a potential concern.The accuracy of rate-responsive features, given that sensors are intracardiac, is not well understood. And last, as noted earlier, optimal management at the time of battery depletion is not known.

Nonetheless, given the lack of a surgical wound, absence of post-implant arm restrictions, and reduced rate of complications, leadless pacemakers represent a paradigm shift that will likely be clinically transformative. Dual-chamber systems are currently under active development; design challenges include device–device communication and fixation in the thin-walled right atrium.

Multicomponent leadless pacing

The WiSE-CRT system (EBR Systems, Sunnyvale, California) uses a multicomponent strategy to provide leadless cardiac resynchronization. A tiny (9.1 mm × 2.7 mm, 0.05 cm3) receiver electrode composed of polyester-covered titanium is implanted endocardially in the LV. A subcutaneous pulse generator is placed in the left lateral thorax and generates ultrasound pulses, which are converted to electrical pacing stimuli by the endocardial seed . All patients in the WiSE-CRT study had a traditional pacemaker or defibrillator; the subcutaneous WiSE-CRT pulse

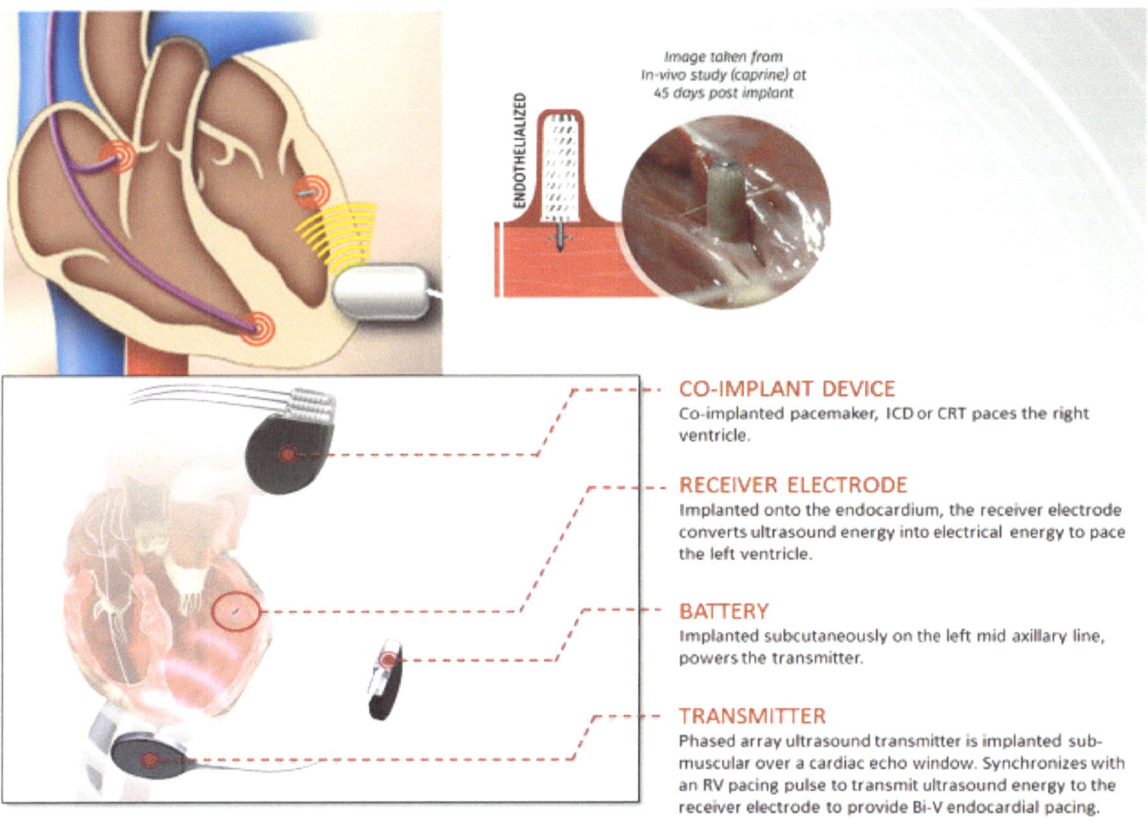

Fig.12.13 **Multicomponent Leadless Pacing System** The battery/transmitter unit detects the pacing stimulus from the coimplant, and an ultrasound pulse is sent to the receiver electrode, which converts the ultrasound energy to a pacing pulse. ICD = implantable cardioverter-defibrillator.

generator detected the RV pacing pulse from the standard system, which triggered endocardial LV pacing. In the initial trial, patients with failed coronary sinus lead placement, nonresponse to CRT, or need for an upgrade to CRT were enrolled. Data from small studies demonstrated significant QRS narrowing, absolute EF improvements of 5%, and improvements in composite clinical scores at 6 months . The initial WiSE-CRT study was stopped for safety reasons: 3 patients (18%) developed pericardial effusions associated with seed delivery . Following delivery system redesign, early data from 14 patients demonstrated no implant-related adverse events . Leadless endocardial LV pacing holds promise in that it may be more physiological, afford greater opportunities for LV pacing site selection, lead to a greater CRT response with lower risk of proarrhythmia, eliminate phrenic nerve stimulation, and mitigate against the risks of mitralregurgitation and lead-related thrombus. However, the technology is early in its development, and there are many unknowns. Challenges may include identification of acoustic windows in a subset of patients, energy inefficiency and early battery depletion, theoretical hazards of chronic sonification of cardiac tissues, and uncertain susceptibility to environmental interference. Other mechanisms for 2-stage leadless pacing are under early exploration. Pre-clinical experiments have been performed using magnetic induction rather than ultrasound to drive an endocardial seed . Other multicomponent leadless systems including the integration of a subcutaneous ICD with a leadless pacemaker are under development, allowing for antibradycardia pacing and antitachycardia pacing in conjunction with a subcutaneous ICD

Batteryless pacing

Battery depletion and pulse generator exchanges represent sources of complications for transvenous systems and uncertainty in leadless systems. Cardiac and pulmonary motion provide an inexhaustible source of energy during the life of a patient. Piezoelectric nanowires have been deployed on flexible devices to generate voltages as large as 1 to 2 V and currents up to 100 nA, sufficient to power the microelectronics of a pacemaker . Motion harvesting pacemakers remain in the realm of research, although devices have been built and tested in animal models.

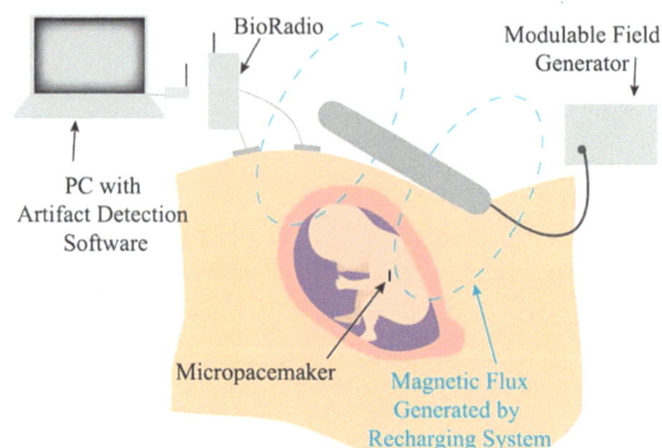

Fig 12.15 Fetal Pacemaker Ready for Human Trial The first-of-its-kind fetal pacemaker boasts a wireless recharging system

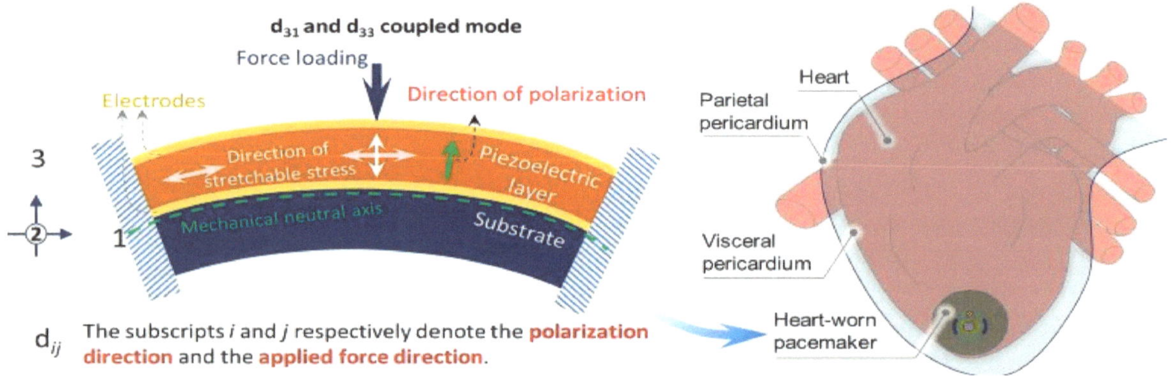

Fig 12.14 Batteryless pacing System. Cardiac and pulmonary motion provide an inexhaustible source of energy during the life of a patient. Piezoelectric nanowires have been deployed on flexible devices to generate voltages as large as 1 to 2 V and currents up to 100 nA, sufficient to power the microelectronics

Biological pacemaker

Biological pacemakers modify nonpacemaker myocytes to provide automaticity using gene therapy technologies, or add pacemaker syncytia to the heart through adult or embryonic stem cell therapies . Biological pacemakers are in the early stages of development, and current challenges include difficulty ensuring long-term engraftment and potential for proarrhythmia.

Percutaneously Implantable Fetal Pacemaker

A miniaturized, self-contained pacemaker that could be implanted with a minimally invasive technique would dramatically improve the survival rate for fetuses that develop hydrops fetalis as a result of congenital heart block.

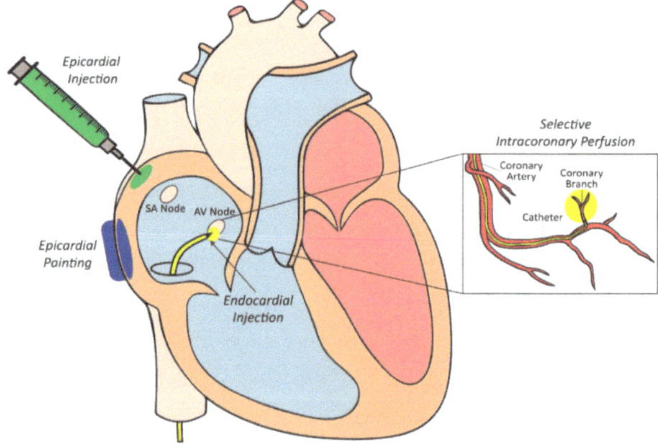

Fig.12.16 Biological pacemakers. Vector delivery approaches targeting the different sites of the myocardium.

Scientists develop wireless pacemaker that dissolves in body

A wireless pacemaker that can dissolve in the body has been created for patients who need only temporary help to regulate their heartbeat.Since the first pacemaker was implanted in 1958, millions of people have benefited from the devices. According to the national audit for cardiac rhythm management, 32,902 pacemakers were implanted for the first time in the UK in the year 2018-19 alone. But while some people require permanent pacemakers, others need them for days or weeks – for example after open-heart surgery. "After a critical risk period, the pacing functionality is no longer needed," said Prof John A Rogers of Northwestern University in Illinois, US, a co-author of the study revealing the new model. While pacemakers can already be used for temporary periods, experts say there are problems, including that leads placed through the skin can pose an infection risk. The external power supply and control system can become accidentally dislodged, and heart tissue can be damaged when the device is removed.Now researchers say they have developed a battery-free pacemaker that can be implanted directly on to the surface of the heart and absorbed by the body when no longer needed. The device – which Rogers said would cost about $100 (£70) – is free of leads and can be controlled and programmed from outside the body.

"With further modifications, it eventually may be possible to implant such bioresorbable pacemakers through a vein in the leg or arm," he added. "In this instance, it also may be possible to provide temporary pacing to patients who have suffered a heart attack or to patients undergoing catheter-based procedures, such as trans-catheter aortic valve replacement."

Modern AI-Enabled Pacemakers

A cardiac pacemaker is a medical equipment that generates impulses within the heart in case of an abnormal heart rhythm and coordinates the electrical signaling between the heart's chambers. Since the development of the first cardiac pacemaker in 1958, this therapeutic device has undergone several modifications. Every year, thousands of surgeries are performed in cardiac patients for pacemaker placement or revision. Although a pacemaker is commonly indicated in patients over 60 years old, it is placed in infants and children if indicated.

There are two types of pacemakers- permanent and temporary. While temporary pacemakers are used in situations where arrhythmias are anticipated to be temporary, permanent pacemakers are often recommended for patients with bradyarrhythmia or tachyarrhythmia. Advancements in implantable pacemakers have resulted in several modifications, such as reducing the size of the device, remote

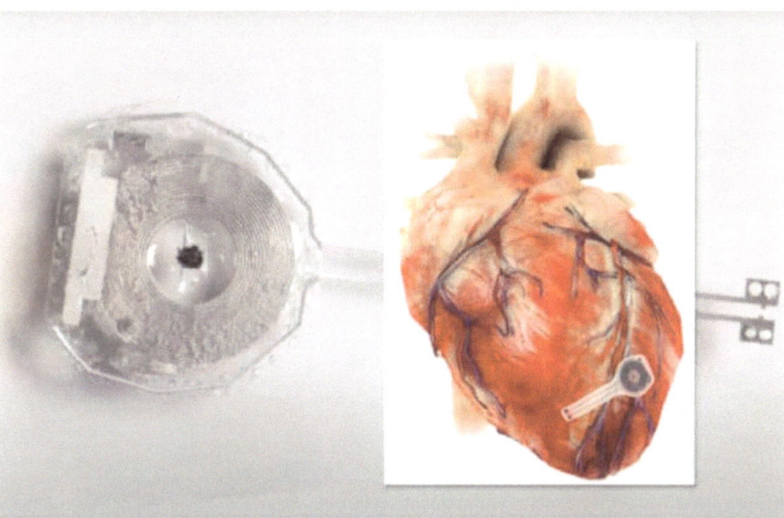

Fig.12.17 Researchers have developed the first-ever transient pacemaker — a wireless, battery-free, fully implantable pacing device that disappears after it is no longer needed.

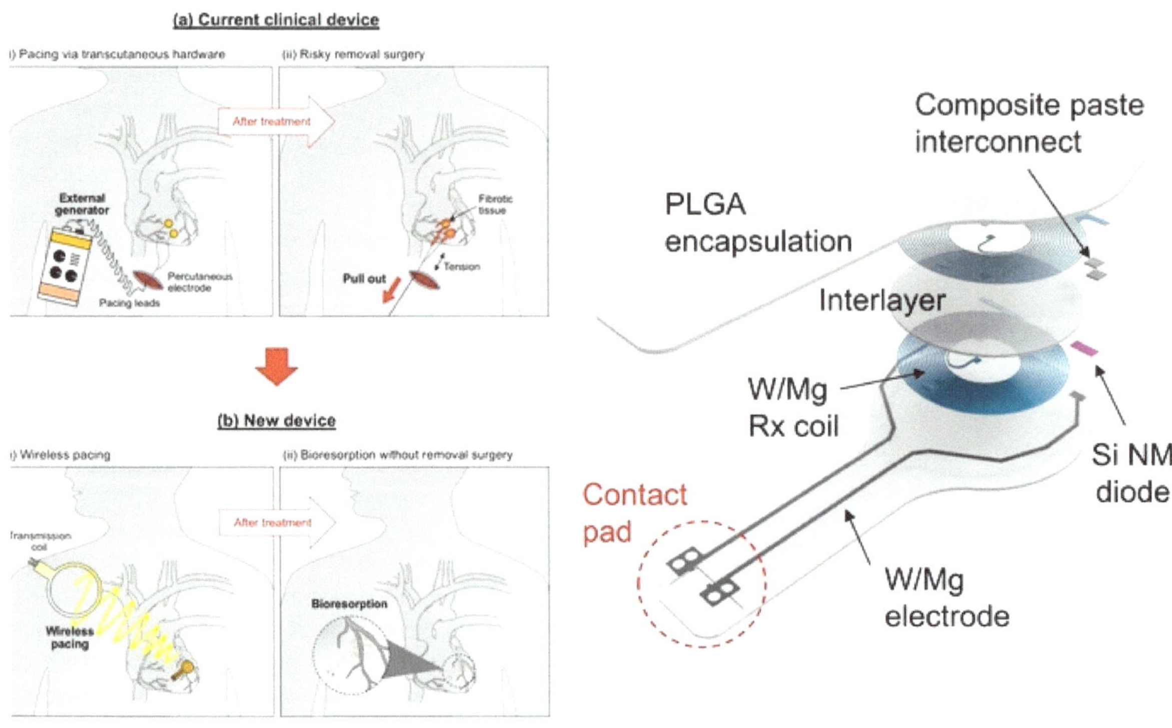

Fig. 12.18 A World's First: Biodegradable Wireless Transient Pacemaker images/Current-vs-New-Transient-Pacemaker

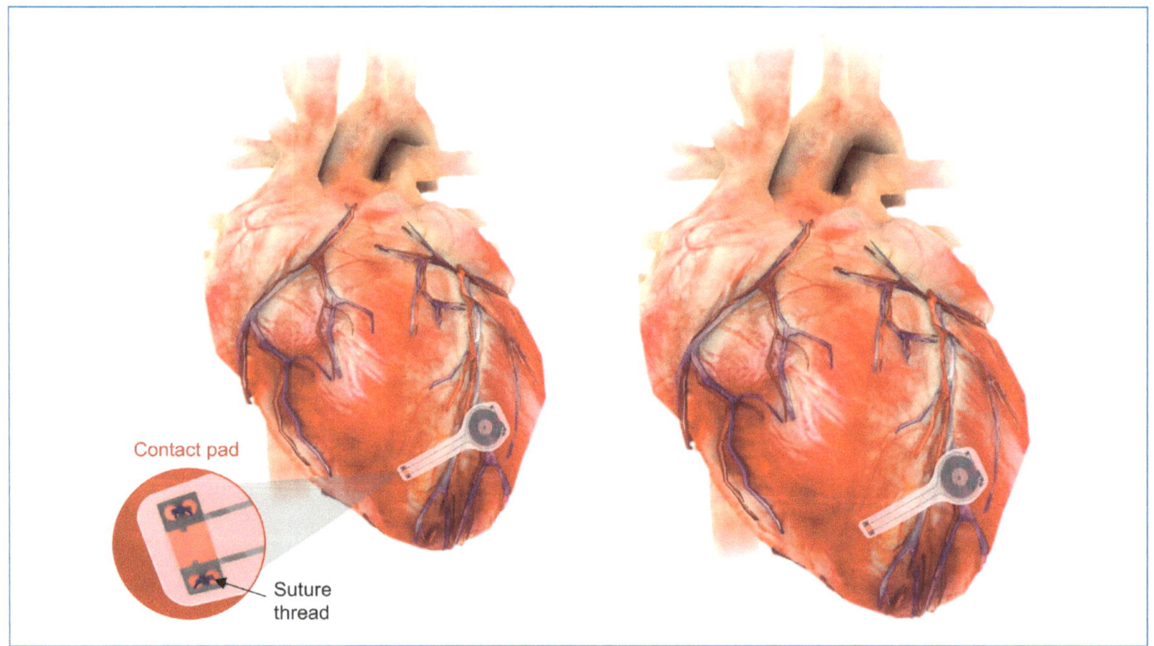

Fig. 12.19 First-ever transient pacemaker harmlessly dissolves in the body

monitoring using the internet, and a considerable increase in battery longevity.

France based Implicity is a startup that can monitor implanted cardiac-connected devices remotely with artificial intelligence. Their product connects with pacemakers and implanted defibrillators to facilitate heartbeat at a regular pace and also treat in cases of emergency such as heart attack. All devices being connected also enables to transmit the data back to the server and the physician. The technology at Implicity examines the patients' data from the implanted pacemaker and from the patient's medical record to identify high-risk patients that would require modifications in medication or change in the treatment plan.

A research team at Bios leverages machine learning to identify patterns of neural biomarkers and then synchronize them based on other organ functions to develop an algorithm. Towards this, they record raw neural data through neural interfaces. They compare with the recordings of physiological signals such as heart rate, blood pressure, glucose levels, body temperature, and physical activity levels.Usually, patients with pacemakers have certain contraindications while undergoing medical and dental treatments. One such contraindication is undergoing MRI imaging. But the recent FDA-approved MRI pacemakers have revolutionized the way cardiac patients undergo imaging examinations without adverse effects, and Biotronik is one such example.

Shallow Blue is a startup that deals with pacemaker predictive analytics. Their system can predict the onset of cardiac arrest in a person with a pacemaker or ICD so that appropriate intervention can be administered in advance.

Furthermore, scientists at Rice University and the Texas Heart Institute (THI) are working on machine learning algorithms that could improve the current pacemaker algorithm's overall sensitivity. It aims to identify an algorithm that can distribute the pacemaker's effect across several areas in the heart in a synchronized and accurate manner with the help of machine learning algorithms and validate the machine learning algorithm to classifydifferent pathophysiology. Another application of implantable pacemaker is the detection of an electrical storm (ES) that is a dangerous arhythmic condition with increased mortality and morbidity. There is ongoing research to construct and validate machine learning models to predict ES based on an intracardiac device's remote monitoring possibility (ICD).

A recent study by Professor Saeed Shakibfar from the University of Copenhagen showed that in patients with ICD, the occurrence of ES could be predicted one day in advance based on the data stored in ICD summaries with good diagnostic accuracies.

Professor Truong and the team at the Linder Research Centre, Ohio, investigated the feasibility of predicting pacemaker risk following transcatheter aortic valve replacement using ECG data and comparing the traditional logistic regression with machine learning approaches. It was found that machine learning methodology is significantly more robust than conventional logistic regression in predicting permanent pacemaker implantation risk following transcatheter aortic valve replacement with good diagnostic accuracy.

Bioelectronic devices are revolutionizing the pacemaker industry primarily by replicating neural signals. These control the activity of abnormal neural circuits that possibly cause the disease. But there is a need for a better understanding of neural biomarkers to receive signals and deliver appropriate treatment autonomously.

There is a need to develop a more efficient implantable device for improved interpretation of neural data. But it may not be as easy as it sounds because the human heart does not function alone in conjunction with other organs. Impulses from different organs and activities heavily affect the functioning of the heart.

What's more, machine learning can also utilize medical data to support patients' personalized clinical decisions after running validated models.

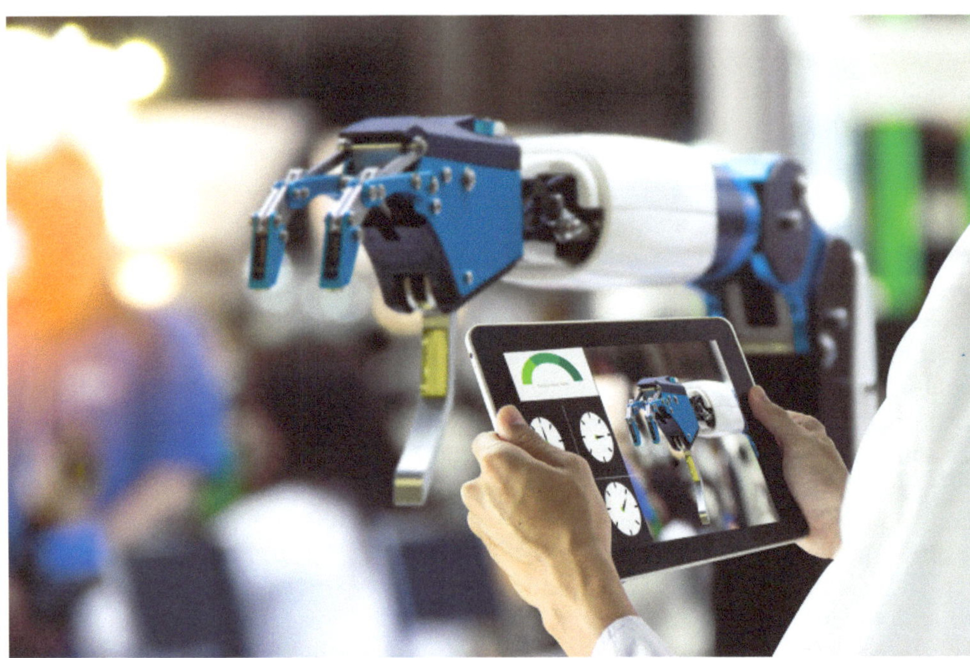

Fig.12.20 Artificial intelligence (AI) is sweeping the industrial manufacturing sector, its adoption and integration across manufacturing facilities spreading incredibly quickly. AI is revolutionizing a host of different processes, including generative design in product development, production forecasting in inventory management, and production processes like machine vision, defect inspection, production optimization, and predictive maintenance.

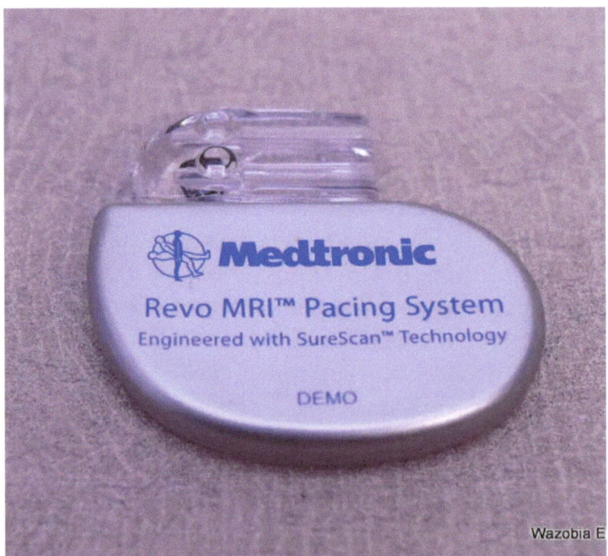

Fig. 12.21 The Food and Drug Administration just approved the first pacemaker in the U.S. that's good to go inside an MRI machine. Medtronic makes the gizmo, called the Revo MRI SureScan Pacing System. In a clinical test that included nearly 500 patients, none of had any MRI-related complications. Though it must be said there were four mild MRI-related reactions including some tingly numbness and palpitations.

Bibliography And Acknowledgement

- Ansalone G., Giannantoni P., Ricci R., et al. "Doppler myocardial imaging to evaluate the effectiveness of pacing sites in patients receiving biventricular pacing". J Am Coll Cardiol 2002;39:489-499.
- Auricchio A., Delnoy P.P., Regoli F., et al.for the Collaborative Study Group. "First-in-man implantation of leadless ultrasound-based cardiac stimulation pacing system: novel endocardial left ventricular resynchronization therapy in heart failure patients". Europace 2013;15:1191-1197.
- Austin, J. L., Preis, L. K., Crampton, R. S., Beller, G. A. & Martin, R. P. Analysis of pacemaker malfunction and complications of temporary pacing in the coronary care unit. Am. J. Cardiol. 49, 301–306 (1982).
- Behar J.M., Bostock J., Ginks M., et al. "Limitations of chronic delivery of multi-vein left ventricular stimulation for cardiac resynchronization therapy". J Interv Card Electrophysiol 2015;42:135-142
- Bernstein, V., Rotem, C. E. & Peretz, D. I. Permanent pacemakers: 8-year follow-up study. Incidence and management of congestive cardiac failure and perforations. Ann. Intern. Med. 74, 361–369 (1971).
- Beshai J.F., Grimm R.A., Nagueh S.F., et al.for the RethinQ Study Investigators. "Cardiac-resynchronization therapy in heart failure with narrow QRS complexes". N Engl J Med 2007;357:2461-2471.
- Betts T.R., Gamble J.H., Khiani R., et al. "Development of a technique for left ventricular endocardial pacing via puncture of the interventricular septum". Circ Arrhythm Electrophysiol 2014;7:17-22
- Biton Y., Zareba W., Goldenberg I., et al.for the MADIT-CRT Executive Committee. "Sex differences in long-term outcomes with cardiac resynchronization therapy in mild heart failure patients with left bundle branch block". J Am Heart Assoc 2015;4:e002013.
- Böhm M., Drexler H., Oswald H., et al. "Fluid status telemedicine alerts for heart failure: a randomized controlled trial". Eur Heart J 2016;37:3154-3163.
- Bristow M.R., Saxon L.A., Boehmer J., et al. "Cardiac-resynchronization therapy with or without an implantable defibrillator in advanced chronic heart failure". N Engl J Med 2004;350:2140-2150.
- C. Xiao, D. Cheng, and K. Wei, "An LCC-C compensated wireless charging system for implantable cardiac pacemakers: theory, experiment, and safety evaluation," IEEE Transactions on Power Electronics, vol. 33, no. 6, pp. 4894–4905, 2018.
- Cheng A., Landman S.R., Stadler R.W. "Reasons for loss of cardiac resynchronization therapy pacing: insights from 32 844 patients". Circ Arrhythm Electrophysiol 2012;5:884-888.
- Choo, M. H. et al. Permanent pacemaker infections: characterization and management. Am. J. Cardiol. 48, 559–564 (1981).
- Crossley G.H., Chen J., Choucair W., et al.for the PREFER Study Investigators. "Clinical benefits of remote versus transtelephonic monitoring of implanted pacemakers". J Am Coll Cardiol 2009;54:2012-2019
- Crossley G.H., Poole J.E., Rozner M.A., et al. "The Heart Rhythm Society (HRS)/American Society of Anesthesiologists (ASA) expert consensus statement on the perioperative management of patients with implantable defibrillators, pacemakers and arrhythmia monitors: facilities and patient management". Heart Rhythm 2011;8:1114-1154.
- Curtis A.B. "Biventricular pacing for atrioventricular block and systolic dysfunction". N Engl J Med 2013;369:579.
  Curtis, J. J. et al. A critical look at temporary ventricular pacing following cardiac surgery. Surgery 82, 888–893 (1977).
- Dagdeviren C., Yang B.D., Su Y., et al. "Conformal piezoelectric energy harvesting and storage from motions of the heart, lung, and diaphragm". Proc Natl Acad Sci U S A 2014;111:1927-1932.
- Dandamudi G., Vijayaraman P. "How to perform permanent His bundle pacing in routine clinical practice". Heart Rhythm 2016;13:1362-1366
- Dendy K.F., Powell B.D., Cha Y.M., et al. "Anodal stimulation: an underrecognized cause of nonresponders to cardiac resynchronization therapy". Indian Pacing Electrophysiol J 2011;11:64-72.
- Epstein A.E., DiMarco J.P., Ellenbogen K.A., et al. "2012 ACCF/AHA/HRS focused update incorporated into the ACCF/AHA/HRS 2008 guidelines for device-based therapy of cardiac rhythm abnormalities: a report of the American College of Cardiology Foundation/American Heart Association Task Force on Practice Guidelines and the Heart Rhythm Society". J Am Coll Cardiol 2013;61:e6-e75
- Ganesan A.N., Brooks A.G., Roberts-Thomson K.C., et al. "Role of AV nodal ablation in cardiac resynchronization in patients with coexistent atrial fibrillation and heart failure: a systematic review". J Am Coll Cardiol 2012;59:719-726.
- Garrigue S., Jaïs P., Espil G., et al. "Comparison of chronic biventricular pacing between epicardial and endocardial left ventricular stimulation using Doppler tissue imaging in patients with heart failure". Am J Cardiol 2001;88:858-862.
- Gold M.R., Singh J.P., Ellenbogen K.A., et al. "Interventricular electrical delay is predictive of response to cardiac resynchronization therapy". J Am Coll Cardiol EP 2016;2:438-447.
- Gorcsan J., Abraham T., Agler D.A., et al. "Echocardiography for cardiac resynchronization therapy: recommendations for performance and reporting—a report from the American Society of Echocardiography Dyssynchrony Writing Group endorsed by the Heart Rhythm Society". J Am Soc Echocardiogr 2008;21:191-213.
- Hara H., Oyenuga O.A., Tanaka H., et al. "The relationship of QRS morphology and mechanical dyssynchrony to long-term outcome following cardiac resynchronization therapy". Eur Heart J 2012;33:2680-2691.
- Hartstein, A. I., Jackson, J. & Gilbert, D. N. Prophylactic antibiotics and the insertion of permanent transvenous cardiac pacemakers. J. Thorac. Cardiovasc. Surg. 75, 219–223 (1978).
- Hauser R.G., Hayes D.L., Kallinen L.M., et al. "Clinical experience with pacemaker pulse generators and transvenous leads: an 8-year prospective multicenter study". Heart Rhythm 2007;4:154-160.
- Hayes D.L., Boehmer J.P., Day J.D., et al. "Cardiac resynchronization therapy and the relationship of percent biventricular pacing to symptoms and survival". Heart Rhythm 2011;8:1469-1475
- Healey J.S., Connolly S.J., Gold M.R., et al.for the ASSERT Investigators. "Subclinical atrial fibrillation and the risk of stroke". N Engl J Med 2012;366:120-129

- Heist E.K., Fan D., Mela T., et al. "Radiographic left ventricular-right ventricular interlead distance predicts the acute hemodynamic response to cardiac resynchronization therapy". Am J Cardiol 2005;96:685-690.
  Imparato, A. M. & Kim, G. E. Electrode complications in patients with permanent cardiac pacemakers. Arch. Surg. 105, 705–710 (1972).
- J. Yoo, L. Yan, S. Lee, Y. Kim, and H.-J. Yoo, "A 5.2 mW self-configured wearable body sensor network controller and a 12 $ \mu$W wirelessly powered sensor for a continuous health monitoring system," IEEE Journal of Solid-State Circuits, vol. 45, no. 1, pp. 178–188, 2010.
- Khan F.Z., Virdee M.S., Palmer C.R., et al. "Targeted left ventricular lead placement to guide cardiac resynchronization therapy: the TARGET study: a randomized, controlled trial". J Am Coll Cardiol 2012;59:1509-1518.
- Kutyifa V., Zareba W., McNitt S., et al. "Left ventricular lead location and the risk of ventricular arrhythmias in the MADIT-CRT trial". Eur Heart J 2013;34:184-190.
- Lakkireddy D., Di Biase L., Ryschon K., et al. "Radiofrequency ablation of premature ventricular ectopy improves the efficacy of cardiac resynchronization therapy in nonresponders". J Am Coll Cardiol 2012;60:1531-1539
- Leclercq C., Gadler F., Kranig W., et al.for the TRIP-HF (Triple Resynchronization In Paced Heart Failure Patients) Study Group. "A randomized comparison of triple-site versus dual-site ventricular stimulation in patients with congestive heart failure". J Am Coll Cardiol 2008;51:1455-1462
- Leyva F., Foley P.W., Chalil S., et al. "Cardiac resynchronization therapy guided by late gadolinium-enhancement cardiovascular magnetic resonance". J Cardiovasc Magn Reson 2011;13:29.
- Linde C., Leclercq C., Rex S., et al. "Long-term benefits of biventricular pacing in congestive heart failure: results from the MUltisite STimulation in cardiomyopathy (MUSTIC) study". J Am Coll Cardiol 2002;40:111-118.
- Link M.S. "Achilles' lead: will pacemakers break free?"N Engl J Med 2016;374:585-586.
- Lumia, F. J. & Rios, J. C. Temporary transvenous pacemaker therapy: an analysis of complications. Chest 64, 604–608 (1973).
- Mabo P., Victor F., Bazin P., et al. "A randomized trial of long-term remote monitoring of pacemaker recipients (the COMPAS trial)". Eur Heart J 2012;33:1105-1111
- Marban E., Cho H.C. "Biological pacemakers as a therapy for cardiac arrhythmias". Curr Opin Cardiol 2008;23:46-54.
- Marek J.J., Saba S., Onishi T., et al. "Usefulness of echocardiographically guided left ventricular lead placement for cardiac resynchronization therapy in patients with intermediate QRS width and non-left bundle branch block morphology". Am J Cardiol 2014;113:107-116.
- McLeod C.J., Boersma L., Okamura H., Friedman P.A. "The subcutaneous implantable cardioverter defibrillator: state-of-the-art review". Eur Heart J 2015Oct29. [E-pub ahead of print].
- Miller M.A., Neuzil P., Dukkipati S.R., et al. "Leadless cardiac pacemakers: back to the future". J Am Coll Cardiol 2015;66:1179-1189.
- Mullens W., Grimm R.A., Verga T., et al. "Insights from a cardiac resynchronization optimization clinic as part of a heart failure disease management program". J Am Coll Cardiol 2009;53:765-773.
- Neuzil P., Reddy V.Y., Sedivy P., et al. "AB 17-01: wireless LV endocardial stimulation for cardiac resynchronization: long-term (12 month) experience of clinical efficacy and clinical events from two centers (abstr)". Heart Rhythm 2016;13:S38.
- Pappone C., Ćalović Z., Vicedomini G., et al. "Multipoint left ventricular pacing improves acute hemodynamic response assessed with pressure-volume loops in cardiac resynchronization therapy patients". Heart Rhythm 2014;11:394-401
- Parthiban N., Esterman A., Mahajan R., et al. "Remote monitoring of implantable cardioverter-defibrillators: a systematic review and meta-analysis of clinical outcomes". J Am Coll Cardiol 2015;65:2591-2600
- Pluijmert M., Lumens J., Potse M., et al. "Computer modelling for better diagnosis and therapy of patients by cardiac resynchronisation therapy". Arrhythm Electrophysiol Rev 2015;4:62-67.
- R. Fensli, J. G. Dale, P. O'Reilly, J. O'Donoghue, D. Sammon, and T. Gundersen, "Towards improved healthcare performance: examining technological possibilities and patient satisfaction with wireless body area networks," Journal of Medical Systems, vol. 34, no. 4, 2010.
- Reddy V., Cantillon D.J., Ip J., et al. "A comparative study of acute and mid-term complications of leadless vs transvenous pacemakers [LBCT02-04]". Paper presented at: 37th Annual Meeting of the Heart Rhythm Society; May6, 2016; San Francisco, CA.
- Reddy V.Y., Exner D.V., Cantillon D.J., et al.for the LEADLESS II Study Investigators. "Percutaneous implantation of an entirely intracardiac leadless pacemaker". N Engl J Med 2015;373:1125-1135.
- Reddy V.Y., Neuzil P., Riahi S., et al. "Presentation of leadless LV endocardial stimulation for CRT: final outcomes of the Safety and Performance of Electrodes Implanted in the Left Ventricle (SELECT-LV) study". Paper presented at: Heart Rhythm Society 37th Annual Scientific Sessions; May4–7, 2016; San Francisco, CA.
- Reynolds D., Duray G.Z., Omar R., et al.for the Micra Transcatheter Pacing Study Group. "A leadless intracardiac transcatheter pacing system". N Engl J Med 2016;374:533-541.
- Robinson R.B. "Engineering a biological pacemaker: in vivo, in vitro and in silico models". Drug Discov Today Dis Models 2009;6:93-98.
- Ruschitzka F., Abraham W.T., Singh J.P., et al.for the EchoCRT Study Group. "Cardiac-resynchronization therapy in heart failure with a narrow QRS complex". N Engl J Med 2013;369:1395-1405.
- Saxon L.A., Hayes D.L., Gilliam F.R., et al. "Long-term outcome after ICD and CRT implantation and influence of remote device follow-up: the ALTITUDE survival study". Circulation 2010;122:2359-2367.
- Saxon L.A., Olshansky B., Volosin K., et al. "Influence of left ventricular lead location on outcomes in the COMPANION study". J Cardiovasc Electrophysiol 2009;20:764-768.
- Sharma A.D., Rizo-Patron C., Hallstrom A.P., et al.for the DAVID Investigators. "Percent right ventricular pacing predicts outcomes in the DAVID trial". Heart Rhythm 2005;2:830-834.

- Sharma P.S., Dandamudi G., Naperkowski A., et al. "Permanent His-bundle pacing is feasible, safe, and superior to right ventricular pacing in routine clinical practice". Heart Rhythm 2015;12:305-312.
- Singh J.P., Fan D., Heist E.K., et al. "Left ventricular lead electrical delay predicts response to cardiac resynchronization therapy". [Erratum in Heart Rhythm 2006;3:1515]Heart Rhythm 2006;3:1285-1292.
- Sipahi I., Carrigan T.P., Rowland D.Y., et al. "Impact of QRS duration on clinical event reduction with cardiac resynchronization therapy: meta-analysis of randomized controlled trials". Arch Intern Med 2011;171:1454-1462.
- Sipahi I., Chou J.C., Hyden M., et al. "Effect of QRS morphology on clinical event reduction with cardiac resynchronization therapy: meta-analysis of randomized controlled trials". Am Heart J 2012;163:260-267.e3.
- Slotwiner D., Varma N., Akar J.G., et al. "HRS expert consensus statement on remote interrogation and monitoring for cardiovascular implantable electronic devices". Heart Rhythm 2015;12:e69-e100.
- Sohal M., Shetty A., Niederer S., et al. "Mechanistic insights into the benefits of multisite pacing in cardiac resynchronization therapy: the importance of electrical substrate and rate of left ventricular activation". Heart Rhythm 2015;12:2449-2457
- Sweeney M.O., van Bommel R.J., Schalij M.J., et al. "Analysis of ventricular activation using surface electrocardiography to predict left ventricular reverse volumetric remodeling during cardiac resynchronization therapy". Circulation 2010;121:626-634.
- Tang A.S., Wells G.A., Talajic M., et al.for the Resynchronization–Defibrillation for Ambulatory Heart Failure Trial (RAFT) Investigators. "Cardiac-resynchronization therapy for mild-to-moderate heart failure". N Engl J Med 2010;363:2385-2395.
- Thibault B., Harel F., Ducharme A., et al.for the LESSER-EARTH Investigators. "Cardiac resynchronization therapy in patients with heart failure and a QRS complex <120 milliseconds: the Evaluation of Resynchronization Therapy for Heart Failure (LESSER-EARTH) trial". Circulation 2013;127:873-881
- Tompkins C., Kutyifa V., McNitt S., et al. "Effect on cardiac function of cardiac resynchronization therapy in patients with right bundle branch block (from the Multicenter Automatic Defibrillator Implantation Trial With Cardiac Resynchronization Therapy [MADIT-CRT] trial)". Am J Cardiol 2013;112:525-529.
- Turakhia M.P., Cao M., Fischer A., et al. "Reduced mortality associated with quadripolar compared to bipolar left ventricular leads in cardiac resynchronization therapy". J Am Coll Cardiol EP 2016;2:426-433
- van Gelder B.M., Houthuizen P., Bracke F.A. "Transseptal left ventricular endocardial pacing: preliminary experience from a femoral approach with subclavian pull-through". Europace 2011;13:1454-1458.
- Varma N., Piccini J.P., Snell J., et al. "The relationship between level of adherence to automatic wireless remote monitoring and survival in pacemaker and defibrillator patients". J Am Coll Cardiol 2015;65:2601-2610.
- Vijayaraman P., Naperkowski A., Ellenbogen K.A., et al. "Electrophysiologic insights into site of atrioventricular block: lessons from permanent His bundle pacing". J Am Coll Cardiol EP 2015;1:571-581
- Waldo, A. L., Wells, J. L. J., Cooper, T. B. & MacLean, W. A. Temporary cardiac pacing: applications and techniques in the treatment of cardiac arrhythmias. Prog. Cardiovasc. Dis. 23, 451–474 (1981).
- Wieneke H., Rickers S., Velleuer J., et al. "Leadless pacing using induction technology: impact of pulse shape and geometric factors on pacing efficiency". Europace 2013;15:453-459.
- Wilhelm, M. J. et al. Cardiac pacemaker infection: surgical management with and without extracorporeal circulation. Ann. Thorac. Surg. 64, 1707–1712 (1997).
- Wilton S.B., Leung A.A., Ghali W.A., et al. "Outcomes of cardiac resynchronization therapy in patients with versus those without atrial fibrillation: a systematic review and meta-analysis". Heart Rhythm 2011;8:1088-1094.
- Yu C.M., Wang L., Chau E., et al. "Intrathoracic impedance monitoring in patients with heart failure: correlation with fluid status and feasibility of early warning preceding hospitalization". Circulation 2005;112:841-848.
- Z. J. Zhu, X. M. Wu, and Z. X. Fang, “The development of programming and telemetery system for cardiac pacemaker,” Progress in Biomedical Engineering, vol. 32, 2011
- Zhang Q., Zhou Y., Yu C.M. "Incidence, definition, diagnosis, and management of the cardiac resynchronization therapy nonresponder". Curr Opin Cardiol 2015;30:40-49.

Zoll, P. M. et al. External noninvasive temporary cardiac pacing: clinical trials. Circulation 71, 937–944 (1985).

CHAPTER

Robotic Assisted Cardiac Interventions

The Minimally Invasive Cardiac Surgery was invented by Francis Duhaylongsod, a Filipino heart surgeon in Hawaii. The first minimally invasive heart cardiac surgery was performed in the United States on January 21, 2005 at The Heart Institute at Staten Island University Hospital in Staten Island, New York by a team led by Dr. Joseph T. McGinn. This technique is an off-pump coronary artery bypass surgery. The procedure is much less invasive than traditional bypass surgery because it's performed through three small incisions rather than the traditional sternotomy. Since its first procedure, over 600 MICS CABG procedures have been performed at The Heart Institute amongst many more around the world.

Minimally invasive heart surgery (also called keyhole surgery) is performed through small incisions, sometimes using specialized surgical instruments. The incision used for minimally invasive heart surgery is about 3 to 4 inches instead of the 6- to 8-inch incision required for traditional surgery.

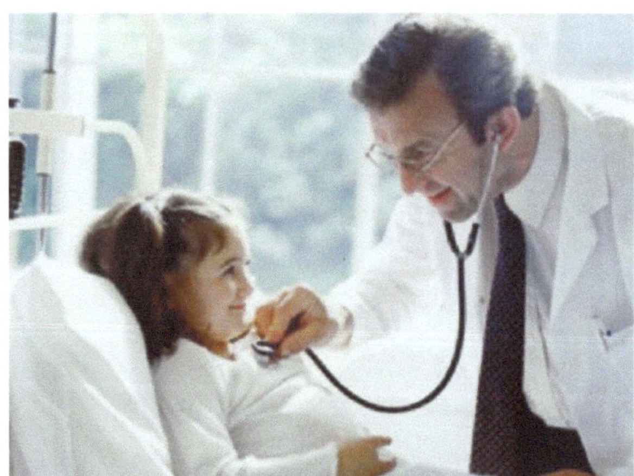

Fig. 13.1: *A young child is being examined by the cardiac surgeon for cardiovascular fitness prior to Robotic heart surgery*

Selection of Patients for Minimally Invasive or Robotic Surgery

Your surgeon will review the results of your diagnostic tests before your scheduled surgery to determine if you are a candidate for a minimally invasive or robotic surgery technique. The surgical team will carefully compare the advantages and disadvantages of these techniques with those of traditional surgery.

The type of treatment recommended for your condition depends on several factors, including the type and severity of heart disease, age, medical history and lifestyle.

The Procedure

MICS CABG is performed through one window incision that stretches 5–7 cm in the 4th intercostal space (ICS). In some cases the thoractomy may be necessary in the 5th ICS instead. A soft tissue refractor is used to allow for greater visibility and access.

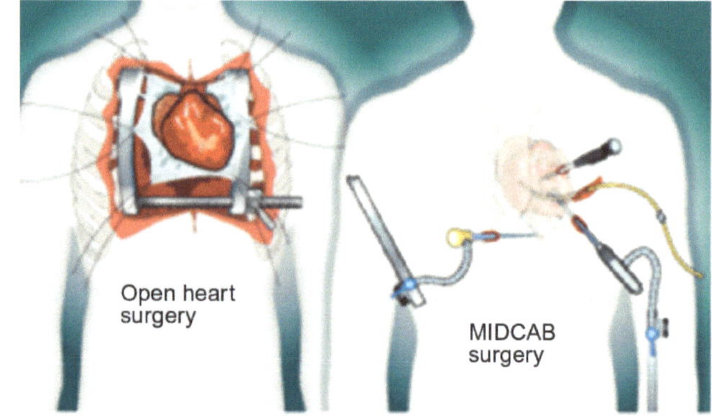

Fig. 13. 2: *Cardiac surgeons are operating on the heart through tiny openings in the chest, eliminating the need for sternotomy-- a large incision through the breastbone (sternum). This method of surgery, called minimally invasive cardiac surgery, is a remarkable improvement over traditional, open-chest procedures.*

Two access incisions are also made at the 6th intercostal space and xphoid process to allow for operative Medtronic® instruments to pass through.

The McGinn Technique (Proximal Anastomoses)

The McGinn Proximal Technique is performed with blood pressure lowered to 90–100 systolic which reduces stress to the aorta, reducing the risk of damage. A series of tools are used to position and stabilize vessels. The technique uses devices developed by Medtronic® to support the surrounding heart tissues while vital surgery takes place. The devices are managed externally and access the heart through small incisions between the ribs.

Pump-Assisted Beating Heart Bypass

A cannula with a pump and vacuum action is fed up through an artery in the groin to reduce the stress on the heart so that it may still function during the operation. This pump flows at 2–3L per minute to support circulation and eliminates the need for a heart-lung bypass machine.

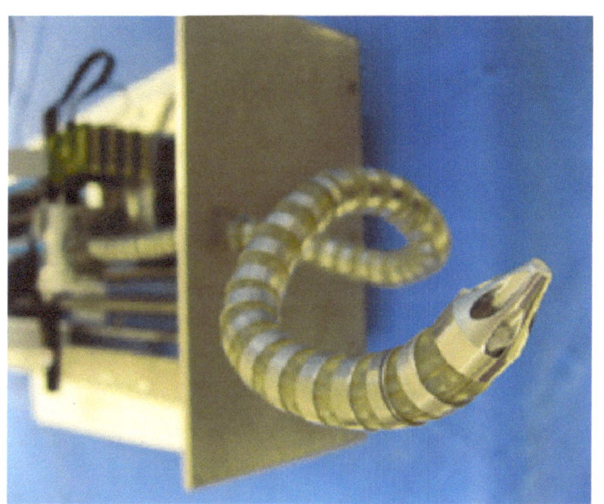

Fig. 13.3: Serpentine Robots in Heart Surgery. Robotic Probe (HARP) to enter the thorax through a subxiphoid port and reach regions of the pericardium that are inaccessible with traditional techniques. It is believed that HARP's functionality will eventually lead to application such as multiple intrapericardial therapies (e.g. cell transplantation by intramyocardial injection, epicardial ablation, epicardial lead placement for resynchronization, etc)."

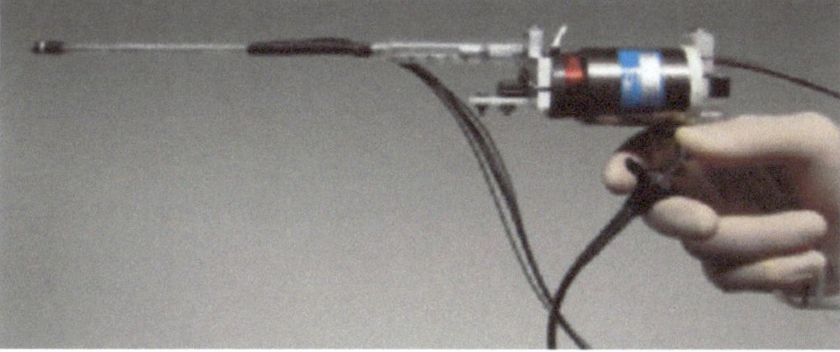

Fig.13.4: *Biorobotics and its role in minimal-invasion cardia surgery (Image courtesy of Harvard SEAS)*

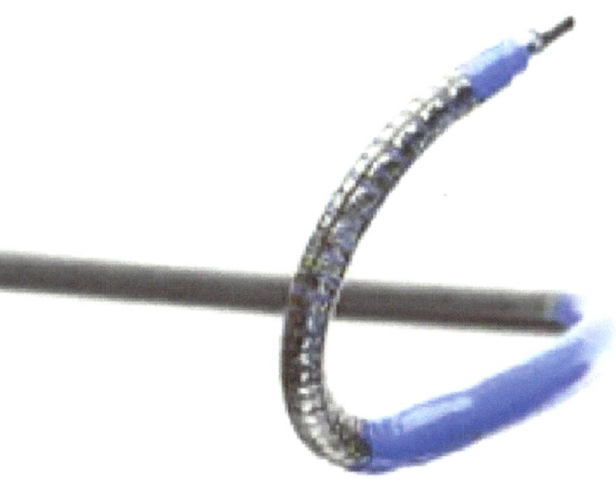

Fig. 13.5: *Hansen Medical's Robotic Catheter Control System for EP Study*

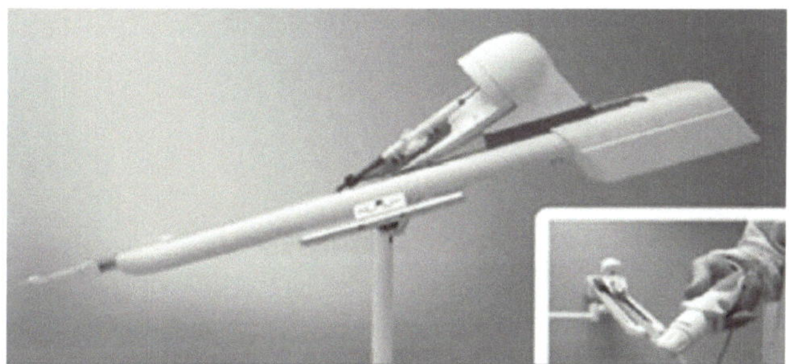

Fig. 13.6: *World's first remote heart rhythm treatment procedure using a Robotic Arm. The world's first remote robotic heart rhythm treatment procedure was conducted at the University Hospitals of Leicester. It was performed using the Catheter Robotics Remote Catheter Manipulation System. A patient with atrial fibrillation had a catheter ablation controlled by a robotic arm, while the cardiologist- sitting in a separate room - used remote control to steer the catheter endovascularly into the heart*

ROBOTICALLY ASSISTED HEART SURGERY

Robotically assisted heart surgery, also called closed-chest heart surgery, is a type of minimally invasive surgery. The cardiac surgeon uses a specially designed computer console to control surgical instruments on thin robotic arms. Robotically assisted technology allows surgeons to perform certain types of complex heart surgeries with smaller incisions and precise motion control, offering patients excellent outcomes. In robotic surgery, small incisions—less than 2 inches—are used, compared with the 3- to 4-inch incision used in traditional minimally invasive heart surgery.

Types of Robotically assisted Heart Surgeries

1. Robotic assisted CABG

2. Robotic assisted coronary angioplasty
3. Mitral valve repair and replacement surgery
4. Tricuspid valve repair and replacement surgery
5. Combined mitral and tricuspid valve surgery
6. Ablation of atrial fibrillation
7. Atrial septal defect (ASD) and PFO repair
8. Removal of cardiac tumors
9. Lead placement
10. Robot implant

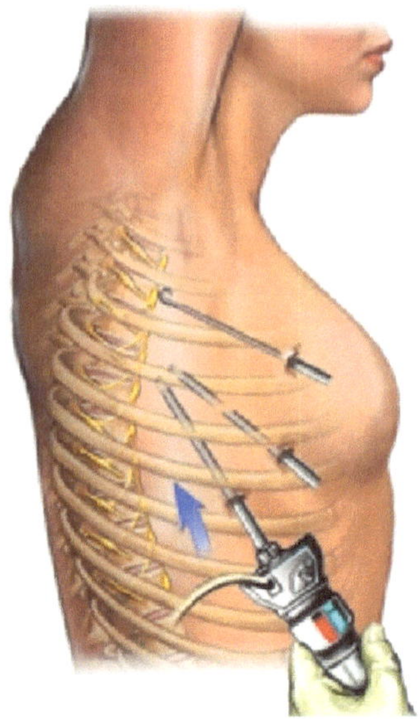

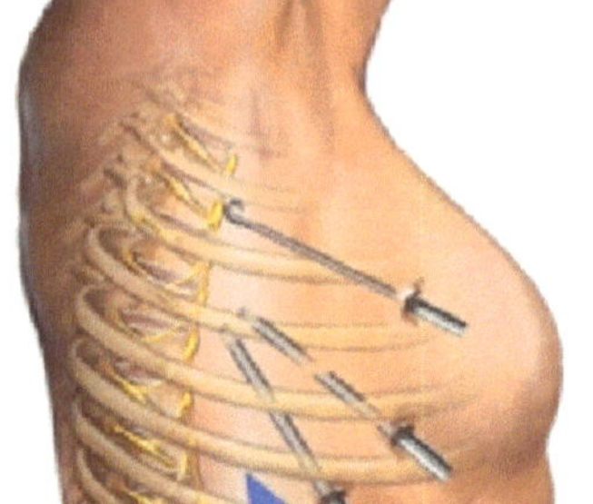

Fig. 13.7: Sites of incisions endoscopes practiced in a operation theatre in conducting Robotic valve heart surgery

Benefits of Minimally Invasive Surgical Techniques

The benefits of minimally invasive and robotic heart surgery techniques include:

1. Small incisions
2. Small scars
3. *Shorter hospital stay after surgery:* The average stay is 3 to 5 days after minimally invasive surgery, while the average stay after traditional heart surgery is 7 to 10 days
4. Low risk of infection
5. Low risk of bleeding and blood transfusion
6. Shorter recovery time and faster return to normal activities/work:

Fig.13.8 : *Robotic arms are performing coronary bypass with robot-assisted heart surgery, In this procedure a surgeon controls small surgical instruments attached to robotic arms*

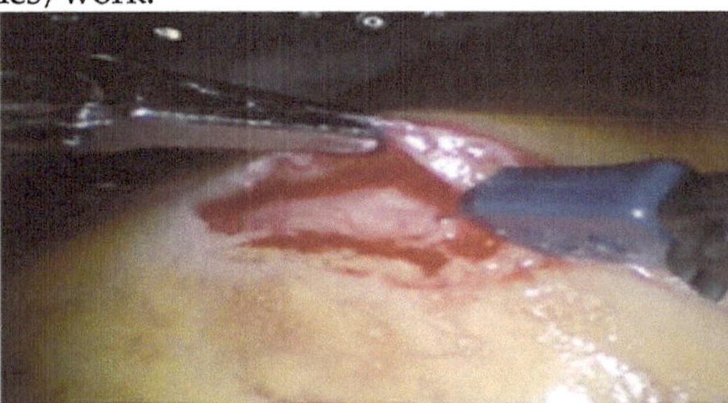

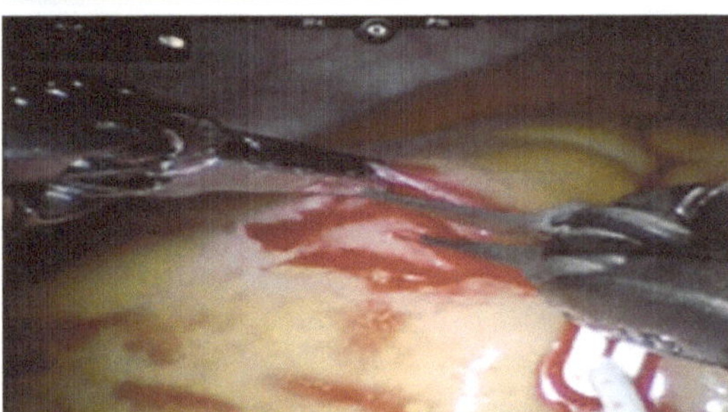

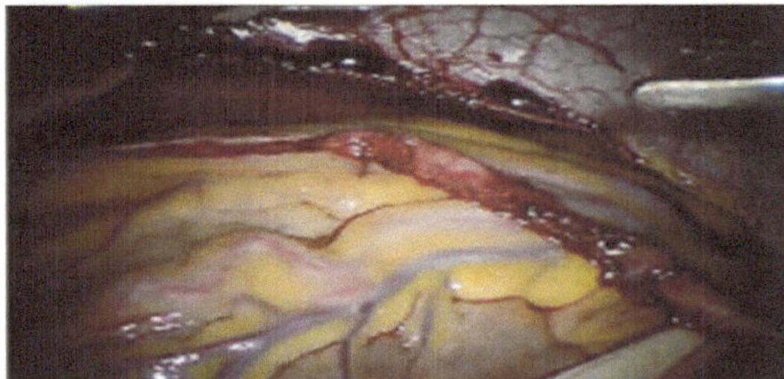

Fig.13.9: A. Opening of coronary with endoscopic knife. B. Coronary arteriotomy with endoscopic Pott scissors. C. Final result.in robotic coronary bypass surgery

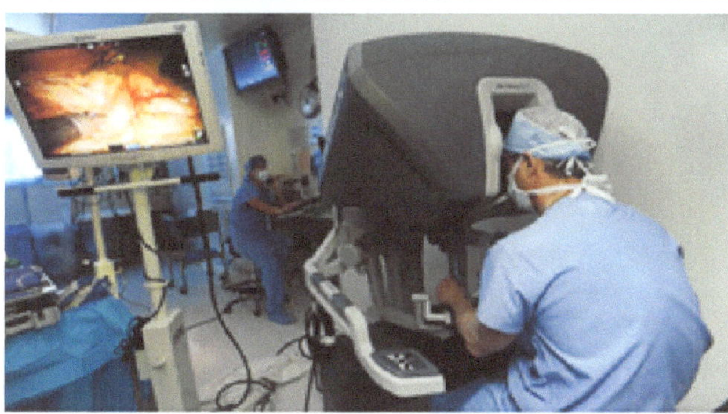

Fig. 13.10: *Surgeon is operating on patient with the help of the da Vinci's arms through the system's console (right)*

The average recovery time after minimally invasive surgery is 1 to 4 weeks, while the average recovery time after traditional heart surgery is 6 to 8 weeks. The recovery time and return to regular activities is shorter for patients who undergo robotically assisted heart surgery. Division of the breastbone is not needed for robotically assisted heart surgery. Important note: Not everyone is a candidate for these surgical techniques. Your surgeon will review the results of your diagnostic tests before your scheduled procedure to determine if you are a candidate for minimally invasive surgery. The surgical team will carefully compare the advantages and disadvantages of minimally invasive techniques versus traditional surgery techniques.

Types of Minimally Invasive Heart Surgeries

Minimally Invasive Valve Surgery

Valve surgeries, including valve repairs and valve replacements, are the most common type of minimally invasive surgery, accounting for 87 percent of all minimally invasive cardiac surgeries performed at Cleveland Clinic.

Minimally Invasive CABG Surgery

Minimally invasive direct coronary artery bypass graft (MIDCABG) surgery is an option for some patients who require a left internal mammary artery bypass graft to the left anterior descending artery.

Saphenous (leg) vein harvest also may be performed using small incisions.

Several techniques for minimally invasive CABG surgery are being explored at Cleveland Clinic, including surgeries performed on a beating (off-pump) or non-beating (on-pump) heart.

Off-pump/beating heart bypass surgery allows surgeons to perform surgery on the heart while it is still beating. A medication may be given to slow the heart during surgery, but the heart keeps beating during the procedure. This type of surgery may be an option for patients with single-vessel disease (such as disease of the left anterior descending artery or right coronary artery).

Traditionally, CABG surgery is performed using a heart-lung bypass machine. This machine allows the heart's beating to be stopped, so the surgeon can operate on a surface that is blood-free and still. The heart-lung bypass machine maintains life despite the lack of a heartbeat, removing carbon dioxide from the blood and replacing it with oxygen before pumping it around the body.

During off-pump/beating heart surgery, the heart-lung machine is not used. The surgeon uses advanced operating equipment to stabilize (hold) portions of the heart and bypass the blocked artery in a highly controlled operative environment. Meanwhile, the rest of the heart keeps pumping and circulating blood to the body.

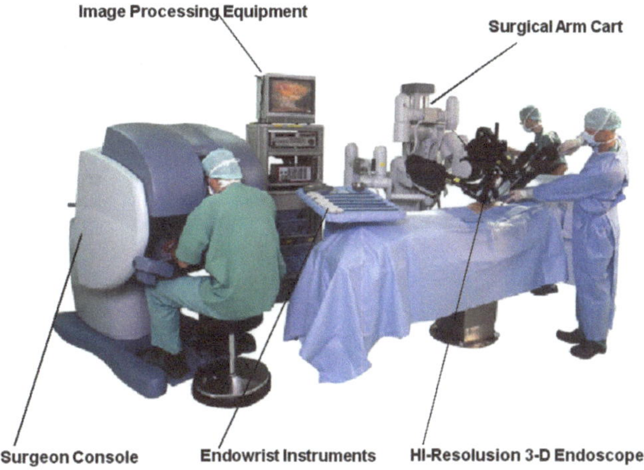

Fig. 13.11: *Different equipments in a operation theatre utilized in conducting Robotic heart surgery*

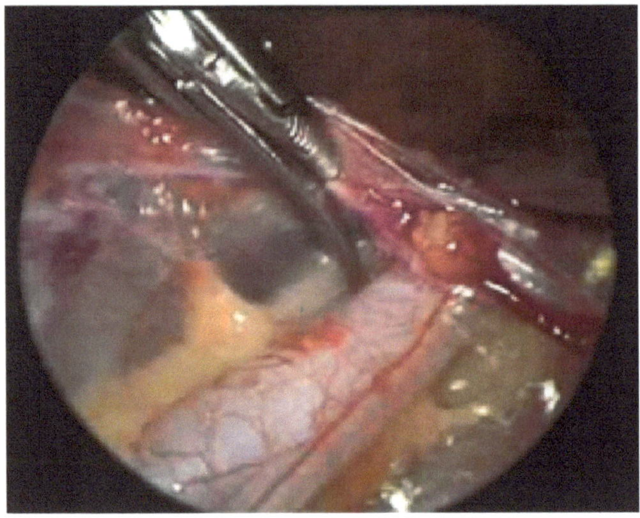

Fig.13.12: *Videoscopic photograph taken from one of the patients undergoing Robotic heart surgery*

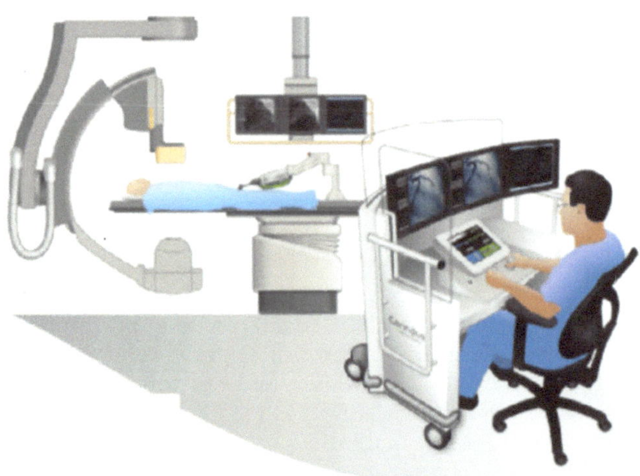

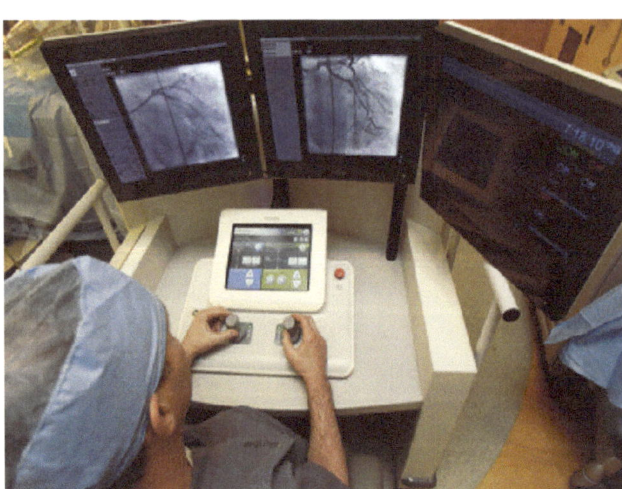

Fig.13.13: *The method of performing robot-assisted coronary angioplasty*

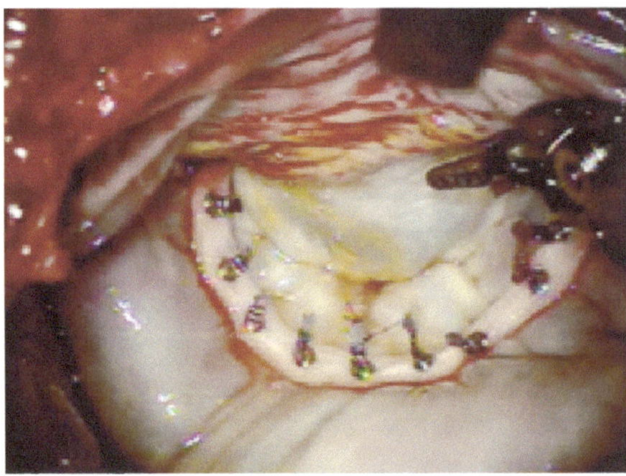

Fig.13.14: *Intraoperative view of a competent mitral valve repaired using robotic assistance*

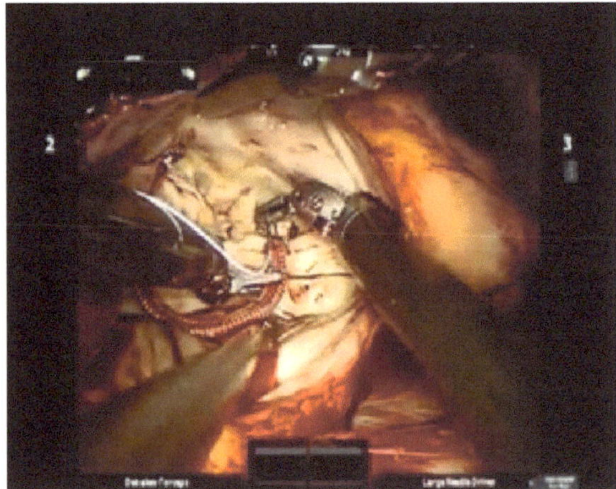

Fig.13.15: *Robotic assisted mitral and tricuspid valve repair*

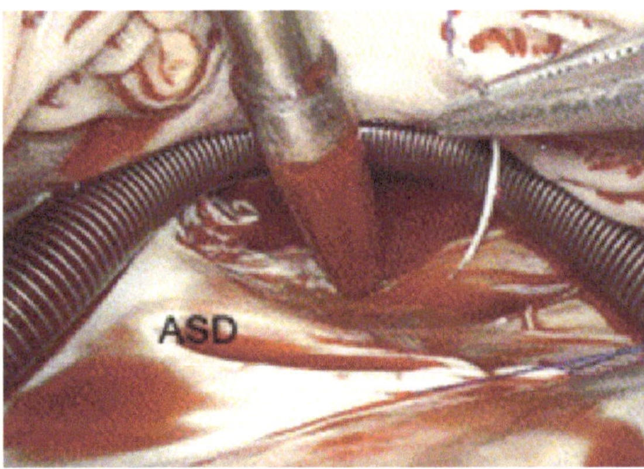

Fig.13.16: *An intraoperative view of atrial septal defect (ASD that was closed by sutures?*

Types of Robotically Assisted Heart Surgeries

Robotically Assisted CABG Surgery

Robotically assisted CABG surgery can be performed without opening the sternum (breastbone). Robotically

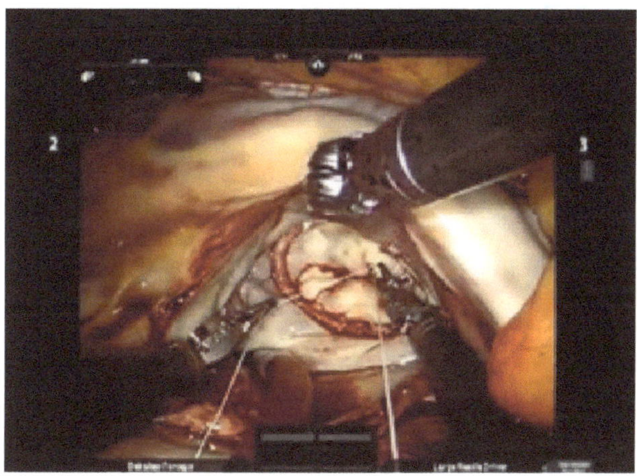

Fig. 13.17: *Robotic repair of mitral valve and PFO closure*

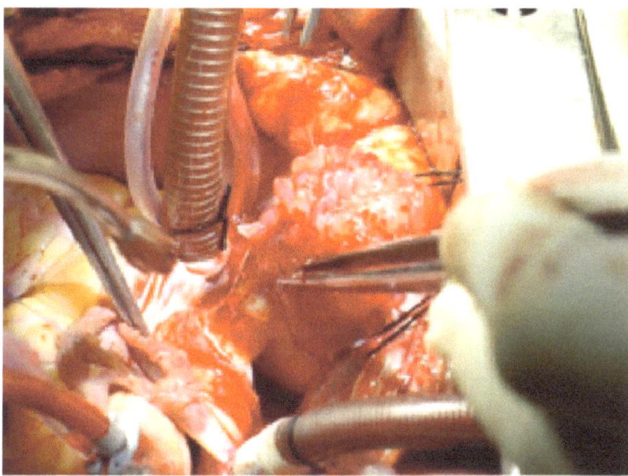

Fig. 13.18: *Intraoperative robotic surgery showing LA Myxoma on stalk*

assisted CABG surgery also can be performed "off pump," which means the surgery can be performed on a beating heart, without using the heart-lung bypass machine.

Robotically Assisted Valve Surgery

Robotically assisted mitral valve repair can be used to treat mitral valve regurgitation. Tricuspid valve surgery also can be performed using the robotically assisted surgical technique.

Robotically Assisted ASD and PFO Repair

Robotically assisted atrial septal defect (ASD) and patent foramen ovale (PFO) repair surgeries can be performed using a robotically assisted approach. Robotic instruments are used to harvest a small patch of pericardial tissue (the sac that surrounds the heart). The patch is then sutured (sewn) over the defect.

Robotically Assisted Removal of Cardiac Tumors

The most common benign tumor of the heart is a myxoma, which most frequently occurs in the left atrium. This type of tumor increases the risk of stroke. Removal of these tumors almost always cures the problem and greatly reduces the risk of stroke. During the robotically assisted tumor removal procedure, the surgeon's hands control the movement and placement of the endoscopic instruments through small incisions in the chest wall, and the instruments are used to remove the tumor.

Robotically assisted heart surgery is performed through a small working incision and three small incisions (ports) that are made in the spaces between the ribs . The surgical instruments (attached to the robotic arms) and one tiny camera are placed through these ports. Motion sensors are attached to the robotic "wrist," so the surgeon can control the movement and placement of the surgical instruments to perform the procedure

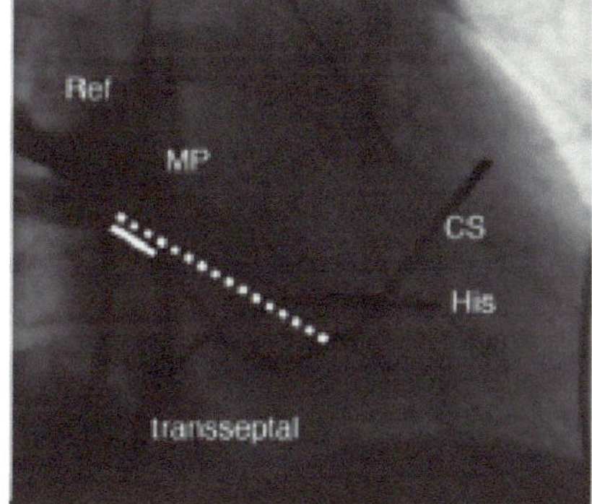

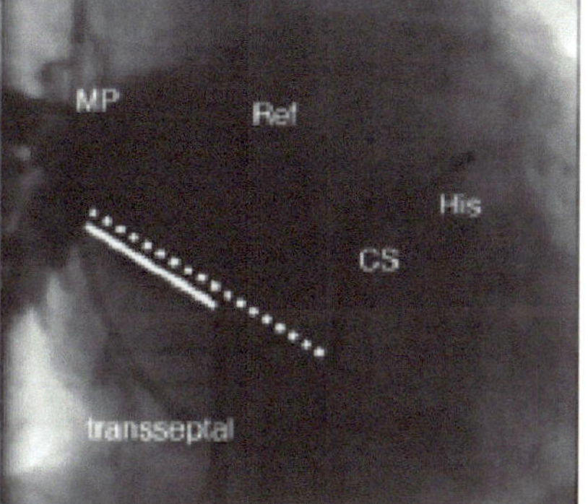

Fig.13.19 :*Remote Robotic Navigation and Electroanatomical Mapping for Ablation of Atrial FibrillationSelective angiographies of the RIPV (RAO 30°). The distance between the anterior border of the RPV ostium and the coronary sinus catheter (dCS, dotted line) and the transseptal puncture site (dTS, full line) were measured. The left panel shows a patient with a posterior transseptal puncture (ratio dCS:dTS, 0.12). The right panel shows a patient with an antero-medial transseptal puncture (ratio dCS:dTS, 0.68). CS indicates coronary sinus catheter; His, multipolar catheter at the His bundle; Ref, Reference catheter on the back of the patient; MP, multi-purpose catheter for angiography*

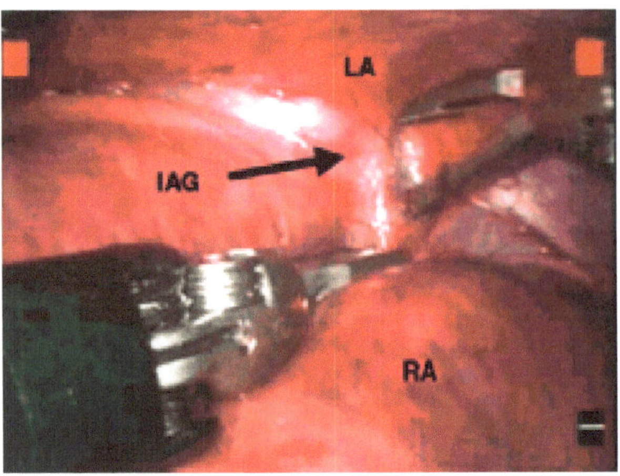

Fig. 13.20: *Atrial fibrillation. Robot-assisted ablation of the PVs Opening of the transverse and oblique sinus was performed robotically. Opening of the pericardial reflections between the superior right PV and the superior caval vein, and between the inferior right PV and the inferior caval vein, and development of the inter-atrial groove were also performed robotically.*

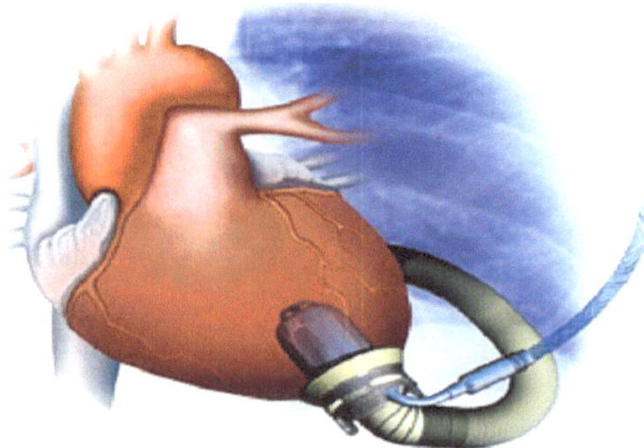

Fig. 13.21 *:This type of Robot implant is to be used on a permanent basis rather than a more common temporary artificial heart*

During robotically assisted surgery, the sternum (breastbone) does not need to be opened to perform the procedure. Depending on the technique, the surgeon may choose to perform surgery on a "beating heart," in which case the patient is not placed on the heart-lung bypass machine (this is called"off-pump" surgery).

In comparison, traditional valve and CABG surgery involve using the heart-lung bypass machine to circulate the patient's oxygenated blood during surgery and stopping the heart in order to stabilize the blood vessels; creating a 6- to 8-inch incision through the sternum; and spreading the ribs to view the heart.

Robotically Assisted Atrial Fibrillation Surgery

During the robotically assisted ablation procedure for atrial fibrillation (an irregular heart rhythm that begins in the upper chambers of the heart), the surgeon's hands control the movement and placement of the endoscopic instruments to open the pericardium (thin sac that surrounds the heart). The instruments are used to precisely place the catheter for ablation, in which energy is applied to correct the abnormal heart rhythm

Robotically Assisted Device Implant for Heart Failure

During the robotically assisted biventricular pacemaker or defibrillator implant procedure, the surgeon's hands control the movement and placement of the endoscopic instruments through small incisions in the chest wall. This surgical technique can be used to place leads on the surface of the left ventricle. The leads then are attached to the biventricular device (defibrillator or pacemaker) to "resynchronize" the heartbeat and improve heart failure symptoms.

Patient's Health after Surgery

You may feel some discomfort at the incision site after surgery. You can take medications to help relieve this discomfort. Ask your doctor which medication you should take for pain relief. If you have discomfort in your chest

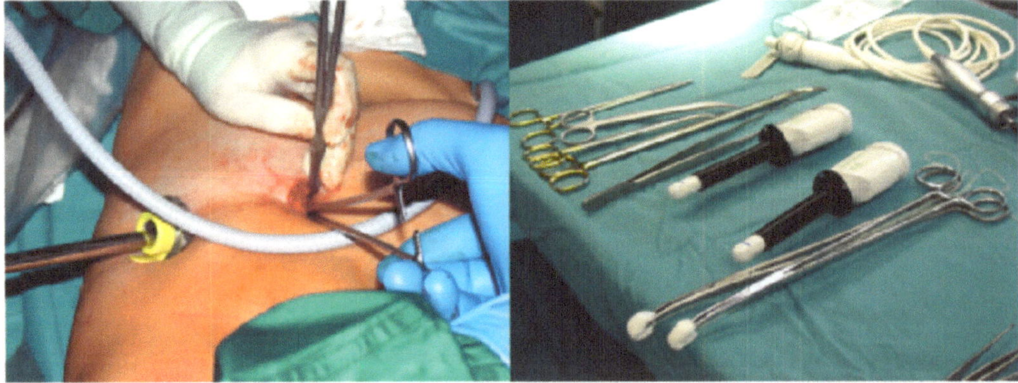

Fig. 13.22: *Instruments for epicardial lead implantation using the VATS two ports techniqueas done in resynchronization therapy in chronic heart failure*

that is similar to the symptoms you had before your surgery, call your doctor.

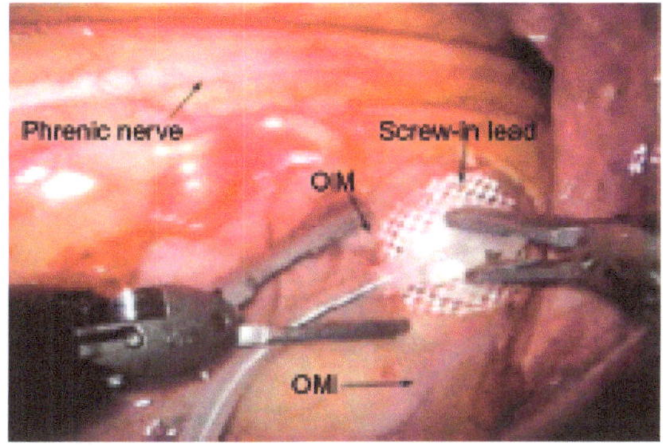

Fig.13.23: Robot-enhanced thoracoscopic approach may provide greater maneuverability in placement of an LV pacing lead on the lateral wall through small chest wall incisions

Recovery of Patient after Surgery

Patients who have minimally invasive or robotic surgery may be able to go home 2 to 5 days after surgery. Your healthcare team will follow your progress and help you recover as quickly as possible.

Your healthcare team will provide specific instructions for your recovery and return to work, including guidelines for activity, driving, incision care and diet.

Recovery after Minimally Invasive Heart Surgery

In general, you may be able to return to work (if you have a sedentary job), resume driving and participate in most non-strenuous activities within 1 to 4 weeks after traditional minimally invasive heart surgery. You can resume heavy lifting and other more strenuous activities within 5 to 8 weeks after surgery. Your healthcare team will provide specific guidelines based on your rate of recovery.

Recovery after Robotically assisted Heart Surgery

The recovery time after robotically assisted heart surgery is shorter than traditional minimally invasive heart surgery. Most patients can resume normal activities, drive and return to work as soon as they feel up to it—usually within 2 to four weeks after surgery. Your healthcare team will provide specific guidelines based on your rate of recovery.

Recovery for All Patients after Heart Surgery

To maintain your cardiovascular health after surgery, we strongly encourage you to make lifestyle changes and take your medications as prescribed. Heart-healthy lifestyle changes that are important to your recovery include:

- Quitting smoking
- Treating high cholesterol
- Managing high blood pressure and diabetes
- Exercising regularly

BIBLIOGRAPHY AND ACKNOWLEDGEMENT

- Argenziano M, Katz M, Bonatti J, et al. Results of the prospective multicenter trial of robotically assisted totally endoscopic coronary artery bypass grafting. Ann Thorac Surg. 2006;81(5):1666–1675. [PubMed]
- Aris A, Cámara ML, Montiel J, Delgado LJ, Galán J, Litvan H. Ministernotomy versus median sternotomy for aortic valve replacement: a prospective, randomized study. Ann Thorac Surg. 1999;67(6):1583–1588.
- Bonatti J, Schachner T, Bernecker O, et al. Robotic totally endoscopic coronary artery bypass: program development and learning curve issues. J Thorac Cardiovasc Surg. 2004;127(2):504–510.
- Bonatti J, Schachner T, Bonaros N, et al. How to improve performance of robotic totally endoscopic coronary artery bypass grafting. Am J Surg. 2008;195(5):711–716.
- Bonatti J, Schachner T, Bonaros N, et al. Robotic totally endoscopic double-vessel bypass grafting: a further step toward closed-chest surgical treatment of multivessel coronary artery disease. Heart Surg Forum. 2007;10:E239– E242.
- Brinkman WT, Hoffman W, Dewey TM, et al. Aortic valve replacement surgery: comparison of outcomes in matched sternotomy and PORT ACCESS groups. Ann Thorac Surg. 2010;90(1):131–135.
- Carpentier A, Loulmet D, Aupècle B, et al. Computer assisted open heart surgery First case operated on with success. CR Acad Sci III. 1998;321:437– 42.
- Carpentier A, Loulmet D, Carpentier A, et al. Open heart operation under videosurgery and minithoracotomy First case (mitral valvuloplasty) operated with success. CR Acad Sci. 1996;319(3):219–223
- Casselman FP, Van Slycke S, Wellens F, et al. Mitral valve surgery can now routinely be performed endoscopically. Circulation. 2003;108(Suppl 1):II48–II54.
- Chitwood WR, Jr, Elbeery JR, Chapman WH, et al. Videoassisted minimally invasive mitral valve surgery: the 'micromitral' operation. J Thorac Cardiovasc Surg. 1997;113(2):413– 414.
- Chitwood WR, Jr, Elbeery JR, Moran JF. Minimally invasive mitral valve repair: using a minithoracotomy and transthoracic aortic occlusion. Ann Thorac Surg. 1997;63:1477–1479.
- Chitwood WR., Jr Current status of endoscopic and robotic mitral valve surgery. Ann Thorac Surg. 2005;79(6):S2248–S2253
- Cohn LH, Adams DH, Couper GS, Bichell DP. Minimally invasive aortic valve replacement. Semin Thorac Cardiovasc Surg. 1997;9(4):331–336.

- Cohn LH, Adams DH, Couper GS, et al. Minimally invasive cardiac valve surgery improves patient satisfaction while reducing costs of cardiac valve replacement and repair. Ann Surg. 1997;226(4):421 428. [PMC free article].
- Cohn LH. Fifty years of open-heart surgery. Circulation. 2003;107(17):2168–2170.
- Cohn WE. Advances in surgical treatment of acute and chronic coronary artery disease. Tex Heart Inst J. 2010;37(3):328–330.
- Corbi P, Rahmati M, Donal E, et al. Prospective comparison of minimally invasive and standard techniques for aortic valve replacement: initial experience in the first hundred patients. J Card Surg. 2003;18(2):133–139.
- Cosgrove DM, 3rd, Sabik JF, Navia JL. Minimally invasive valve operations. Ann Thorac Surg. 1998;65(6):1535–1538.
- Cosgrove DM, 3rd, Sabik JF. Minimally invasive approach for aortic valve operations. Ann Thorac Surg. 1996;62(2):596–597.
- de Canniere D, Wimmer-Greinecker G, Cichon R, et al. Feasibility, safety, and efficacy of totally endoscopic coronary artery bypass grafting: Multicenter European experience. J Thorac Cardiovasc Surg. 2007;134:710–716.
- de Vaumas C, Philip I, Daccache G, et al. Comparison of minithoracotomy and conventional sternotomy approaches for valve surgery. J Cardiothorac Vasc Anesth. 2003;17(3):325–328.
- Detter C, Reichenspurner H, Boehm DH, et al. Minimally invasive direct coronary artery bypass grafting (MIDCAB) and off-pump coronary artery bypass grafting (OPCAB), two techniques for beating heart surgery. Heart Surg Forum. 2002;5:157–162.
- Estrera AL, Reardon MJ. Current approaches to minimally invasive aortic valve surgery. Curr Opin Cardiol. 2000;15(2):91–95.
- Falk V, Walther T, Autschbach R, Diegeler A, Battellini R, Mohr FW. Robot-assisted minimally invasive solo mitral valve operation. J Thorac Cardiovasc Surg. 1998;115(2):470–471.
- Farhat F, Lu Z, Lefevre M, et al. Prospective comparison between total sternotomy and ministernotomy for aortic valve replacement. J Card Surg. 2003;18(5):396–402.
- Galloway AC, Schwartz CF, Ribakove GH, et al. A decade of minimally invasive mitral repair: long-term outcomes. Ann Thorac Surg. 2009;88:1180–1184.
- Gammie JS, Bartlett ST, Griffith BP. Small-incision mitral valve repair: safe, durable, and approaching perfection. Ann Surg. 2009;250(3):409–415.
- Gammie JS, Zhao Y, Peterson ED, O'Brien SM, Rankin JS, Griffith BP. Less-invasive mitral valve operations trends and outcomes from the society of thoracic surgeons adult cardiac surgery database. Ann Thorac Surg. 2010;90:1401–1410.
- Gaudiani VA, Grunkemeier GL, Castro LJ, Fisher AL, Wu Y. Mitral valve operations through standard and smaller incisions. Heart Surg Forum. 2004;7(4):E337–E342.
- Greenspun HG, Adourian UA, Fonger JD, Fan JS. Minimally invasive direct coronary artery bypass (MIDCAB), surgical techniques and anesthetic considerations. J Cardiothorac Vasc Anesth. 1996;10:507–509.
- Grossi EA, Galloway AC. Minimally invasive mitral valve surgery: a 6-year experience with 714 patients. Ann Thorac Surg. 2002;74(3):660–664
- Grossi EA, LaPietra A, Ribakove GH, et al. Minimally invasive versus sternotomy approaches for mitral reconstruction: comparison of intermediate-term results. J Thorac Cardiovasc Surg. 2001;121(4):708–713.
- Holzhey DM, Jacobs S, Mochalski M, et al. Seven-year followup after minimally invasive direct coronary artery bypass: experience with more than 1300 patients. Ann Thorac Surg. 2007;83(1):108–114.
- Iribarne A, Karpenko A, Russo MJ, et al. Eight-year experience with minimally invasive cardiothoracic surgery. World J Surg. 2010;34(4):611–615.
- Iribarne A, Russo MJ, Easterwood R, et al. Minimally invasive versus sternotomy approach for mitral valve surgery: a propensity analysis. Ann Thorac Surg. 2010;90(5):1471–1477.
- Iribarne A, Russo MJ, Moskowitz AJ, Ascheim DD, Brown LD, Gelijns AC. Assessing technological change in cardiothoracic surgery. Semin Thorac Cardiovasc Surg. 2009;21(1):28–34.
- Kiaii B, McClure RS, Stewart P, et al. Simultaneous integrated coronary artery revascularization with long-term angiographic follow-up. J Thorac Cardiovasc Surg. 2008;136:702–708
- Korach A, Shemin RJ, Hunter CT, Bao Y, Shapira OM. Minimally invasive versus conventional aortic valve replacement: a 10-year experience. J Cardiovasc Surg (Torino) 2010;51(3):417–421.
- Kronzon I, Matros TG. Intraoperative echocardiography in minimally invasive cardiac surgery and novel cardiovascular surgical techniques. Am Heart Hosp J. 2004;2(4):198–204.
- Lapierre H, Chan V, Ruel M. Off-pump coronary surgery through mini-incisions: is it reasonable? Curr Opin Cardiol. 2006;21(6):578–583..
- Loulmet DF, Carpentier A. Less invasive techniques for mitral valve surgery. J Thorac Cardiovasc Surg. 1998;115(4):772–779.
- Machler HE, Bergmann P. Minimally invasive versus conventional aortic valve operations: a prospective study in 120 patients. Ann Thorac Surg. 1999;67(4):1001–1005.
- Mathew JP, Parks R, Savino JS, et al. Atrial fibrillation following coronary artery bypass graft surgery: predictors, outcomes, and resource utilization MultiCenter Study of Perioperative Ischemia Research Group. JAMA. 1996;276:300–306.
- Mihaljevic T, Cohn LH, Unic D, Aranki SF, Couper GS, Byrne JG. One thousand minimally invasive valve operations: early and late results. Ann Surg. 2004;240(3):529–534.

- Mohr FW, Falk V, Diegeler A, Walther T, van Son JA, Autschbach R. Minimally invasive port-access mitral valve surgery. J Thorac Cardiovasc Surg. 1998;115(3):567–576.
- Morgan JA, Thornton BA, Peacock JC, et al. Does robotic technology make minimally invasive cardiac surgery too expensive? A hospital cost analysis of robotic and conventional techniques. J Card Surg. 2005;20(3):246–251.
- Morishita A, Shimakura T, Miyagishima M, et al. Minimally invasive direct redo coronary artery bypass grafting. Ann Thorac Cardiovasc Surg. 2002;8(4):209–212.
- Navia JL, Cosgrove DM. Minimally invasive mitral valve operations. Ann Thorac Surg. 1996;62:1542–1544.
- Novick RJ, Fox SA, Kiaii BB, et al. Analysis of the learning curve in telerobotic, beating heart coronary artery bypass grafting: a 90 patient experience. Ann Thorac Surg. 2003;76(3):749–753.
- Pascucci S, Gunkel L, Zietak T, et al. Use of MIDCAB procedure for redo coronary artery bypass. J Cardiovasc Surg. 2002;43(2):143–146
- Pisano GP, Bohmer RM. Organizational differences in rates of learning: evidence from the adoption of minimally invasive cardiac surgery. Manag Sci. 2001;47(6):752–768.
- Plass A, Scheffel H, Alkadhi H, et al. Aortic valve replacement through a minimally invasive approach: preoperative planning, surgical technique, and outcome. Ann Thorac Surg. 2009;88(6):1851–1856.
- Puskas J, Cheng D, Knight J, et al. Off-pump versus conventional coronary artery bypass grafting: a metaanalysis and consensus statement from the 2004 ISMICS consensus conference. Innovations. 2005;1(1):3–27
- Reichenspurner H, Boehm DH, Gulbins H, et al. Threedimensional video and robot-assisted port-access mitral valve operation. Ann Thorac Surg. 2000;69(4):1176–1181.
- Riess FC, Lower C, Bleese N. Prevention of potential complications after minimal access aortic valve replacement. Ann Thorac Surg. 1998;66(5):1866.
- Robicsek F. Robotic cardiac surgery: time told! J Thorac Cardiovasc Surg. 2008;135(2):243–246.
- Schmitto JD, Mokashi SA, Cohn LH. Minimally-invasive valve surgery. J Am Coll Cardiol. 2010;56(6):455–462.
- Schwartz DS, Ribakove GH, Grossi EA, et al. Minimally invasive mitral valve replacement: port-access technique, feasibility, and myocardial functional preservation. J Thorac Cardiovasc Surg. 1997;113(6):1022–1030.
- Sellke FW, Chu LM, Cohn WE. Current state of surgical myocardial revascularization. Circ J. 2010;74(6):1031–1037.
- Sellke FW, DiMaio JM, Caplan LR, et al. Comparing on-pump and off-pump coronary artery bypass grafting: numerous studies but few conclusions: a scientific statement from the American Heart Association council non cardiovascular surgery and anesthesia in collaboration with the interdisciplinary working group on quality of care and outcomes research. Circulation. 2005;111:2858–2864.
- Shapira OM, Natarajan V, Kaushik S, et al. Off-pump versus on-pump reoperative CABG via a left thoracotomy for circumflex coronary artery revascularization. J Cardiac Surg. 2004;19(2):113–118.
- Srivastava S, Gadasalli S, Agusala M, et al. Use of bilateral internal thoracic arteries in CABG through lateral thoracotomy with robotic assistance in 150 patients. Ann Thorac Surg. 2006;81:800–806.
- Srivastava SP, Patel KN, Skantharaja R, et al. Off-pump complete revascularization through a left lateral thoracotomy (ThoraCAB), the first 200 cases. Ann Thorac Surg. 2003;76(1):46–49.
- Stamou SC, Hill PC, Dangas G, et al. Stroke after coronary artery bypass: incidence, predictors, and clinical outcome. Stroke. 2001;32:1508–1513.
- Stevens JH, Burdon TA, Peters WS, et al. Port-access coronary artery bypass grafting: a proposed surgical method. J Thorac Cardiovasc Surg. 1996;111(3):567–573.
- Stover EP, Siegel LC, Parks R, et al. Variability in transfusion practice for coronary artery bypass surgery persists despite national consensus guidelines: a 24-institution study Institutions of the Multicenter Study of Perioperative Ischemia Research Group. Anesthesiology. 1998;88:327–333.
- Subramanian VA, Patel NU. Current status of MIDCAB procedure. Curr Opin Cardiol. 2001;16:268–270.
- Svensson LG, Atik FA, Cosgrove DM, et al. Minimally invasive versus conventional mitral valve surgery: a propensity-matched comparison. J Thorac Cardiovasc Surg. 2010;139(4):926–932.
- Svensson LG, D'Agostino RS. J incision minimal-access valve operations. Ann Thorac Surg. 1998;66(3):1110–1112.
- Vanermen H, Farhat F, Wellens F, et al. Minimally invasive video-assisted mitral valve surgery: from port-access towards a totally endoscopic procedure. J Card Surg. 2000;15:51–60.
- Vleissis AA, Bolling SF. Mini-reoperative mitral valve surgery. J Cardiac Surg. 1998;13(6):468–470.
- Walther T, Falk V, Metz S, et al. Pain and quality of life after minimally invasive versus conventional cardiac surgery. Ann Thorac Surg. 1999;67:1643–1647.
- Walther TS. Midterm results after stentless mitral valve replacement. Circulation. 2003;108(Suppl 1):II85–II89.
- Wang D, Wang Q. Mitral valve replacement through a minimal right vertical infra-axillary thoracotomy versus standard median sternotomy. Ann Thorac Surg. 2009;87(3):704–708.
- Wong MC, Clark DJ, Horrigan MC, Grube E, Matalanis G, Farouque HM. Advances in percutaneous treatment for adult valvular heart disease. Intern Med J. 2009;39(7):465–474.
- Yamada T, Ochiai R, Takeda J, Shin H, Yozu R. Comparison of early postoperative quality of life in minimally invasive versus conventional valve surgery. J Anesth. 2003;17(3):171–176

CHAPTER

Recent Advances In The Diagnosis And Treatment of Chronic Heart Failure

After a decade without successful development of novel heart failure therapeutics, the PARADIGM-HF trial and the SHIFT trial demonstrated significant reductions in cardiovascular death and heart failure hospitalization for sacubitril-valsartan and in heart failure hospitalization alone for ivabradine. Since the market introduction of these two therapies, several heart failure therapies have received or stand on the verge of market approval. In light of the rapid advances in the care of adults living with chronic heart failure, it was therefore advocated to update the general practitioner on heart failure therapies in the light of successful drug development.

Implementation of sacubitril-valsartan

Two clinical trials have tested novel strategies for the safe and effective implementation of sacubitril-valsartan in 498 patients with heart failure and a reduced ejection fraction. The TITRATION study compared the safety and efficacy of conservative and condensed up-titration schedules for sacubitril-valsartan in ambulatory patients 1. All patients received sacubitril-valsartan 24/26 mg twice daily for 5 days during an open-label, run-in period followed by randomization and two additional treatment periods. At randomization, patients in the conservative arm continued sacubitril-valsartan at 24/26 mg twice daily whereas patients in the condensed arm were titrated to 49/51 mg twice daily. After 2 weeks, the conservative arm increased to 49/51 mg twice daily and the condensed arm increased to the maximal dose of 97/103 mg twice daily. The condensed arm then continued the maximal 97/103 mg twice dailyfor the remaining 9 weeks of the study, whereas the conservative arm continued the 49/51 mg twice-daily regimen for 3 weeks before increasing to the maximal 97/103 mg twice daily for 6 weeks In aggregate, the condensed arm reached the maximal dose with one fewer visit than the conservative arm and increased from 24/26 mg to 49/51 mg 2 weeks earlier than the conservative arm and from 49/51 mg to 97/103 mg 3 weeks earlier than the conservative arm.

The proportion of patients experiencing any hypotension (9.7% vs. 8.4%; P = 0.57) and systolic blood pressure less than 95 mm Hg (8.9% vs. 5.2%; P = 0.10) was not significantly different between the conservative and condensed arms. Serum potassium of more than 5.5 mmol/L occurred in 7.3% of condensed and 4% of conservative patients (P = 0.10). There was no significant difference in renal dysfunction between the two arms (7.3% vs. 7.6%; P = 0.99). Adverse effects occurred most frequently in patients who switched to sacubitril-valsartan from a low dose of an angiotensin-converting enzyme inhibitor (≤10 mg of enalapril or equivalent) or angiotensin receptor blocker (≤160 mg of valsartan or equivalent) and those who had baseline systolic blood pressure of 100 to 110 mm Hg. Less than one fifth of patients with heart failure reach target doses of renin–angiotensin–aldosterone inhibitors

The randomized, double-blind PIONEER-HF trial compared in-hospital initiation of sacubitril-valsartan to initiation or enalapril among 881 patients with stabilized decompensated heart failure . Change in N-terminal pro B-type natriuretic peptide (NT-proBNP) from baseline to week 8 was significantly greater in

the sacubitril-valsartan group than the enalapril group (geometric mean ratio vs. baseline: 0.53 for sacubitril-valsartan vs. 0.75 for enalapril; between-group percent change: −47% vs. −25%; P <0.001). Sacubitril-valsartan had no effect on a secondary 7-point composite clinical endpoint but was associated with a reduced risk of rehospitalization for heart failure [8%] vs. 61 [14%]; hazard ratio [HR] 0.56,
95% confidence interval [CI] 0.37 to 0.84; P = not reported). Of note, the trial protocol aimed to achieve maximal sacubitril-valsartan doses within 1 week if tolerated. Slightly more patients experienced worsening renal function (13.6% vs. 14.7%), hyperkalemia (11.6% vs. 9.3%), and symptomatic hypotension (15.0% vs. 12.7%) but these differences did not reach statistical significance.These important trials provide clinicians with structured protocols to maximize sacubitril-valsartan doses in hemodynamically stable, normokalemic patients with heart failure and a reduced ejection fraction and relatively intact renal function (estimated glomerular filtration rate of at least 30 mL/min per 1.73 m 2).

Sacubitril-valsartan for the treatment of heart failure with preserved ejection fraction

The PARAGON-HF trial tested the hypothesis that sacubitril-valsartan lowers the rate of a composite outcome of total heart failure hospitalizations and cardiovascular death compared with valsartan alone in patients with heart failure and preserved ejection fraction .In addition to a left ventricular ejection fraction (LVEF) of at least 45%, patients were required to have additional objective criteria of heart failure, including an elevated natriuretic peptide level, structural heart disease (left atrial enlargement or increased left ventricular wall thickness), and diuretic use. Patients were ineligible if they had a previous LVEF of less than 40%. After a single-blind run-in phase, 4796 patients were randomly assigned to sacubitril-valsartan (target dose of 97/103 mg twice daily) or valsartan (target dose of 160 mg twice daily) and followed for a median of 35 (interquartile range of 30 to 41) months.The number of composite heart failure hospitalizations or cardiovascular deaths was nominally lower in the sacubitril-valsartan arm than in the valsartan arm (526 vs. 1009; rate ratio 0.87,

Sacubitril-Valsartan Dose Titration Schedules for Ambulatory Patients

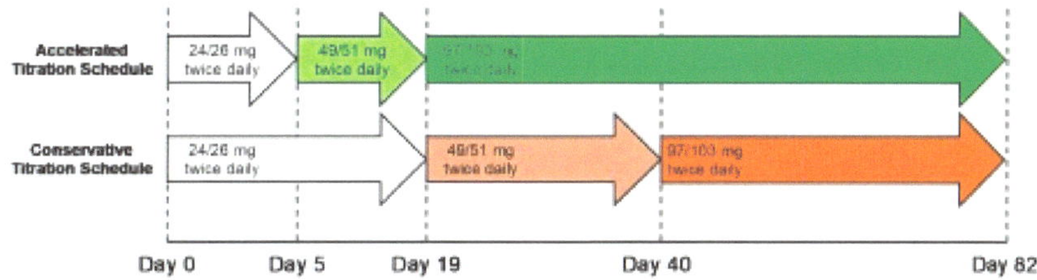

Sacubitril-Valsartan Dose Titration Schedules for Stable, Hospitalized Patients

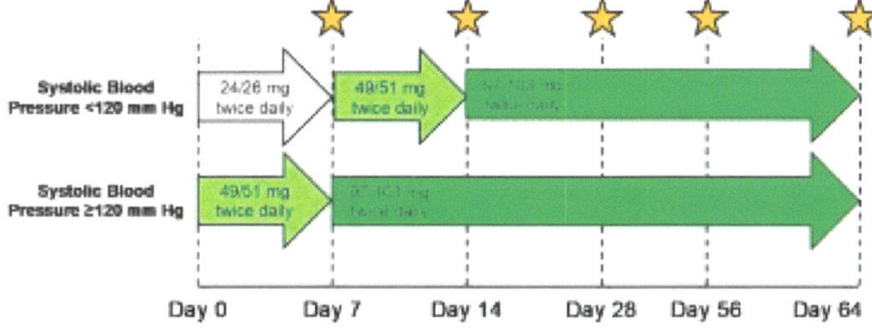

Titration guidelines: Ensure washout period of 36 hours for patients taking an angiotensin-converting enzyme inhibitor. Check systolic blood pressure prior to each dose increase. Doses should not be increased for patients with systolic blood pressure < 110 mm Hg at Day 7 or <100 mm Hg at Day 14 or thereafter. Clinicians should also consider serum potassium and renal function when determining dose adjustments.

Fig. 14.1 Titration schedules for ambulatory and hospitalized patients initiating sacubitril-valsartan.

95% CI 0.75 to 1.01; P = 0.06) but did not achieve statistical significance. Randomization to sacubitril-valsartan was associated with a smaller total number of heart failure hospitalizations (690 vs. 797; rate ratio 0.85, 95% CI 0.72 to 1.00) but no difference in death due to cardiovascular causes (204 [8.5%] vs. 212 [8.9%] in the sacubitril-valsartan and valsartan arms respectively) or due to any cause (342 [14.1%] vs. 349 [14.6%]). Although New York Heart Association functional class remains unchanged at 8 months in most patients, more sacubitril-valsartan patients than valsartan patients appeared to have investigator-assessed improvements in functional class (347 [15%] vs. 289 [12.6%]; P = not reported due to hierarchical analysis plan). Hypotension with systolic blood pressure of less than 100 mm Hg and elevations in serum creatinine of at least 2.0 mg/dL occurred less frequently in the sacubitril-valsartan arm, whereas angioedema occurred more frequently in the sacubitril-valsartan arm ([0.6%] vs. 4 [0.2%], P = 0.02).The investigators concluded that sacubitril-valsartan did not reduce the rate of a composite outcome of total heart failure hospitalizations and cardiovascular deaths compared with valsartan in patients with heart failure and preserved ejection fraction. Furthermore, any potential beneficial treatment effect appeared restricted to heart failure hospitalization and not cardiovascular mortality. The use of valsartan as an active comparator was consistent with most participants' pre-enrollment treatment regimens but may have diminished any potential between-group differences.

In pre-specified subgroup analyses, significant heterogeneity of effect was observed by qualifying LVEF and gender. Sacubitril-valsartan reduced the primary composite outcome in patients with an ejection fraction below the median of 57% (rate ratio 0.78, 95% CI 0.64 to 0.95) but not those with an ejection fraction above the median of 57% (rate ratio 1.00, 95% CI 0.81 to 1.23) and among women (rate ratio 0.73, 95% CI 0.59 to 0.90) but not men (rate ratio 1.03, 95% CI 0.85 to 1.25). Although the results of pre-specified subgroup analyses in an overall neutral trial must be considered with caution, the intriguing interactions by LVEF and gender may prove to be significant for several reasons. Patients who have a preserved but modestly depressed ejection fraction may be phenotypically more similar to those with a markedly reduced than robustly preserved ejection fraction 4. Sacubitril-valsartan has proven benefits in patients with an ejection fraction of less than 40% 5. Moreover, post-hoc analyses of spironolactone 6 and candesartan 7 clinical trials suggest a benefit for these therapies in patients with a mid-range ejection fraction. The effect modification of gender merits further research. Although this unexpected finding may be attributable to chance, the known biological differences between men and women provide multiple potential explanations for future investigation. In addressing one question, PARAGON-HF has not only advanced our understanding of heart failure with preserved ejection fraction but also highlighted several areas for future research. It will be interesting to see whether guidelines incorporate the results of PARAGON-HF in a manner consistent with TOPCAT, as American guidelines give spironolactone a IIb recommendation for decreasing hospitalizations

Treatment of secondary mitral regurgitation

Although secondary mitral regurgitation due to left ventricular dysfunction confers an increased risk of hospitalization and death, treatment options remain limited as surgical repair or replacement does not improve clinical outcomes 9, 10. The MitraClip is a percutaneous device that reduces mitral regurgitation severity by facilitating approximation of the anterior and posterior mitral valve leaflets 11. The efficacy and safety of mitral valve repair with the MitraClip were studied in two clinical trials with similar designs MITRA-FR (N = 304) and COAPT (N = 614) were randomized comparisons of mitral valve repair with the MitraClip plus guideline-directed medical therapy versus guideline-directed medical therapy alone Although both trials enrolled patients with at least moderate to severe regurgitation, COAPT targeted a population of patients with a larger effective orifice regurgitant area (≥30 vs. ≥20 mm 2) or a larger regurgitant volume (>45 vs. >30 mL) and less severe left ventricular dysfunction (LVEF 20 to 50% vs. 15 to 40% and left ventricular end-systolic diameter of not more than 70 mL in COAPT vs. no restriction in MITRA-FR). Thus, the contribution of mitral regurgitation to heart failure symptoms relative to myocardial dysfunction may have been greater in COAPT than MITRA-FR. In addition, COAPT patients were enrolled after optimization of guideline-directed medical therapy.In MITRA-FR, mitral valve repair with the MitraClip had no significant effect on the primary endpoint of all-cause death or heart failure hospitalization at 12 months (54.6% vs. 51.3% for repair vs. usual care; HR 1.16, 95% CI 0.73 to 1.83; P = 0.53). In contrast, in the COAPT trial, mitral valve repair with the MitraClip significantly reduced the risk of the primary endpoint of heart failure hospitalization at 24 months (35.8% vs. 67.9%; HR 0.53, 95% CI 0.40 to 0.70; P <0.001) and the composite of all-cause death or heart failure hospitalization (P <0.001).

Pharmacologic treatment with sacubitril-valsartan may also reduce mitral valve regurgitation, although the effects on clinical outcomes remain unclear. In the PRIME trial, patients with heart failure and mitral valve regurgitation who were randomly assigned to sacubitril-valsartan had significantly greater reductions in effective orifice regurgitant area (−0.06 ± 0.10 vs. −0.02 ± 0.10 cm 2; P = 0.03) and regurgitant volume (−4.3 ± 15.1 vs. −11.6 ± 14.4 mL; P = 0.009) than those randomly assigned to valsartan. One (2%) death and three (5%) heart failure events occurred in the sacubitril-valsartan group versus zero and five (9%) in the valsartan group (P >0.49 for each).

SGLT-2 inhibitors and heart failure

The risk of incident heart failure in patients with type 2 diabetes mellitus (T2DM) is twofold greater than that of patients without T2DM . Moreover, the presence of T2DM is associated with a poor prognosis among patients with heart failure About 90% of tubular glucose reabsorption occurs through the tubular sodium-glucose co-transporter-2 (SGLT-2) . SGLT-2 inhibitors therefore lower blood glucose concentrations by enhancing glucosuria. SGLT-2 inhibition also induces durable weight loss (primarily a reduction in fat mass and not in lean mass) and lowers blood pressure. Secondary and post-hoc analyses of three clinical trials provide strong evidence that SGLT-2 inhibitors modulate heart failure outcomes in patients with T2DM. Three SGLT-2 inhibitors (empagliflozin, canagliflozin, and dapagliflozin) significantly reduce the composite of heart failure hospitalization or cardiovascular death Whereas the beneficial effects of empagliflozin were consistent between patients with and without a history of heart failure at baseline , canagliflozin and dapagliflozin demonstrated larger effect sizes in patients with a history of heart failure Small observational studies suggest that treatment of T2DM (with or without heart failure) with SGLT-2 inhibitors improves left ventricular filling pressure, as measured by E/e′ ratio and left atrial volume index . The molecular mechanisms through which SGLT-2 inhibition may modulate cardiac structure and function remain under investigation. Hypothesized mechanisms include altered myocardial metabolism and energetics, glucosuria-induced diuresis without concomitant renin–angiotensin–aldosterone system activation, and inhibition of the myocardial sodium-hydrogen transporter Most recently, the DAPA-HF trial extended the benefits of SGLT-2 inhibitors from patients with T2DM to heart failure with reduced LVEF patients without T2DM . This trial randomly assigned 4744 patients with symptomatic heart failure and an ejection fraction of less than 40% to receive dapagliflozin 10 mg once daily or placebo, in addition to background heart failure therapy. The primary endpoint was hospitalization or urgent visit for heart failure or cardiovascular death. Most patients (58%) did not have a history of diabetes mellitus at baseline. The mean LVEF and the median NT-proBNP level at baseline were approximately 31 ± 7% and 1400 (857 to 2650) pg/mL, respectively. Use of guideline-directed medical therapy was high, including angiotensin-converting enzyme inhibitor (56%), angiotensin receptor blocker (27%) or sacubitril-valsartan (11%), a beta-blocker (96%), and mineralocorticoid receptor antagonist (71%). After a median follow-up duration of 18.2 months, patients randomly assigned to dapagliflozin experienced significantly fewer primary composite events than those randomly assigned to placebo (16.3% vs. 21.2%; HR 0.74, 95% CI 0.65 to 0.85; P <0.001). Dapagliflozin also reduced the incidence of each of the individual components of the primary outcome.Furthermore, the benefits of dapagliflozin did not significantly differ between patients with (HR 0.75, 95% CI 0.63 to 0.90) and without (HR 0.73, 95% CI 0.60 to 0.88) T2DM at baseline (P interaction = not reported). As expected, hypoglycemia requiring intervention occurred infrequently (4/2368 [0.2%]) in the dapagliflozin arm. There were no significant differences in amputations, diabetic ketoacidosis, or renal adverse events. These exciting results have re-positioned SGLT-2 inhibitors as a complete cardiometabolic, rather than glucose-lowering, therapy.

Transthyretin amyloid cardiomyopathy

Aggregation of misfolded transthyretin monomers into amyloid fibrils and subsequent tissue deposition lead to tissue dysfunction . Myocardial infiltration of amyloid fibrils can cause heart failure by interfering with cardiac contractility and relaxation as well as through direct toxicity of the amyloid fibrils. Transthyretin amyloid cardiomyopathy may represent up to 12% of all cases of heart failure with preserved ejection fraction . Until the development of transthyretin stabilizers and RNA therapeutics, transthyretin amyloid cardiomyopathy treatment focused on symptom palliation and there was minimal impetus to diagnose this debilitating condition.

Tafamidis

Tafamidis is a synthetic small molecule that binds to the thyroxine-binding sites on transthyretin 29. In adults with either wild-type or hereditary transthyretin amyloid cardiomyopathy, tafamidis significantly reduced the risk of all-cause mortality and cardiovascular hospitalization in the randomized, double-blind, placebo-controlled ATTR-ACT study 30. Of the 441 patients of ATTR-ACT, 71% (n = 186) of tafamidis patients were living compared with 57% (n = 101) of placebo patients at 32 months (win ratio 1.70, 95% CI 1.26 to 2.29; P <0.001). Cardiovascular hospitalization occurred in 138 tafamidis patients (52%; 0.48 per patient-year) compared with 107 placebo patients (61%; 0.70 per patient-year) (relative risk ratio 0.68, 95% CI 0.56 to 0.81; P = not reported).The effects of tafamidis were consistent across transthyretin genotypes
(for those with hereditary transthyretin amyloid cardiomyopathy) and both the 80 mg and 20 mg tafamidis doses. Delayed worsening heart failure symptoms and declining exercise capacity were observed in the tafamidis arms as early as 6 months, whereas the mortality benefit emerged after 18 months. ATTR-ACT was not powered to detect statistically significant improvements in left ventricular structure and function, although favorable trends were observed in left ventricular wall thickness and left ventricular global longitudinal strain. The incidence of serious adverse events was not significantly different between tafamidis and placebo.

Patisiran

Patisiran is a small, interfering RNA 31 encapsulated within a liposome that targets a conserved sequence in the 3′ untranslated region of wild-type and mutant transthyretin mRNA, thereby suppressing gene expression via the RNA-induced silencing complex. Patisiran 0.3 mg/kg every 3 weeks decreased serum transthyretin levels by 81% and improved neuropathy, as measured by the modified Neuropathy Impairment Score + 7 in 225 patients with hereditary transthyretin amyloidosis enrolled in the randomized, double-blind, placebo-controlled APOLLO study (N = 225) .
Transthoracic two-dimensional echocardiography was performed in 126 (56%) APOLLO patients with left ventricular wall thickness of at least 13 mm and no history of aortic valve disease or hypertension . Mean left ventricular wall thickness (least squares mean difference [LSMD] ± standard error of the mean [SEM], −0.9 ± 0.4; P = 0.017) and left ventricular end-diastolic volume (LSEM ± SEM, −5.1 ± 1.9 vs. −13.4 ± 3.4; P = 0.036) each decreased to a greater extent in the patisiran arm compared with placebo at 18 months. Patisiran improved left ventricular absolute global longitudinal strain by 1.4% (95% CI 0.3 to 0.5%; P = 0.02) versus placebo. Absolute basal, midwall and apical longitudinal strains also improved with patisiran treatment with basal longitudinal strain reaching statistical significance. In an exploratory post-hoc analysis of clinical outcomes, patisiran was associated with a trend toward lower risk of cardiac death or hospitalization compared with placebo (10.1 vs. 18.7 events per 100 patient-years; HR 0.54, 95% CI 0.28 to 1.01).

Clinical implementation

Tafamidis was approved by the US Food and Drug Administration for the treatment of wild-type or hereditary transthyretin-mediated amyloid cardiomyopathy in 2019, whereas patisiran was approved for the treatment of hereditary transthyretin amyloid polyneuropathy, but not amyloid cardiomyopathy, in 2018. Both agents have a considerable cost of tens or hundreds of thousands of dollars annually. Thus, patisiran is unlikely to be covered by payers for the treatment of amyloid cardiomyopathy and tafamidis is unlikely to be covered for the treatment of polyneuropathy. Tafamidis is the preferred agent for patients with amyloid cardiomyopathy The effects of a second RNA therapeutic, inotersen 36, and a second transthyretin tetramer stabilizer, AG10 , on cardiac structure and function in adults with transthyretin amyloid cardiomyopathy are unclear.

Iron deficiency

Depending upon the definition, iron deficiency (with or without anemia) affects up to 50% of adults with chronic heart failure and is associated with poor prognosis , impaired exercise capacity and skeletal muscle function , and worse quality of life . Patients with heart failure have decreased myocardial iron content , and iron-deficient cardiomyocytes have impaired contractility and mitochondrial dysfunction . Iron repletion with intravenous iron improves quality of life and may prevent heart failure hospitalizations in patients with heart failure and iron deficiency, irrespective of anemia status In 2017, three clinical trials addressed important unanswered questions related to iron repletion in adults with heart failure, namely the effect of iron repletion on exercise capacity as measured by peak oxygen consumption 50, the effect of iron repletion on peripheral skeletal muscle function , and the role of oral iron supplements in patients with heart failure and iron deficiency

Effect of ferric carboxymaltose on exercise capacity in patients with iron deficiency and chronic heart failure (EFFECT-HF)

EFFECT-HF randomly assigned 172 adults with symptomatic heart failure with reduced ejection fraction and iron deficiency (defined as serum ferritin of less than 100 ng/mL or serum ferritin 100 to 300 ng/mL with a transferrin saturation of less than 20%) to receive ferric carboxymaltose, dose-adjusted to target hemoglobin, ferritin, and transferrin saturation levels, or usual care for 24 weeks At 24 weeks, peak oxygen consumption decreased to a greater extent in the usual care arm than the ferric carboxymaltose arm (LSMD ± SEM, 1.0 ± 0.4 mL •kg −1 •min −1; P = 0.02). There were no between-group differences in ventilatory efficiency, as measured by the slope of the carbon dioxide–minute ventilation relationship, or treatment effect differences between patients with and without concomitant anemia.

Thus, EFFECT-HF was the first trial to demonstrate an improvement in exercise capacity using gas-exchange variables rather than the 6-minute walk test. In their joint 2017 focused update of the Guideline for the Management of Heart Failure, the American College of Cardiology Foundation and the American Heart Association gave intravenous iron replacement to improve function status and quality of life a weak recommendation (IIb) based upon moderate-quality evidence (B-R) EFFECT-HF was not included in the focused guideline update.

Ferric iron in heart failure II (FERRIC-HF II)

FERRIC-HF was a randomized, double-blind, placebo-controlled clinical trial of 40 patients with symptomatic heart failure with reduced ejection fraction, iron deficiency (defined as serum ferritin of less than 100 ng/mL or serum ferritin 100 to 300 ng/mL with a transferrin saturation of less than 20%), and normal folate and vitamin B 12 levels . Patients randomly received iron isomaltoside (the total dose was calculated by using the Ganzoni formula) or matching placebo. The primary endpoint was phosphocreatine recovery half-time on dynamic 31P magnetic resonance spectroscopy during submaximal exercise, where a shorter half-life indicates faster phosphocreatine recovery and improved mitochondrial oxidative function.

At 2 weeks, phosphocreatine half-time was −6.8 seconds (95% CI −11.5 to −2.1; P = 0.006) shorter in the iron isomaltoside group than the placebo group. Iron isomaltoside also improved adenosine diphosphate recovery half-time but had no effect on resting or end-exercise phosphocreatine or adenosine diphosphate half-time. This study provides important mechanistic insight into the pleiotropic effects of iron repletion in heart failure.

Iron repletion effects on oxygen uptake in heart failure (IRONOUT HF)

In IRONOUT HF, 225 patients with symptomatic heart failure with reduced ejection fraction and iron deficiency (defined as serum ferritin of less than

100 ng/mL or serum ferritin 100 to 300 ng/mL with a transferrin saturation of less than 20%) were randomly assigned to receive iron polysaccharide 150 mg twice daily for 16 weeks Oral iron supplementation with iron polysaccharide had no effect on peak oxygen consumption, ventilatory efficiency, 6-minute walk distance, or heart failure symptoms. Notably, iron polysaccharide had minimal effects on serum ferritin (median change from baseline of 18 ng/mL, 95% CI −8 to 38) and transferrin saturation (median change from baseline of 2%, 95% CI −3 to 7%). Subgroup analyses suggest that iron repletion was greater among patients with lower levels of hepcidin, an iron regulatory protein that decreases enteral iron absorption and sequesters iron intracellularly.ng/mL or serum ferritin 100 to 300 ng/mL with a transferrin saturation of less than 20%) were randomly assigned to receive iron polysaccharide 150 mg twice daily for 16 weeks 52. Oral iron supplementation with iron polysaccharide had no effect on peak oxygen consumption, ventilatory efficiency, 6-minute walk distance, or heart failure symptoms. Notably, iron polysaccharide had minimal effects on serum ferritin (median change from baseline of 18 ng/mL, 95% CI −8 to 38) and transferrin saturation (median change from baseline of 2%, 95% CI −3 to 7%). Figure 2 compares changes in serum ferritin and transferrin saturation between oral and intravenous iron repletion regimens in patients with heart failure at multiple time points. Subgroup analyses suggest that iron repletion was greater among patients with lower levels of hepcidin, an iron regulatory protein that decreases enteral iron absorption and sequesters iron intracellularly.

Biomarker-guided heart failure therapy

The natriuretic peptide B-type natriuretic peptide (BNP) and its congener N-terminal-proBNP (NT-proBNP) provide considerable diagnostic and prognostic value in heart failure . Yet the value of natriuretic peptide–guided heart failure management remains unclear. A meta-analysis of 2000 participants across 11 clinical trials demonstrated significant reductions in all-cause mortality (HR 0.62, 95% CI 0.45 to 0.86; P = 0.004), heart failure hospitalization (HR 0.80, 95% CI 0.67 to 0.94; P = 0.009), and cardiovascular hospitalization (HR 0.82, 95% CI 0.67 to 0.99; P = 0.048) with natriuretic peptide–guided heart failure management. In contrast, the GUIDE-IT trial (N = 894) found no difference in time to first heart failure hospitalization or cardiovascular death between patients randomly assigned to an NT-proBNP–guided strategy and usual care .

An exploratory, post-hoc analysis of the neutral TIME-CHF trial used the gap-time method to compare ***NT-proBNP–guided therapy*** with usual care to account for recurrent events. While NT-proBNP–guided therapy was associated with reduced second all-cause hospitalizations, there was no effect on the second heart failure hospitalization. In the subgroup of patients younger than 75 years, guided therapy was associated with reduced first and second all-cause and heart failure hospitalizations. Current guidelines do not recommend natriuretic peptide–guided therapy ***Carbohydrate antigen 125*** is a glycoprotein associated with prognosis in acute heart failure. In a multicenter clinical trial of 380 patients, carbohydrate antigen 125–guided therapy significantly reduced the composite of death or heart failure hospitalization at 1 year. Replication of these results would provide compelling support for carbohydrate antigen 125–guided therapy.

Remote hemodynamic monitoring-guided heart failure therapy

Titration of guideline-recommended medical therapy to a target pulmonary artery diastolic pressure, estimated using an implantable hemodynamic monitor, reduces heart failure hospitalizations by 28% in patients with reduced and preserved ejection fraction Recent analyses have provided additional insights into the efficacy and safety of remote hemodynamic monitoring. First, the findings of the CHAMPION trial have been replicated in two separate analysis of routinely collected clinical data Second, review of medication titration patterns during the CHAMPION trial has demonstrated that diuretic adjustments and (among patients with heart failure and a reduced ejection fraction) guideline-directed medical therapy adjustments contributed to the reduced hospitalization rates. Third, individual practices have begun to report their experience with the implementation and maintenance of a remote hemodynamic monitoring program. These practice-based insights will prove useful as additional remote monitoring devices reach the market. Last, comparative effectiveness studies suggest that remote hemodynamic monitoring meets currently accepted thresholds for cost-effectiveness but the overall budget impact may be difficult to absorb. Ongoing research is investigating the role of remote hemodynamic monitoring in patients with mechanical circulatory support devices and the effects of novel heart failure therapies on pulmonary artery pressure

Conclusions

After more than a decade of relatively modest advancements, heart failure therapeutic development has accelerated and led to several advances in the treatment of chronic heart failure. Some of these new technologies improved clinical outcomes, whereas others improve functional or patient-reported outcomes.

Artificial intelligence for the diagnosis of heart failure

The prevalence of heart failure (HF) has been increasing1,2. HF is associated with high morbidity and mortality3. Because HF is a complex syndrome that can result from structural and functional cardiac disorder, rather than a single disease entity, its correct diagnosis can be challenging even for HF specialists. Currently, HF is classified according to ejection fraction, i.e., HF with reduced ejection fraction (HFrEF), HF with mid-range ejection fraction (HFmrEF), and HF with preserved ejection fraction (HFpEF)4. A correct diagnosis is mandatory before proper treatment can be initiated4,5. Furthermore, present-day physicians are challenged by rapidly changing scientific evidences, new drugs, and the complexity of guidelines for HF management, especially in outpatient clinic. With enormous advancements in information and communication technologies, such as easy storage, acquisition, and recovery of big data and knowledge, artificial intelligence (AI) has been gaining an important role in cardiology.

Two types of AI decision systems are available: a white-box-based and a black-box-based one. A white-box AI-based decision system involves correlations and transparency among rules for the analysis of accumulated data, and is mainly constructed using supervised algorithms such as decision tree algorithm7. On the contrary, a black-box-based AI has opaque algorithms and its process and reasoning applied in providing the respective conclusions are difficult to clarify. IBM Watson for Oncology (WFO) is black-box AI-based decision systems. WFO demonstrated a concordance rate of 93% for the treatment recommendation in breast cancer. However, WFO cannot disclose the recommendation processes for the final clinical decision Clinical Decision Support System (CDSS) is a health information technology that assists physicians in clinical decision making. The concept of computer-based clinical decision has been developed for informatics six decades ago9. In spite of the enthusiasm for evolving CDSS which is assisted with the potential of AI, the realities and complexities of real clinical practice limit the rapid evolution of CDSS. An effective CDSS requires CDSS to match the individual patient's characteristics to the clinical knowledge base, provides patient-centric assessments and recommendations, and finally presents recommendations in white-box manner to the physicians for their final decision

A study was conducted assessing the level of agreement with respect to the HF diagnosis to identify the three types of HF, i.e. HFrEF, HFmrEF, and HFpEF, between HF specialists and AI-CDSS at a tertiary center in Korea. First, we created an AI-CDSS using a hybrid approach of expert-driven knowledge acquisition and ML-driven rule generation. Second, we evaluated the diagnosis concordance (degree of agreement) of AI-CDSS in a test set of patients with and without HF as a pilot clinical study. Third, we prospectively tested the diagnostic performance of AI-CDSS in consecutive patients presenting with dyspnea to the outpatient clinic.

Development of cardiovascular AI-CDSS

Using the training dataset of 600 patients with and

without HF, the AI-CDSS was created using predefined steps including expert-driven knowledge acquisition, machine learning (ML)-driven rule generation, and hybridization of both types of knowledge.

Development of cardiovascular AI-CDSS was studied under the following headings;-

1.Expert-driven knowledge acquisition

2.ML-driven rule generation

3.Hybrid knowledge

Correct diagnosis of HF can be challenging for physicians, even for HF specialists. In this study, we first created AI-CDSS by using the data of 1198 patients with and without HF and showed that AI-CDSS had very high diagnostic accuracy in these patients. In a prospective cohort of patients presenting with dyspnea to the outpatient clinic, AI-CDSS consistently showed a remarkably high diagnostic accuracy. By contrast, non-HF specialists showed a relatively low diagnostic accuracy for HF. Therefore, AI-CDSS may be useful for the diagnosis of HF, especially when HF specialists are not available.CDSS has been applied in clinical diagnosis11, preventive care12, and chronic disease management13, among others. It provides a proficient decision-making service to improve the quality of healthcare, but has several complexities and limitations8. Generally, AI-CDSS acquires knowledge from structured and unstructured data using ML and natural language processing techniques. The amalgamation of ML-driven rule generation with expert-driven knowledge acquisition enhances the system accuracy10. Therefore, we chose the hybrid approach for the knowledge acquisition of AI-CDSS, which includes three distinct steps: expert-driven knowledge acquisition, ML-driven rule generation, and hybridization of both types of knowledge.

In expert-driven knowledge acquisition, we first built CKM by transforming expert-driven knowledge into a mind map and decision tree10. Finally, the decision tree was validated with the PM of ML-driven knowledge.

In ML-driven knowledge acquisition, we created a PM with an available big dataset. Various ML algorithms can be used to analyze and extract the hidden patterns in the form of knowledge models. In our study, we used white box AI and causal machine algorithms such as decision tree, random forest, CHAID (Chi-squared Automatic Interaction Detector), , and CART/CRT. White-box model AI are selected for their transparency, which enables easily determining all attributes for classification and verification of new patient data

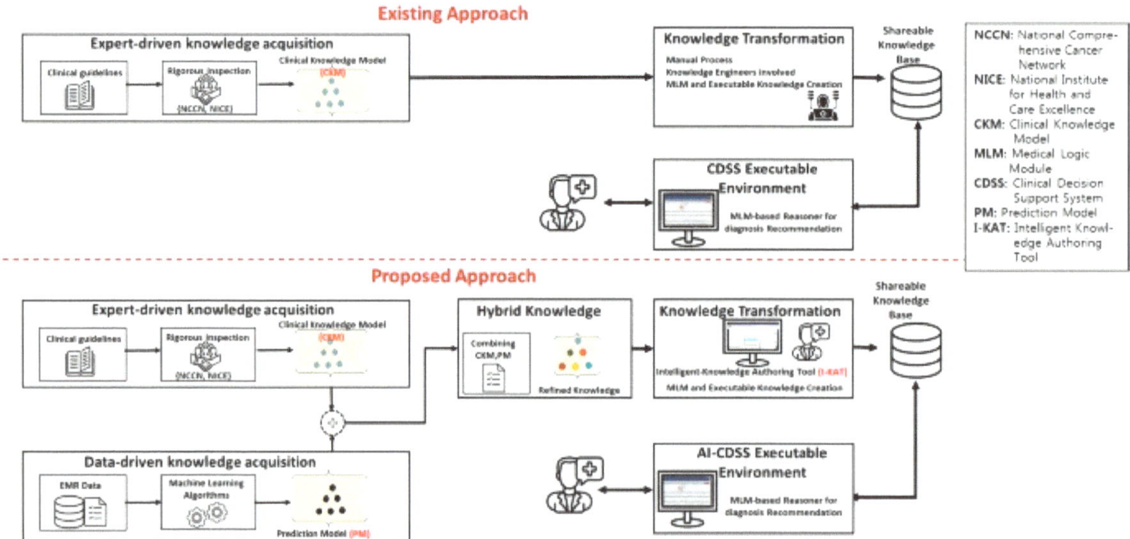

Fig.14.2: Comparison of existing CDSSs and our proposed artificial intelligence-CDSS. CDSS Clinical Decision Support System, CKM clinical knowledge model, I-KAT Intelligent Knowledge Authoring Tool, NCCN National Comprehensive Cancer Network, NICE National Institute for Health and Care Excellence, PM prediction model

They also increase the physicians' satisfaction level, because the rationale for a decision is also provided to the physician using the features contributing to the final decision. In addition, the computational complexity of the decision tree constructing algorithms (white box) is relatively low. By contrast, black box algorithms have no transparency in knowledge modeling owing to difficulty in interpreting the inner working layers of the models.

In the hybridization of the both knowledge types, we validated the PM from the ML-driven approach against the mind map of CKM from the expert-driven approach to produce the final hybrid knowledge in form of R-CKM.

Finally, we developed a web-based application in the form of cardiovascular AI-CDSS for use of physicians in real clinical practice. For this purpose, the R-CKM knowledge was transformed into MLM for knowledge shareability and computer-executable format using I-KAT, which had been developed by our team7. The resultant knowledge can be easily shared and integrated into various formats of HF diagnosis systems, because the resultant knowledge was built with consolidation of the standard data model vMR (Virtual Medical Record) and the standard terminology SNOMED CT (Systematized Nomenclature of Medicine—Clinical Terms).Because HF is a syndrome with various clinical features, its diagnosis can be very challenging even for HF specialists. In patients with HF, pulmonary congestion can develop because of congestion in the left heart, causing dyspnea. However, dyspnea as a symptom can also arise from lung disease, anemia, and mental disorders17. Leg swelling is a typical sign of congestion in the right heart. However, it also has many differential diagnoses, including kidney disease, adverse effect of drugs, and chronic venous insufficiency, among others18. In clinical practice, many patients are diagnosed as having HF even if they do not have HF, and vice versa.A correct diagnosis of HF is crucial because patients with HF have a grave prognosis that is comparable to that of oncologic malignancies19, and there exist therapy that can improve survival in patients with HF4,6. Consequently, misdiagnosis of HF can hinder the chance of improving the outcomes. AI-CDSS is a tool that helps in making better medical decisions, thereby reducing clinical errors and improving the quality of life. It has the potential to generate alerts and reminders, diagnostic assistance, therapy critiquing and planning, and image recognition and interpretation.

Currently, HF is classified according to LVEF into HFrEF, HFmrEF, and HFpEF. With respect to HFrEF, a decrease in LVEF may alert physicians to the possible diagnosis of HF. By contrast, for HFpEF >50%, the normal systolic function may "blind" the physicians and HFpEF may remain undiagnosed. We showed that AI-CDSS showed acceptably high concordance for diagnosing HF regardless of type, whereas non-HF specialists misdiagnosed HFpEF in almost half of the patients.

In medicine, IBM WFO demonstrated high concordance with oncologists in treatment recommendations14. In the field of cardiology, our study presents the clinical feasibility of AI for diagnosing HF.

There are several limitations in this study. The intervention of the physicians is crucial in knowledge creation and validation. However, the level of expertise varies from physician to physician, so that the CKM developed by physicians in a hospital may differ from that developed in another hospital. Similarly, because the attributes in the PM depend on the patient data used, they may also differ from variables recommended in the guidelines. Therefore, further studies are necessary to validate the AI-CDSS in other study populations.

Generation of cardiovascular AI-CDSS

The traditional CDSSs usually focus on the expert-driven approach with collaboration between physicians and knowledge engineers, where the knowledge engineer is an expert in AI language who investigate the underlying problems, develop the main concepts, and efficiently represent the knowledge in the domain. The fundamental knowledge resource is the clinical practice guidelines and physicians' expertise.All images were obtained using a standard ultrasound machine with a 2.5-MHz probe. Standard techniques were used to obtain M-mode, two-dimensional, and Doppler measurements in accordance with the American Society of Echocardiography guidelines. Tissue-Doppler-derived peak systolic, early, and late diastolic velocities of the septal mitral annulus were recorded.

In conclusions, AI-CDSS showed high diagnostic accuracy for HF, independent of HF types. Therefore, AI-CDSS may be useful for the diagnosis of HF, especially when HF specialists are not available.

BIBLIOGRAPHY AND ACKNOWLEDGEMENT

- Abraham J, Bharmi R, Jonsson O, et al.: Association of Ambulatory Hemodynamic Monitoring of Heart Failure With Clinical Outcomes in a Concurrent Matched Cohort Analysis. JAMACardiol.2019;4(6):556–563.
- Abraham WT, Adamson PB, Bourge RC, et al.: Wireless pulmonary artery haemodynamic monitoring in chronic heart failure: A randomised controlled trial. Lancet. 2011;377(9766):658–66.
- Adams D, Gonzalez-Duarte A, O'Riordan WD, et al.: Patisiran, an RNAi Therapeutic, for Hereditary Transthyretin Amyloidosis. N Engl J Med. 2018;379(1):11–21.
- Adamson PB, Abraham WT, Bourge RC, et al.: Wireless pulmonary artery pressure monitoring guides management to reduce decompensation in heart failure with preserved ejection fraction. Circ Heart Fail. 2014;7(6):935–44.
- Ali, T. et al. Multi-model-based interactive authoring environment for creating shareable medical knowledge. Comput. Methods Prog. Biomed. 150, 41–72 (2017).
- Asgar AW, Mack MJ, Stone GW: Secondary mitral regurgitation in heart failure: pathophysiology, prognosis, and therapeutic considerations. J Am Coll Cardiol. 2015;65(12):1231–1248.
- Benson MD, Waddington-Cruz M, Berk JL, et al.: Inotersen Treatment for Patients with Hereditary Transthyretin Amyloidosis. N Engl J Med. 2018;379(1):22–31.
- Berliner, D., Schneider, N., Welte, T. & Bauersachs, J. The differential diagnosis of dyspnea. Dtsch. Arzteblatt Int. 113, 834–845 (2016).
- Bleumink, G. S. et al. Quantifying the heart failure epidemic: prevalence, incidence rate, lifetime risk and prognosis of heart failure The Rotterdam Study. Eur. Heart J. 25, 1614–1619 (2004).
- Buckley LF, Cooper IM, Navarro-Velez K, et al.: Burden of nursing activities during hemodynamic monitoring of heart failure patients. Heart Lung. 2018;47(4):304–307.
- Bulawa CE, Connelly S, Devit M, et al.: Tafamidis, a potent and selective transthyretin kinetic stabilizer that inhibits the amyloid cascade. Proc Natl Acad Sci U S A. 2012;109(24):9629–34.
- Carbone S, Dixon DL, Buckley LF, et al.: Glucose-Lowering Therapies for Cardiovascular Risk Reduction in Type 2 Diabetes Mellitus: State-of-the-Art Review. Mayo Clin Proc. 2018;93(11):1629–1647.
- Charles-Edwards G, Amaral N, Sleigh A, et al.: Effect of Iron Isomaltoside on Skeletal Muscle Energetics in Patients With Chronic Heart Failure and Iron Deficiency. Circulation. 2019;139(21):2386–2398.10.1161
- Choi, D. J. et al. Characteristics, outcomes and predictors of long-term mortality for patients hospitalized for acute heart failure: a report from the Korean Heart Failure Registry. Korean Circ. J. 41, 363–371 (2011).
- Ciocon, J. O., Fernandez, B. B. & Ciocon, D. G. Leg edema: clinical clues to the differential diagnosis. Geriatrics 48, 34–40, 45 (1993).
- Coelho T, Adams D, Silva A, et al.: Safety and efficacy of RNAi therapy for transthyretin amyloidosis. N Engl J Med. 2013;369(9):819–29.
- Costanzo MR, Stevenson LW, Adamson PB, et al.: Interventions Linked to Decreased Heart Failure Hospitalizations During Ambulatory Pulmonary Artery Pressure Monitoring. JACC Heart Fail. 2016;4(5):333–44. 10.1016/j.jchf.2015.11.011
- Davarzani N, Sanders-van Wijk S, Karel J, et al.: N-Terminal Pro-B-Type Natriuretic Peptide-Guided Therapy in Chronic Heart Failure Reduces Repeated Hospitalizations-Results From TIME-CHF. J Card Fail. 2017;23(5)
- DeFronzo RA, Norton L, Abdul-Ghani M: Renal, metabolic and cardiovascular considerations of SGLT2 inhibition. Nat Rev Nephrol. 2017;13(1):11–26. 10.1038/nrneph.2016.170
- Dunlay SM, Givertz MM, Aguilar D, et al.: Type 2 Diabetes Mellitus and Heart Failure, A Scientific Statement From the American Heart Association and Heart Failure Society of America. J Card Fail. 2019;25(8):584–619.
- Enjuanes C, Klip IT, Bruguera J, et al.: Iron deficiency and health-related quality of life in chronic heart failure: Results from a multicenter European study. Int J Cardiol. 2014;174(2):268–75.
- Feldman T, Foster E, Glower DD, et al.: Percutaneous repair or surgery for mitral regurgitation. N Engl J Med. 2011;364(15):1395–406.
- Felker GM, Anstrom KJ, Adams KF, et al.: Effect of Natriuretic Peptide-Guided Therapy on Hospitalization or Cardiovascular Mortality in High-Risk Patients With Heart Failure and Reduced Ejection Fraction: A Randomized Clinical Trial. JAMA. 2017;318(8):713–720. 10.1001/jama.2017.10565
- Figtree GA, Rådholm K, Barrett TD, et al.: Effects of Canagliflozin on Heart Failure Outcomes Associated With Preserved and Reduced Ejection Fraction in Type 2 Diabetes Mellitus. Circulation. 2019;139(22):2591–2593. 10.1161/
- Fire A, Xu S, Montgomery MK, et al.: Potent and specific genetic interference by double-stranded RNA in Caenorhabditis elegans. Nature. 1998;391(6669):806–11.
- Fitchett D, Zinman B, Wanner C, et al.: Heart failure outcomes with empagliflozin in patients with type 2 diabetes at high cardiovascular risk: results of the EMPA-REG OUTCOME® trial. Eur Heart J. 2016;37(19):1526–34.
- Givertz MM, Stevenson LW, Costanzo MR, et al.: Pulmonary Artery Pressure-Guided Management of Patients With Heart Failure and Reduced Ejection Fraction. J Am Coll Cardiol. 2017;70(15):1875–1886.
- González-López E, Gallego-Delgado M, Guzzo-Merello G, et al.: Wild-type transthyretin amyloidosis as a cause of heart failure with preserved ejection fraction. Eur Heart J. 2015;36(38):2585–94. 10.1093/
- Haddad S, Wang Y, Galy B, et al.: Iron-regulatory proteins secure iron availability in cardiomyocytes to prevent heart failure. Eur Heart J. 2017;38(5):362–372
- Heywood JT, Jermyn R, Shavelle D, et al.: Impact of Practice-Based Management of Pulmonary Artery Pressures in 2000 Patients Implanted With the CardioMEMS Sensor. Circulation. 2017;135(16):1509–1517.
- Hinton, G. Deep learning—a technology with the potential to transform health care. JAMA 320, 1101–1102 (2018).
- Hoes MF, Grote Beverborg N, Kijlstra JD, et al.: Iron deficiency impairs contractility of human cardiomyocytes through decreased mitochondrial function. Eur J Heart Fail. 2018;20(5):910–919.

- Hsu JJ, Ziaeian B, Fonarow GC: Heart Failure With Mid-Range (Borderline) Ejection Fraction: Clinical Implications and Future Directions. JACC Heart Fail. 2017;5(11):763–771. 10.1016/j.jchf.2017.06.013 [PMC free article] [PubMed] [CrossRef] [Google Scholar]
- Hussain, M. et al. Data-driven knowledge acquisition, validation, and transformation into HL7 Arden Syntax. Artif. Intell. Med. 92, 51–70 (2018).
- Jankowska EA, Rozentryt P, Witkowska A, et al.: Iron deficiency: an ominous sign in patients with systolic chronic heart failure. Eur Heart J. 2010;31(15):1872–80. 10.1093/eurheartj/ehq158 [PubMed] [CrossRef] [Google Scholar]
- Jankowska EA, Tkaczyszyn M, Suchocki T, et al.: Effects of intravenous iron therapy in iron-deficient patients with systolic heart failure: A meta-analysis of randomized controlled trials. Eur J Heart Fail. 2016;18(7):786–95. 10.1002/ejhf.473 [PubMed] [CrossRef] [Google Scholar]
- Jermyn R, Alam A, Kvasic J, et al.: Hemodynamic-guided heart-failure management using a wireless implantable sensor: Infrastructure, methods, and results in a community heart failure disease-management program. Clin Cardiol. 2017;40(3):170–176. 10.1002/clc.22643 [PMC free article]
- Johnson, K. W. et al. Artificial intelligence in cardiology. J. Am. Coll. Cardiol. 71, 2668–2679 (2018).
- Judge DP, Heitner SB, Falk RH, et al.: Transthyretin Stabilization by AG10 in Symptomatic Transthyretin Amyloid Cardiomyopathy. J Am Coll Cardiol. 2019;74(3):285–295. 10.1016/j.jacc.2019.03.012 [PubMed] [CrossRef] [Google Scholar]
- Kato ET, Silverman MG, Mosenzon O, et al.: Effect of Dapagliflozin on Heart Failure and Mortality in Type 2 Diabetes Mellitus. Circulation. 2019;139(22):2528–2536. 10.1161/CIRCULATIONAHA.119.040130 [PubMed] [CrossRef] [Google Scholar] F1000 Recommendation
- Khan Z, Gholkar G, Tolia S, et al.: Effect of sacubitril/valsartan on cardiac filling pressures in patients with left ventricular systolic dysfunction. Int J Cardiol. 2018;271:169–173. 10.1016/j.ijcard.2018.03.093 [PubMed] [CrossRef] [Google Scholar]
- Kilic A, Katz JN, Joseph SM, et al.: Changes in pulmonary artery pressure before and after left ventricular assist device implantation in patients utilizing remote haemodynamic monitoring. ESC Heart Fail. 2019;6(1):138–145. 10.1002/ehf2.12373 [PMC free article] [PubMed] [CrossRef] [Google Scholar]
- Kim, M. S. et al. Korean guidelines for diagnosis and management of chronic heart failure. Korean Circ. J. 47, 555–643 (2017).
- Kline, J. A., Zeitouni, R. A., Hernandez-Nino, J. & Jones, A. E. Randomized trial of computerized quantitative pretest probability in low-risk chest pain patients: effect on safety and resource use. Ann. Emerg. Med. 53, 727–735. e721 (2009).
- Klip IT, Comin-Colet J, Voors AA, et al.: Iron deficiency in chronic heart failure: an international pooled analysis. Am Heart J. 2013;165(4):575–582.e3. 10.1016/j.ahj.2013.01.017 [PubMed] [CrossRef] [Google Scholar]
- Kucher, N. et al. Electronic alerts to prevent venous thromboembolism among hospitalized patients. N. Engl. J. Med. 352, 969–977 (2005).
- Lang, R. M. et al. Recommendations for cardiac chamber quantification by echocardiography in adults: an update from the American Society of Echocardiography and the European Association of Cardiovascular Imaging. J. Am. Soc. Echocardiogr. 28, 1–39. e14 (2015).
- Ledley, R. S. & Lusted, L. B. Reasoning foundations of medical diagnosis; symbolic logic, probability, and value theory aid our understanding of how physicians reason. Science 130, 9–21 (1959).
- Lewis GD, Malhotra R, Hernandez AF, et al.: Effect of Oral Iron Repletion on Exercise Capacity in Patients With Heart Failure With Reduced Ejection Fraction and Iron Deficiency: The IRONOUT HF Randomized Clinical Trial. JAMA. 2017;317(19):1958–1966. 10.1001/jama.2017.5427 [PMC free article] [PubMed] [CrossRef] [Google Scholar] F1000 Recommendation
- Lund LH, Claggett B, Liu J, et al.: Heart failure with mid-range ejection fraction in CHARM: characteristics, outcomes and effect of candesartan across the entire ejection fraction spectrum. Eur J Heart Fail. 2018;20(8):1230–1239. 10.1002/ejhf.1149 [PubMed] [CrossRef] [Google Scholar]
- Martens P, Verbrugge FH, Nijst P, et al.: Limited contractile reserve contributes to poor peak exercise capacity in iron-deficient heart failure. Eur J Heart Fail. 2018;20(4):806–808. 10.1002/ejhf.938 [PubMed] [CrossRef] [Google Scholar]
- Matsutani D, Sakamoto M, Kayama Y, et al.: Effect of canagliflozin on left ventricular diastolic function in patients with type 2 diabetes. Cardiovasc Diabetol. 2018;17(1):73. 10.1186/s12933-018-0717-9 [PMC free article] [PubMed] [CrossRef] [Google Scholar]
- Maurer MS, Schwartz JH, Gundapaneni B, et al.: Tafamidis Treatment for Patients with Transthyretin Amyloid Cardiomyopathy. N Engl J Med. 2018;379(11):1007–1016. 10.1056/NEJMoa1805689 [PubMed] [CrossRef] [Google Scholar] F1000 Recommendation
- McMurray JJ, Packer M, Desai AS, et al.: Angiotensin-neprilysin inhibition versus enalapril in heart failure. N Engl J Med. 2014;371(11):993–1004. 10.1056/NEJMoa1409077 [PubMed] [CrossRef] [Google Scholar]
- McMurray JJV, Solomon SD, Inzucchi SE, et al.: Dapagliflozin in Patients with Heart Failure and Reduced Ejection Fraction. N EnglJMed.2019;381(21):1995–2008.
- Melenovsky V, Petrak J, Mracek T, et al.: Myocardial iron content and mitochondrial function in human heart failure: a direct tissue analysis. Eur J Heart Fail. 2017;19(4):522–530. 10.1002/ejhf.640 [PubMed] [CrossRef] [Google Scholar]
- Minamisawa M, Claggett B, Adams D, et al.: Association of Patisiran, an RNA Interference Therapeutic, With Regional Left Ventricular Myocardial Strain in Hereditary Transthyretin Amyloidosis: The APOLLO Study. JAMA Cardiol. 2019;4(5):466–472. 10.1001/jamacardio.2019.0849 [PMC free article] [PubMed] [CrossRef] [Google Scholar]
- Moretti D, Goede JS, Zeder C, et al.: Oral iron supplements increase hepcidin and decrease iron absorption from daily or twice-daily doses in iron-depleted young women. Blood. 2015;126(17):1981–9.
- Neal B, Perkovic V, Mahaffey KW, et al.: Canagliflozin and Cardiovascular and Renal Events in Type 2 Diabetes. N Engl J Med. 2017;377(7):644–657.
- Nishimura RA, Otto CM, Bonow RO, et al.: 2017 AHA/ACC Focused Update of the 2014 AHA/ACC Guideline for the Management of Patients With Valvular Heart Disease: A Report of the American College of Cardiology/American Heart Association Task Force on Clinical Practice Guidelines. J Am Coll Cardiol. 2017;70(2):252–289.

- Rådholm K, Figtree G, Perkovic V, et al.: Canagliflozin and Heart Failure in Type 2 Diabetes Mellitus. Circulation. 2018;138(5):458–468. CIRCULATIONAHA.118.034222 [PMC free article] [PubMed] [CrossRef] [Google Scholar]
- Redfield, M. M. et al. Burden of systolic and diastolic ventricular dysfunction in the community: appreciating the scope of the heart failure epidemic. JAMA 289, 194–202 (2003).
- Romero, C., Olmo Ortiz, J. L. & Ventura, S. A meta-learning approach for recommending a subset of white-box classification algorithms for moodle datasets. Proc. Educational Data Mining, Memphis, TN, USA (2013).
- Roumie, C. L. et al. Improving blood pressure control through provider education, provider alerts, and patient education: a cluster randomized trial. Ann. Intern. Med. 145, 165–175 (2006).
- Ruberg FL, Grogan M, Hanna M, et al.: Transthyretin Amyloid Cardiomyopathy: JACC State-of-the-Art Review. J Am Coll Cardiol. 2019;73(22):2872–2891. 10.1016/j.jacc.2019.04.003 [PMC free article] [PubMed] [CrossRef] [Google Scholar]
- Sandhu AT, Goldhaber-Fiebert JD, Owens DK, et al.: Cost-Effectiveness of Implantable Pulmonary Artery Pressure Monitoring in Chronic Heart Failure. JACC Heart Fail. 2016;4(5):368–75. 10.1016/j.jchf.2015.12.015 [PMC free article] [PubMed] [CrossRef] [Google Scholar]
- Senni M, McMurray JJ, Wachter R, et al.: Initiating sacubitril/ valsartan (LCZ696) in heart failure: results of TITRATION, a double-blind, randomized comparison of two uptitration regimens. Eur J Heart Fail. 2016;18(9):1193–202.
  Shortliffe, E. H. & Sepulveda, M. J. Clinical decision support in the era of artificial intelligence. JAMA 320, 2199–2200 (2018).
- Singh R, Varjabedian L, Kaspar G, et al.: CardioMEMS in a Busy Cardiology Practice: Less than Optimal Implementation of a Valuable Tool to Reduce Heart Failure Readmissions. Cardiol Res Pract. 2018;2018:4918757.
- Soga F, Tanaka H, Tatsumi K, et al.: Impact of dapagliflozin on left ventricular diastolic function of patients with type 2 diabetic mellitus with chronic heart failure. Cardiovasc Diabetol. 2018;17(1):132.
- Solomon SD, Adams D, Kristen A, et al.: Effects of Patisiran, an RNA Interference Therapeutic, on Cardiac Parameters in Patients With Hereditary Transthyretin-Mediated Amyloidosis. Circulation.2019;139(4):431–443.10.1161/
- Solomon SD, Claggett B, Lewis EF, et al.: Influence of ejection fraction on outcomes and efficacy of spironolactone in patients with heart failure with preserved ejection fraction. Eur Heart J. 2016;37(5):455–62.
- Solomon SD, McMurray JJV, Anand IS, et al.: Angiotensin-Neprilysin Inhibition in Heart Failure with Preserved Ejection Fraction. N Engl J Med. 2019;381(17):1609–1620.
- Somashekhar, S. P. et al. Watson for oncology and breast cancer treatment recommendations: agreement with an expert multidisciplinary tumor board. Ann. Oncol.: Off. J. Eur. Soc. Med. Oncol. 29, 418–423 (2018
- Tkaczyszyn M, Drozd M, Węgrzynowska-Teodorczyk K, et al.: Depleted iron stores are associated with inspiratory muscle weakness independently of skeletal muscle mass in men with systolic chronic heart failure. J Cachexia Sarcopenia Muscle. 2018;9(3):547–556.10.1002/jcsm.12282
- Troughton RW, Frampton CM, Brunner-La Rocca HP, et al.: Effect of B-type natriuretic peptide-guided treatment of chronic heart failure on total mortality and hospitalization: An individual patient meta-analysis. Eur Heart J. 2014;35(23):1559–67.
- van Veldhuisen DJ, Ponikowski P, van der Meer P, et al.: Effect of Ferric Carboxymaltose on Exercise Capacity in Patients With Chronic Heart Failure and Iron Deficiency. Circulation. 2017;136(15):1374–1383.10.1161/
- Veenis JF, Manintveld OC, Constantinescu AA, et al.: Design and rationale of haemodynamic guidance with CardioMEMS in patients with a left ventricular assist device: the HEMO-VAD pilot study. ESC Heart Fail. 2019;6(1):194–201. 10.1002
- Velazquez EJ, Morrow DA, DeVore AD, et al.: Angiotensin-Neprilysin Inhibition in Acute Decompensated Heart Failure. N Engl J Med. 2019;380(6):539–548. 10.1056/NEJMoa1812851
- von Haehling S, Gremmler U, Krumm M, et al.: Prevalence and clinical impact of iron deficiency and anaemia among outpatients with chronic heart failure: The PrEP Registry. Clin Res Cardiol. 2017;106(6):436–443.10.1007/s00392-016-1073-yr]
- Wiviott SD, Raz I, Bonaca MP, et al.: Dapagliflozin and Cardiovascular Outcomes in Type 2 Diabetes. N Engl J Med. 2019;380(4):347–357.
- Yancy CW, Jessup M, Bozkurt B, et al.: 2013 ACCF/AHA guideline for the management of heart failure: a report of the American College of Cardiology Foundation/American Heart Association Task Force on practice guidelines. Circulation. 2013;128(16):e240–327.
- Yancy CW, Jessup M, Bozkurt B, et al.: 2017 ACC/AHA/HFSA Focused Update of the 2013 ACCF/AHA Guideline for the Management of Heart Failure: A Report of the American College of Cardiology/American Heart Association Task Force on Clinical Practice Guidelines and the Heart Failure Society of America. J AmCollCardiol.2017;70(6):776–803.
- Yeo TJ, Yeo PSD, Ching-Chiew Wong R, et al.: Iron deficiency in a multi-ethnic Asian population with and without heart failure: prevalence, clinical correlates, functional significance and prognosis. Eur J Heart Fail. 2014;16(10):1125–1132.
- Zinman B, Wanner C, Lachin JM, et al.: Empagliflozin, Cardiovascular Outcomes, and Mortality in Type 2 Diabetes. N Engl J Med. 2015;373(22):2117–28.

Special Procedures In The Management Of Critical Heart Diseases. A Review

CHAPTER

1.The Impella Device:

In 1968, Dr. Adrian Kantrowitz and colleagues at Maimonides Medical Center in New York reported the first successful use of a novel mechanical circulatory support system, intra-aortic balloon pump counter pulsation (IABP), in the treatment of a patient with cardiogenic shock. Subsequently, this technique was rapidly accepted as a valuable treatment in cardiogenic shock, as well as, later, in the treatment of refractory angina pectoris. Indeed, by 1980, over 50,000 IABP procedures had been performed. Bregman and Casarella at Columbia/Presbyterian Center in New York reported successful percutaneous placement of the IABP in 1980. This simplified technical approach soon became the standard with consequent even greater use of the IABP. As coronary angioplasty (PCI) developed in the 1980s and 1990s, interventional cardiologists began performing this procedure in increasingly challenging patient subgroups (such as depressed left ventricular function and multivessel coronary artery disease). Awareness of the potential of IABP to reduce the ischemic burden during such high-risk PCI procedures led to its use to increase the efficacy and safety of high-risk PCI (so-called facilitated PCI). Remarkably, 50 years after the initial report of the device by Kantrowitz et al , the IABP remains the most commonly used method of mechanical circulatory support in the cardiac catheterization laboratory and in the intensive care units.However, in recent years, large scale, randomized clinical trials have failed to demonstrate a clinically useful role for the IABP in the treatment of patients with acute myocardial infarction complicated by cardiogenic shock and in patients undergoing high-risk PCI. This has resulted in increased attention to other available forms of mechanical circulatory support systems: the Impella device (Abiomed, Danvers, Massachusetts), the Tandem Heart system (Cardiac Assist, Pittsburgh, PA), and ECMO (percutaneous extracorporeal cardiopulmonary support).

The Impella device is a catheter-based miniaturized ventricular assist device that pumps blood from left ventricle (LV) into ascending aorta and responsible for systemic circulation at an upper rate between 2.5 and 5.0 L/min. It is notable that, in his initial clinical paper on IABP, Kantrowitz et al emphasized that, for widespread use of a mechanical circulatory support system, simplicity of initiation and maintenance are crucial requirements. As will be explained later in this review, the Impella system admirably fulfills these requirements.

Setup and Hemodynamic Effects of the Impella

The current left sided Impella devices comprise the Impella 2.5, Impella CP, Impella 5.0, and Impella 5.0/ LD (left direct). The Impella 2.5 and Impella CP models are generally inserted via a retrograde femoral arterial approach, similar to the technique used for placement of an IABP . The larger sized Impella 5.0 model requires an arteriotomy for placement. The Impella 5.0/LD can be placed directly into the proximal aorta via an end-to-end anastomotic conduit. All models are placed across the aortic valve using fluoroscopic or echocardiographic guidance. The pigtail shape of the catheter facilitates crossing of the aortic valve and promotes a stable position. Once in a satisfactory position within the LV, the Impella catheter is connected distally to a portable mobile console that displays invasive pressures with the actual revolutions per minute of the pump, thus guiding the correct positioning of the device. Once activated, the Impella continuously draws blood from the LV via the inlet port and then expels it into the ascending aorta via the outlet port . The Impella 2.5, Impella CP, and Impella 5.0 can provide

A

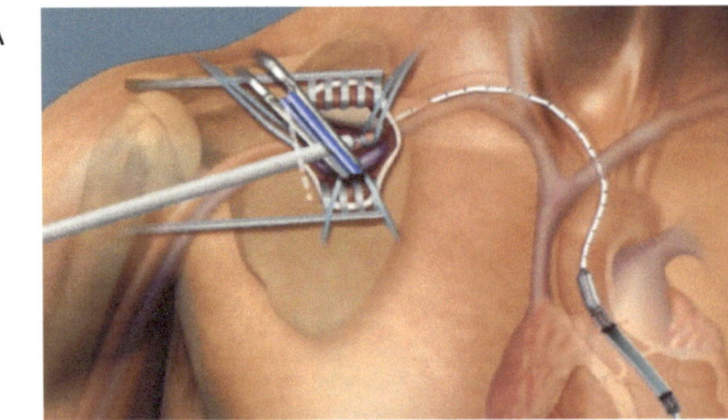

B

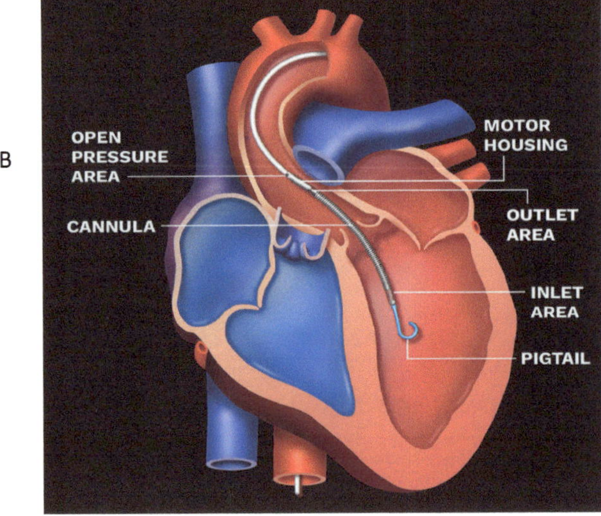

Fig.15.1 (A) Impella, the world's smallest heart pump, temporarily assists with the pumping function of a heart during a high-risk coronary intervention. The difference in this new procedure is that the access point is near the shoulder as opposed to the groin. It is estimated that less than one percent of interventional cardiologists have developed the meticulous skill set to use this new access point, which offers many benefits and advantages to the patient.(B) Illustrations showing important features and its passage from aorta to left ventricle

antegrade flow up to 2.5 L/min, 4.0 L/min, and 5.0 L/min, respectively. In comparison, the ability of the IABP to augment cardiac output is very modest; no more than 0.5 L/min. By continuously drawing blood from the LV, the Impella unloads the LV, thereby decreasing LV work and myocardial oxygen demand. In addition, by delivering large volumes of blood to the aorta, Impella operation results in an increase in mean arterial pressure and cardiac output, resulting, in turn, in improved systemic perfusion and increased coronary flow. Finally, Impella leads to a decrease in pulmonary wedge pressure and a secondary reduction in right ventricular afterload.

Indications for Impella Use

The most common indications for using Impella are in the treatment of ;-

- Acute myocardial infarction complicated by cardiogenic shock (AMICS) and to facilitate high risk PCI.
- Treatment of cardiomyopathy with acute decompensation,
- Postcardiotomy cardiogenic shock (PCCS),
- off-pump coronary bypass surgery

Cardiogenic Shock

For nearly 50 years, cardiologists and cardiac surgeons viewed the IABP as an often vital aid in the treatment of patients with cardiogenic shock. Accordingly, the publication in 2012 of the landmark randomized controlled IABP-SHOCK II trial left many of these physicians feeling quite bewildered. The results of this large scale, rigorously executed and meticulously analyzed study concluded that IABP did not reduce mortality in AMICS. 7 Indeed, such was the influence of this trial that use of IABP in AMICS fell from a class I to a class II-a indication in the United States and from a class I to a class II-b indication in Europe. Even when treated with an invasive approach (cardiac catheterization, PCI, or coronary bypass surgery) AMICS is associated with an in-hospital mortality approaching 40%. Accordingly, in recent years investigators have directed their attention to other forms of mechanical circulatory support systems that may reduce mortality in this challenging condition. The superior hemodynamic effects of the Impella system, as well as its relative ease of insertion, have led to considerable focus on this device as a possible way of making some dent on the frustratingly high mortality rate associated with cardiogenic shock.In recent years, there has been increasing evidence for the importance of early (i.e., prior to PCI) Impella implantation in improving survival in patients with AMICS. 36 Equally, routine performance of right and left heart catheterization (to allow calculation of measurements, such as cardiac power) has been advocated to optimize management of patients receiving Impella for AMICS. O'Neill et al designed a trial (the Detroit Cardiogenic Shock Initiative) in which both of these practices were routinely employed in AMICS patients. 35 Between July 2016 and April 2017, 41 patients with cardiogenic shock presenting to four metro Detroit sites were enrolled. Survival to explant for the entire cohort was 85%, a significant improvement from institutional historical controls (85 vs. 51%; $p < 0.001$). Moreover, survival to discharge was an impressive 76%. 37 These encouraging observations resulted in the launch of a national, multicenter, quality initiative entitled the National Cardiogenic Shock Initiative. This initiative will track metrics that have been associated with improved survival in AMICS. Included among these metrics are:

(1) Impella use prior to PCI,

(2) duration of shock to Impella support time of ≤90 minutes,

(3) attainment of cardiac power output > 0.6 W after completion of therapy. It is hoped that with optimal Impella use, survival rates of ≥80% can eventually be achieved in AMICS.

High-Risk Nonemergent PCI

Patients with multivessel or left main coronary artery disease and severely depressed left ventricular function are generally considered for mechanical revascularization by coronary artery bypass graft surgery, particularly if disabling anginal symptoms are present. However, in some of these patients, adverse clinical and angiographic features, such as multiple comorbidities, advanced age, or poor distal targets make surgery an unattractive option. Such patients may be considered for high-risk PCI. This option, of course, is also potentially hazardous as transient ischemia caused by coronary balloon or stent inflation may result in hemodynamic collapse or lethal dysrhythmias. Timely and effective mechanical circulatory support, initiated prior to intervention, may allow complex PCI without abrupt circulatory deterioration during coronary occlusion, thus allowing for more complete revascularization. 21 A large, contemporary, RCT examining the effects of IABP insertion prior to high-risk PCI, showed no reduction in the occurrence of major adverse cardiac events, such as death, stroke, or myocardial infarction. 8 As regards Impella supported PCI, feasibility and safety as well as registry studies have demonstrated that the Impella 2.5 system is safe, easy to implant, and provides excellent hemodynamic support during high-risk PCI. There has been one randomized controlled trial (the PROTECT II study) with regard to the potential benefits of Impella support in high-risk PCI. The 30-day incidence of major adverse events (the primary end point of the study) was not different for patients with IABP or Impella 2.5 hemodynamic support. However, trends for improved outcomes were observed for Impella 2.5-supported patients at 90 days

Impella Support for Other Indications

A growing indication for Impella use is to provide hemodynamic support during ablation of ventricular tachycardia (VT). It has been noted that 50 to 80% of patients with structural heart disease referred for VT ablation have unstable VT, thus making electrophysiological testing a considerable hemodynamic challenge. In the PERMIT 1 study Miller et al evaluated the hemodynamic support provided by the Impella 2.5 device during scar-related VT ablation in 20 patients.. During fast simulated VT, the device provided a considerably more favorable hemodynamic profile compared with pharmacological agents alone. The authors concluded that Impella supported scar-VT ablation was safe and feasible.

Suradi and Breall have reported use of the Impella device as a bridge to permanent LVAD placement. They described a patient who presented with cardiogenic shock secondary to giant cell myocarditis. The patient was supported hemodynamically with the Impella recover LP 2.5 device until a permanent LVAD could be surgically implanted. The Impella device has also been used to provide temporary mechanical circulatory support in patients with acute heart failure secondary to a variety of conditions, including postpartum cardiomyopathy, Takotsubo cardiomyopathy, and nonischemic cardiomyopathy.

Severe aortic stenosis has traditionally been viewed as a relative contraindication to use the Impella device. However, there have been a growing number of reports regarding successful and safe use of the device to support high risk aortic valvuloplasty and PCI. In addition, emergency use of the Impella device to treat acute circulatory collapse following transaortic valve replacement has been described.

Contraindications to the Impella Placement

The presence of thrombus in the LV is an important contraindication to the placement of the device. Thrombus may be sucked up by the Impella screw, blocking it and causing it to stop working. In addition, as with any other catheter placed in the LV, the Impella catheter has the potential to dislodge thrombus, thus potentially causing systemic embolization. Accordingly, if time permits, prior echocardiographic visualization of the LV to exclude thrombus is advised in all patients being considered for Impella placement. Moderate to severe aortic valve regurgitation is another important contraindication. In such patients, Impella support will increase aortic pressure and thus worsen aortic regurgitation and LV dilation. Severe peripheral vascular disease will preclude attempting Impella placement via the femoral artery. In such cases, consideration should be given to an axillary artery approach.

Complications

The main complications associated with the Impella device are related to vascular access site issues. Percutaneous femoral arterial access for the Impella 2.5 device is obtained with a 14F sheath. This is considerably bigger than the sheath size used for an angioplasty guide catheter (6F) or for an IABP (8F). Vascular complications include hematoma formation, bleeding requiring transfusion, and vascular injury requiring surgical intervention. Meticulous attention should be paid to selection and management of the access site for Impella support to reduce the complications associated with large bore sheaths.

Future Directions

A key future development will be decreasing the size of the Impella catheters so that they can be inserted percutaneously through smaller sized arterial sheaths. This will likely lead to a reduction in vascular complications and make the procedure more widely acceptable to operators.It is likely that there will soon be increasing adoptionof a strategy of early Impella placement in the treatment of patients with cardiogenic shock, as proposed in the National Cardiogenic Shock Initiative. In turn, it is hoped that this strategy will result in improved survival.

Conclusions

A growing body of registry and observational data suggest an important role for the Impella system in the treatment of cardiogenic shock. Recently, it has been appreciated that a strategy of early use of Impella (i.e., prior to performance of PCI) in shock patients is associated with improved survival. Equally, routine performance of right heart catheterization during an Impella-supported PCI helps to guide the therapy and may improve outcomes. There has, however, been, to date, a lack of evidence based on RCT to support a clear role for Impella in the treatment of cardiogenic shock. Equally, while there is much evidence for a useful place for Impella in facilitating selected high-risk PCI procedures, there are no definitive RCT data to support this. Accordingly, RCT examining these issues are urgently needed

Bibliography and Acknowledgement

- Abiomed Impella Quality (IQ) Database AbiomedDanvers, Massachusetts Abiomed surpasses 50,000 Impella patients treatedintheUnitedStates.DAIC,2017.
- Bangalore S, Gupta N, Guo Y et al.Outcomes with invasive vs conservative management of cardiogenic shock complicating acute myocardial infarction. Am J Med. 2015;128(06):601–608
- Cena M, Karam F, Ramineni R, Khalife W, Barbagelata A. New Impella cardiac power device used in patient with cardiogenic shock due to nonischemic cardiomyopathy. Int J Angiol. 2016;25(04):258–262
- Dixon S R, Henriques J P, Mauri L et al.A prospective feasibility trial investigating the use of the Impella 2.5 system in patients undergoing high-risk percutaneous coronary intervention (the PROTECT I trial): initial U.S. experience. JACC Cardiovasc Interv.2009;2(02):91–96
- Flaherty M P, Khan A R, O'Neill W W. Early initiation of Impella in acute myocardial infarction complicated by cardiogenic shock improves survival: a meta-analysis. JACC Cardiovasc Interv. 2017;10(17):1805–1806
- Glazier J J, Kaki A. Improving survival in cardiogenic shock: is Impella the answer? Am J Med. 2018;131 Siess T, Nix C, Menzler F. From a lab type to a product: a retrospective view on Impella's assist technology. Artif Organs. 2001;25(05):414–421

coronary intervention with the Impella 2.5 device the Europella registry. J Am Coll Cardiol. 2009;54(25):2430–2434

2. Extracorporeal Shock Wave Therapy for Coronary Artery Disease:

The current management of coronary artery disease (CAD) relies on three major therapeutic options, namely medication, percutaneous coronary intervention (PCI), and coronary artery bypass grafting (CABG). However, severe CAD that is not indicated for PCI or CABG still bears a poor prognosis due to the lack of effective treatments. In 2006, extracorporeal cardiac shock wave (SW) therapy reported on human for the first time. This treatment resulted in better myocardial perfusion as evaluated by dipyridamole stress thallium scintigraphy, angina symptoms, and exercise tolerance. Cardiac shock wave therapy (CSWT) is a newly developed method that utilizes a non-invasive application of low-intensity shock waves (SW), which induce the release of angiogenic factors such as endothelial nitric oxide synthase, vascular endothelial growth factor, and proliferating cell antinuclear antigen

Technique of SW therapy

As shown in Fig the patient should lay down on the bed in a supine position. No anesthesia was used during the therapy. Additionally, electrocardiography and the monitoring of blood pressure, respiration, and blood oxygen saturation were performed during the SW therapy each time. The machine is equipped with a shock wave generator and in-line echocardiography. The shock wave generator is attached to the chest wall of the patient. The shock wave pulse was easily focused on the ischemic myocardium under the guidance of echocardiography. There was no need of anesthesia or sedatives. The target myocardial regions and ischemic area were located by the echocardiography and single-photon emission computed tomography (SPECT), respectively. The SW was applied in an R-wave triggered manner to avoid inducing ventricular arrhythmias. In addition, 12-lead electrocardiography, blood chemistry testing (including troponin I and N-terminal pro-brain natriuretic peptide [NT-pro BNP]), and hematological analysis were performed before and after each session

All the patients are followed for three months after the SW therapy to evaluate any change in myocardial ischemia based on symptoms, adenosine stress thallium scintigraphy, transthoracic echocardiography, and blood biochemistry examinations.The patients continued their oral medications throughout the study period. Time course of symptoms are evaluated with the CCS class scores (i.e., 1: ordinary physical activity, 2: slight limitation of ordinary activity, 3: marked limitation of ordinary activity, 4: inability to perform any activity without angina or angina at rest).

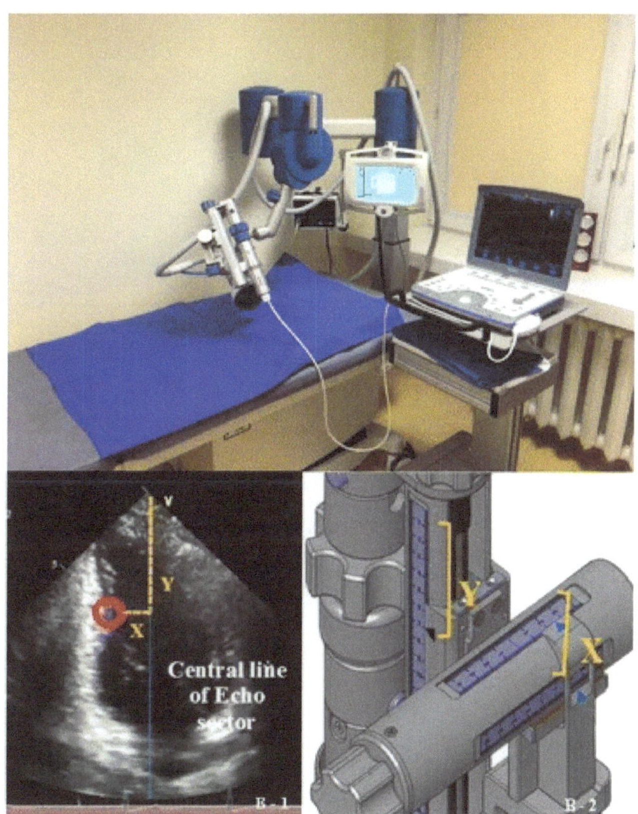

Fig.15.2 The methodology of cardiac shock wave therapy. a Shock wave generator system (Medispec, Germantown, MD, USA) and cardiac imaging system (Vivid i, GE Healthcare, Horten, Norway). b Shock wave focal zone alignment: Position of the sub-segment on the 2-dimensional image determined by X and Y coordinates . The shockwave applicator position is identically adjusted along X- and Y-axes corresponding to the X and Y coordinates of the ultrasound image.

How Can shockwave therapy affect your heart?

Cardiac shockwave therapy improves myocardial function in patients with refractory coronary artery disease by promoting VEGF and IL-8 secretion to mediate the proliferation of endothelial progenitor cells.

The various studies have demonstrated the potential efficacy and safety of cardiac SW therapy in CAD patients. After cardiac SW therapy, ischemic symptoms, and perfusion of CAD patients were significantly improved, and no SW complications were observed. As the findings revealed, symptom amelioration was associated with the improvement of ischemia in the CAD patients using extracorporeal SW therapy.

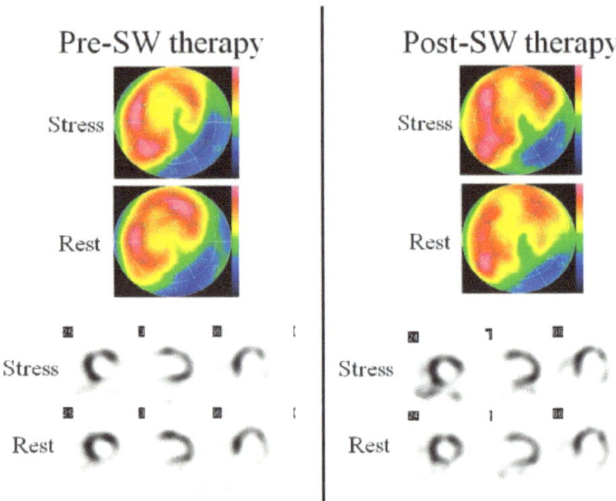

Fig.15.3 Stress myocardial perfusion scintigraphy in an elderly person had a history of myocardial infarction in the inferior wall. He suffered from diabetes mellitus, hypertension, and dyslipidemia. He was taking aspirin, angiotensin receptor blocker, calcium channel blocker, beta blocker, statin and nitrate. He was also ex-smoker. He had stenotic lesions in diagonal branch and periphery of the right coronary artery and left circumflex. From one month ago, chest pain at the time of exercise was recognized, and new lateral wall area ischemia and inferior wall infarction were confirmed by adenosine stress thallium scintigraphy His test results were CCS class II, SSS of 15, SRS of 11, SDS of 4, LVWMSI of 1.308, NT-proBNP of 113 pg/mL, and troponin I of less than 0.006 ng/mL. Due to the lack of indication for existing treatments, he underwent SW therapy for the lateral wall with ischemia. After SW therapy, both chest pain and lateral wall ischemia were improved. His test results after treatment were CCS class I, SSS of 10, SRS of 6, SDS of 4, LVWMSI of 1.182, NT-proBNP of 77 pg/mL, and troponin I of less than 0.006 ng/mL

What is coronary shockwave therapy?

Shockwave IVL, which harnesses the power of sonic pressure waves historically used to break up kidney stones through lithotripsy, is bringing new hope to individuals with severely calcified coronary artery disease and can eliminate the need for open heart surgery in some cases

Indications of coronary shockwave therapy

1. Patients with stable CAD proven by coronary angiography or computed tomography
2.Angiography, not amenable to revascularization,
3.Angina class II-IV (Canadian Cardiology Society, CCS), despite OMT,
4. Documented stress induced myocardial ischemia. Severly calcified coronary artery disease

Effect of SWT on clinical variables such as;-

1.Cardiac shock wave therapy has shown positive effect on exercise capacity
2.Cardiac shock wave therapy has demonstrated significant improvement in LV function
3.Cardiac SWT has demonstrated beneficial changes of myocardial perfusion associated with increase of LVEF
4.Cardiac shock wave therapy effect on angiogenesis markers Kikuchi et al. found that the number of circulating progenitor cells (CD 34+/ KDR+ and CD 34+/KDR+/c-kit+) in peripheral blood remained unchanged Cai et al. observed significant increase in the number of circulating progenitor cells (CD45low/CD34+/VEGFR2) in peripheral blood

Mechanism of generation of shock waves and cardiac shock wave treatment.-

Shock waves (SW) belong to acoustic waves that can be transmitted through a liquid medium and focused with a precision of several millimetres to any intended treatment area inside the body
In CAD patients, SW can be delivered to the border of the ischemic area to potentially induce neovascularization from the healthy area to the ischemic zone. Shock waves can be generated by discharge of a high-voltage spark under water or electromagnetic impulse. CSWT is performed using a SW generator system coupled with a cardiac ultrasound imaging system that is traditionally used to target the treatment to area with previously documented ischemia . SW are delivered via a special applicator through the anatomical acoustic window to the treatment area under electrocardiographic R-wave gating. For optimal therapy, the treatment area is divided into target zones corresponding to the size of the focal zone of the SW applicator

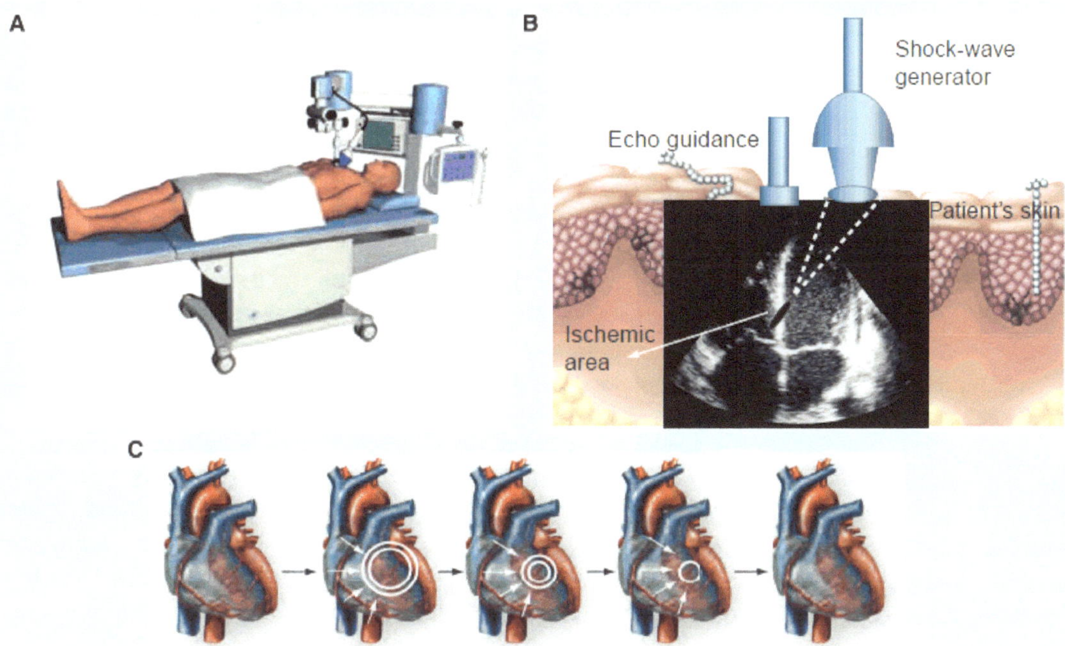

Fig.15.4: Extracorporeal cardiac shock-wave therapy. (A) The patient under electrocardiographic monitoring (B) receives, in the ischemic zones localized with ultrasound guidance, the shock waves produced by the generator that is attached to the chest wall. (C) At each session, cardiac shock-wave therapy is applied to the border of the ischemic area to potentially induce neovascularization from the healthy region to the ischemic area.

The Coronary Intravascular Lithotripsy System

The amount of coronary artery calcification increases with age and the presence of cardiovascular risk factors and comorbidities. Up to 20% of percutaneous coronary intervention (PCI) procedures are challenged by severe calcifications, and coronary calcifications have been shown to be an independent predictor of PCI failure and future adverse cardiac events. Lesion calcification increases procedural complexity and time. More specifically, calcium localisation (superficial or deep), distribution (focal, circumferential and longitudinal extension) and thickness influence procedural success, stent delivery and deployment.Several techniques to treat calcified lesions in native coronary arteries are available, including high-pressure and super-high pressure non-compliant balloons, cutting/scoring balloons, atherectomy devices, both rotational and orbital, and excimer lasers.

These devices rely on tissue compression and or tissue debulking, and have higher rates of procedural complications, such as dissections, perforations and distal embolisation. Moreover, their success rate is reduced when deep, thick or eccentric calcifications are present, and the induced tissue injury might accelerate uncontrolled neointimal growth and restenosis. So far, neither specialty balloons nor atherectomy devices have been proved to be superior to high-pressure non-compliant balloons in improving clinical outcome Recently, an alternative way to disrupt calcium has been developed that is based on the lithotripsy concept used to treat kidney and ureteral stones. The Intravascular Lithotripsy (IVL) System (Shockwave Medical) transforms electrical energy into mechanical energy during low-pressure balloon inflation.The technology does not rely on direct vascular tissue injury for plaque modification but on sonic waves, which travel from the balloon-based catheter to the surrounding tissue with the intention of safely and selectively breaking both superficial and deep calcium deposits with minimal soft tissue impairment, while improving vessel compliance.In contrast to debulking techniques, the calcium fragments resulting from the IVL therapy remain in situ, reducing the likelihood of distal embolisation.

Technical considerations

The Coronary IVL System consists of a portable, rechargeable generator, a connector cable with a push button to allow manually controlled delivery of electric pulses, and a 6 Fr compatible, rapid-exchange, semi-compliant balloon catheter to be used following standard angioplasty practice over a 0.014" guidewire.The semi-compliant balloon integrates two radiopaque lithotripsy emitters 6 mm apart and two conventional markers at the proximal and distal edges of the balloon. These emitters receive electrical pulses from the generator vaporising the fluid (a standard mixture of 50% NaCl 0.9% and 50% radiopaque contrast) within the balloon and creating a rapidly expanding and collapsing bubble. This bubble can transmit unfocused circumferential pulsatile mechanical energy into the vessel wall, in the form of sonic pressure waves equivalent to approximately 50 atmospheres (atm). The balloons are available in diameters ranging from 2.5 mm to 4.0 mm with a standard length of 12 mm their crossing profiles range from 0.043" to 0.046" The IVL therapy consists of a series of 10 pulses (1 cycle) or 10 seconds (1 pulse per second). The number of therapies needed per lesion will depend on lesion resistance; however, the maximum number of pulses to be delivered by each individual catheter is limited to 80 pulses (eight cycles)

Intravascular Lithotripsy Procedure

The IVL procedure does not require high level additional training for interventional cardiologists. The shockwave balloon must be sized accordingly to the reference vessel diameter (ratio 1:1), placed in the target calcified lesion and inflated up to 4 atm to ensure apposition to the vessel wall; the lithotripsy emitters are then activated to deliver the acoustic pulses by pushing the button on the connector cable. Once a cycle of 10 pulses has been delivered, the balloon can be inflated up to 6 atm (nominal pressure) to increase balloon compliance and to assess symmetrical expansion, confirming calcium modification.

Next, the balloon is deflated carefully to allow small air bubbles to escape. The previous steps must be repeated for each intended IVL cycle and at least two IVL cycles are recommended to treat the target area. For the treatment of lesions longer than 12 mm, the catheter needs to be repositioned and overlapping treatment areas might occur. Due to the slightly higher profile of the shockwave catheter, pre-dilatation with standard balloons might be necessary in some cases to facilitate deliverability and positioning, especially when lumen reduction is severe. Notwithstanding this, the balloon allows the use of guide-catheter extenders and buddy-wire support. Furthermore, although the system is labelled 6 Fr compatible, it could be used with a 5 Fr guiding catheter where the radial artery is small..The use of dilatation with non-compliant balloons after IVL, although not mandatory, could be considered to expand the lumen further. Moreover, aggressive plaque modification devices such as cutting/scoring balloons or atherectomy could be used as adjuvant therapy in challenging lesions to improve results

Potential Uses

At present, the instructions for use of the Shockwave Coronary IVL System restrict its use to lesion preparation in native coronary arteries . Given it is assumed to be safer than previous approaches, the number of case reports and small case series reporting on its use in more challenging scenarios is increasing.

1.Acute Coronary Syndromes

Calcified lesions in culprit vessels are common in patients presenting with acute coronary syndromes (moderate calcification is found 26.1% of these patients and severe calcification in 5.9%), and their presence is a strong predictor of definite stent thrombosis (HR 1.62; 95% CI [1.14–2.30]; p=0.007) and target lesion revascularisation (HR 1.44; 95% CI [1.17–1.78]; p<0.001). The Disrupt CAD study included only patients with stable and unstable angina. Although there is not enough evidence to support the use of the IVL during primary PCI, early experience has shown favourable results.

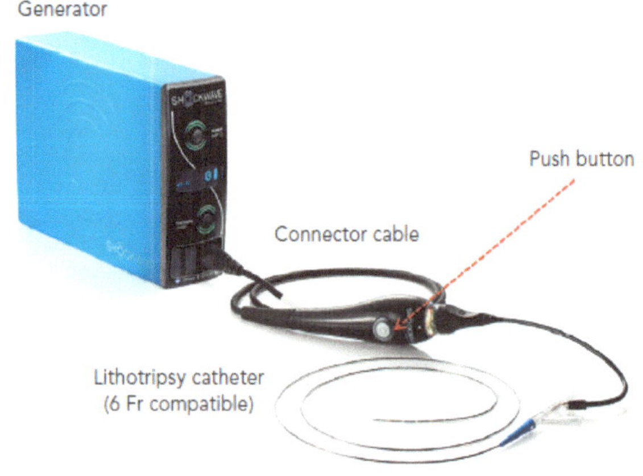

Fig. 15.5 Shockwave coronary intravascular lithoplasty system

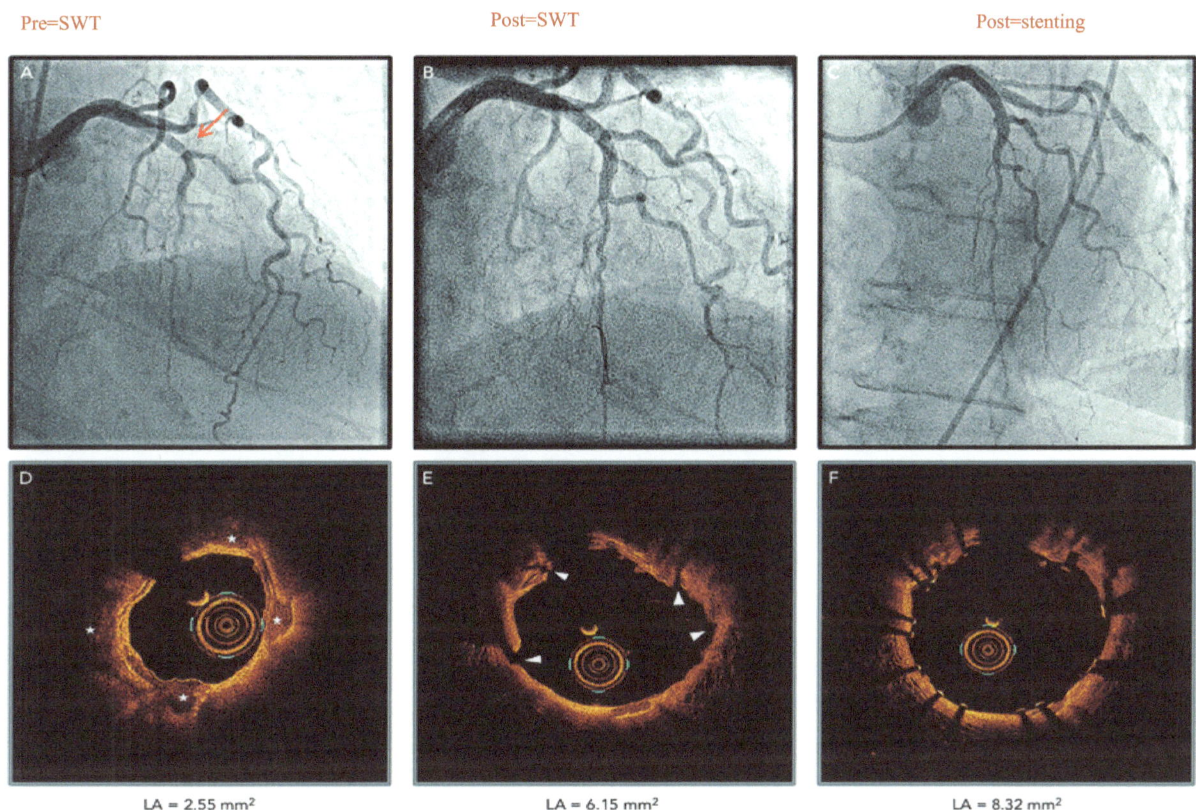

Fig 15.6. Intravascular Lithoplasty Therapy: Effect on Heavy Calcified Coronary Lesions

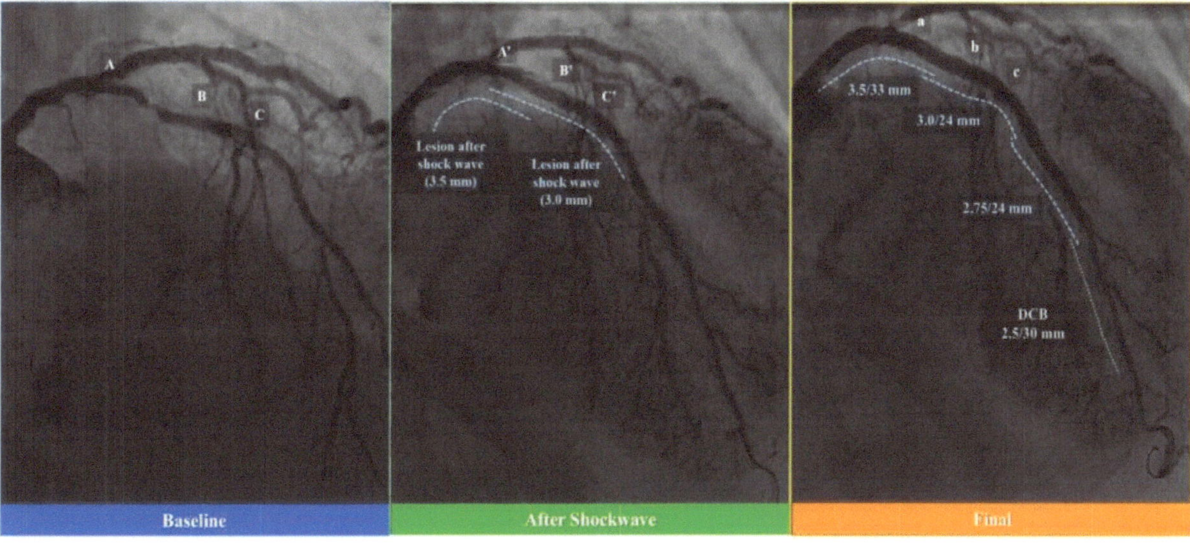

Fig.15.7 Serial coronary angiograms of the representative case treated with shockwave intravascular lithotripsy

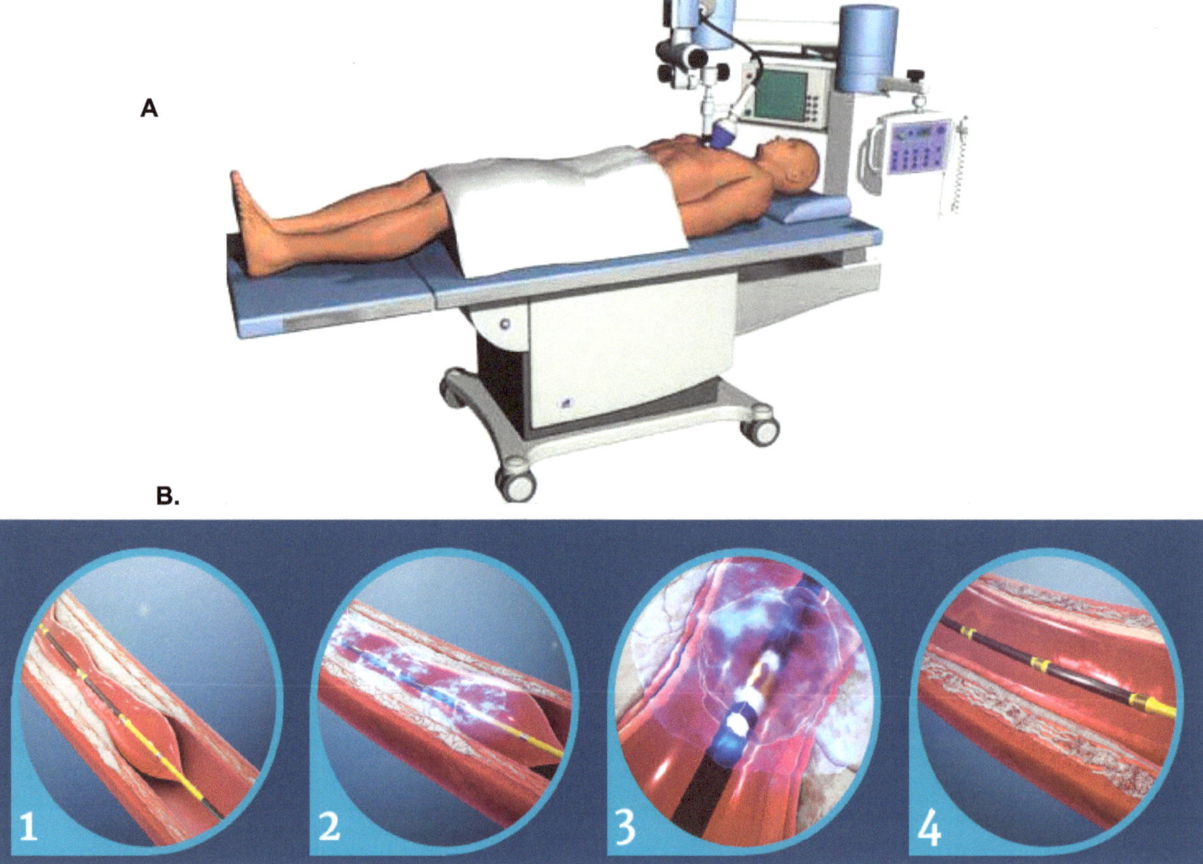

Fig 15.8 **Shockwave IVL** **(A)** Shockwave IVL Machine with table . **(B)**The device is composed of a fine 0.014-inch guidewire with an array of lithotripsy emitters enclosed in an integrated balloon. This enables clinicians to use the same minimally invasive technique as balloon angioplasty to get directly to the site of calcified lesions and transmit the sonic pressure waves to the blood vessel wall, to fracture calcium and make the arteries easier to dilate.

2.Unprotected Left Main Calcified Stenosis

PCI has become an option for the treatment of left main (LM) disease, with a class IA recommendation for patients with a SYNTAX score ≤22 and class IIA for a SYNTAX score 23–32. Calcification increases procedural complexity and therefore the risk of complications. Although atherectomy has previously been proposed as a valid and feasible option, the high-risk profile of those patients means safer approaches would be welcome.The Coronary IVL System, with controlled pulses delivered under low pressure, might potentially improve plaque modification with a lower risk of vessel closure, perforation or embolisation.

3.Chronic Total Occlusions

Moderate to severe calcification is frequently found in chronic total occlusions, and debulking devices are usually avoided because the procedure is difficult and has a high risk of complications; where standard balloons fail, the Coronary IVL System might be useful in facilitating lumen dilatation and communication with the subintimal space.

4.Stent Underexpansion due to Underlying Calcification

Although the technique has been developed to treat calcified lesions in native coronary arteries before stenting, patients with severe stent underexpansion because of heavy calcification are at a higher risk of stent failure and future adverse events. Until now, undilatable lesions in previously stented segments have been courageously approached with debulking devices such as cutting balloons and atherectomy, with unpredictable results and risks of procedural complications and stent damage.Of note, the effectiveness of those techniques is limited by the presence of metallic struts, and deeper calcifications therefore remain unaffected. The circumferential sonic waves of the Coronary IVL System, conversely, have the advantage of extending beyond strut layers and fracture deeper calcium deposits.Several case reports have supported the use of the technology for optimising stent expansion without complications.The efficacy of the system in segments with multiple layers of stents has not been demonstrated and its impact on stent backbone/polymer integrity and drug elution is still unknown. Nonetheless, at present, there are no alternative percutaneous options for patients left with underexpanded stents due to heavy calcification.

5.Effects on Cardiac Rhythm

Electric signals similar to pacing spikes on the electrocardiogram (ECG) tracing during pulse-delivery have been described.17,40–42 These so-called 'shocktopics' and asynchronous cardiac pacing have been reported in up to 77.8% of the cases, with a 16-fold increased risk in patients with a heart rate <65 BPM. Cardiac pacing has not been linked to any specific number of IVL cycles or coronary artery anatomy, although its frequency is higher when either the left anterior descending artery or the right coronary artery are treated. The exact mechanism behind this phenomenon is still unclear. A potential explanation might be that the transformed mechanical energy reaches and couples with the cardiac conduction system producing ectopic atrial and or ventricular captures

Although no relevant clinical events have been reported, it warrants paying special attention to ECG and aortic pressure waveforms changes during IVL administration; the resulting VOO pacing mode is theoretically pro-arrhythmic (potential R on T phenomenon) and, until further data become available, pacemaker carriers should be assessed for inappropriate device sensing during the IVL cycles and to ensure correct pacing function post-procedure. Further investigation in the matter will be provided by the substudies in the Disrupt CAD III trial.

Challenging Lesions

Some lesions might respond better to IVL therapy than to other plaque modification approaches. Reports have pointed out the usefulness of the IVL therapy on creating calcium fractures as assessed with intravascular ultrasound, and achieving optimal stent expansion in undilatable lesions that have been resistant to specialty balloons and rotational atherectomy.

In contrast, some lesions might not be suitable for IVL treatment or may remain resistant after the application of all 80 pulses. Severe tortuosity or angulation, critical lumen reduction, plaque indentation into the lumen and a very low vessel expansion compliance (small vessels and multiple stent layers present), could impact balloon deliverability and positioning. Up to 46% of the lesions might also require dedicated lesion pre-dilatation and/or post-dilatation with non-compliant balloons or could benefit from adjuvant lesion preparation with conventional devices such as specialty balloons or atherectomy to either facilitate balloon delivery or increase calcium compliance after lithotripsy therapy

While balloon rupture is uncommon, it can cause vessel complications. Case reports have described sudden IVL balloon burst during lithotripsy therapy with important vessel dissection; however, it is fair to highlight that either critical stenosis or severe vessel tortuosity were present, which suggests that, in some anatomies, the IVL system might not be suitable or should be used with caution Furthermore, vessels with a diameter >4 mm (maximum shockwave balloon size) or important plaque eccentricity preclude appropriate IVL balloon apposition to the vessel wall, and may reduce the efficacy of the therapy. More data are needed on the specific efficacy of IVL in concentric versus eccentric lesions. In the Disrupt CAD study, 22% of the patients had eccentric plaques; nevertheless, overall device success was 98%

Moreover, performing intracoronary imaging where important coronary calcification is suspected during the angiographic assessment could help to accurately assess calcium distribution, localisation and thickness. The use of intracoronary imaging before and after lithotripsy therapy could not only assist the appropriate selection of IVL balloon sizes but also potentially help to identify IVL responders and identify patients who might need adjuvant therapy from other plaque-modification devices .

Conclusion

The Coronary IVL System is a promising new treatment modality to tackle moderate to severe calcified coronary lesions, with a high rate of success .

Bibliography and Acknowledgement

- Caspari GH, Erbel R: Revascularization withextracorporeal cardiac shock wave therapy:first clinical results. Circulation100(Suppl. 19), 84 (1999).
- Capaccio P, Torretta S, Pignataro L:Extracorporeal lithotripsy techniques forsalivary stones. Otolaryngol. Clin. North Am.42, 1139–1159 (2009).
- Fukumoto Y, Ito A, Uwatoku T et al.:Extracorporeal cardiac shock wave therapyameliorates myocardial ischemia in patientswith severe coronary artery disease. Coron.Artery Dis. 17, 63–70 (2006).
- Gutersohn A, Marlinghaus E: Comparision of cardiac shock wave therapy and percutanousmyocardial laser revascularization therapy inendstage CAD patient with refractory angina.Eur. Heart J. 27(Suppl. 1), 351 (2006).Haupt G, Haupt A, Ekkernkamp A, GeretyB, Chvapil M: Influence of shock waves onfracture healing. Urology 39, 529–532(1992).
- Khattab AA, Brodersen B,Schuermann-Kuchenbrandt D et al.:Extracorporeal cardiac shock wave therapy:first experience in the everyday practice fortreatment of chronic refractory anginapectoris. Int. J. Cardiol. 121, 84–85(2007).
- Kikuchi Y, Ito K, Ito Y et al.: Double-blindand placebo-controlled study of theeffectiveness and safety of extracorporealcardiac shock wave therapy for severeangina pectoris. Circ. J. 74, 589–591(2010).
- Manganotti P, Amelio E: Long-term effect ofshock wave therapy on upper limb hypertoniain patients affected by stroke. Stroke 36,1967–1971 (2005).
- Nishida T, Shimokawa H, Oi K et al.:Extracorporeal cardiac shock wave therapymarkedly ameliorates ischemia-inducedmyocardial dysfunction in pigs in vivo.Circulation 110, 3055–3061 (2004).
- Parsi MA, Stevens T, Lopez R, Vargo JJ:Extracorporeal shock wave lithotripsy forprevention of recurrent pancreatitis caused byobstructive pancreatic stones. Pancreas. 39,153–155 (2010).
- Prinz C, Lindner O, Bitter T et al.:Extracorporeal cardiac shock wave therapyameliorates clinical symptoms and improvesregional myocardial blood flow in a patientwith severe coronary artery disease andrefractory angina. Case Report Med. 2009,639594 (2009).
- Seitz C, Fajkovic H, Waldert M et al.:Extracorporeal shock wave lithotripsy in thetreatment of proximal ureteral stones: doesthe presence and degree of hydronephrosisaffect success? Eur. Urol. 49, 378–383(2006).
- Sems A, Dimeff R, Iannotti JP:Extracorporeal shock wave therapy in thetreatment of chronic tendinopathies. J. Am.Acad. Orthop. Surg. 14, 195–204 (2006).
- Song J, Qi M, Kaul S, Price RJ: Stimulationof arteriogenesis in skeletal muscle bymicrobubble destruction with ultrasound.Circulation 106, 1550–1555 (2002).
- Tandan M, Reddy DN, Santosh D et al.:Extracorporeal shock wave lithotripsy of largedifficult common bile duct stones: efficacyand analysisof factors that favor stonefragmentation. J. Gastroenterol. Hepatol. 24,1370–1374 (2009).
- Wang CJ, Huang HY, Pai CH: Shockwave-enhanced neovascularization at thetendon-bone junction: an experiment indogs. J. Foot Ankle Surg. 41, 16–22(2002).
- Young SR, Dyson M: The effect oftherapeutic ultrasound onangiogenesis. Ultrasound Med. Biol. 16,261–269 (1990).
- Zelle BA, Gollwitzer H, Zlowodzki M,Buhren V: Extracorporeal shock wavetherapy: current evidence. J. Orthop. Trauma24(Suppl. 1) S66–S70 (2010).

Transmyocardial revascularization with a carbon dioxide laser

Transmyocardial laser revascularization (TMR or TMLR) is a procedure used to improve the flow of oxygen-rich blood to the heart muscle. It reduces the effects of angina (chest pain), a symptom of coronary artery disease. The heart needs oxygen-rich blood to survive, which the coronary arteries deliver. Coronary artery disease causes clogged coronary arteries, resulting in decreased blood flow to the heart. A lack of oxygen-rich blood to the heart leads to ischemia, increasing the risk of angina and heart attack.

People who have coronary artery disease are treated with either medication, angioplasty, stenting, or coronary artery bypass surgery to enhance blood flow to the heart muscle. Some may remain symptomatic, such as angina, even after conventional therapies have been exhausted. TMR is often the safest and most effective alternative for such people.

What is transmyocardial laser revascularization?

Transmyocardial laser revascularization (TMR) is a type of surgery that uses a laser to make tiny channels through the heart muscle into the lower-left chamber of the heart to improve oxygen-rich blood flow.

TMR can do the following:

- Improve myocardial oxygenation
- Eliminate or reduce angina
- Improve the cardiovascular function
- Relieve chest pain
- Improve the quality of life
- Reduce the frequency of hospital admissions

How does transmyocardial laser revascularization work?

Transmyocardial laser revascularization is based on the use of a high-powered carbon dioxide laser. The laser interjects a strong energy pulse into the left ventricle, vaporizing the ventricular muscle and creating a transmural channel with a 1-mm diameter.

- This eventually improves the blood flow to the heart.
- The tiny channels act as bloodlines. The pumping of the ventricle sends oxygen-rich

- The tiny channels act as bloodlines. The pumping of the ventricle sends oxygen-rich blood through these channels, restoring blood flow to the heart muscle.
- The procedure promotes angiogenesis (the growth of new capillaries or blood vessels that help supply blood to the heart muscle).

What are the indications for transmyocardial laser revascularization?

Although coronary artery bypass grafting is effective in most people, transmyocardial laser revascularization (TMR) is a treatment option for:

- Severe angina (that limits daily activities or causes sleep disruption despite medications)
- Ischemia (decreased blood supply to the heart muscle), which is identified using nuclear perfusion scan
- Coronary artery disease, which does respond to or is not eligible for other traditional procedures
- People with a history of bypass surgery or angioplasty

TMR is contraindicated for people with:

- Severely damaged heart muscle is due to heart attacks
- No areas of ischemia in the heart muscle
- Infarcted or scarred heart tissues
- Severe adhesions due to prior coronary artery bypass surgery

What tests determine the need for transmyocardial laser revascularization?

Apart from a thorough medical history and physical examination, tests required before transmyocardial laser revascularization include:

- Cardiac catheterization
- Other tests to determine the blood flow and the pumping ability of the heart
- Echocardiogram
- Positron emission tomography scan
- Dobutamine echocardiography
- Cardiac MRI

How is a transmyocardial laser revascularization performed?

Before the procedure

Let your cardiologist know all medications including prescription, over-the-counter, and supplements that you are taking.

- You may undergo certain tests, such as an electrocardiogram, blood tests, urine tests, and a chest X-ray, to analyze your current health condition.
- Avoid smoking at least two weeks before the surgery, which may help reduce the risk of excessive bleeding.
- Do not eat or drink anything after midnight the night before the surgery

During the procedure

An electrocardiogram machine monitors your heart's rhythm and electrical activity. It is attached to your chest through small metal disks called electrodes.

- An intravenous line is established to administer anesthesia during surgery.
- A mild tranquilizer is administered to help you relax before entering the operating room.
- After you are completely asleep, a tube is inserted down the trachea and connected to a respirator, which will allow breathing.
- Another tube is inserted through the nose and throat and into your stomach to stop liquid and air from collecting in the stomach.
- The surgeon makes an incision in the left side of the chest to access the left ventricle and uses a special carbon dioxide laser to make 20 to 40 tiny channels (1 mm wide) in the heart muscle to achieve complete blood flow to the heart.
- The entire transmyocardial laser revascularization procedure typically takes about two hours.

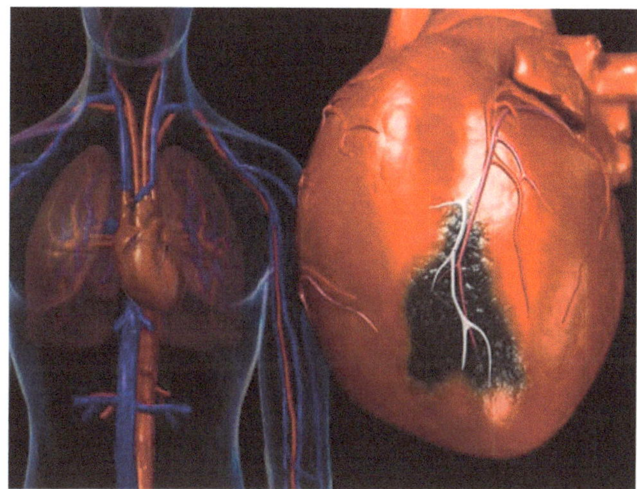

Fig.15.9 Restricted flow in a coronary artery causing decreased oxygen supply. Courtesy MedicineNet.

How does TMR work?

Transmyocardial revascularization (TMR) remedies this by using laser to create vascular tissues to supply blood to the the outer walls of the heart. The method was called "snake heart procedure" for sometime, in

Transmyocardial revascularization (TMR) remedies this by using laser to create vascular tissues to supply blood to the the outer walls of the heart. The method was called "snake heart procedure" for sometime, in analogy with reptilian hearts that supply blood to the heart muscle through channels that extend from heart chambers.

In a transmyocardial procedure, high energy pulsed laser beams are used to create 20 to 40 incisions from the outer wall to the left ventricle. Each incision is about a millimeter in diameter. The incisions allow blood to carry oxygen to the outer walls of the heart. The holes in the heart are clotted to be sealed shut and heal within days. Over the months, these incisions promote angiogenesis, which is the formation of new vascular tissue on the outer walls of the heart.

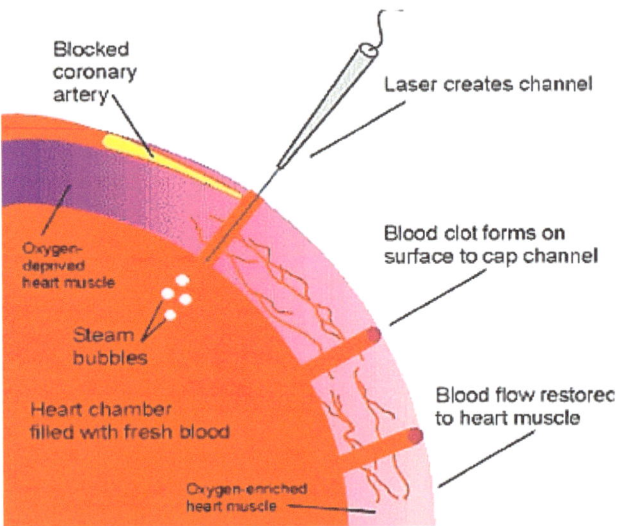

Fig.15.10 Cross section of Tranmyocardial incisions. Courtesy UWHealth.

Transmyocardial procedure has several advantages compared to other procedures. Most importantly, the heart is not stopped as in a bypass surgery, and the procedure is a lot less invasive compared with an open heart surgery. The procedure does however require an incision between the patients ribs to reach to the heart

Not surprisingly, TMR has also a faster recovery time compared to a bypass surgery. Medicinal researchers are currently exploring the use of so-called percutaneous TMR (PTMR) to prevent the need of a chest incision to reach the heart. In PTMR, the laser energy is delivered through a catheter inserted through an artery to reach the heart.

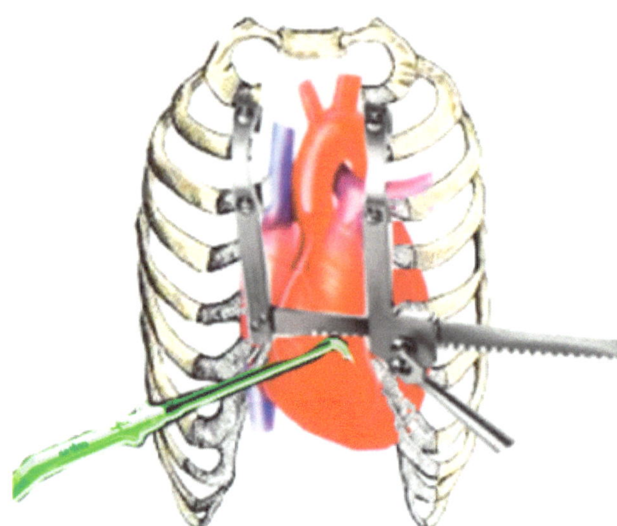

Fig.15.11 showing open sternum ,with retractor and heart underneath for laser energy livery in TMR. Courtesy Medscape.

Laser Doppler Flowmetry for Transmyocardial Surgery

TMR procedure requires monitoring the blood flow in the newly formed vascular tissue and reading flow levels right below the clotted region. Laser doppler flowmetry (LDF) is the primary technique for this purpose. To measure the flow rate, doctors use emitting and receiving fibers to register the reflected from hemoglobin light. The received Doppler shifted wavelength provides information about the velocity of the blood cells. The image below shows a simple setup using LDF during such a heart surgery.

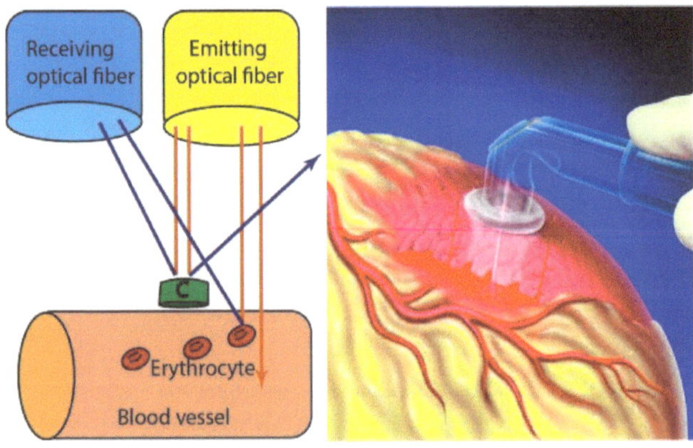

Fig 15.12 showing Laser Doppler Flowmetry for Transmyocardial Surgery.

The most effective lasers for TMR are CO2 and Ho:YAG. Other lasers such as Nd:YAG, Eb:YAG have been explored experimentally, but none have been pursed on a significant scale for clinical applications. At the moment, only CO2 and Ho:YAG are clinically approved for transmyocardial incisions. CO2 operates at a wavelength of 10.6 um, and Ho:YAG at 2.12 um. The primary mechanism of tissue ablation for both of these lasers is the absorption of light by the water contained in the heart tissue. Since water absorbs strongly at these wavelengths, the transfer of energy is very efficient. Care must be taken while using the Ho:YAG laser in the pulsed mode. If significant time is not present between two pulses, accumulated heat can cause tissue to explode under pressure. The operation parameters for Ho:YAG is 6-8 W/pulse. The CO2 laser for TMR operates at a slightly higher pulse energy.

After the procedure

- Stay in the hospital for four to seven days.
- Rest and limit your activities for at least four to six weeks.
- Though the symptoms of coronary artery disease and angina get better, it may take three months or more for complete improvement.

Post-Surgery Effects

Most of the laser drilled channels are closed soon after the surgery. However, the short-lived flow of the blood through the channels continues to stimulate oxygen supply to the heart wall. Even though the theoretical details of why new blood vessels appear in TMR are not clear, its practical efficacy has been demonstrated. Since its FDA approval in 1998, it has been the only procedure for treating patients with severe coronary problems, with only patients with unstable angia or reduced left ventricular function not benefiting from this procedure.

What are the complications of TMR?

The potential complications of transmyocardial laser revascularization include:

- Supraventricular tachycardia
- Pleural effusion
- Incisional pain from the thoracotomy
- Postoperative myocardial infarctions

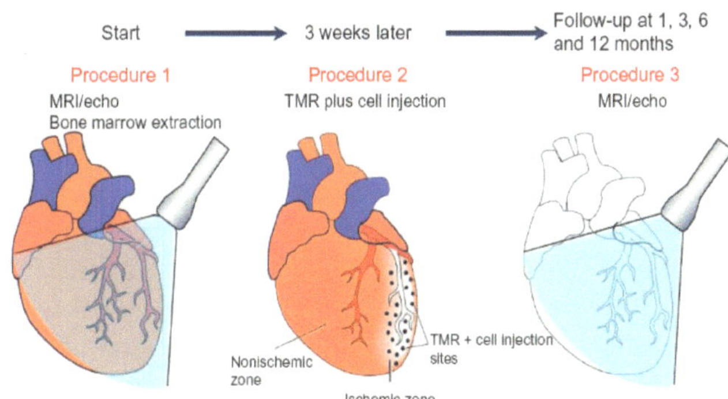

Fig.15.13 **Stages for post-surgery effects.** Over the weeks of the surgery, the formed incisions promote angiogenesis. This is shown in the image below.

Bibliography and Acknowledgement

- AabergeLRootweltKBlomhoffSSaatvedtKAbdelnoorMForfangKContinued symptomatic improvement three to five years after transmyocardial revascularization with CO(2) laser: a late clinical follow-up of the Norwegian Randomized trial with transmyocardial revascularizationJ Am Coll with refractory angina: a randomised controlled trialLancet19993539152519524100289 79
- Babin-EbellJSieversHHCharitosEITransmyocardiallaser revascularization combined with intramyocardial endothelial progenitor cell transplantation in patients with intractable ischemic heart disease ineligible for conventional revascularization: preliminary results in a highly selected small patient cohortThorac Cardiovasc Surg201058111162007 2970
- CampeauLLetter:GradingofanginapectorisCirculation1976543522523947585
- DowlingRDPetracekMRSelingerSLAllenKBTransmyocardial revascularization in patients with refractory, unstable anginaCirculation199898Suppl 19II73II75discussion II75–II769852884
- Eckert SHorstkotteDManagement of angina pectoris: the role of spinal cord stimulationAm J Cardiovasc Drugs200991172819178129
- GasslerNWintzerHOStubbeHMWullbrandAHelmchenUTransmyocardial laser revascularization. Histological features in human nonresponder myocardiumCirculation19979523713759008451
- HorvathKAClinical studies of TMR with the CO2 laserJ Clin Laser Med Surg19971562812859641084
- KadipaşaogluKASartoriMMasaiTIntraoperative arrhythmias and tissue damage during transmyocardial laser revascularizationAnn Thorac Surg1999672423431 10197664
- WeintraubWSJonesELCraverJMGuytonRAFrequency of repeat coronary bypass or coronary angioplasty after coronary artery bypass surgery using saphenous venous graftsAm J Cardiol19947321031128296729
- YanoOJBielefeldMRJeevanandamVPrevention of acute regional ischemia with endocardial laser channelsAnn Thorac Surg19935614653 8328875

Enhanced external counterpulsation (EECP) improves exercise tolerance

Conventional treatments for patients with symptomatic coronary artery disease (CAD) include medication, coronary angioplasty and coronary artery bypass grafting. These conventional treatments have made it possible to successfully treat such patients . However, a number of patients still do not adequately respond to such treatments, and some patients are not candidates for coronary angioplasty or coronary artery bypass grafting for several reasons.

Enhanced external counterpulsation (EECP) may be an alternative nonpharmacologic therapy for patients with symptomatic CAD. Enhanced external counterpulsation involves sequential inflation and deflation of compressive cuffs wrapped around the lower extremities. The cuffs are sequentially inflated from calf to thigh to buttocks proximally during diastole with rapid deflation of all cuffs at the beginning of systole. These sequential events may theoretically result in increased diastolic aortic pressure and cardiac output and decreased cardiac afterload . Recently, it has been shown that EECP is effective in relieving angina and improving exercise tolerance in patients with chronic angina pectoris . Moreover, the beneficial effects of EECP have been shown to last for long-term periods . Some objective improvements of ischemia by EECP have been reported , but they need to be confirmed. And detailed evaluations of hemodynamics have not been reported. Accordingly, this study was designed to uncover objective evidence of improvement of myocardial ischemia by thallium scintigraphy and to obtain detailed hemodynamic and humoral data. We found that EECP reduces myocardial ischemia and improves diastolic filling in patients with CAD. **EECP** Enhanced external counterpulsation equipment (Vasomedical Inc., Westbury, New York) used in this study consisted of an air compressor, a console, a treatment table and two sets of three cuffs. After these cuffs were wrapped around the patient's legs, compressed air pressure was applied via the cuffs to the lower extremities in a sequence synchronized with the cardiac cycle. The diastolic augmentation pressure was progressively increased by increasing external compression. In this study, the pressure applied to the cuffs during EECP was set at 300 mm Hg. Blood pressure changes were continuously monitored by finger plethysmography. To assess the hemodynamic effect of EECP, the diastolic to systolic pressure ratio was calculated. In this study, the mean diastolic to systolic pressure ratio was 1.1 ± 0.4, showing effective diastolic augmentation. There were no major complications during EECP treatment in any of the patients. No other therapeutic interventions were performed during the study.

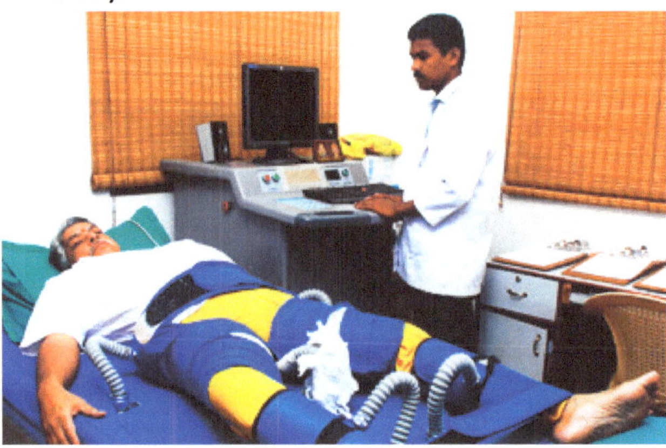

Fig.15.14 The patient with chest pain is undergoing Enhanced external counterpulsation (EECP)

What conditions can EECP therapy treat?

Your healthcare provider may recommend EECP if you have;-

- Chest pain.
- Cough.
- Fatigue.
- Shortness of breath (dyspnea).

EECP can also help other conditions, including:

- Cardiac syndrome X (a type of angina).
- Cerebrovascular disease.
- Heart failure.
- Kidney (renal) failure.
- Left ventricular dysfunction (an early stage of heart failure).
- Lung disease (pulmonary disease).
- Peripheral artery (vascular) disease (PAD).
- EECP cannot treat unstable angina (acute coronary syndrome). This type of angina causes more severe, more frequent and longer-lasting symptoms. Symptoms develop suddenly, even while you rest.

How does EECP therapy work?

EECP treatment applies pressure to blood vessels in your lower limbs. The pressure increases blood flow back to your heart, so your heart works better. When your heart pumps better, symptoms ease.

This type of therapy can also encourage blood vessels to open new pathways for blood to flow to your heart. These pathways eventually become "natural bypass" vessels that help relieve symptoms of angina if your coronary arteries are narrowed or blocked.

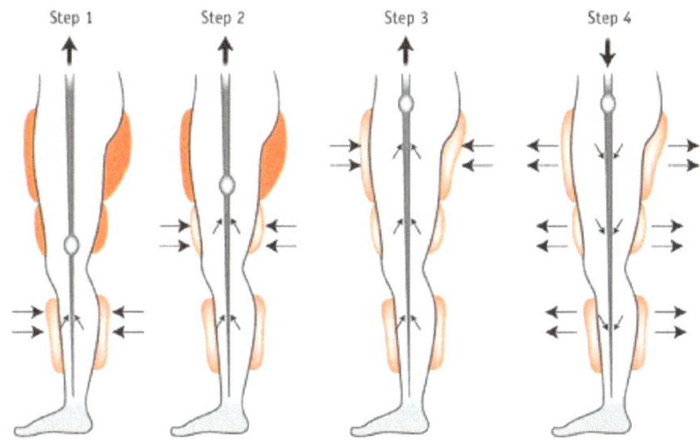

Fig 15.15 Technique of EECP Three pairs of pneumatic cuffs are applied to the calves, lower thighs, and upper thighs. The cuffs are inflated sequentially during diastole, distal to proximal. The compression of the lower-extremity vascular bed increases diastolic pressure and flow and increases venous return. Inflation and deflation are timed according to the R-wave on the patient's cardiac monitor.

Who is eligible for EECP therapy?

You may be eligible for EECP therapy if you:

- Have long-term chest pain or pressure that comes and goes during physical activity or stress.
- No longer experience relief with medication.
- Don't qualify for an invasive procedure like surgery.
- Experience renewed symptoms after an invasive procedure such as bypass surgery, angioplasty or stenting.

Who should not undergo EECP therapy?

Talk to your healthcare provider about whether you qualify for EECP therapy. EECP therapy isn't recommended for people who are pregnant. Providers may recommend other options for people who have pacemakers or conditions such as:

- Aortic insufficiency.
- Atrial fibrillation (Afib).
- Blood clots.
- Congenital heart disease.
- Enlarged heart (cardiomegaly).
- Heart valve disease.
- Hemorrhage.
- High blood pressure (hypertension).
- Irregular heartbeat.
- Fast heart rate (tachycardia).
- Hypertrophic cardiomyopathy.
- Pulmonary hypertension (PH).
- Severe peripheral vascular disease.

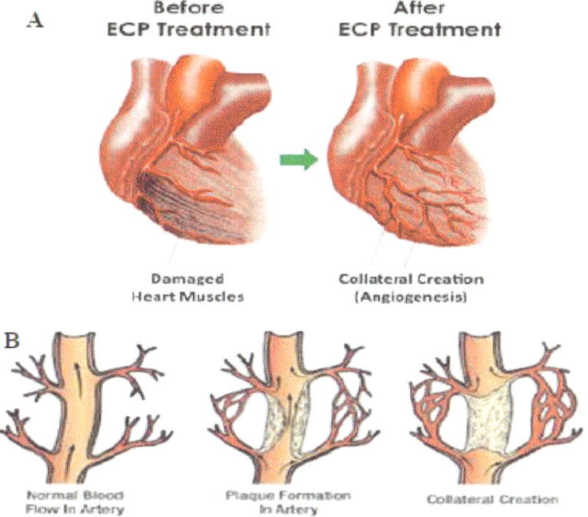

Fig.15.16: (A) Showing damaged heart muscle due to heart attack (left)and multiple natural bypass after EECP(Right) (B) Showing normal blood supply of the heart (left) ,plaque formation (middle)and development of natural collateral circulation after EECP (right)

Is EECP therapy a common procedure?

Hundreds of thousands of people worldwide have received EECP therapy. This treatment relieves heart disease symptoms that can't be controlled by medicine or treated with surgery.

What happens before EECP therapy?

Before you receive EECP therapy, a healthcare provider performs a physical exam and exercise stress test.

Your provider also explains the procedure and equipment involved.

Immediately before treatment, a provider:

- Asks you to empty your bladder and change into special treatment pants.
- Places three electrocardiogram (EKG) patches on your chest and inflatable cuffs around your legs and buttocks. The cuffs connect to air hoses.
- Gives you a finger sensor to check blood oxygen and pressure levels, so providers can adjust therapy for best results.

What happens during EECP therapy?

During EECP therapy, you relax or nap on a padded table while air fills the cuffs around your lower limbs. You'll feel the cuffs grow tighter around your legs and bottom until they reach full treatment pressure. EKG and blood pressure monitors synchronize inflation and deflation with your heartbeat. The cuffs inflate as soon as your heart rests, increasing blood supply to the arteries that deliver blood to your heart. Then they quickly deflate to make it easier for your heart to pump again.Once you get used to the sensation, therapy should be comfortable. It shouldn't cause pain or discomfort. You can return to your regular daily routine after treatment.

How long does EECP therapy last?

EECP therapy is an outpatient treatment. You usually have it for a total of 35 hours: one hour a day, five days a week, for seven weeks.You can also have it twice daily for three and a half weeks. You have a one-hour session, a break and then another session.

How will I feel after EECP therapy?

Responses to EECP therapy vary. You may feel tired for several days after treatment. Most people say symptoms feel improvement in the last couple of weeks of the seven-week treatment.

Can I have EECP therapy more than once?

Talk to your healthcare provider if your symptoms return. About 20% of people need repeat EECP therapy, especially if they didn't complete the initial 35 hour course.

What are the advantages of EECP therapy?

Research shows many people report improved symptoms for up to a few years after EECP treatment. They say they experience:

- Fewer and less frequent symptoms of angina, including chest pain.
- Increased energy.
- More ability to be active or exercise without symptoms.
- Reduced need for medication.

What are the risks or complications of EECP therapy?

Complications from treatment are usually minor. Most people don't experience any major side effects, discomfort or complications. In rare cases, people develop shortness of breath, requiring hospitalization and treatment.

Typical side effects include fatigue or muscle aches. Some people experience blisters or mild skin irritation due to the equipment. Others may have:

- Bruises.
- Edema.
- Fatigue.
- Muscle or joint discomfort.
- Numbness or tingling.
- Pressure sores.

What is the recovery time from EECP?

EECP therapy doesn't require a hospital stay. You can return to your regular routine immediately after treatment. Alert your healthcare provider if you experience any side effects.

Many people experience improved blood flow and reduced symptoms of angina for several years after treatment. In some cases, you may need another course of EECP therapy.

When should I see my healthcare provider?

If you experience frequent chest pain or pressure due to physical activity or stress, talk to your healthcare provider. Together, you can determine if you are eligible for EECP therapy. Call emergency number immediately if you have unexpected chest pain that could lead to a heart attack.

Can I be active when I'm receiving EECP therapy?

Exercise helps keep your heart healthy. Your healthcare provider can help you plan an appropriate exercise program during the treatment weeks. Talk to your provider if you plan to play sports or be sexually active during treatment.

Bibliography and Acknowledgement

- American Heart Association. Angina Pectoris (Stable Angina). (https://www.heart.org/en/health-topics/heart-attack/angina-chest-pain/angina-pectoris-stable-angina) Accessed 3/17/2022.
- EECP.com, Vaso Corporation. VasoMedical EECP® Therapy. (http://www.eecp.com/) Accessed 3/17/2022.
- Gillen C, Goyal A. Stable Angina. Stable Angina. (https://www.ncbi.nlm.nih.gov/books/NBK559016/) [Updated 2021 Jul 7]. In: StatPearls [Internet]. Treasure Island (FL): StatPearls Publishing; 2021 Jan-. Accessed 3/17/2022.
- Sharma U, Ramsey HK, Tak T. The role of enhanced external counter pulsation therapy in clinical practice. (https://www.ncbi.nlm.nih.gov/pmc/articles/PMC3917995/) Clin Med Res. 2013;11(4):226-232. Accessed 3/17/2022.

CHAPTER

Cell And Gene Therapies for Heart Disease. Current and Future State.

Patients have an ongoing unmet need for effective therapies that reverse the cellular and functional damage associated with heart damage and disease. The discovery that > %–2% of adult cardiomyocytes turn over per year provided the impetus for treatments that stimulate endogenous repair mechanisms that augment this rate. Preclinical and clinical studies provide evidence that cell-based therapy meets these therapeutic criteria. Recent and ongoing studies are focused on determining which cell type(s) works best for specific patient population(s) and the mechanism(s) by which these cells promote repair. Here we review clinical and preclinical stem cell studies and anticipate future directions of regenerative medicine for heart disease.

Clinical trials have assessed the safety and feasibility of cell-based therapy, largely testing culture-expanded cells from bone marrow, adipose tissue, or the heart itself. While initial studies demonstrated positive results, some trials have produced little or no functional improvements in cardiac performance. A majority of studies have focused on surrogate primary end points, such as changes in left ventricular ejection fraction (LVEF) and cardiac volumes, but in some studies only small improvements (5% on average) were seen, which has dampened enthusiasm toward the field.. However, substantial efforts continue toward improving cell-based approaches for cardiac repair. Here, we will review clinical trials of cell-based therapy for heart disease and speculate on potential future directions of regenerative cardiovascular medicine.

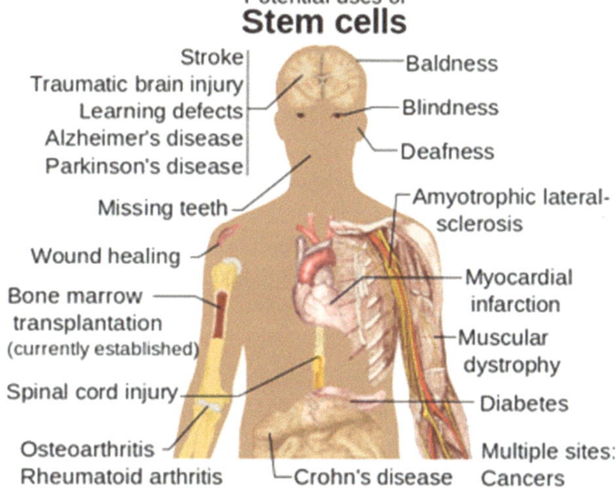

Fig.16.1 Illustration showing various indications of stem cell therapy besides cardiovascular disorders.

Section 1. Types Of Cells Used For Cardiac Transplantation

Several different types of cells have been used in both animal studies and patients to promote the repair of damaged myocardium. The two main sources of stem cells are adult stem and embryonic stem (ES) cells. Embryonic stem (ES) cells ES cells are derived from the inner mass of developing embryos during the blastocyst stage. Characteristic features of ES cells include their proliferative and self-renewing properties and their ability to differentiate into a wide variety of cell types, including cardiac myocytes. The major concerns with their use in human trials include the formation of teratomas when ES cells are injected into immunocompromised animals. This is particularly important because the ES

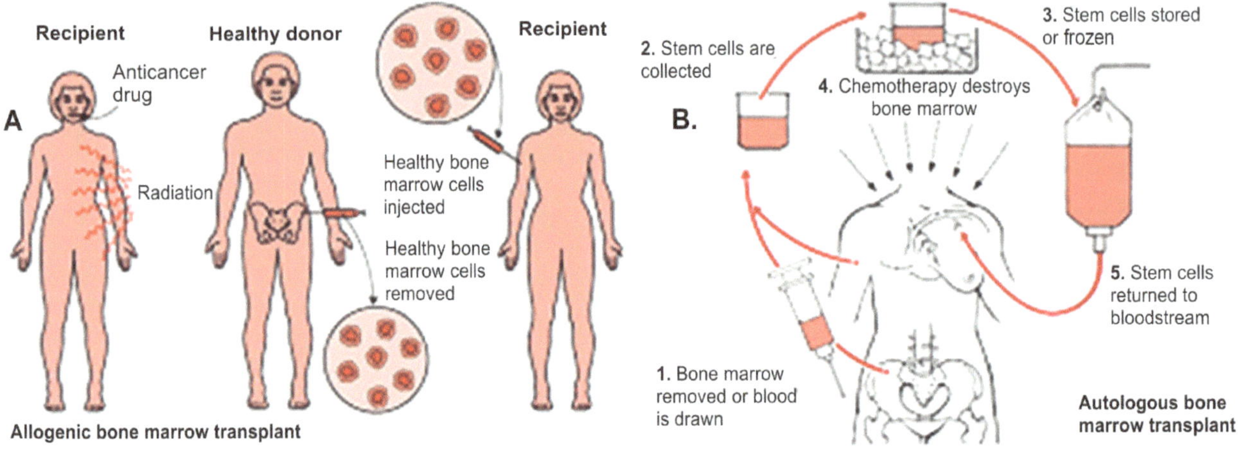

Fig.16.2 Illustrations showing allogenic bone marrow transplant (A) and autologous bone marrow transplant (B).

cells currently available for use in humans would be of allogeneic origin and therefore would require immunosuppression. As nuclear transfer techniques improve, they will provide a way of generating an unlimited supply of histocompatible ES cells using the nuclei of cells obtained directly from the recipient patients with heart disease.

Adult Stem Cells

Bone Marrow–Derived Stem Cells

Several different types of stem cells can be isolated from adult bone marrow. Examples of some of these subpopulations of cells include hematopoietic stem cells, endothelial progenitors, and mesenchymal stem cells. Several investigators have chosen to deliver unfractionated bone marrow–derived cells, a technique that has the advantage of minimizing extensive ex-vivo manipulation of the cells to isolate and expand a selected population of cells. The potential disadvantage of delivering a mixture of cells is that the percentage of cells that are therapeutically useful may be small. An alternative strategy is to isolate purer populations of cells that express specific antigens. For example, endothelial progenitors express the cell surface marker CD133. These cells have a greater potential to promote angiogenesis but are more technically challenging to isolate in significant quantities. Mesenchymal cells represent a rare population of bone marrow–derived cells that do not express CD34 or CD133. Mesenchymal cells can differentiate into bone, cartilage, adipocytes, and, under certain culture conditions, cardiac myocytes. One advantage of using mesenchymal cells is that clones of these cells can easily be expanded in vitro, exhibit relatively low immunogenicity, and might be particularly useful when autologous stem cells are not readily available.

Skeletal Myoblasts

Skeletal myoblasts are a population of progenitor cells that can be isolated from skeletal muscle biopsies and expanded in vitro. These myoblasts can differentiate into myotubes and exhibit skeletal muscle phenotype after transplantation, leading to improvements in left ventricular (LV) systolic and diastolic function. However, the transplanted skeletal myocytes are not electrically coupled to surrounding cardiomyocytes and thus may lead to the development of arrhythmias.

Resident Cardiac Stem Cells

Several investigators have recently identified a population of stem cells within the myocardium that are capable of differentiating into cardiac myocytes. It has recently been reported that these cells can be harvested from cardiac biopsies. Injecting these cells in the setting of myocardial infarction can promote cardiomyocyte formation with associated improvements in systolic function. At present, these cells are limited in number and require ex vivo separation and expansion over several weeks.

Third-generation therapy includes genetic reprogramming, exosomes, microRNA (miRNA), and the use of biomaterials to enhance the differentiation and regenerative capabilities of the cells.40 Exosomes are extracellular bilayer membrane vesicles that contain a diverse collection of proteins, lipids, and mRNAs/miRNAs and are secreted by a multitude of cell types.The exosomes secreted by iPSCs, ESCs, MSCs, and CDCs have different profiles, which ultimately physiologically manifest as increased self-renewal or expansion. Moreover, there is a growing body of evidence that exosome secretion is an important mode of cardiac cell communication

Induced Pluripotent Stem Cells

Due to the ethical concerns of harvesting ESCs, scientists have sought alternative methods to isolate multipotent stem cells. Takahashi and Yamanaka developed a novel protocol to generate pluripotency from murine somatic cell by integrating a variety of transcription factors into the cell's genome via retroviral transduction.104 This technique was then applied to human somatic cells.105 Subsequent studies have demonstrated that these iPSCs have the capacity to differentiate into all three germ layers in addition to somatic cells, including cardiomyocytes and other cardiovascular cells. Furthermore, these cells could also aid in repair of heart valves and vessels.108 A major concern when using these pluripotent cells, as with ESCs, is tumorigenesis. However, this risk can be mitigated by isolating cells or cell lines that have undergone at least some differentiation.109 An initial clinical trial to evaluate safety and efficacy of a patch with 100 million reprogrammed iPSC cardiomyocytes was approved in Japan. Three patients with ICM were treated initially; a further 7–10 patients will be recruited and followed up over the period of 1 year.110 The Treating Heart Failure With hPSC-CMs (HEAL-CHF) Trial (NCT03763136) is an open-label study recruiting 5 patients to receive epicardial injection of allogeneic PSC-CMs. There are as yet no reports from either of these two studies. Continuing studies will have to investigate methods to maintain stable cell lines as well as address scalability for clinical grade production. compares the efficacy of different cell types for increasing LVEF, and reducing EDV and scar size in clinical trials to date.

Placental Stem Cells

The placenta is a novel source of potentially cardio-regenerative cells. Perinatal tissue is a rich source of a variety of stem cells that can be isolated from the amnion, chorion, umbilical cord (e.g. Wharton's jelly) and the placental cotyledons from the fetal side and the decidua from the maternal side. Many of these cells display MSC-like characteristics, such as adherence to plastic and immunomodulation. Furthermore, in vitro, they inhibit cardiomyocyte apoptosis and are pro-angiogenic (reviewed by Bollini et al.).Cells isolated from the murine near-term placenta and expressing the Caudal-type homeobox-2 (Cdx2) were recently reported to form beating cardiomyocytes and vascular lineages ex vivo. Furthermore, these Cdx2+ cells homed to the injured heart and promoted cardiac repair when injected intravenously (1×106 cells) post-MI in a mouse model. Three months post-injection, the cells were found integrated within the myocardium, primarily in the border zone, where they exhibited a cardiomyocyte morphology. Cell-treated hearts exhibited improved LVEF and stroke volume and reduced adverse remodeling compared to placebo-injected mice

Tissue-specific MSCs

Most studies have assessed the therapeutic effects of bone marrow- and adipose tissue-derived MSCs. These cells can be isolated and expanded in large quantities while retaining their immunomodulatory characteristics, but the properties of these MSCs are influenced by their tissue of origin. For example, bone marrow-derived MSCs are highly proangiogenic120 and may be more immunosuppressive than adipose-derived MSCs. Mesenchymal stem cells have also been isolated from other tissues, including umbilical cord (Wharton's jelly), amniotic fluid, peripheral blood, and the heart. Again, the tissue of origin appears to provide MSCs with characteristic properties and secretomes,and for therapeutic use it may be important to determine which MSC source is best for a specific patient.

Exosomes/ Microvesicles

Some studies suggest that exosomes have an (almost) equivalent therapeutic efficacy as intact cells.Other data also demonstrate that the therapeutic effect of cell therapy may not correlate with engraftment, supporting a paracrine mechanism. The discovery of these paracrine mechanisms of repair not only significantly challenges the notion of engraftment-dependent healing, but also opens another avenue of therapy delivery. Engineered exosomes with an ischemic myocardium-targeting peptide can enhance myocardial viability and reduce infarct size after MI in mouse models. Cell-free suspensions containing important reparative exosomes could be used instead

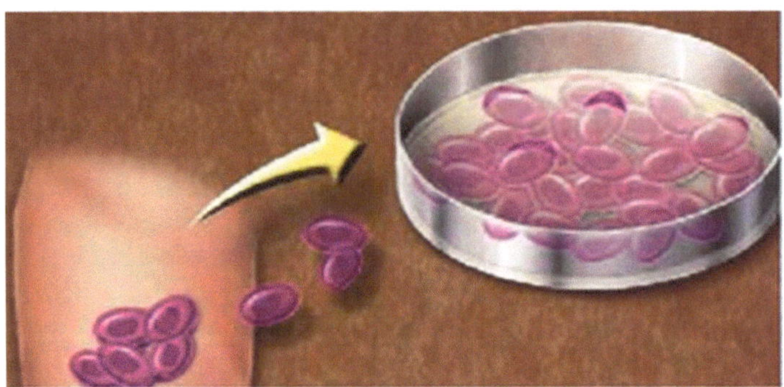

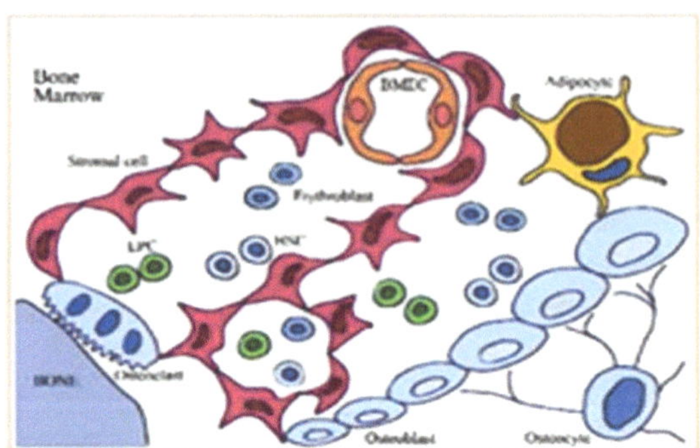

Fig. 16.3 Cell therapy. Left: Stem cells derived from skeletal myoblasts. Right: Schematic drawing of various stem cell populations found in bone marrow.

intact cells, avoiding some of the inherent issues associated with cells, such as ex vivo expansion, tumor formation, and immune rejection. Studies directly comparing the different approaches will provide guidance toward the most therapeutic approach.

Patches/Biomaterials:Bioenglneering In Stem Cell Therapy

Transplantation of viable cells into the harsh environment of necrotic myocardium remains a significant therapeutic challenge resulting in very poor cell retention. To combat this problem, tissue engineering approaches have designed biomaterials as cell retention mediums.

These injectable biomaterials must perform many (often contradictory) functions. They must be biodegradable, biocompatible, provide mechanical support, be of appropriate dimension, allow for precise placement, improve cell survival, and promote tissue regeneration. These polymers can either be synthetic or naturally derived, each having their own advantages and disadvantages. Some polymers can even be specifically tailored to optimize cardiac repair, and 3D-printing has increased the available types of biomaterials, improving cell integration and vascularization. Preclinical studies have demonstrated improved cell viability and cardiac repair when used with human pluripotent stem cells and MSCs. While significant progress has been made, improving polymer compatibility and mechanical properties must occur before clinical studies can begin.

Methods Of Stem Cell Delivery

A major goal of cardiac stem cell therapy is to transplant enough cells into the myocardium atthe site of injury or infarction to maximize restoration of function. Several different approaches currently are being used to deliver stem cells.

1.Transvenous,
2.Endoventricular

An alternative approach is to inject stem cells intravenously. In the setting of myocardial infarction, circulating stem cells have been shown to home to sites of injury, but the number of cells that home to the heart in this way is significantly less than by local injection.

Transvascular Route

A transvascular approach is particularly well suited totreat patients with acutely infarcted and reperfused myocardium. Stem cells can be infused directly into the coronary arteries and have a greater likelihood of remaining in the injured myocardium as a result of the activation of adhesion molecules and chemokines. The advantage of an intracoronary infusion is that the cells can be directed to a particular territory.

Endoventricular (Direct Injection Into the Ventricular Wall)

Direct injection of stem cells is used in patients presenting with established cardiac dysfunction in whom a transvascular approach may not be possible because of total occlusion or poor flow within the vessel of the affected territory. There are 3 different approaches to direct injection. A transendocardial approach can be used in which a needle catheter is advanced across the aortic valve and positioned against the endocardial surface. Cells can then be

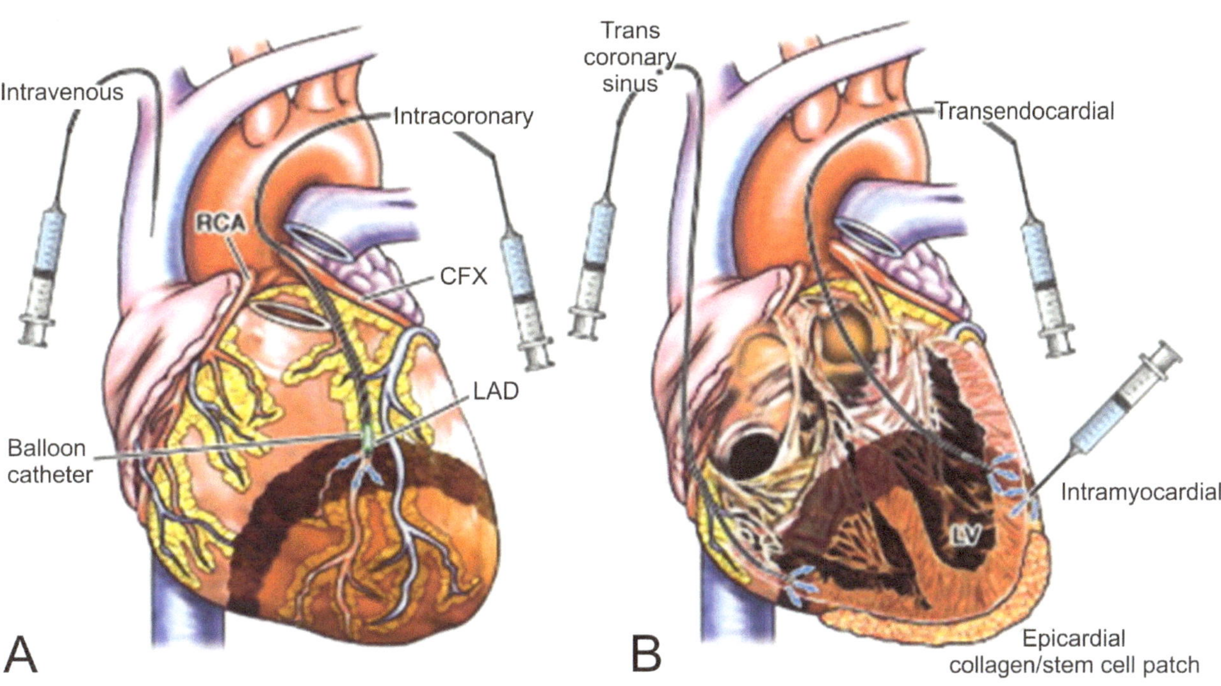

Fig. 16.4 Various Transplantation Methods in Heart Disease (A) Intracoronary and (B) intramyocardial transplantation methods in heart disease. Depicted are clinically used methods for vascular and myocardial cell delivery in cardiac intervention and cardiac surgery. CFX = circumflex artery; LAD = left anterior descending artery; LV = left ventricle; RCA = right coronary artery

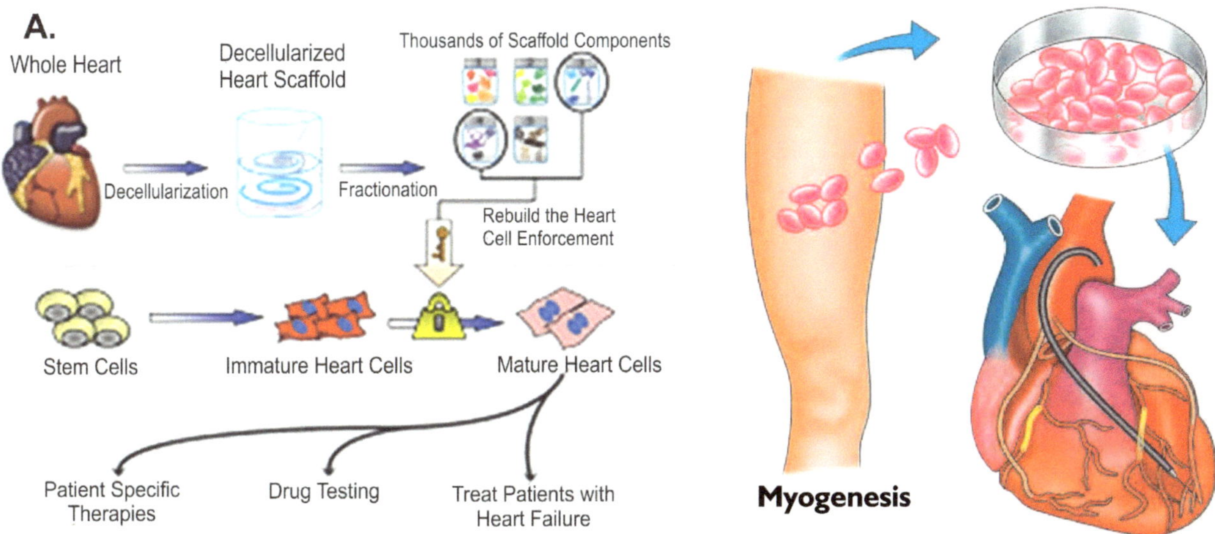

Fig. 16.5 Illustrations. (A) Showing technique of rebuilding of a damaged heart with stem cells. (B) Diagrammatic depiction of myogenesis in the heart muscle derived from bone marrow.

injected directly into the left ventricle. Electrophysiological mapping can be used to differentiate sites of viable, ischemic, or scarred myocardium.In a transepicardial approach, cells are injected during open heart surgery. The advantage of this approach is that it allows direct visualization of the myocardium and easier identification of regions of scar and border zones of infarcted tissues. A third approach involves the delivery of cells through one of the cardiac veins directly into the myocardium. The limitation of this approach is that positioning the catheter within a particular coronary vein may be considerably more time consuming and technically challenging.

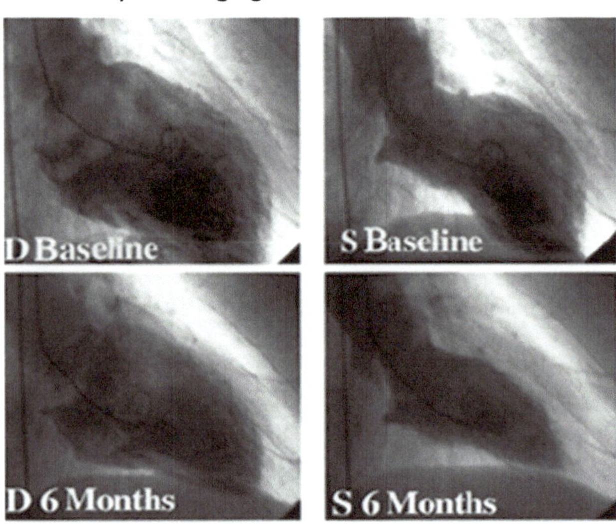

Fig.16.6 Ventriculography at baseline (akinesia in anterior region) and after 6 months (with clear improvement in contractil-ity of anterior region) for patient D indicates diastole; S, systole

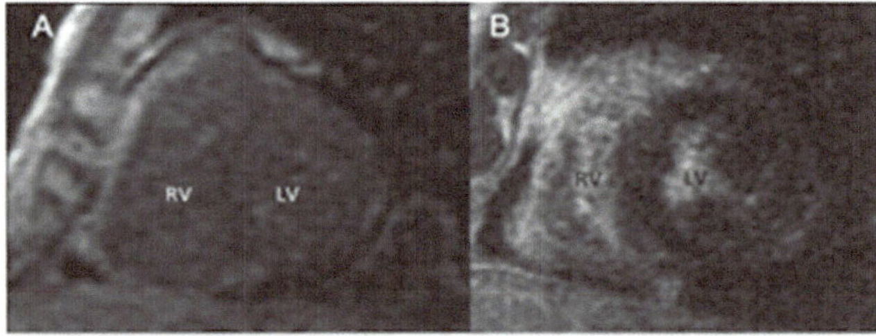

Fig.16.7 (A), Baseline midventricular short axis magnetic resonance imaging (MRI) obtained 10 minutes after administration of intravenous gadolinium shows diffusely abnormal nulling of the myocardium with a characteristic dark blood pool, consistent with cardiac amyloidosis. (B), Three years after stem cell transplant, postgadolinium midventricular short axis MRI image shows normal nulling of the myocardium with faint patchy areas of residual delayed enhancement. RV indicates right ventricle; LV, left ventricle.

Safety Concerns

1.Arrhythmias

Over the past few years, some of the early-phase clinical studies have suggested the possibility of a proarrhythmic effect associated with stem cell transplantation. In study, skeletal myoblasts were injected transepicardially at the time of coronary artery bypass surgery. Four patients had documented ventricular tachycardia at 11, 12, 13, and 22 days after stem cell implantation Interestingly, these events occurred early and were not observed in treated patients later after several months of follow-up. A similar proarrhythmic effect was observed when autologous skeletal myoblasts were delivered via a transvascular route. Other studies have similarly reported an increased frequency of non-sustained ventricular tachycardia in patients treated with skeletal myoblasts, peaking 11 to 30 days after stem cell transplantation. A proposed mechanism for the increased incidence of arrhythmias is that the injected stem cells do not communicate electrically with neighboring cardiac myocytes and/or result in slowed conduction, thereby promoting reentrant arrhythmias. It has recently been suggested that skeletal myoblasts that have been genetically engineered to express gap junction protein connexin exhibited decreased arrhythmogenicity. Although proarrhythmic effects have been observed predominantly in patients receiving skeletal myoblast transplantation, they also have been observed recently in two patients shortly after transplantation of CD133+ cells.

2.Restenosis, Accelerated Atherosclerosis, and Coronary Obstruction

There have been conflicting reports regarding the potential for increased restenosis after stem cell transplantation. In 1 study, a high rate of restenosis was observed after intracoronary delivery of peripheral blood stem cells mobilized with granulocyte colony-stimulating factor in the setting of myocardial infarction and stent placement. In another study, CD133+ cells were delivered via intracoronary injection in the setting of myocardial infarction, with in-stent restenosis rates of 37% and reocclusion rates of 11%. Relatively low rates of restenosis were observed in earlier studies using bone marrow–derived stem cells. In addition to restenosis, it is also possible that stem cell transplantation may promote the formation of de novo lesions or atherosclerotic plaque progression. In 2 recent studies, there was a fairly high proportion of new lesions identified in the non-stented vessels after stem cell transplantation. It is also possible that if the cells are delivered at a high enough concentration via the coronary circulation, they may adhere to each other, form aggregates, and thereby lead to the occlusion of microvessels. In 1 study in which mesenchymal stem cells were administered by intracoronary injection in pigs, there was associated occlusion of microvessels and macrovessels.

3. Abnormal Cellular Differentiation

Fortunately, no clinical trials to date that have used stem cells to promote cardiac tissue regeneration have demonstrated an increased frequency of tumor formation. However, most of the clinical trials have been conducted on small numbers of patients. Furthermore, it is not clear how adequate testing would be conducted to monitor for this potential side effect. Because stem cells are known to migrate to several other organs after delivery to the heart, it is conceivable that aberrant cellular differentiation with the potential of tumor formation could occur in any of these organs.

Tracking Of Stem Cells

One of the major concerns regarding the delivery of stem cells is determining which cells remain in the heart and which cells ultimately end up in other organs as a result of a washout effect. Within a few hours after transplantation, stem cells injected locally within the heart also are observed within the lungs, spleen, liver, and kidney. One day after transplantation of neonatal cardiac myocytes into rat hearts, only 24% of the originally injected cells remained in the heart. Given the small fraction of stem cells that remain within the heart after injection and the multiple organs to which the stem cells migrate, it is imperative that better methods of tracking stem cells be developed to determine the fate of these cells after transplantation. Several potential methods have been developed to label and track stem cells in animal models,including scintigraphy, PET, and MRI PET scanning and MRI also have been tested recently in humans to track stem cells. One hour after injection of 18F-fluorodeoxyglucose–labeled CD34+ cells, only 5.5% of the cells were detectable in the heart by PET scanning. Unfortunately, because of the short half-life of F-fluorodeoxyglucose, other isotopes with a longer half-life may need to be evaluated for optimal long-term tracking of stem cells.

Evidence for Tissue Regeneration

The ultimate goal of stem cell therapy is to promote cardiac tissue regeneration so that the regenerated cardiac tissue leads to improvements in cardiac function in a fashion that is synchronized with the rest of the functioning heart in the absence of proarrhythmic or other adverse effects. More recently, however, there is evidence that stem cells may lead to improvements in cardiac function that are independent of tissue regeneration. Although early studies supported the ability of bone marrow–derived mononuclear cells to differentiate into cardiac myocytes, subsequent studies failed to support these initial observations It has been suggested that the locally injected cells can act in a paracrine fashion to improve ventricular function through the release of growth factors or other paracrine mediators.

These mediators may act to directly augment systolic function, prevent apoptosis of ischemic myocardial cells, or limit injury by promoting angiogenesis. The locally injected stem cells would promote the salvage of injured myocardium rather than tissue regeneration. Additional long-term studies are needed to determine whether the improvements observed after weeks to a few months are generally sustained over onger periods of time. These paracrine effects are more likely to be useful in patients with acute myocardial ischemia or with hibernating myocardium and less likely to be beneficial in patients with chronically infarcted myocardium with significant scar formation. Significant challenges remain with regard to cardiac tissue regeneration. Future studies areneeded to identify the best stem cell type to use. To promote cardiac tissue regeneration, sufficient numbers of cells will need to be delivered and maintained within the heart at the site of LV dysfunction, and the new tissue needs to be vascularized, electrically and mechanically coupled with the rest of the myocardium. The hope is that the strategies will include ways of replacing scarred or fibrotic tissue in regions of LV dysfunction. Unless autologous cells can be used to generate the cardiac tissue, potential graft rejection needs to be addressed. Real progress toward this goal will require the collaborative interaction of investigators with expertise in tissue engineering, molecular biology, electrophysiology, cardiac physiology, immunology, and vascular biology.

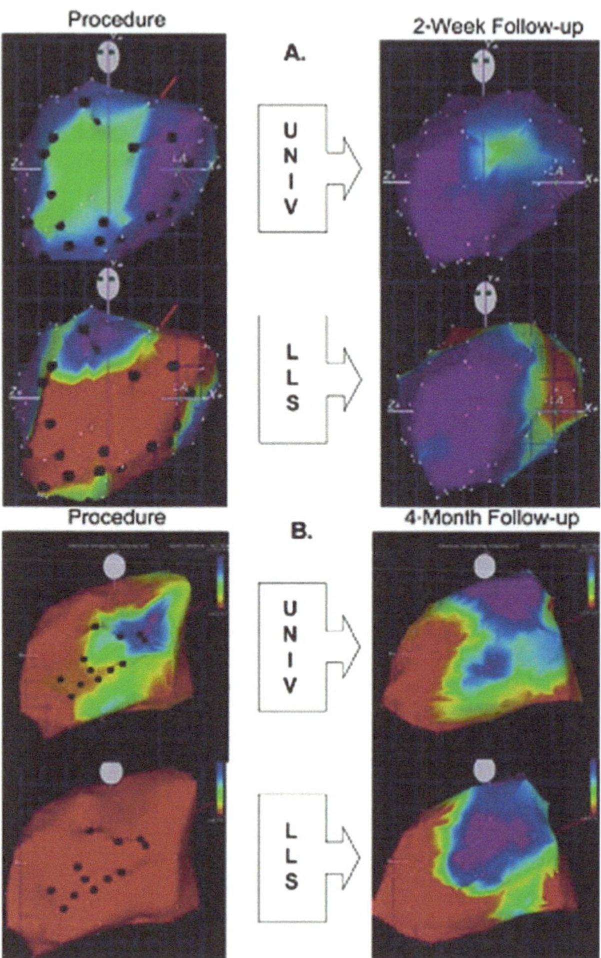

Fig.16.8 (A) NOGA™ electrical (UNIV, at top) and mechanical (LLS, at bottom) maps from a canine in the stem cell treatment group. Maps at left are those performed at the time of injection and maps at right are those at 2-week follow-up. The green area in the top left denotes infarcted myocardium with decreased electrical signal. The red area in the bottom left denotes impaired mechanical function corresponding to the infarct. Maps at right show improvement in both electrical and mechanical function. B. NOGA™ electrical (UNIV, at top) and mechanical (LLS, at bottom) maps from a human patient in the stem cell treatment group. Maps at left are those performed at the time of injection and maps at right are those at 4-month follow-up. An area of viability, showing normal electrical activity, can be noted on the upper-right map. Maps at the right show improvement in both electrical and mechanical function. LLS = linear local shortening; UNIV = unipolar voltage

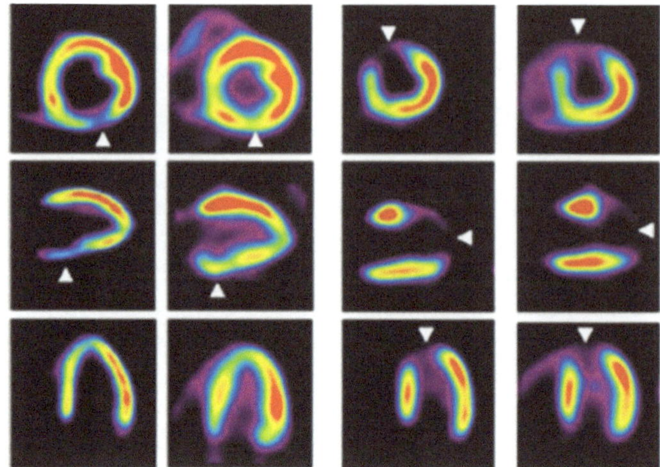

Fig.16.9 F-18-fluorodeoxyglucose (FDG) positron emission tomography (PET) imaging. The left-hand panel corresponds to the PET image in a post-myocardial infarction patient. The arrowheads point to a deficit of FDG uptake that would indicate an image of necrosis. At 3 months after revascularization surgery and autologous myoblasts implantation, a highly significant improvement in FDG uptake can be seen which would indicate greater viability. The right-hand panel corresponds to a patient who underwent revascularization surgery without cell transplantation and in whom improved tissue viability cannot be seen.

Section11 Gene Therapy for Cardiovascular Disease

The field of cardiovascular gene transfer has developed rapidly during the past 5 years. Important advances have been made in vector development, in vivo gene delivery, and definition of potential therapeutic targets. Despite substantial progress, a number of technical issues need to be addressed before gene therapy is applied safely and broadly to cardiovascular diseases. In this review, major advances in cardiovascular gene transfer are summarized. In addition, technical issues required for translation of preclinical studies of gene transfer into clinical protocols are discussed. Advances in recombinant DNA technology, including gene transfer, have stimulated hope that this technology can be used to improve the practice of cardiovascular medicine. Applications of this technology that affect the clinical management of patients include the development of new therapeutic products, engineered by the overexpression of genes, such as recombinant tissue-type plasminogen activator. Recombinant DNA technology has also provided techniques that have been used to create animal models of cardiovascular diseases. These models permit definition of the role of specific

Table 16.1. Optimization of Gene Delivery Technology

Myocardial Preconditioning	Creation of Closed Loop System	Enhancement of Transgene Expression	Coronary Sinus Infusion	Minimizing Collateral Expression
Temporary Ischemia	Catheter Based	Increasing Transcapillary Gradient	Normal	Enhancing Vector Tropism
Concomitant Venous Blockade	Cardiopulmonary Bypass Based	A. Pharmacological B. Physical	Selective Pressure	Removal of Residual Vector

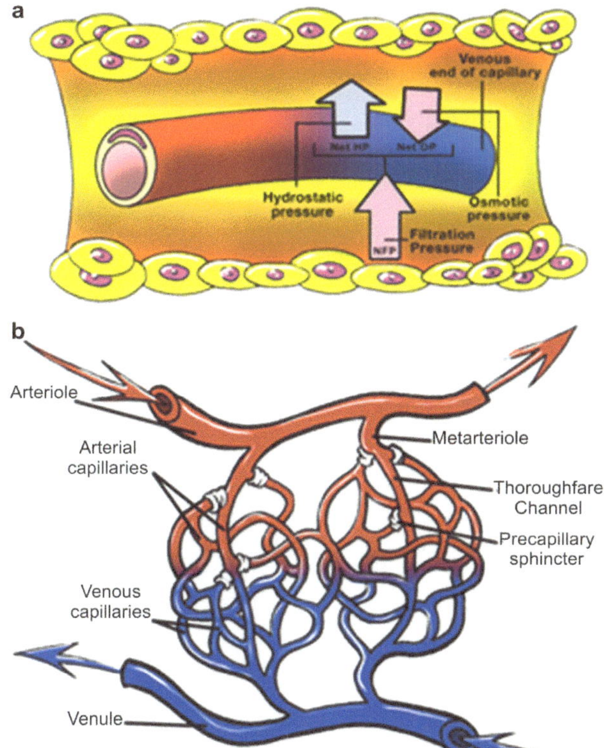

Fig 16.10 (a) The movement of fluid between capillaries and the interstitial fluid. The direction of fluid with vector movement across the capillary wall depends on the difference between two opposing forces: hydrostatic and osmotic pressure. With retro-grade perfusion, hydrostatic pressure increases at the venous end of the capillaries and therefore gene filtration and transduction are also increased. (b) Coronary capillary net. After the tissue has been perfused through the coronary sinus, capillaries join to become arterioles and metarterioles which return blood to the aorta. A capillary net consist of two types of vessels: true capillaries which provide exchange between cells and thoroughfare (shunts) channels which directly connects the arterioles and venules. Pre-capillary sphincters are rings of smooth muscles at the origin of arterial capillaries that regulate blood flow through a tissue. The advantage of the retrograde delivery is its ability to overcome the resistance of precapillary sphincters proximally located on the arterial side of the capillary bed. Thus, less blood is shunted through the thoroughfare channels into the cardiac chambers.

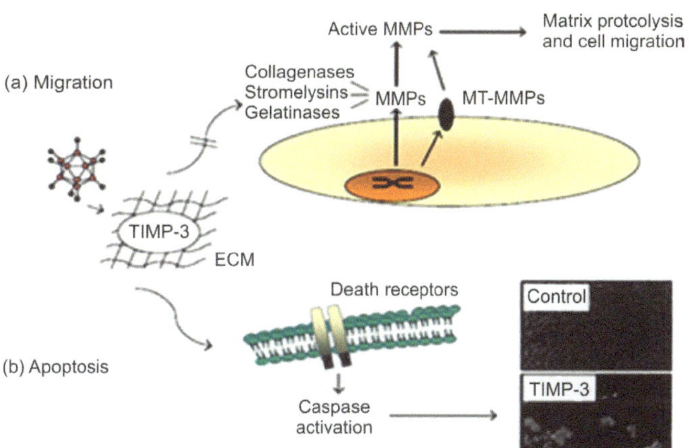

Fig.16.11 Gene therapy by overexpression of TIMP-3. Following Ad-mediated gene delivery to vascular smoth muscle cells, TIMP-3 is secreted and is found located with the extracellular matrix (ECM). From here, TIMP-3 is available to exert two distinctly different phenotypes through its metalloproteinase inhibitory effects. (a) Matrix metalloproteinases (MMPs, including collagenases, stromelysins, gelatinases, and membrane-type metalloproteinases [MT-MMPs]) are upregulated following vascular injury. TIMPs, through their native MMP inhibitory activity, are able to bind to and retard pro-MMP-to-active enzyme conversion and combined with the ability to block active MMP activity, matrix proteolysis and hence cell migration is inhibited (b) TIMP-3, uniquely amongst the TIMP family, is also able to promote smooth muscle cell death through death receptor-induced caspase activation and induction of apoptosis. Micrographs courtesy of Mark Bond, Bristol Heart Institute, UK.

gene products in the pathogenesis of cardiovascular diseases. Characterization of its molecular basis has led to a more precise definition of diseases and the potential for relevant clinical treatments. The development of molecular genetic interventions to treat cardiovascular diseases depends on technical advances in the development of methods of gene delivery; achievement of long-term, highly efficient, and targeted expression to relevant cells of the cardiovascular system; and design of vectors that are safe for long-term human administration

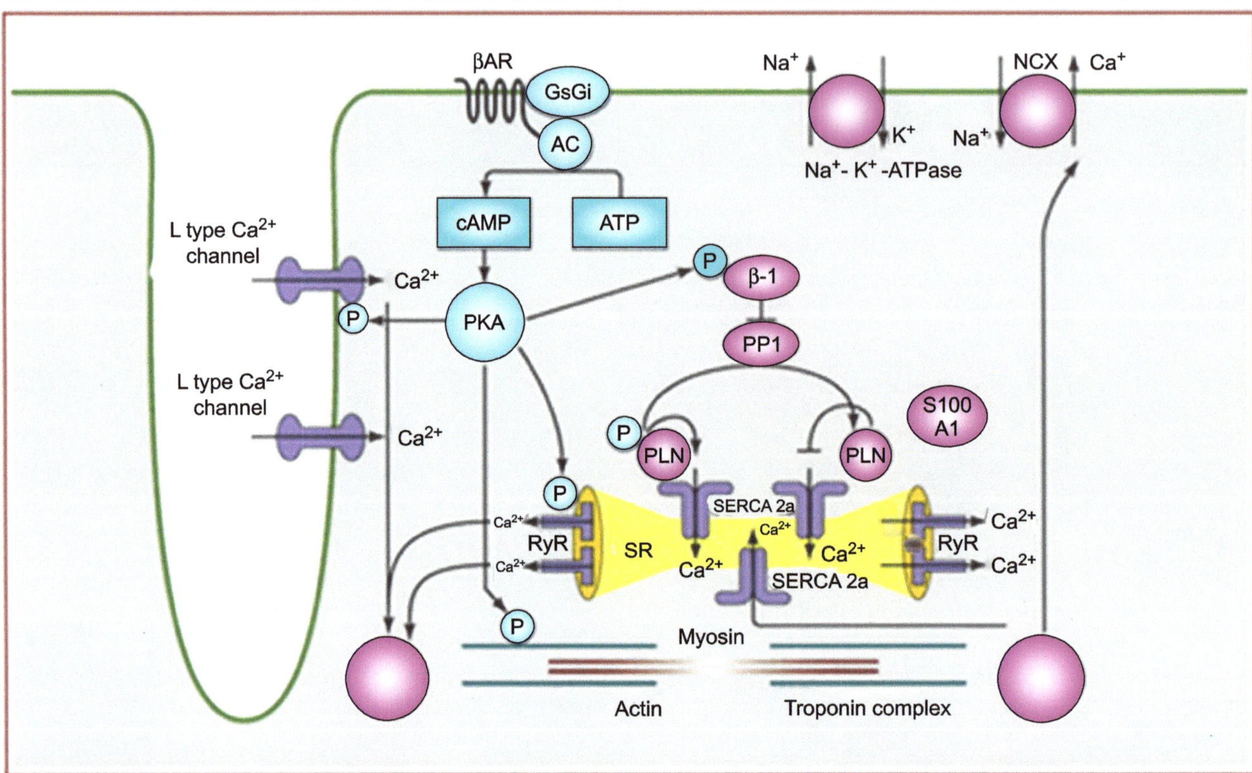

Fig. 16.12 Excitation-contraction signaling in cardiomyocytes with emphasis on targets for gene therapy. Interplay between calcium handling (purple) and adrenergic (blue) systems is illustrated. AC: adenylyl cyclase; ATP: adenosine triphosphate; AR: beta adrenergic receptor; I-1: (protein phosphatase) inhibitor-1; cAMP: cyclic adenosine monophosphate; Gs: stimulatory G protein; Gi: inhibitory G protein; NCX: sarcolemnal sodium/calcium exchanger; PKA: protein kinase A; PLN: phospholamban; PP: protein phosphatase; RyR: ryanodine receptor; SERCA:sarcoplasmic/endoplasmic reticulum calcium ATPase; SR: sarcoplasmic reticulum

Table 16.2 Comparison of gene delivery system used for in vivo cardiovascular gene transfer.

	Effective (in vivo)	*DNA integration*	*Target cells*	*Gene size (max)*	*Duration of expression*	*Host response*	*Potential side effects*
Viral							
Retrovirus	+	Yes	Replicating and non-replicating*	~6 kb	Weeks to months	+	Oncogenesis Virla mutation
Andenovirus	++++	No	Replicating and non-replicating	~7.5 kb	7-14 days	++++	Cytotoxicity Viral mutation
AAV	+	Sometimes	Replicating and non-replicating	~4 kb	Weeks to months	+	Oncogenesis Viral mutation Viral contamination
Non-viral							
Liposomes	+	No	Replicating and non-replicating	Unlimited	7-14 days	+	Cytotoxic at high concentrations
Fusigenic liposome	++	No	Replicating and non-replicating	Unlimited	7-14 days	+	Cytotoxic at high concentrations
Pressure	++	No	Replicating and non-replicating	Unlimited	7-14 days	+	None known
Naked plasmid	+	No	Replicating and non-replicating	Unlimited	7-14 days	+	None known

*Lentivirus.

+, lowest, ++++, highest, AAV, adeno-associated virus

Methods of Gene Delivery

The transduction and expression of genes in appropriate cell types represent important steps in the development of gene therapy. Therefore, investigations have focused on the development of methods to deliver and express genes in vascular cells and cardiac myocytes. Viral vectors (retroviruses and adenoviruses), viral conjugate vectors (adenovirus-augmented receptor-mediated vectors and hemagglutinating virus of Japan [HVJ] liposomes), and nonviral vectors (cationic liposomes, polymers, and injection of plasmid DNA) have been used. To optimize gene delivery to target cells, characteristics of the cell must be considered, such as proliferative capacity and location within the target tissue. Vascular cells (endothelial and smooth muscle cells) and cardiac myocytes differ particularly in proliferation features, and therefore different strategies have been used to transduce these cells.

- **Vascular Cells**
- **Retroviral Vectors**

Because vascular cells are accessible through the blood stream, percutaneous, site-specific gene delivery was developed for local arterial segments. Retroviral vectors were initially used in in vivo vascular gene transfer studies. Interest in retrovirus-mediated gene transfer was based on the use of these vectors in gene transfer to other organ systems, including bone marrow stem cells,liver,and the skin, where in some target cells, these vectors transduce a large proportion of target cells. In the case of retroviral vectors, the viral vector stably integrates into chromosomal DNA of the target cell, resulting in potentially stable gene expression, although integration into chromosomal DNA could potentially result in insertional mutagenesis. These vectors are most appropriate for ex vivo gene transfer for cardiovascular disease,which involves removal of the relevanttarget cells, ie, endothelial cells or hepatocytes from the host, transfection of the cells in vitro, and subsequent reintroduction of the modified cells into the animal of patient. It is unknown whether stable high-level gene expression in vivo will be achieved with retrovirally transduced cells. Several features of retroviral gene transfer may limit its application to cardiovascular medicine, particularly with respect to direct in vivo gene therapy.

Replication of target cells is necessary for proviral integration. Recent studies suggest that viral integration may depend on mitosis, not just DNA synthesis. Successful retrovirus-mediated gene transfer to vascular cells may require induction of proliferation in target endothelial or smooth muscle cells, at least for short periods of time. In uninjured arteries, endothelial and smooth muscle cell proliferation occurs slowly, and therefore retroviral integration would occur at a low frequency. After vascular injury or stimulation, such as with a balloon catheter, injured vascular cells may be transduced at higher rates. Previous studies have suggested that retroviral transduction of vascular cells can be used successfully in vivo. Limitations of this gene delivery vector include its low frequency of gene transfer and the relative lability of retroviral particles compared with other viruses. Retroviral particles are rapidly inactivated in vivo in primates, presumably by the presence of complement in serum. Because of the instability of retroviral particles and the inability of retroviruses to integrate in nonreplicating cells, retroviral vectors may have limited use for direct gene transfer in vivo, although there may be a role for these vectors for ex vivo gene transfer to vascular stents or prosthetic grafts.

Adenoviral Vectors

To improve the frequency of direct gene transfer into arteries, recent investigations have focused on adenoviral vectors. The adenovirus genome is composed of linear, double-stranded DNA of approximately 36 kb in length . The gene products are organized into early (E1-E4) and late (L1-L5) regions, based on expression before or after initiation of DNA replication. Expression of viral genes depends on cellular transcription factors and expression of the adenoviral E1 region, which encodes a transactivator of viral gene expression. The E3 region encodes viral proteins that regulate immunosurveillance in vivo. Adenoviruses have a lytic life cycle, characterized by attachment to an adenoviral glycoprotein receptor on mammalian cells and cell entry by receptor-mediated endocytosis. Adenoviruses escape degradation in lysosomes due to adenoviral capsid proteins, and viral DNA is transported to the nucleus. In the nucleus, adenoviral genome persists in an unintegrated form. During the lytic infection, viral genome replicates to several

Table 16.3 Key features of gene therapy viral vector

Viral vectors	*Integration*	*Long-term gene expression*	*Immune response*	*Comments*
Adenovirus	-	-	+	Broad tropism, easy to produce high titre stocks, widely characterized in vivo
Adeno-associated virus (AAV)	+	+	-	Limited cloning capacity, non-pathogenic, integrate randomly in the absence of the rep gene
Lentivirus	+	+	-	Retrovirus-derived, pseudotyping with heterologus coat proteins improves biosafety
Retrovirus	+	+	-	Only infects dividing cells

thousand copies per cell. Adenovirus serotypes 2 (Ad-2) and 5 (Ad-5) have been developed as viral vectors for gene transfer the E1A and E1B genes from the viral genome. Vectors are produced by homologous recombination in 293 cells or any cell line that contains an integrated copy of the adenoviral E1 gene. A foreign cDNA with eukaryotic regulatory sequences is introduced into a bacterial plasmid containing a region of the left adenoviral genome that is deleted of the E1 gene. This plasmid is cotransfected into 293 cells with an incomplete adenoviral genome. Homologous recombination between the two DNAs generates a recombinant genome in which the E1 gene is replaced by the foreign DNA. Viral stock is propagated in 293 cells to high titer, approximately 10 to 10 particles per millilitre.

Adenoviruses effectively infect mammalian cells, including non-dividing cells in vitro and in vivo. Physiological levels of recombinant proteins have been secreted into the circulation after adenoviral infection of skeletal muscle. The virus particle is relatively stable and amenable to purification and concentration at a high titer. Integration of adenoviral DNA sequences into chromosomal DNA of the target cell occurs at a low frequency, and adenoviral DNA is maintained in an extrachromosomal form. Extrachromosomal replication of the vector reduces the likelihood of mutation by random integration and dysregulation of cellular genes.Despite these advantages, there are limitations to current, or "first-generation," adenoviral vectors. In most models, gene expression is transient after adenoviral infection, generally less than 3 weeks, and inflammation is observed in organs expressing the transgene. Gene expression in vascular cells is transient as well, usually persisting for only several weeks. Although transient gene expression may be well suited tovascular therapies requiring expression of a gene product over a short period of time, development of an immune response to adenoviral proteins is a major limitation to the use of these vectors. Recent studies in genetically defined strains of mice have demonstrated that viral proteins, expressed from the E1-deleted adenoviral genome, are presented as foreign antigens and lead to the generation of cytolytic T lymphocytes that destroy adenovirus-infected cells. Insertion of a temperature-sensitive mutation within the E2A region of E1-deleted adenoviral vectors results in lack of expression of late viral gene products at nonpermissive temperatures, resulting in prolonged gene expression (e"70 days) and blunted cytolytic T-cell infiltration in mouse liver.

In arterial gene transfer studies using first-generation adenoviral vectors, mononuclear cell infiltrates have been occasionally observed in the adventitia of peripheral and pulmonary arteries of pigs, but medial and intimal inflammation, necrosis, and aneurysm formation have not been observed. Further studies are required to examine the use of first-generation adenoviral vectors for vascular gene transfer studies. It is likely that further modifications in these vectors, including deletions in the E2 and E4 regions and modifications in the E3 region, will diminish host immune responses.

Adenovirus-Augmented, Receptor-Mediated Gene Delivery

Viral vector conjugate systems may have application in vascular gene therapy and include adenovirus-augmented, receptor-mediated gene delivery. This vector uses inactivated adenovirus complexed to a receptor ligand to facilitate entry of DNA to a cell.

This vector consists of two components. DNA condenses with polylysine, which in turn is bound to inactivated virus. The virus is coupled to a ligand such as transferrin. The transferrin ligand binds to a transferrin receptor in a cell, and the transferrin viral polylysine DNA complex enters the cell by receptor-mediated endocytosis. The inactivated adenovirus functions to disrupt lysosomes in the host cell, reducing DNA degradation and releasing DNA into the cytoplasm. The use of these vectors for vascular gene transfer is being investigated.

Cationic Liposomes

Most nonviral methods of gene transfer rely on normal mechanisms used by cells for the uptake and cellular transport of macromolecules. These methods rely on receptor-mediated endocytotic pathways or fusion of cell membranes. One example is cationic liposomes, which are positively charged artificial lipid vesicles that incorporate negatively charged DNA and deliver nucleic acid to cells through fusion with cell membranes or receptor-mediated endocytosis. Plasmid DNA is released in the cytoplasm and transported to the nucleus where it is maintained in an unintegrated form. Cationic liposomes interact spontaneously and rapidly with polyanions, such as DNA and mRNA, to form liposome complexes. Cationic liposome reagents used in vascular gene transfer studies include DOTMA/DOPE (Lipofectin), DC-cholesterol ,DOSPA/DOPE (Lipofectamine),and DMRIE/DOPE.Expression of recombinant genes in vivo after liposomal transfection has been reported in rats,rabbits,dogs, and pigs . Cationic liposomes produce more efficient gene delivery compared with neutrally charged or anionic liposomes,but current formulations, including DOSPA/DOPE, are less efficient than adenoviral vectors. Further modifications in plasmids and chemical formulations of liposomes appear to have promise in improving transfection efficiency. Cationic liposomes have a favorable safety profile for in vivo administration. Liposome vectors contain no viral sequences, and there are no cDNA size constraints in vector construction. In addition, this vector is straightforward to prepare for clinical use. Cell division is not required for liposome transfection, although the efficiency appears to be increased in proliferating cells.

HVJ Liposome Conjugates

Recent studies suggest that complexing inactivated HVJ with liposomes improves transfection efficiencies of vascular smooth muscle cells in in vitro and in vivo models of vascular injury, including the injured rat carotid artery.These vectors have also been successfully used for hepatic and renal in vivo gene transfer. It is likely that further modifications to vectors used for vascular gene transfer will include components of viral and nonviral vectors that optimize delivery, improve gene expression, and minimize toxic side effects.

Polymers

Additional strategies for the local delivery of therapeutic agents include impregnating oligonucleotides into polymer gels and applying the polymer to the external surfaces of arteries. Although pharmacokinetics of oligonucleotide delivery and retention have not been precisely defined, the data suggest that there is sufficient retention of oligonucleotide to inhibit c-myb and PCNA RNA expression within 24 hours after balloon injury and inhibit intimal thickening after 2 weeks.Plasmid DNA and adenoviral vectors have been applied directly to polyethylene balloons coated with a hydrogel polymer. Although there is some loss of plasmid DNA from the balloon during transit through the circulation, DNA is distributed transmurally after inflation of the balloon. Modifications in polymers to provide slow release of therapeutic agents hold promise for site-specific delivery of oligonucleotides and vectors to arterial segments.

Myocyte Gene Transfer

Dissection of molecular mechanisms governing myocardial differentiation has been performed in neonatal cardiac myocytes in culture, in part because these cells are relatively amenable to gene transfer with plasmid-based transfections. Recombinant gene expression in adult myocardium in vivo requires an expression vector with high-level activity in adult cardiac myocytes and a method for introducing this vector into myocardial cells. Because cardiac myocytes are terminally differentiated cells, they require a vector that is not dependent on cell replication for delivery and expression. The analysis of foreign genes within intact adult myocardium has been performed by direct injection of plasmid DNA. Although direct injection of genes is a simple procedure and permits examination of the behaviour of genes in vivo, this technique is limited by transfection of a small number of cells within several millimetres around the injection site. Expression of recombinant genes is temporally limited as well, withexpression peaking within several weeks and declining rapidly thereafter. Episomal persistence of the introduced DNA and the postmitotic state of adult cardiac myocytes, which prevent integration of genes into chromosomes, limit stability of the transgene.

Some limitations of in vivo plasmid DNA injection have been addressed by adenoviral vectors. Adenoviruses effectively infect nonreplicating mammalian cells, including skeletal and cardiac myotubes. These viruses are grown and purified in high titer. These properties result in highly efficient gene transfer into adult cardiac myocytes in vitro and in vivo. Quantitative comparisons of chloramphenicol acetyltransferase (CAT) activity resulting from injection of a CAT plasmid or an adenoviral vector encoding CAT revealed that the amount of CAT activity resulting from adenovirus infection was 10- to 100-fold higher compared with plasmid DNA. Similar findings were observed comparing adenoviral vectors and plasmids encoding lacZ.Although adenoviral vectors produce efficient gene transfer into the myocardium, expression is transient, peaking at 1 to 2 weeks. Acute inflammatory responses have been observed in hearts injected with adenovirus, although inflammation along the injection path has also been noted after injection of plasmid DNA. Further investigations will identify factors that account for the transient nature of gene expression and will characterize potential proinflammatory effects of this vector.

Animal Models Of Gene Transfer

Vascular Gene Transfer

In the past 5 years, there has been great interest in expressing recombinant DNA and other nucleic acids in blood vessels in vivo. The goals of these studies have been to define gene function and to develop new therapeutic strategies for vascular diseases. The feasibility of direct gene transfer to arteries in vivo was demonstrated using viral (retrovirus) and nonviral (liposomes) vectors in several animal species, including pigs, rabbits, and dogs. These studies reported a low efficiency of gene transfer, generally 1% or less of vascular cells in vivo.More recent studies have suggested that the efficiency of gene transfer into arteries can be improved with adenoviral vectors; increased expression of reporter genes has been reported in sheep,rat,rabbit, and pig vessels. Endothelial cells of normal arteries and endothelial and smooth muscle cells in injured arteries have been transduced at efficiencies approximately 10- to 100-fold higher than reported for retroviral and liposome vectors. A major limitation to adenoviral gene transfer in the vasculature has been transient expression; in most studies, expression of reporter gene has been observed for 7 to 14 days and is diminished or lost by 28 days. Lack of persistence of gene expression may result from cytolytic responses directed against infected cells. Transient gene expression, however, may be desirable for vascular diseases, like restenosis after angioplasty, which are characterized by cellular proliferation peaking in the first several weeks after arterial injury.

Several observations concerning the delivery of recombinant genes and patterns of gene expression can be drawn from these studies. Infusion of vector into normal arteries with an intact endothelium results in transfection of intimal cells (primarily endothelial cells). Injury to the vessel and/or application of pressure to the vector infusate results in delivery of DNA transmurally and gene expression in the media.Several catheters have been used in gene transfer studies, including double-balloon catheters, porous balloon catheters, and hydrogel catheters, and the patterns of gene expression within an artery may differ depending on the design of the catheter, animal species, and type of artery transduced.

Direct gene transfer has been used to create somatic transgene models to define gene function in arteries. In this system, genes can be expressed within arterial segments, and their biological function can be investigated. This approach has proved useful for investigation of genes whose direct in vivo effects have been difficult to analyze. For example, transfection of a recombinant angiotensin-converting enzyme gene into rat arteries using HVJ liposomes promotes angiotensin II–mediated vascular hypertrophy. After transfer of a recombinant endothelial cell–type nitric oxide (NO) synthase (ec-NOS) gene into balloon-injured rat carotid arteries, NO production was associated with a reduction in intimal thickening.Gene transfer approaches have also proved useful in the analysis of atrial natriuretic peptide, type 2 angiotensin II receptor, and VCAM-1.Growth factors and cytokines stimulate vascular cell proliferation and vessel formation in vivo. Although the genes encoding many factors have been cloned and their mechanism of action defined in vitro, definition of their role in vivo has been more difficult to analyze. Several recombinant growth factor genes, including platelet-derived growth factor–B (PDGF-B), a secreted form of acidic fibroblast growth factor (FGF-1), and an active form of transforming growth factor–^{2}1 (TGF-^{2}1) have been expressed by direct gene transfer in porcine arteries, and the function of these gene products has been analyzed. Expression of a PDGF-B gene in porcine arteries stimulated intimal hyperplasia characterized by smooth muscle cell proliferation.

Synthesis and secretion of FGF-1 were associated with expansion of the intima as well as intimal angiogenesis. Arteries transfected with a TGF-^{2}1 gene demonstrated increased procollagen synthesis in the intima and media as early as 4 days after gene transfer compared with control arteries transfected with a reporter gene. Although these recombinant genes stimulate vascular cell proliferation in vivo, they exert otherwise distinct effects on smooth muscle cell proliferation, angiogenesis, and extracellular matrix formation. These studies suggest that intimal thickening may represent a common response to gene expression of multiple growth factors, which in turn exert different effects on vessel repair.

Another approach to investigating the pathogenesis of vascular cell proliferation in vivo is to examine gene products that inhibit cell proliferation. Local delivery of an antiproliferative agent during the peak of smooth muscle cell proliferation or extracellular matrix synthesis after balloon injury might limit expansion of the intima. Several approaches have been explored in this setting, including recombinant chimeric toxins, antisense oligonucleotide strategies,and gene transfer.One approach to the selective elimination of dividing cells is to express a herpes virus thymidine kinase (HSV-tk) gene in smooth muscle cells after balloon injury. Thymidine kinase, when expressed in transduced cells, converts ganciclovir, a nucleosideanalogue, into an active toxic form, and subsequent in corporation of phosphorylated ganciclovir into cellular DNA induces chain termination in dividing cells, causing cell death. A bystander effect, demonstrated in smooth muscle and endothelial cells, confers susceptibility to ganciclovir in neighbouring dividing cells, leading to inhibition of cell growth in nontransduced neighbouring cells as well. Adenoviral vectors encoding a HSV-tk gene or no cDNA insert were introduced into porcine arteries immediately after balloon injury, and a course of ganciclovir or saline was initiated. Three weeks after balloon injury and adenoviral infection, a significant reduction in intima-to-media area ratios (54% to 59%) was observed. A reduction in intimal BrdC (5-bromo-deoxycytosine) incorporation of 40% was observed in HSV-tk ganciclovir-treated animals compared with HSV-tk saline-treated animals 7 days after gene transfer, indicating that inhibition of smooth muscle cell proliferation contributed to this effect. A significant reduction in intima-to-media area ratios in the HSV-tk ganciclovir-treated animals was observed 6 weeks after treatment, suggesting that the decrease in intimal hyperplasia was stable. In addition, no major systemic toxicities were observed associated with adenoviral infection and ganciclovir treatment. These data suggest that expression of an enzyme that catalyzes the formation of a cytotoxic drug locally within an artery may limit smooth muscle cell proliferation after balloon injury.

In balloon-injured rat carotid arteries, introduction of adenoviral vectors encoding HSV-tk immediately after balloon injury or 7 days later and treatment with ganciclovir also result in significant reductions in intima-to-media area ratios. Reendothelialization was present in rat and porcine arteries infected with HSV-tk adenoviral vectors and treated with ganciclovir, and significant toxicities were not observed in treated arteries or systemic organs. Additional approaches to limiting smooth muscle cell proliferation after vascular injury include targeting of nuclear cell cycle regulatory pathways, including the retinoblastoma gene product (Rb). Studies in injured rat carotid and porcine femoral artery models suggest that expression of a nonphosphorylatable, constitutively active form of Rb after adenoviral infection limits intimal smooth muscle proliferation for at least 3 weeks after vascular injury.

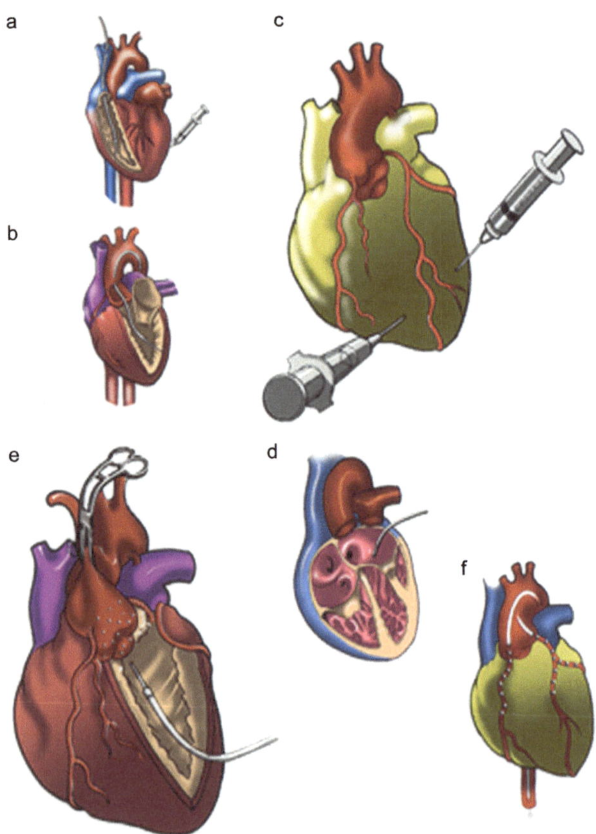

Fig.16.13 Direct and transvascular techniques of gene delivery. (a) Intramyocardial injection via the intracavitary catheter in right ventricle. (b) Intramyocardial injection via the intracavitary catheter in left ventricle. (c) Intramyocardial injection via the syringe. (d) Transvascular intracavitary delivery. (e) Transvascular nonselective intracoronary delivery with aortic cross-clamping.(f) Transvascular selective antegrade intracoronary delivery.

Myocardial Gene Transfer

Recent exciting developments hold promise for transduction of adult myocytes in vivo. Initial studies demonstrated the feasibility of expression of reporter genes in rat and canine myocardium by direct injection of plasmid DNA, but these studies were limited by low efficiencies that hindered investigations of gene expression in myocytes. The observation that adenoviruses infect nondividing cells has heightened interest in these vectors for gene transfer to adult myocardium. Indeed, recent studies have demonstrated higher levels of gene expression in rat myocardium after direct injection of adenovirus vectors compared with injection of plasmid DNA alone. Adult myocardium in vivo has also been transduced by intravascular administration of adenoviral vectors encoding reporter genes. Gene expression was observed in both the coronary vasculature and the adjacent myocardium. Levels of gene expression in the myocardium were 10- to 50-fold higher compared with direct DNA plasmid injection. Although adenoviral vectors provide efficient gene transfer, gene expression in the myocardium is transient. In most studies, reporter gene expression peaked at 1 week, diminished at 2 weeks, and was present at low levels after 1 month in adult myocytes. The mechanisms for loss of gene expression, including immune responses, are not completely understood.

Gene transfer to the myocardium has proven to be a useful tool in understanding cardiac gene regulation in vivo. For example, transcriptional elements regulating basal and thyroid hormone–responsive cardiac ±-myosin heavy chain (±-MHC) gene expression in adult rat hearts in vivo have been studied; Sequences upstream of the rat ±-MHC gene linked to a luciferase reporter were injected into adult rat hearts, and thyroid hormone responsiveness was evaluated. The thyroid hormone–responsive element was necessary, but not sufficient, to confer positive and negative regulation of thyroid hormone. Direct injection of constructs into the myocardium is a model system for investigating DNA elements and regulatory pathways that control gene expression and growth in the heart.

An additional promising area is the direct injection of adenoviral vectors into skeletal muscle for production of secreted proteins. Myoblasts, transduced by retroviral vectors expressing human growth hormone, injected into skeletal muscle produced physiological levels of human growth hormone in the serum. Recent studies suggest that physiological levels of recombinant erythropoietin are secreted into the circulation after intramuscular injection of adenovirus into skeletal muscle of neonatal mice or adult SCID mice.Neonatal and adult SCID mice injected once with 10 to 10 plaque-forming units demonstrated significant dose-dependent elevations in serum human erythropoietin levels and increased hematocrit levels that were stable over the 4-month time course of the experiments, and no evidence of a localized inflammatory response or systemic infection was present. Intramuscular injection of adenoviral vectors may be useful for the treatment of inherited disorders of deficient serum proteins.

Lipoprotein Metabolism

Direct gene transfer has been a promising tool for investigations of hepatic regulation of lipoprotein metabolism. Initial approaches used ex vivo transduction of hepatocytes to express an LDL receptor (LDLR). Hypercholesterolemia in the Watanabe rabbit was reversed after infusion of LDLR-expressing hepatocytes into the liver. This approach has been used in a human gene therapy trial of familial hypercholesterolemia. Recently, adenoviral vectors have been used to reconstitute LDLR function in Watanabe rabbits and in homozygous mice lacking LDLRs produced by homologous recombination. In this latter study, adenoviral vectors encoding a human LDL cDNA were injected intravenously into the tail vein of mice, and the hypercholesterolemic effects of the LDLR deficiency were reversed at 4 days. Adenoviral targeting to hepatocytes has also been demonstrated in healthy mice, where transient gene expression was observed.

Hepatic chylomicron remnant uptake has been studied by adenovirus-mediated gene transfer. The hypothesis that LDLR-related protein (LRP) mediates the uptake of dietary lipoprotein into hepatocytes in concert with LDLR was tested by transferring a dominant negative regulator of LRP function into livers of homozygous mice lacking LDLR. Inhibition of LRP was associated with accumulation of chylomicron remnants in these mice, suggesting a role for LRP and LDLR in chylomicron remnant clearance. Intravenous injection of an adenoviral vector encoding an apolipoprotein A-I gene results in transient hepatic production of HDL and total cholesterol. These studies demonstrate the usefulness of genetically engineered animal models for the study of lipoprotein metabolism.

Gene therapy in the cardiovascular system: an update

Two years ago a focus on cardiovascular gene therapy was published in which several reviews were presented on different fields of cardiovascular medicine, where gene therapy was emerging as a novel potential treatment modality. While somedomains, including therapeutic angiogenesis,

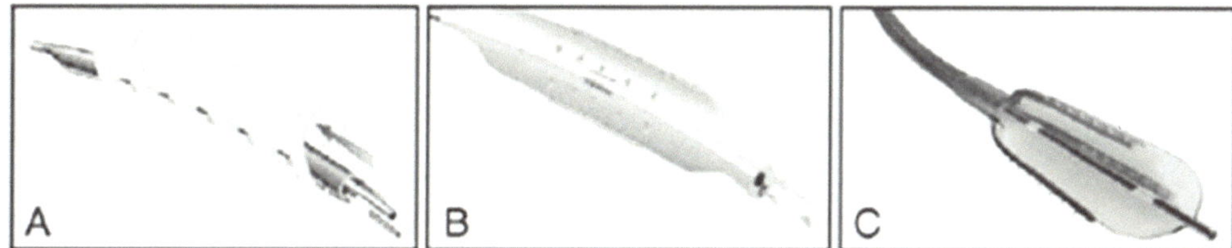

Fig. 16.14 Three types of endovascular local gene delivery devices. (A) Passive diffusion device (Dispatch catheter; SciMed Life/Boston Scientific). (B) Pressure-driven device (Remedy balloon catheter; SciMed Life/Boston Scientific). (C) Mechanically enhanced device (Infiltrator; Inter Ventional Technologies/Boston Scientific).

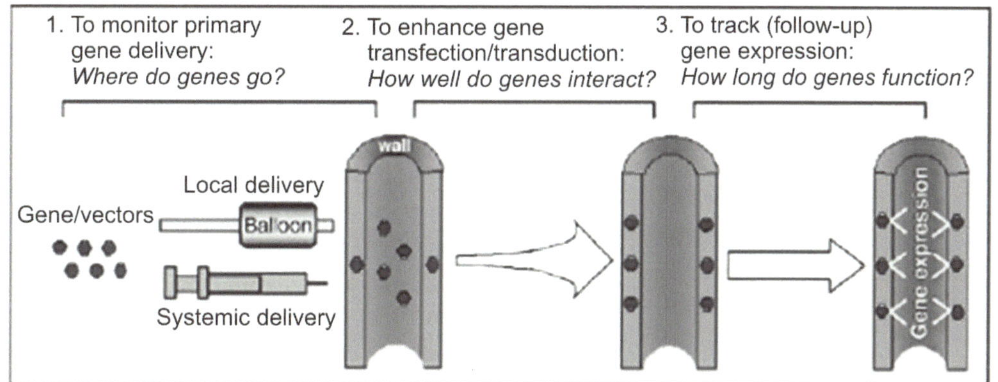

Fig. 16.15 Clinical imaging of vascular gene therapy includes three components: monitoring of primary gene or vector delivery procedure (1), enhancement of vascular gene transfection and transduction (2), and tracking of vascular gene expression (3).

have progressed at a remarkable pace, other areas are still in the phase of in vitro and small animal research. On the other hand, the powerful gene therapy technology has contributed significantly to a better understanding of cardiovascular biology. Yet many hurdles remain before gene therapy will make a noticeable impact on the treatment of cardiovascular disease: vector-related inflammation, limited expression span, suboptimal delivery systems, and gene expression levels are among the major concerns. Moreover, treatment strategies are often based on mechanisms identified in small animal models, the relevance of which for patient care needs careful consideration.

Cancer patients for whom conventional treatment failed, might be more eager to try novel, and still incompletely validated treatments, while many patients with cardiovascular diseases and their doctors hesitate to consider gene therapy. From this view point, patients suffering from cardiac diseases with few or no therapeutic options, including cardiomyopathies and end-stage heart failure, might be better candidates for gene-based treatments in the near future. Also, in some areas where gene therapy appeared as a promising alternative for failing pharmacological approaches, novel strategies are emerging. For instance, the introduction of brachytherapy in the prevention and treatment of restenosis and the advances in percutaneous revascularization procedures might bear on possible applications of gene therapy in its current state.

This update is not intended as a comprehensive overview of current research in cardiovascular gene therapy, but rather as a concise update on new developments in areas that were highlighted in a former focused issue of Cardiovascular Research in 1997 and with special emphasis on recent developments in gene therapy for angiogenesis and vasculoproliferative diseases.

1 Angiogenesis

The therapeutic implications of angiogenic growth have been clearly identified in recent years in different animal models , and have led to the initiation of clinical trials in patients with coronary and peripheral vascular insufficiency. Intramuscular injection of naked plasmid DNA encoding the 165 amino acid isoform of human vascular endothelial growth factor (VEGF) induced angiogenesis and decreased ischemia in patients with ischemic ulcers due to peripheral vascular disease In a landmark study, patients with refractory stable angina who were not amenable to classical revascularization received direct intramyocardial injections of VEGF plasmid via a mini-thoracotomy Patients had reduced clinical symptoms of angina and objective evidence of reduced ischemia as documented by dobutamine single photon emission computed tomography (SPECT) imaging.

However, the results of these studies have to be considered cautiously because of the absence of a control group. Furthermore, inflammation caused by the vector or even the needle injections might have contributed to formation of new capillaries. The need for a control group was also illustrated by the VIVA trial In this trial, patients with ischemic heart disease received placebo or intracoronary recombinant VEGF protein followed by an IV infusion. Both in the treated and the placebo group the patients' clinical status and treadmill tests improved, but the absence of a positive effect led to the premature termination of the study. Catheter-based interventional techniques will undoubtedly provide an easier way to achieve myocardial delivery and will facilitate inclusion of a control group. In this respect, successful gene transfer was obtained using a transmyocardial injection catheter.Pericardial delivery using a transatrial or transmyocardial approach has also been considered for diffusable angiogenic gene products, with the pericardial space serving as a sustained-release reservoir. An alternative approach could be to use the percutaneous PerDUCER device , allowing for safe access to the pericardial space via a minimal subxiphoid incision.

To date, the majority of gene-based experiments have been conducted in small animal models, predominantly in the murine ischemic hindlimb model. Decreased angiogenesis in diabetic mice could be overcome by intramuscular injection with adenovirus encoding VEGF . New angiogenic growth factors are also being investigated, including hepatic growth factor (HGF) , leptin [and thrombopoietin . Of interest, local overexpression of a hypoxia-inducible transcription factor has been shown to augment blood flow to an ischemic hindlimb. Hypoxia-inducible factor 1 (HIF-1) is a post-transcriptionally regulated transcription factor, controlling several hypoxia-inducible genes . Overexpression of HIF 1-

related proteins might therefore induce a broader angiogenic response than overexpression of a single angiogenic factor. Nitric oxide synthase (NOS), the enzyme responsible for endothelial NO production, might also be considered as a potential angiogenic factor, as both VEGF and FGF have been shown to modulate angiogenesis in part through the activation of NOS. Despite these exciting results two major caveats remain. First, the proof of concept of therapeutic angiogenesis in large animal models is a prerequisite for future gene therapy protocols in patients. Second, potential side effects associated with untoward angiogenesis need careful investigation.

Neoangiogenesis is indeed implicated in physiological as well as pathological processes including tumor and metastatic growth, diabetic retinopathy, and atherosclerotic plaque rupture . Inoue et al. demonstrated that expression of VEGF and its receptors flt-1 and flk-1 correlated with the severity of atherosclerosis in human coronary arteries. Furthermore, inhibition of angiogenesis by specific anti-angiogenic molecules reduced plaque growth in an atherosclerotic mouse model , whereas local administration of FGF contributed to unfavorable arterial remodeling in injured coronary arteries , possibly due to enhanced adventitial angiogenesis and increased cellular proliferation. Another safety concern is the use of angiogenic factors in diabetic patients, who commonly suffer from diffuse coronary artery disease and are potential candidates for therapeutic angiogenesis. VEGF concentrations are increased in ocular liquid of patients suffering from diabetic retinopathy , and VEGF inhibition in an experimental model of ischemic retinopathy in mice was associated with less retinopathy . Significant circulating levels of recombinant VEGF are detected after intramuscular and intramyocardial administration which may modulate unwanted angiogenesis at remote sites.

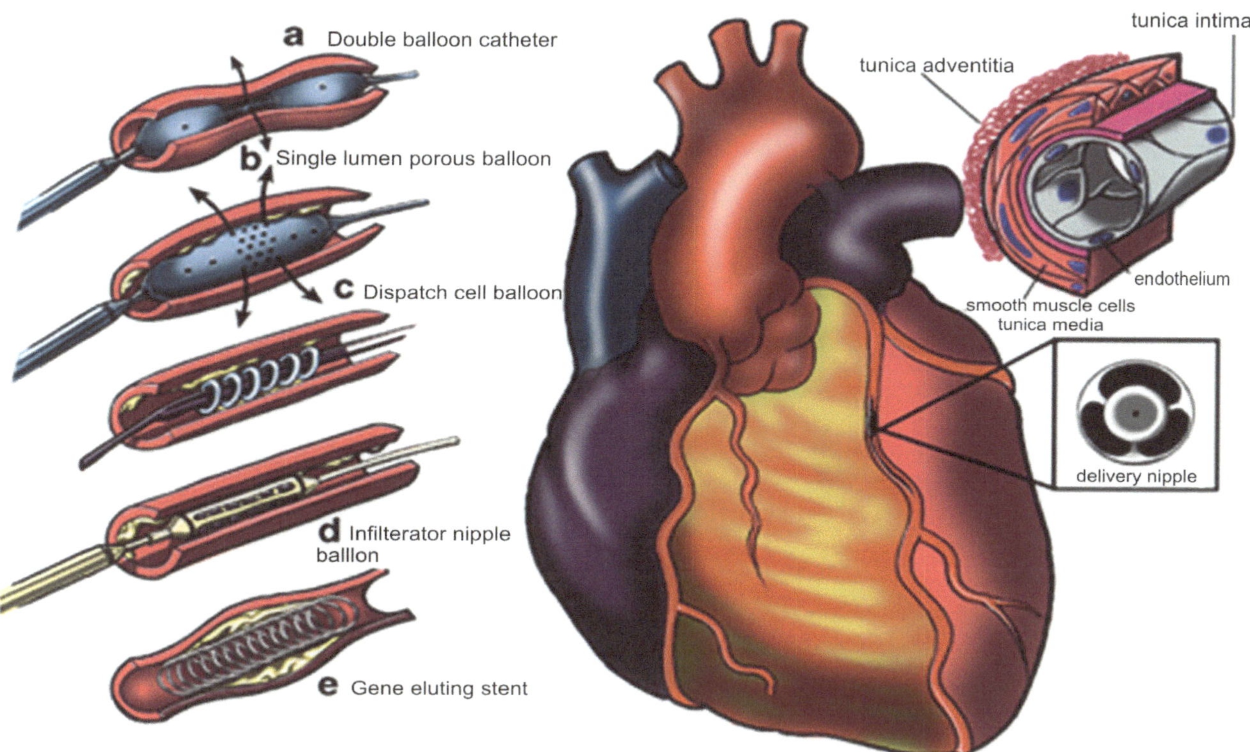

Fig. 16.16 Showing different catheters and stent for transvascular intracoronary wall gene delivery.

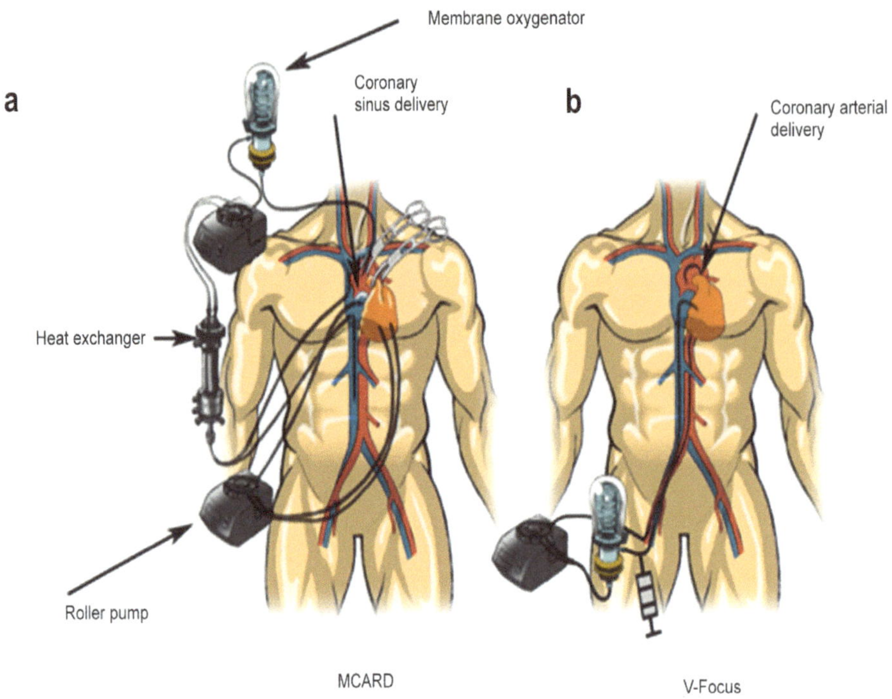

Fig 16.17 Closed-loop recirculatory systems. (a) Cardiopulmonary bypass-based technology e.g., molecular cardiac surgery with recirculating delivery (MCARD). After initiating systemic bypass, the vent cannulas were placed into left and right ventricles and connected to the venous limb of the circuit. The arterial limb is connected to the coronary sinus catheter. After stopping the heart with cardioplegia, recirculation commences for 20 min and then coronary circuit flashed. (b) Catheter-based technology (V-Focus). Coronary venous blood was drained from the coronary sinus. Following oxygenation the blood is returned to the left main coronary artery via a roller pump. Gene of interest was delivered into the antegrade limb of the circuit. Time of recirculation is 10 min. To minimize systemic expression coronary venous blood collection continued for 2 min, and the blood was diverted to a drainage bag. Main differences between V-Focus and MCARD: (i) beating vs stopping heart; (ii) direction of recirculation (coronary arteries to coronary sinus vs coronary sinus to coronary arteries); (iii) time of recirculation (10 vs 20 min); (iv) percutaneous catheter- based methodology vs cardiopulmonary bypass-based.

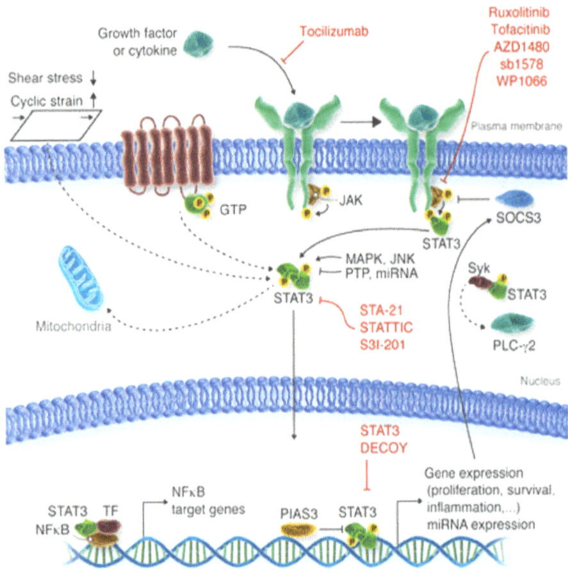

Fig.16.18. Physiological regulation and pharmacological inhibition of the STAT3 signalling pathway. STAT3 is a key player in cell signalling and transcription in response to a wide range of stimuli and in various ways. The most relevant STAT3 signalling pathways in vascular diseases are indicated with continuous lines; less well-investigated STAT3 signalling pathways are indicated with broken lines. GTP, guanosine triphosphate; JAK, janus kinase; JNK, c-Jun N-terminal kinase; MAPK, mitogen-activated protein kinase; miRNA, microRNA; NFKB, nuclear factor 'kappa-light-chain-enhancer' of activated B-cells; P, phosphate residue; PIAS3, protein inhibitor of activated STAT; PLC-g2, phospholipase C, g2 isoform; PTP, protein tyrosine phosphatase; SOCS3, suppressor of cytokine signalling; Syk, spleen tyrosine kinase; TF, transcription factor.

Clearly, further basic research needs to clarify these safety issues, and expand our knowledge of therapeutic angiogenesis and vasculogenesis as new strategies for postnatal neovascularization.

2.Vasculo-Proliferative Diseases

Gene therapy for restenosis also progressed from the experimental phase to the first clinical trials. To investigate if VEGF overexpression can accelerate re-endothelialization and thus reduce neointima after local vascular injury, as demonstrated in a rabbit model VEGF plasmid was locally delivered to patients after PTCA using the dispatch catheter . Although no final results have been reported, the method seems feasible and safe in the short term. In another trial, antisense oligonucleotides against c-myc were used to prevent coronary restenosis in stented patients (ITALICS trial) Although successful in experimental porcine studies , the results could not be reproduced in patients in part due to methodological limitations. The delivery device could have been suboptimal for effective gene transfer in the vessel wall, and both dose–response and pharmacokinetic characteristics need a more detailed evaluation.Two recent reviews have extensively covered the pros and the cons of gene therapy for restenosis. Despite major advances that have led to the first clinical trials, many hurdles remain. The difficulties to translate the excellent effect of many gene-based approaches in small animal models of vascular injury to larger, more relevant animal models and to patients relate to suboptimal delivery systems, and vector-associated toxicity.

Essential cell-cycle regulatory proteins have been targeted to prevent neointima formation, because smooth muscle cell (SMC) proliferation is a key component in the narrowing process in injured arteries In contrast, restenosis in patients is a complex biological phenomenon involving not only SMC proliferation, but also SMC migration and apoptosis, and matrix formation and degradation, which contribute to remodeling. Proteins with pleiotropic effects on vascular cell functions might have an advantage to better target the response to vascular injury in patients than is the case with cell-cycle further investigation. inhibitory proteins. In this respect, overexpression of NOS , heme oxygenase (H01) and C-type natriuretic peptide (CNP) have shown promising initial results, and deserve further investigation.

Local delivery via conventional interventional techniques remains the Achilles' heel of vascular gene therapy because of low transfection efficacy. Surgical methods, including local dwelling, are cumbersome or impossible to perform routinely. Adventitial delivery of adenoviral vectors may cause less medial inflammation than intraluminal delivery , potentially reducing vector-induced inflammation, but requires surgical procedures or perforating needle catheters . Few novel devices have emerged since a previous review in this journal more than 2 years ago. Different approaches to optimize local gene delivery have been tested. In a comparative study, three intramural pressure-driven catheters and one mechanical intramural catheter were compared in a porcine coronary artery balloon-angioplasty model . Three of the four catheters tested (Infusasleeve Crescendo and Infiltrator) demonstrated comparable efficiency as reflected by vascular luciferase gene expression levels. Clearly, further development of interventional devices is essential to increase intracoronary gene transfer and to test the role of gene therapy for restenosis.Another question relates to gene transfer efficacy and safety in complex, lipid rich atherosclerotic arteries. Adenovirus-mediated gene transfer of the marker gene human placental alkaline phosphatase was found equally effective in human atherosclerotic vessels and in normal vessels in organ culture Anti-neointimal strategies have been successful in atherosclerotic rabbits . However, there might be some concern that adenoviral vectors may induce thrombosis in atherosclerotic arteries. Lafont et al. found that adenoviral gene transfer induced thrombosis in atherosclerotic rabbit arteries, but not in normal arteries, although transfection efficiency was similar. Although NOS overexpression in balloon-injured porcine arteries reduces neointima local NOS overexpression could paradoxically contribute to neointima formation in diseased or balloon-injured atherosclerotic arteries via the generation of toxic peroxynitrite In contrast, NOS overexpression in atherosclerotic rabbit arteries might reduce mural inflammation

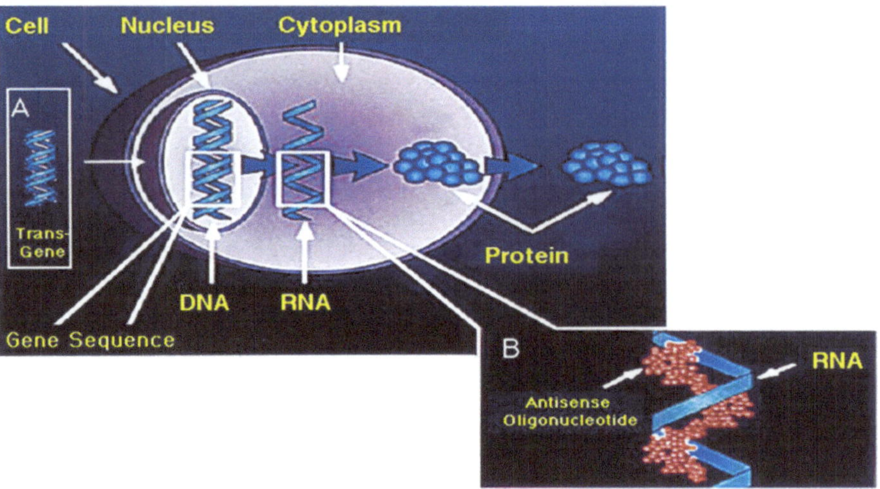

Fig. 16.19 Gene therapy strategies. (A) Gene transfer involves delivery of an entire gene, either by viral infection or by non-viral-vectors, to the nucleus of a target cell. Expression of the gene via transcription into mRNA and translation into a protein geneproduct yields a functional protein that either achieves a therapeutic effect within a transduced cell or is secreted to act on othercells. (B) Gene blockade involves the introduction into the cell of short sequences of nucleic acids that block gene expression,such as antisense oligonucleotide that bind mRNA in a sequence-specific fashion and prevent translation into protein.

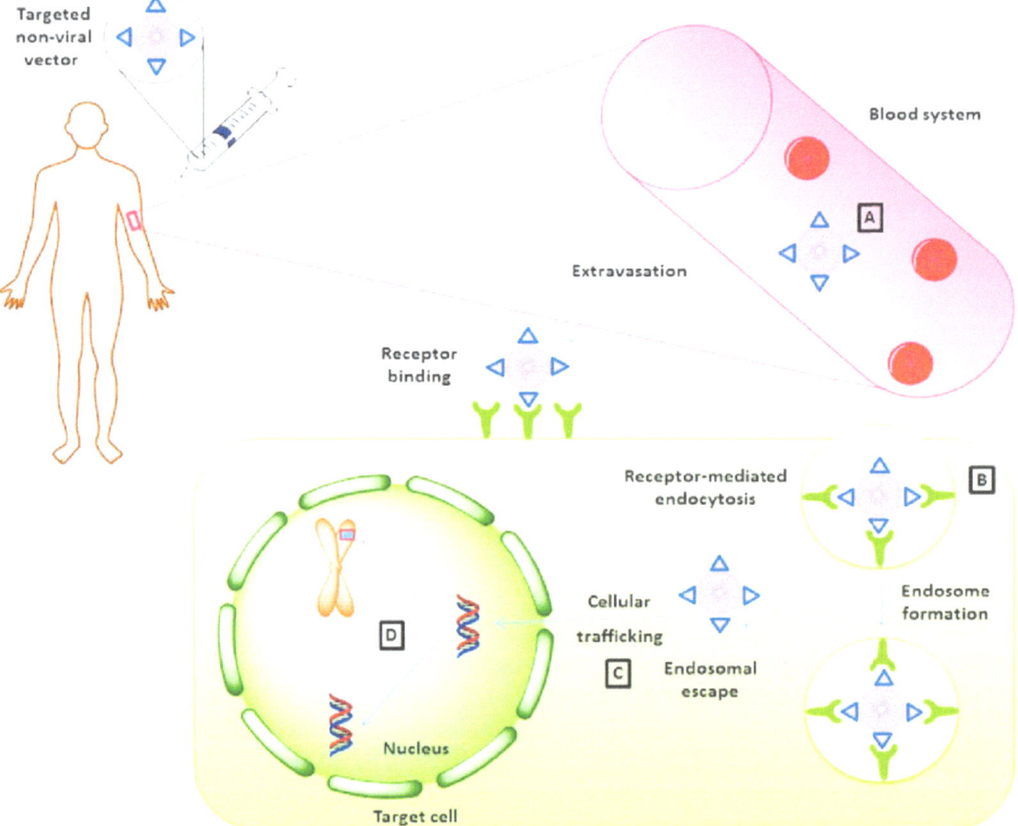

Fig. 16.20 Therapeutic gene delivery mediated by non-viral vectors. Successful gene delivery mediated by non-viral vectors

and lipid accumulation , and there are indications that NO reduces neointimal hyperplasia after balloon angioplasty in hypercholesterolemic rabbits .

The current widespread use of stents has virtually eliminated the problem of late constrictive remodeling, but remains associated with in-stent restenosis. In-stent restenosis is mainly caused by a SMC hyperproliferative response and overexpression of NOS or GAX and chimeric DNA–RNA hammerhead ribozyme to proliferating cell nuclear antigen [were capable of significantly inhibiting stenosis in a porcine coronary injury model. Coating stents with DNA or viruses may provide an interesting alternative for local vascular gene transfer, obviating the need for sophisticated and expensive delivery devices. High transfection efficiencies were reported with a DNA-eluting polymer-coated stent in porcine coronary arteries Furthermore, bioresorbable microporous intravascular stents can be impregnated with virus or DNA, providing a sustained-release local reservoir while still serving as an effective scaffold to the artery . A few years ago, seeding of genetically modified cells on stents was proposed as a promising technique , but no intracoronary applications of this approach have been reported so far.

Preventing neointimal growth in venous bypass grafts or cardiac allografts might be a particularly attractive objective for gene therapy, mainly because of the easy surgical access during tissue prelevation . Two years ago, the authors of a review on gene therapy for the prevention of vein graft failure regretted the lack of interest for gene therapy in this field. Since then, pressure-mediated delivery of E2F decoy oligonucleotide was tested in vein grafts , and was associated with decreased primary vein graft failure Reduction of neointimal growth in vein grafts has also been reported after overexpression of a constitutively active retinoblastoma protein A different approach is to reduce SMC migration in vein grafts by overexpressing tissue inhibitors of metalloproteinases (TIMP) 1 and 2 the elastase inhibitor elafin , or the senescent cell-derived inhibitor sdi-1 Coronary arteriosclerosis in a mouse cardiac transplantation model was prevented by transfer of antisense oligonucleotides against cyclin-dependent kinase CDK-2 .Further insight in the arterial response to balloon-angioplasty and stent implantation in patients will be necessary to identify the best targets to reduce restenosis. Continuous improvements in PTCA and stent implantation procedures, and the availability of intracoronary radiation will need to be balanced against the added benefit of gene therapy for restenosis. Possible candidates for gene therapy in vasculoproliferative disease include in-stent restenosis, vein graft disease and transplant atherosclerosis.

3. Hypercholestrolemia And Atherosclerosis

Atherosclerotic cardiovascular disease remains the leading cause of death in western countries. Inherited disorders of lipoprotein metabolism often lead to lipid levels that are difficult to control with conventional lipid-lowering drugs, making them particularly attractive targets for gene therapy. Four years ago, the first clinical study using ex vivo gene therapy for familial hypercholesterolemia was published. Although significant reductions of LDL levels in three out of five patients tested were observed for four months after gene transfer, to date no other clinical studies have been initiated.

Gene therapy for atherosclerosis and hyperlipidemia has been focusing on modulating lipoprotein metabolism. Successful attempts have been made to elevate HDL and to decrease LDL , VLDL , and triglyceride levels The effect of gene therapy on lipid profiles in transgenic or knock-out mice lacking key components of the lipoprotein metabolism has been amply reviewed . Gene-based techniques have also contributed to a better understanding of the pathogenesis of atherosclerosis. More recently, research has shifted to explore the effect of lipoprotein gene transfer on the development of the atherosclerotic process itself . Although larger animal models for atherosclerosis are under investigation, a proper interpretation of the effects of local genetic interventions on the atherosclerotic process, plaque stability and plaque progression remains very difficult. This is mainly due to the large variation and the unpredictability of lesions in these animals. Nevertheless, gene-based strategies for atherosclerosis and its complications will require experimental scrutiny in relevant animal models before they can be considered for clinical applications. Alternative approaches to reduce atherosclerosis and its complications include the reduction of risk factors, e.g. the inhibition of apolipoprotein(a) expression, a known risk factor for atherosclerosis . Novel non-lipoprotein-based strategies, including overexpression of NOS with subsequent reduction of inflammatory cell infiltration and lipid accumulation, might also be of interest . The use of gene therapy to stabilize arterial plaques might be a promising approach. However, intravascular administration of the gene encoding galactosidase to brachial arteries of hypercholesterolemic monkeys increased vessel wall inflammation and was associated with progression of early atherosclerotic lesions.

This might have been caused by the vector itself, or by an immunological reaction to the transgene product. Gene transfer into the atherosclerotic wall to reduce plaque progression or plaque rupture may therefore require less immunogenic vectors.

4. Myocardial Diseases

The incidence of congestive heart failure is increasing and despite advances in pharmacological treatment, the associated morbidity and mortality remain high. Therefore, gene-based strategies to improve cardiac function and overall clinical outcome might be particularly useful for these patients.

Gene-based approaches for heart failure are focusing on proteins with a positive inotropic effect. Adenoviral gene transfer of a vasopressin receptor in cardiomyocytes

Table 16.4 Potential gene therapy targets for heart failure

System	*Gene*	*Mechanism*	*Outcome*	*Clinical trials*
β-adrenergic system	β2-AR	Increases a denylyl cyclase activity	Positive inotropic effect	No
	GRK2	Abolishing GRK2 reverses agonist-dependent desensitization of β-βRs	Positive inotropic effect and improved ventricular remodeling (inconsistent results)	No
	ACVI	Full mechanism remains unclear	Positive inotropic effect	No
		Increases AMP generating	Improved ventricular remodeling	
		capacity improves phosphorylation of cTnI	Reduced apoptosis	
Ca^{2+} cycling proteins	SERCA2a	Improves cytosloic Ca^{2+} regulation	Positive inotropic effect	In proress
			Improved ventricular remodeling	
			Decreased oxygen cost of LV contractility	
			Decreased incidence of ischemic ventricular arrhythmias	
	PLN	PLN inhibition of relieves inhibitory effect of SERCA2a expression	Improved systolic and diastolic function (inconsistent results)	No
	I-1	Inhibits PP_1 leading to phosphorylation of PLN and increased SERCA2a activity	Positive inotropic effect Improves diastolic function Ameliorates ischemia reperfusion-induced injury	
	S100AI	Enhances the activity of ryanodine receptors and SERCA2a	Positive inotropic effect Improved ventricular remodeling	No
Cell death	βcl-2	Enhances cell survival	Anti-apoptotic and positive inotropic effect in ischemia/reperfusion	No
	I-1, S100 A_1	Regulation of calcium handling and decreased endoplasmic reticulum stress	Anti-apoptotic effect	No
	β2-AR	Gi-mediated pathway	Anti-α poptotic effect	No

potentiated myocardial contraction by bypassing the desensitized ²-adrenergic receptor signaling , and overexpression of phospholamban or ²2-adrenergic receptor improved ventricular function in rodent hearts. Gene transfer vectors with extended transgene expression profiles are required to effectively target heart failure. In this respect, intramyocardial or intracoronary injection of recombinant adenovirus-associated vector encoding ²-galactosidase resulted in significant transgene expression levels for up to 8 weeks after the intervention, without evidence of myocardial inflammation or necrosis Myocardial infarction is a recent target for gene-based strategies, and reduction of reperfusion injury by overexpressing antioxidative proteins might be a valuable approach. Overexpression of extracellular superoxide dismutase (ec-SOD) attenuated stunning in ischemic rabbit hearts , and adenovirus-mediated cardiac gene transfer of the antioxidant proteins SOD and catalase reduced contractile dysfunction after ischemic reperfusion in the neonatal mouse heart . Delivery of decoy double stranded DNA against NFºB, a transcriptional factor that regulatescytokine and adhesion genes, reduced the extent of myocardial infarction after reperfusion in the rat .

However, gene transfer directly into infarcted myocardium suffers of low transfection efficiency when compared to non-infarcted normal myocardium.Further experiments will have to determine the optimal delivery method and time of delivery of candidate genes for the reduction of necrosis after myocardial infarction.

A completely different genetic approach to the treatment of heart failure and myocardial infarction, is transfer of ex vivo modified cells to the myocardium, as reviewed before . Primary cells were forced to differentiate into muscle cells after overexpression of MyoD, a transcription factor that drives myogenesis in non-muscle cells. This could in theory modify the phenotype of the failing heart, provided that a sufficient number of cells can be implanted without prohibitive toxicity. These obstacles have thus far limited the applicability of the technique in large animal models.

Table 16.5 Candidate genes for antithrombotic gene therapy

Antithrombotic genes	*Biological activity*	*Mechanism of action*	*Gene therapy results*
Genes with antiplatelet activity			
Cyclooxygenase-1	Conversion of arachidonic acid into prostaglandin I_2	Antiplatelet, antimitogenic for VSMC, vasodilator	Decreased thrombosis and neointima formation in injured porcine carotid arteries
Prostacyclin synthase	Conversion of prostaglandin I2 into prostacyclin	Antiplatelet, antimitogenic for VSMC, vasodilator	–
Endothelial NO synthase (eNOS)	Endothelial NO synthesis	Antiplatelet, antimitogenic for VSMC, vasodilator	Decreased neointima formation in injured rat carotid arteries
Inducible NO synthase (iNOS)	Inducible NO synthesis in VSMC	Antiplatelet, antimitogenic for VSMC, vasodilator	Decreased neointima formation in injured rat carotid arteries
Genes with anticoagulant activity			
Hirudin	Thrombin inhibition	Anticoagulant, antiplatelet, antimitogenic for VSMC	Decreased neointima formation in injured rat carotid arteries
Thrombomodulin	Activation of protein C	Anticoagulant	Decreased clot formation in an in vitro model
Tissue factor pathway inhibitor (TFPI)	Regulation of tissue factor-induced coagulation	Anticoagulant	–
Antistasin (AST)	Factor Xa inhibition	Anticoagulant, potentiates fibrinolysis	–
Genes with fibrinolytic activity			
Tissue-type plasminogen activator (t-PA)	Plasminogen activation	Fibrinolytic	Decreased platelet deposition and fibrinogen accumulation on AV femoral shunts seeded with genetically modified cells in baboons
Urokinase-type plasminogen activator (u-PA)	Plasminogen activation	Fibrinolytic	Decreased platelet deposition and fibrinogen accumulation on AV femoral shunts seeded with genetically modified cells in baboons

• VSMC=vascular smooth muscle cells; NO=nitric oxide; AV=arteriovenous.

Gene therapy for inherited myocardial diseases still suffers from many of the obstacles pointed out 2 years ago . Targeting a sufficient number of myocytes remains a challenge, and several approaches are being contemplated to improve efficacy. Intracoronary injection is a fairly straightforward approach, but leads only to very limited transduction, with only 0.3% of the cells transfected with an adenoviral vector . Pericardial delivery is under investigation and has been combined with matrix degrading proteins which facilitate the penetration of the visceral pericardial barrier and markedly increase efficiency . Also, retrograde delivery via the sinus venosus during occlusion of the LAD has been shown to transduce 30–50% of cardiomyocytes in the LAD region .

Recently, gene-based approaches have also been proposed for the treatment of arrhythmias, both for acquired rhythm abnormalities (e.g. in heart failure or myocarditis and for inherited diseases (e.g. the long QT syndromes and familial atrial fibrillation). Improved delivery systems and vectors with longer and more stable expression patterns will allow future investigations in this field.

5. Thrombosis

In a review on gene therapy for arterial thrombosis , the first experiments to deliver antithrombotic genes (including hirudin, urokinase and cyclooxygenase) in injured arteries were described. To date, several new genes have been studied for their ability to reduce thrombosis. Adenoviral mediated overexpression of tPA , thrombomodulin , or tissue factor pathway inhibitor reduced arterial thrombosis in injured rabbit arteries. These genetic approaches need to be weighed against developments in antithrombotic molecules (GP IIbIIIa antagonists), which have significantly improved the safety/ efficacy profile of these drugs in patients suffering from acute coronary events . Certainly, if local overexpression of antithrombotic gene products will further decrease bleeding complications associated with current systemic therapy and retain therapeutic efficiency, this approach might be a valuable alternative.

6. Hypertension

Genetic strategies based on inhibition of components of the renin–angiotensin system are currently emerging to treat systemic hypertension . Intravenous injection of the gene encoding atrial natriuretic peptide (ANP) not only attenuated hypertension in rats, but also decreased cardiac hypertrophy and renal injury . While gene transfer is certainly feasible and has shown proof of principle , it seems nevertheless unlikely that it will replace pharmacological therapy in the near future, given the multifactorial etiology of the disease and the very effective pharmacological therapy.

In contrast, gene therapy for pulmonary hypertension might offer novel perspectives as pharmacological treatment options are often limited. Adenovirus-mediated delivery of constitutive NO Synthase via aerosol decreased both acute and chronic hypoxia-induced pulmonary hypertension in rats . As extended transgene expression is required for the treatment of chronic pulmonary hypertension, and because of uncertainties surrounding inflammatory reactions and immunogenicity of current vectors, improvements in vector design are necessary before considering clinical applications.

7. New Vectors

To date, DNA and oligonucleotide-based treatments have been very popular, probably due to less safety concerns as compared with viral vectors, and have been used in the first clinical trials. However, at least one clinical trial has shown negative results, possibly because of very low transduction rates. Nevertheless, oligonucleotide-based gene therapy strategies might have a future . Transfer of double stranded DNA that binds essential transcription factors inhibits the activation of endogenous gene transcription by these factors . This strategy has been successfully used in a clinical trial of prevention of vein graft failure . New oligonucleotide design can improve vector performance. Ribozymes for instance not only bind to complementary RNA sequences, but also cleave the sequence enzymatically, thereby amplifying their effect, in contrast with conventional oligonucleotides. This novel method has been successfully used in experimental models of in-stent restenosis

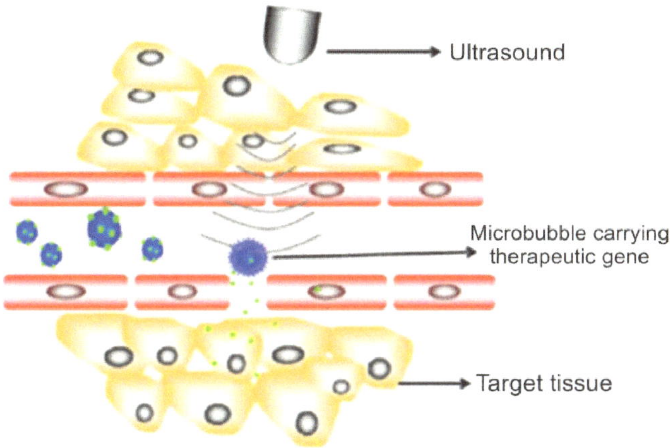

Fig. 16.21 Schematic diagram of gene therapy mediated by UTMD. Microbubbles carrying therapeutic gene are destroyed at the site of the target tissue, resulting in sonoporation and delivery of the drug directly to the target cell. The process of sonoporation induced by US application leads to transiently holes in cell membrane and capillary, which facilitates the uptake of therapeutic gene.

Although clearly more effective than naked DNA, viral vectors still suffer from local and systemic toxicity. Replication-defective adenoviruses are generated using a helper cell-line that provides the missing E1gene function. Due to possible recombination events between sequences in the vector and in the packaging helper cell-line, this method does not entirely exclude the generation of replication-competent adenoviral clones (RCA) during the manufacturing process. As RCA may contribute significantly to adenovirus-related local and systemic toxicity, the development of a new helper cell-line for the generation of virus batches free of RCA has been a major step towards future clinical use of these vectors. Because RCA have been implicated in the genesis of cardiomyopathies, previous caveats on the use of viral vectors in myocardial disease will need to be reconsidered. Thus vectors with additional deletions of adenoviral gene sequences (E2A/E4 , E1/E4 , E1/E3/E4) or vectors with all of the viral genes deleted ('gutless' vectors) have been constructed and tested in animals,often with conflicting results. However, proper engineering of viral genes will likely result in adenoviral vectors with low toxicity and immunogenicity, and which will allow prolonged expression and repeated administration.Adenovirus-associated virus (AAV)-derived vectors have been proposed as a valuable alternative for cardiovascular gene therapy. AAV-derived vectors have some advantages over adenoviral vectors, mainly because of their non-pathogenic nature and absence of inflammation, allowing stable, long-term expression . Expression of a reporter gene was observed in rat carotid arteries up to 6 months after infection with AAV . On the other hand, the AAV genome is small, only allowing room for about 4.8 kb of added DNA, and the difficulties of reproducible amplification procedures to yield high titer AAV-derived vectors have limited this far the introduction of this vector in cardiovascular disease models. Nevertheless, efforts to improve infectious titer and yield have initiated the first AAV cardiovascular gene therapy protocols in vitro and in vivo .

Retroviral vectors integrate into the host cell's genome and result in a more stable and longer expression. They can only infect dividing cells and can theoretically induce malignant transformation by their random integration in the host cell DNA. As for adenoviruses, one of the major concerns with retroviral vectors is the possibility that a replication-competent retrovirus is generated during the manufacturing process. Nevertheless, retroviral vectors are currently used for cardiovascular gene therapy protocols , and the advent of lentiviral vectors, which can infect non-dividing cells is expected to facilitate its application for cardiovascular diseases.

This is of particular interest for cardiovascular gene therapy where long term expression is desirable. An alternative to increase retroviral vector transfer efficiency is to stimulate cell proliferation in the target tissue. A limited partial liver resection to stimulate the rate of hepatocyte turn-over was performed in combination with portal vein injection of cytotoxic thymidine kinase gene followed by ganciclovir treatment. This combined suicidal gene transfer and surgical intervention resulted in improved hepatic uptake and expression of the desired transgene .Directing gene transfer vectors to the target cells exclusively might also reduce toxicity and increase efficiency.

This can be done physically with microspheres carrying vectors. Intravenous administration of oligonucleotides against c-myc bound to microbubbles, followed by transthoracic ultrasound-mediated destruction of these bubbles, prevented stenosis in balloon-injured porcine arteries . Another approach is the construction of new vectors with specific promoters which regulate transgene expression, as already described two years ago. These new promoters may include cell-specific promoters including the smooth muscle actin promotor or the ±-myosin heavy chain promoter to target the vascular SMCs and cardiomyocytes respectively. Alternatively, vectors can incorporate promoters with conditional expression including hypoxia-induced or shear stress-sensitive promoter sequences, or the viral vector envelope can be modified to increase tissue specificity. The retroviral envelope has been modified to incorporate the high affinity collagen-binding domain from von Willebrand factor , targeting the infection to the subendothelial matrix. As vascular injury exposes collagen in the vessel wall, this vector might be particularly interesting to target damaged arteries.

8.Biologic Pacemaker - Role Of GeneAnd Cell Therapy In Cardiac Arrhythmias

Researchers say they've found a way to transform ordinary pig heart muscle cells into a "biological pacemaker," a feat that might one day lead to the replacement of electronic pacemakers in humans. "Rather than having to undergo implantation with a metallic device that needs to be replaced regularly and can fail or become infected, patients may some day be able to undergo a single gene injection and be cured of slow heart rhythm forever," said senior study author Dr. Eugenio Cingolani, director of the Cedars-Sinai Heart Institute's Cardiogenetics-Familial Arrhythmia Clinic, in Los Angeles. Using gene therapy, the researchers altered a peppercorn-sized area in the heart muscle of pigs to create a new "sino-atrial node"—the bundle of neurons that normally serves as the heart's natural pacemaker.The technique kept alive a handful of pigs suffering from complete heart block, a condition in which the heart beats very slowly or not at all due to problems in the heart's electrical system. The biological pacemaker also appeared to function as well as an original sino-atrial node and better than typical electronic pacemakers, said study co-author Dr. Eduardo Marban, director of the Cedars-Sinai Heart Institute, in Los Angeles. "When we exercise, our hearts go faster. When we rest, our hearts slow down," Marban said. "The pigs with the biological pacemaker faithfully reproduced these responses, which were absent in 'control' pigs that had been treated only with an electronic pacemaker." About 300,000 electronic pacemakers are placed in humans in the United States each year, at an annual cost of $8 billion, Marban said. They work by sending electrical pulses to the heart if it is beating too slowly or if it misses a beat. The key to the new procedure is a gene called TBX18, which converts ordinary heart cells into specialized sino-atrial node cells, Marban said.

The heart's sino-atrial node initiates the heart beat like a metronome, using electric impulses to time the contractions that send blood flowing through people's arteries and veins, the scientists explained. People with abnormal heart rhythms suffer from a defective sino-atrial node.

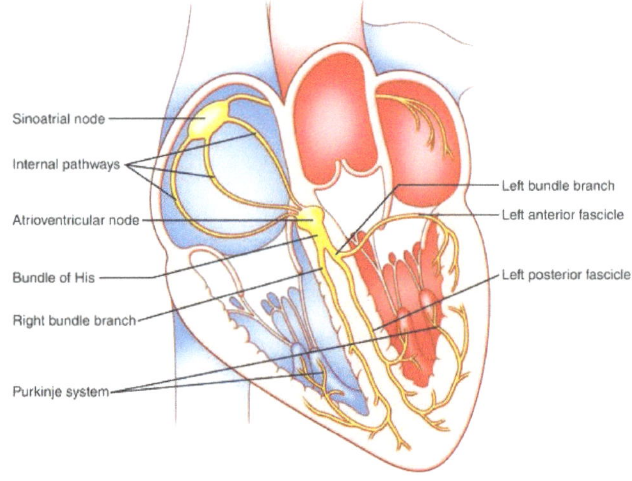

Fig 16.22 Illustration showing native physiological pacemaker at sinoatrial node for generating conventional cardiac impulse.

Researchers injected the gene into a very small area of the pumping chambers of pigs' hearts. The gene transformed the heart cells into a new pacemaker. "In essence, we create a new sino-atrial node in a part of the heart that ordinarily spreads the impulse, but does not originate it," Marban said. "The newly created node then takes over as the functional pacemaker bypassing the need for implanted electronics and hardware." Pigs were used in the research because their hearts are very similar in size and shape to those of humans, said lead study author Dr. Yu-Feng Hu, a fellow at the Cedars-Sinai Heart Institute. Within two days of receiving the gene injection, pigs had significantly stronger heartbeats than pigs that did not receive the gene. The effect persisted for the duration of the 14-day study. Toward the end of the two weeks, the treated pigs' heart rates began to falter somewhat, but remained stronger than that of the pigs who did not receive the gene injection. The research team hopes to advance to human trials within three years, Cingolani said. However, results from animal trials often can't be duplicated in humans. If the approach does work in humans, one expert said biological pacemakers could have several uses. They could be used as a "bridge" to help patients whose electronic pacemaker has to be removed or replaced, said Dr. David Friedman, chief of heart failure services at North Shore-LIJ's Franklin Hospital in Valley Stream, N.Y. Many people with electronic pacemakers that help maintain normal heart rhythm experience short periods when their pacemaker is compromised due to infection or other problems that render it non-functional," Friedman explained. "This gene therapy may someday fill that gap, expanding the arsenal of currently experimental gene and stem cell therapies that symbolize the 'holy grail' of treatments for a wide array of heart conditions."Cingolani said the therapy could also be used to treat fetuses with congenital heart block, who cannot receive a traditional pacemaker because they are still in the womb. This condition affects one out of every 20,000 fetuses.

In mammalian heart, the sino-atrial (SA) node is the pacemaker region, which contains a family of ionic currents that contributes to the pacemaker

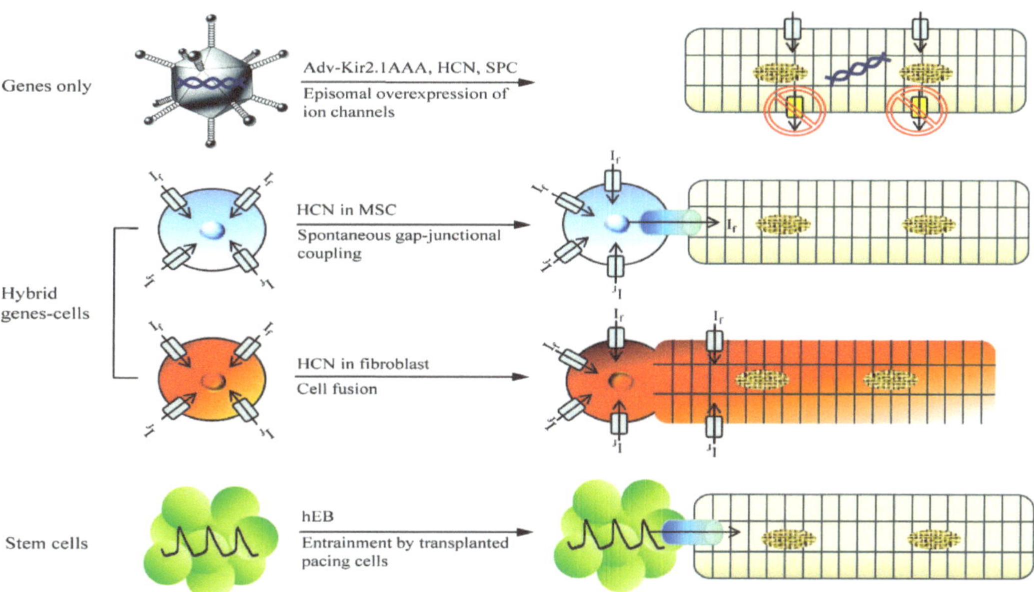

Fig 16.23 A summary of different approaches to creating a biological pacemaker. First approach (top row) is a strict gene therapy in which Kir2.1AAA, HCN, or synthetic pacemaker channel genes are overexpressed in myocytes via adenoviral delivery. Kir2.1 dominant negative proteins suppress repolarizing, outward currents whereas pacemaker channels directly contribute to diastolic membrane potential depolarization. Delivering If by MSCs requires gap-junctional coupling between myocytes and MSCs (second row). In the cell fusion approach (third row), If and the pacemaker activity arise from the HCN channels expressed on the cell membrane of the heterokaryon, without the need for gap-junctional coupling. Spontaneously beating human EBs and cardiospheres transduce their pacemaker activity to cardiomyocytes via electrotonic cell–cell coupling (fourth row).

potential. Using SA nodal cells, experiments have shown that dysrhythmias are easily elicited under conditions involving calcium overload that occur during ischemia and cardiac failure. Clinically these SA nodal dysfunctions cause bradyarrhythmias in general and areassociated with syncope but rarely with death. To initiate pacemaker function an inward current (If) carried by sodium through a family of channels that are hyperpolarization- activate dandcyclic nucleotide-gated (HCN channels).

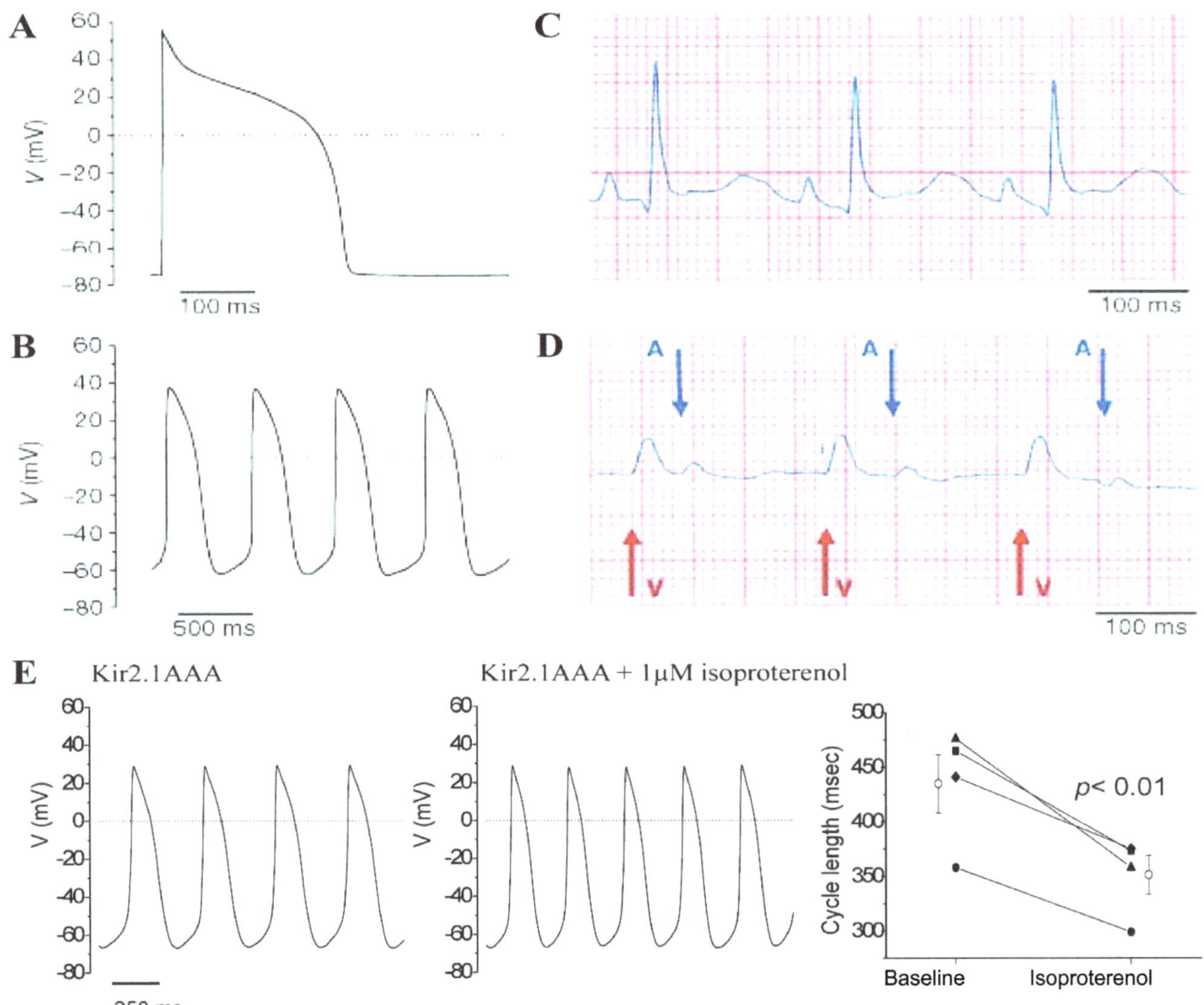

Fig. 16.24 Suppression of Kir2.1 channels unmasks latent pacemaker activity in ventricular cells. (A), APs evoked by depolarizing external stimuli in control ventricular myocytes. (B), Spontaneous APs in Kir2.1AAA-transduced myocytes with depressed IK1. (C), Baseline electrocardiograms in normal sinus rhythm. (D), Ventricular rhythms 72 hours after gene transfer of Kir2.1AAA. P waves (A and arrow) and wide QRS complexes (V and arrow) march through to their own rhythm. A through D are reproduced from Miake et al with permission.37 (E), Guinea pig ventricular myocytes in which Kir2.1AAA was overexpressed (left) and exposed acutely to 1 umol/L isoproterenol (with courtsy from J. Miake, H. B. Nuss, and E.M.)

Recent advances in molecular and cellular biology, specifically in the areas of stem cell biology and tissue engineering have initiated the development of a new field in molecular biology, regenerative medicine, seeks to develop new biological solutions, using the mobilization of endogenous stem cells or delivery of exogenous cells to replace or modify the function of diseased, absent, or malfunctioning tissue. As far as adult cardiomyocytes have limited regenerative capacity it represents an attractive candidate for these emerging technologies. Therefore, dysfunction of the specialized electrical conduction system may result in inefficient rhythm initiation or impulse conduction leading to significant bradycardia that may require the implantation of a permanent electronic pacemaker. Replacement of the dysfunctional myocardium by implantation of external heart muscle cells is emerging as a novel paradigm for restoration of the myocardial electromechanical properties, but has been significantly limited by the paucity of cell sources for human heart cells and by the relatively limited evidence for functional integration between grafted and host cells. Human embryonic stem cell lines may provide a possible solution for the cell sourcing problem. Although electronic pacing is an excellent therapy, still have disadvantage like the need for monitoring and replacement, indwelling catheter-electrodes in the heart, possibility of infection, and lack of autonomic responsiveness, geometric limitations with respect to pediatric patients make it warrant a search for better alternatives The biological pacemaker, a tissue that spontaneously or via engineering confers pacemaker properties to regions of the heart, is an exciting alternative. Several approaches have been taken in attempting to produce biological pacemakers. These can be considered in 3 headings:

1.The use of viral vectors to deliver genes to regions of the heart such that a pacemaker potential resulting in spontaneous impulse initiation evolves in the region of gene administration.
2.The use of embryonic stem cells grown along a cardiac lineage and manifesting the electrophysiologic properties of sinus node cells.
3. The use of mesenchymal stem cells as platforms to carry pacemaker genes to the heart, relying on gap junctional coupling such that the stem cell and a coupled myocyte form a single functional unit to generate pacemaker function.

Why biological pacemakers needed

Although electronic pacemakers reduced mortality associated with complete heart block and morbidity of sinoatrial node dysfunction, still they have disadvantages:

1.The imposed limitations on the exercise tolerance and cardiac rate-response to emotion. Despite the use of para-digms to improve heart rate response during increased physical activity, there is no substitute currently available for the autonomic modulation of heart rate.
2.In pediatrics, patient age and size, the mass of the power pack, and the size and length of the electrode catheter are important considerations. The hardware must be tailored to the growth of the patient.
3.The pacement site of the stimulating electrode in the ventricle and the resultant activation pathway may have beneficial or deleterious effects on electrophysiologic or contractile function.
4.The long-but-limited life battery expectancy, requiring testing and replacement at periodic intervals.
5.Infection may require removal and/or replacement of the pacemaker.
6.Various devices including neural stimulators metal detectors and magnetic resonance imaging equipment have been reported to interfere at times with electronic pacemaker function.
7.So a biological alternative that might last for the life of the patient, respond to physiologic demands for different heart rates at different times, and activate the heart via a pathway tailored to the anatomy of disease in any individual is an exciting possibility. An ideal biological pacemaker should be that which

1.Creates relatively aceepted physiologic rhythm for the life of the individual.
2.Needs no battery or electrode, and no replacement.
3.Effectively compete in direct comparison with electronic pacemakers.

4.Has no inflammatory or infectious potential.
5.Not carcinogenic.
6.Adapts to changes in physical activity and/or emotion with appropriate rapid changes in heart rate.
7.Propagate through an optimal pathway of activation to maximize efficiency of contraction and cardiac output.
8.Not arrythmogenic.
9.Potentially curative.

Strateges For Building a Biological Pacemaker

Three strategies reported till now to create biological pacemaker activity:
1.Up-regulation of adrenergic neurohumoral actions on heart rate
2.Reduction of repolarizing current
3.Increasing inward current during diastole
All three strategies had their foundations in 20th century pharmacology and physiology. In studies of autonomic modulation, increased heart rate via beta-adrenergic catecholamines or sympathetic stimulation through an increase in pacemaker current in the sinus node and in accessory pacemakers, whereas increasing vagal tone or stimulating muscarinic receptors decreased heartrate (Di Francesco et al 1986, Campbell et al 1989). In studies of ionic determinants of pacemaker activity, augmentation of hyperpolarizing, outward currents decreased pacemaker rate (Di Francesco et al 1995), suggesting that the opposite intervention, i.e. decreasing hyperpolarizing, outward currents, would increase rate (Miake et al 2002). Pharmacological experiments demonstrated that suppressing inward current carried by the T-type or L-type Ca channel slows pacemaker rate.(Lasker et al 1997, Robinson, Di Francesco 2001). What are needed are the tools to apply this knowledge to the molecular and genetic determinants of the pacemaker potential.

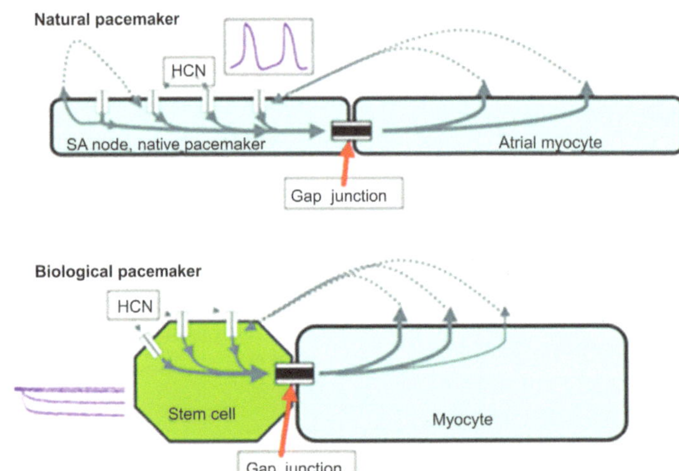

Fig.16.25 Rationale for building a biological pacemaker. Top, Initiation of spontaneous rhythms by sinoatrial (SA) node cells. Here, action potentials (inset) are initiated via inward current flowing through transmembrane HCN channels. These open as the membrane repolarizes toward its maximum diastolic potential and close when the membrane depolarizes during the action potential. Current flowing via gap junctions to adjacent myocytes results in their excitation and the propagation of impulses through the conducting system. Bottom, A stem cell engineered to incorporate HCN channels in its membrane. These channels can only open and carry in-ward current when the membrane is hyperpolarized. This hyperpolarization can be delivered if an adjacent myocyte is tightly coupled to the stem cell via gap junctions. In this setting, the opening of the HCN channels induces local current flow to excite the adjacent myocyte and initiate an action potential that propagates through the conducting system. The depolarization of the action potential will result in the closing of the HCN channels. Hence, the stem cell-myocyte pairing has 2 cells working as a single functional unit whose operation depends on the gap junctions that form between the 2 cell types. From Rosen et al with permission.

The necessary information was provided in part via the identification and cloning of the gene products that determine the beta adrenergic receptors, the inward rectifier current, and the pacemaker current. Also of central importance was the development of tools for; 1- gene therapy, wherein genes encoding the molecular subunits of interest are inserted via plasmids or viral vectors into cells of the myocardium; 2- cell therapy via the use of embryonic stem cells, whose differentiation is directed into myocardial precursors manifesting pacemaker activity, or mesenchymal stem cells used as platforms to implant channels into cardiac myocytes. A critical factor is the development of models in which to test pacemaker constructs. In vitro models of cells in culture are a standard for testing a variety of gene therapies it has been found that infecting neonatal rat ventricular myocytes with replication-deficient adenoviral constructs incorporating the gene of interest (with or without coexpression of GFP) provides a cost-effective and reproducible assay Using a variation on this model for testing the ability of stem cells to transmit the electrical signal of interest .It has been considered that a 100 times or more overexpression of current and a statistically significant effect on beating rate as standards that discriminate efficacy, More research is required to establish uniform guidelines permitting reliable correlation of in vitro and in vivo effectiveness. As an intact animal screen, the use of guinea pig (Miake et al 2002), swine (Edelberg et al 2001), and dog (Qu et al 2003, Plotnikovet al 2004, Potapova et al 2004) has been reported. The use of dog is based on its cardiac size, tractability as a chronic model, and similar electrophysiologic properties to those of man.

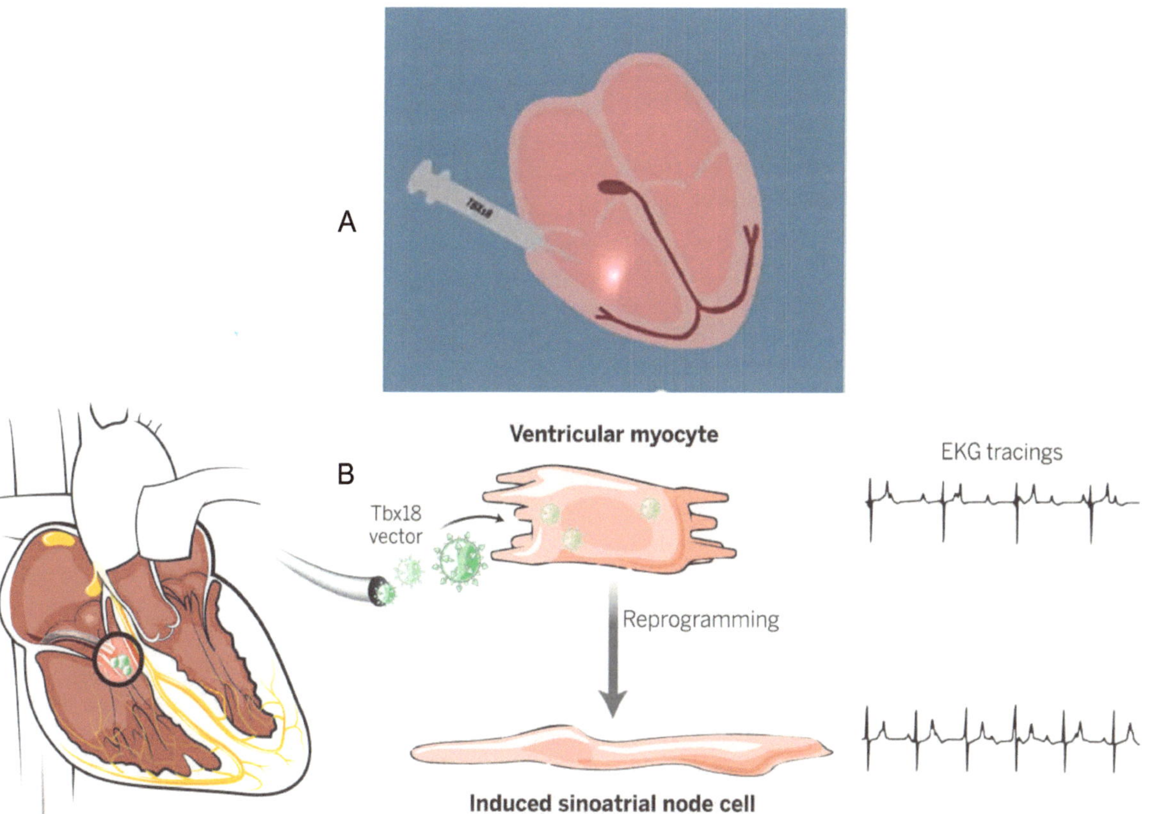

Fig. 16.26 (A&B)Researchers successfully used gene therapy to create a "biological pacemaker" that could one day replace electronic pacemakers currently used to treat human heart conditions.

Cell therapy for the treatment of cardiac arrhythmias

An alternative approach to overcome the shortcomings of gene therapy may be the use of genetically modified cell grafts that can be initially transfected ex vivo with excellent long-term efficiency and then transplanted to the in vivo heart. This will require the following:

1.Establish the proper cell sources for transplantation.
2.Assessment of the phenotypic structural and functional properties of the cell grafts, in vitro.
3.Establish transplantation strategies to deliver the cells to the desired locations.
4.Achieve the desired in vivo effect by assuring the survival of the cell grafts, their integration and interactions with host tissue, and their proper function.

Cell therapy can be applied for the treatment of cardiac arrhythmias at three different levels

1.Replace absent or malfunctioning cells of the conduction system.
2.Modify the myocardial electrophysiological substrate by using cell grafts genetically engineered to express specific ionic channels, which can couple and modify the electrophysiological properties of host tissue through electrotonic interactions.
3.Modify the myocardial environment by local secretion of specific recombinant proteins.

A major limitation for the development of such cell replacement strategies is the paucity of cell sources for human cardiomyocytes. The use of the recently described human embryonic stem cell lines may be solution to this cell-sourcing problem (Gepstein 2002). These unique cell lines have the capability to be propagated in vitro in the undifferentiated state in large quantities and to be coaxed to differentiate to a plurality of cell lineages, including cardiomyocytes (Kehat et al 2001(a). This differentiating system is not limited to the generation of isolated cardiac cells, but rather a functional cardiac syncytium is generated with a stable pacemaker activity and electrical propagation (Kehat et al 2002). that can alsorespond to adrenergic and cholinergic stimuli The ability to generate, ex vivo, different subtypes of human cardiomyocytes (with pacemaking-, atrial-, ventricular-, or Purkinje-like phenotypes) (Mummery et al 2003) that could lend themselves to genetic manipulation may be of great value for future cell therapy strategies aiming to regenerate or to modify the conduction system.

The ability of the grafted cells (pacemaker cells or conductive tissue) to integrate structurally and functionally with host tissue is a sole requirement. The human ES cell derived cardiomyocytes were able to integrate ex vivo both structurally and functionally with preexisting cardiac tissue and to generate a single functional syncytium (Kehat et al 2001 (b). Whereas it is not surprising that cardiomyocyte cell grafts can form intercellular connections with host cells (Isner 2002). Recent studies have demonstrated that other cell types such as fibroblasts (Rook et al 1992, Fast et al 1996,Gaudesius et al 2003) are also capable of forming gap junctions with host cardiomyocytes and that specific electrotonic interactions can be generated between these cells. The feasibility of using genetically engineered fibroblasts, transfected to express the voltage-gated potassium channel Kv1.3, to modify the electrophysiological properties of cardiomyocyte cultures have been examined, in a study, using a high-resolution multi-electrode array mapping technique to assess the electrophysiological and structural properties of primary neonatal rat ventricular cultures. The transfected fibroblasts were demonstrated to significantly alter the electrophysiological properties of the cardiomyocyte cultures. These changes were manifested by a significant reduction in the local extracellular signal amplitude and by the appearance of multiple local conduction blocks (Feld et al 2002). The location of all conduction blocks correlated with the spatial distribution of the transfected fibroblasts as assessed by vital staining and all of the electrophysiological changes were reversed following the application of a specific Kv1.3 blocker Genetically engineered cell grafts, transfected to express potassium channels, can couple with host cardiomyocytes and alter the local myocardial electrophysiological properties by reducing cardiac automaticity and prolonging refractoriness. Investigators studied the ex vivo, in vivo, and computer simulation studies to determine the ability of transfected fibroblasts to express the voltage-sensitive potassium channel Kv1.3 to modify the local myocardial excitable properties. Co-culturing of the transfected fibroblasts with neonatal rat ventricular myocyte cultures resulted in a significant reduction (68%) in the spontaneous beating frequency of the cultures compared with baseline values and co-cultures seeded with naive fibroblasts. In vivo grafting of the transfected fibroblasts in the rat ventricular myocardium significantly prolonged the local effective refractory period from an initial value of 84 +/-8 ms (cycle length, 200 ms) to 154+/-13 ms (P<0.01). Marga toxin partially reversed this effect (effective refractory period, 117 +/-8 ms; P <0.01). In contrast, effective refractory period did not change in nontransplanted sites (86+/-7 ms) and was only mildly increased in the animals injected with wild-type fibroblasts (73 +/-5 to 88+/-4 ms; P<0.05). Similar effective refractory period prolongation also was found during slower pacing drives (cycle length, 350 to 500 ms) after transplantation of the potassium channels expressing fibroblasts (Kv1.3 and Kir2.1) in pigs. (Yankelson et al 2008).The possible utilization of cell grafts (fibroblasts, different stem cell derivatives, or other cell sources) that can be genetically manipulated ex vivo to display specific electrophysiological characteristics and then grafted to the in vivo heart may possess a number of theoretical advantages over direct gene therapy. These advantages may be related to a better efficiency and control of the transfection process ex vivo, the ability to screen the phenotypic properties of the cells before transplantation, and the possible achievement of long-term effect because cardiac cell grafts were demonstrated to survive for prolonged periods following transplantation (Muller-Ehmsen et al 2002). Yet, determining the optimal way for the delivery of the cells, controlling their survival followingtransplantation, assuring appropriate integration of the cells with host tissue, and developing means to control the required electrophysiological effect are all important obstacles for the future use of this approach as a therapeutic strategy.

Ischemic heart disease represents one of the most important conditions predisposing to arrhythmias. A variety of preclinical and clinical studies have demonstrated the potential utility of gene therapy in the management of chronic ischemic patients through the local secretion of angiogenic growth factors such as vascular endothelium growth factor (VEGF) and fibroblast growth factor (Isner 2002). Cell therapy strategies may similarly play a dual role in promoting angiogenesis. First, cells transfected ex vivo may be used for sustained local release of recombinant proteins with angiogenic properties following in vivo grafting. Second, transplantation of specific cell types such as endothelial progenitor cells may contribute directly to the neovascularization process. The improved understanding of the molecular pathways involved in the development of heart failure allow definition of several molecular targets for gene therapy to improve systolic and diastolic properties of failing myocytes. To focus on modulating calcium homeostasis, manipulating the beta-adrenergic receptor signaling pathways, and improving cardiomyocyte resistance to apoptosis need to be looked for in future strategies. Similarly, cellular cardiomyoplasty and tissue engineering approaches to regenerate functional myocardium also represent a novel approach for the treatment of heart failure.

Future prospective in biological pacing system

Improvement in the understanding of the mechanisms underlying many of cardiac arrhythmias and the development of molecular and cellular tools suggest a future role for gene and cell therapies for treatment of different cardiac arrhythmia. Bridging the gap between the proof-of-concept and the clinical application will require important methodological developments as well as extensive animal experiments. Newer refinements in vector development and design are needed to have better transduction in cardiovascular tissue. Cell specific regulatory elements and promoters to to selectively target the cardiac tissue is a potential area of interest (Beck et al 2004). Bacterial gene delivery as an alternative to viral vectors has been proposed (Palffy et al 2006). Hybrid vectors, gutted vectors and new generation non viral vectors may hold the key to future. Evidence from both viral and stem cell approaches state that proof of concept is there. Trials can be designed that permit us to test biological versus electronic pacemakers in relative safety in patients who are protected from failure of the biological unit. Tandem pacing is the proposed way to proceed clinically (patients with chronic atrial fibrillation and complete heart block); i.e. implant both a biological pacemaker and an electronic demand pacemaker in the same individual, this has been tested in dogs in complete heart block an adenoviral HCN2 construct (into the left bundle-branch system) were delivered and an electronic demand unit, the electrode of which was placed in the right ventricular endocardial apex (Bucchi et al 2006). The biological pacemaker fired 70% of the time and was catecholamine responsive. Moreover, when the biological unit slowed, the electronic unit took over; similarly, the electronic unit sensed the biological unit well and discontinued its function when the biological function emerged, the memory function of the electronic unit can track the function of the biological unit, providing a record for the cardiologist.

Given the imperfections that still reside with electronics, the possibility of a system with no wires, no hardware, and a software that is of the body's own ion channels and autonomic nervous system offers something more appealing, if it can be made to function at the level needed and for the time required. As mentioned above, rate responsiveness is here, and improved and leadless systems have arrived as well. Therefore, there are two competitive approaches evolving. Which will dominate,traditional electronics upgraded to achieve still newer levels of success or biologics, is unknown, and the future will answer.

Scientists Created A Pig-Human Hybrid Embryo For Human Organ Transplantation

Scientists at the Salk Institute in California have created a part-human, part-pig embryo.

Bioethicist Arthur Caplan told us about the ethical concerns involved in mixing human and animal DNA.An experiment reported on Thursday in Cell, a peer-reviewed scientific journal, announced a purported break through in bioengineering: the successful creation of an embryo with both human and pig DNA (and to be clear, the artwork above is just a photo of a sculpture). The results, "raise the possibility of xeno-generating transplantable human tissues and organs towards addressing the world-wide short-age of organ donors," according to the paper.

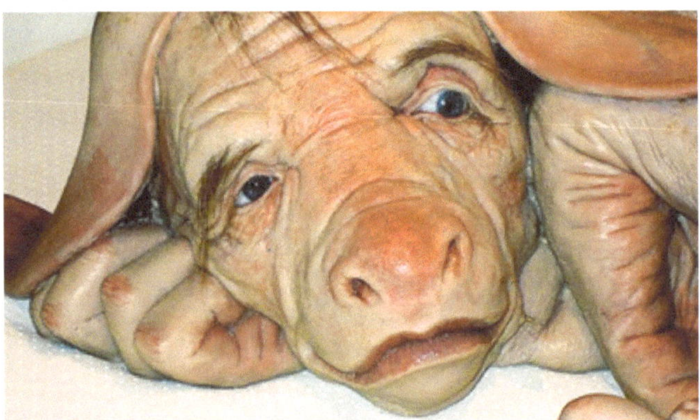

Fig. 16.27 Scientists at the Salk Institute in California have cre-ated a part-human, part-pig embryo.

- New line of pigs do not reject transplants Fig. 80.39 Scientists at the Salk Institute in California have created a part-human, part-pig embryo.
- Will allow for future research on stem cell therapies
- Pigs are much closer to humans than many other test-animalsScientists have successfully transplanted human stem cells into pigs that were genetically modified not to reject them. The cells were able to thrive, raising hopes of potential stem cells treatments for debilitating diseases. The breakthrough could also aid in developing treatments for patients suffering from severe immune deficiency.

Bibliography and Acknowledgement

- Aoki M., Morishita R., Matsushita H., et al.(1998) Benefic angiogenesis induced by over-expression of human hepatocyte growth factor (HGF) in non-infarcted and infarcted myocardium: potential gene therapy for myocardial infarction [abstract] Circulation 98:I321.
- Barr E, Carroll J, Kalynych AM, Tripathy SK, Kozarsky K, WilsoJM, Leiden JM. Efficient catheter-mediated gene transfer into the heart using replication-defective adenovirus. Gene Ther. 1994;1:51-58.
- Baumgartner I., Pieczek A., Manor O., et al.(1998) Constitutive expression of phVEGF165 after intramuscular gene transfer promotes collateral vessel development in patients with critical limb ischemia. Circulation 97:1114–23.
- Berkner KL. Expression of heterologous sequences in adenoviral vectors. Curr Top Microbiol Immunol. 1992;58:39-66.
- Bonanno G, Mariotti A, Procoli A, et al. Human cord blood CD133+ cells immunoselected by a clinical-grade apparatus differentiate in vitro into endothelial- and cardiomyocyte-like cells. Transfusion. 2007;47(2):280-
- Bouloumie A., Drexler H.C., Lafontan M., Busse R.(1998) Leptin, the product of Ob gene, promotes angiogenesis. Circ Res 83:1059–66.
- Brown H.F., Kimura J., Noble D., Noble S.J., Taupignon A.The ionic currents underlying pacemaker activity in rabbit sinoatrial node: experimental results and computer simulations. Proc. R. Soc. Lond. B. Biol. Sci 222:329-347
- Cheng F, Zou P, Handong Y. Induced differentiation of human cord blood mesenchymal stem/progenitor cells into cardiomyocyte-like cells in vitro. J Huazong Univ Sci and Tech. 2003;23(2):154-7.
- Chen SL, Fang WW, Ye F, Liu YH, Qian J, Shan SJ, Zhang JJ, Chunhua RZ, Liao LM, Lin S, Sun JP. Effect on left ventricular function of intracoronary transplantation of autologous bone marrow mesenchymal stem cell in patients with acute myocardial infarction. Am J Cardiol 2004; 94:92-95.
- Cone RD, Mulligan RC. High-efficiency gene transfer into mammalian cells: Generation of helper-free recombinant retrovirus with broad mammalian host range. Proc Natl Acad Sci U S A. 1984;81:6349-53.
- Cornetta K, Moen RC, Culver K, Morgan RA, McLachlin JR, Sturm S, Selegue J. Amphotropic murine leukemia retrovirus is not an acute pathogen for primates. Hum
- Gene Ther. 1990;1:15-30. DeYoung M.B., Dichek D.A (1998) Gene therapy for restenosis: are we ready? Circ Res 82:306–13.
- Di Francesco D. (1981) A study of the ionic nature of the pacemaker current in calf Purkinje fibres. J. Physiol 314:377-93. Di Francesco D. (1982) Block and activation of the pacemaker channel in calf Purkinje fibres: effects of potassium, caesium and rubidium. J. Physiol 329:485-507.
- Engelhardt JF, Simon RH, Yang Y, Zepeda M, Weber-Pendleton S, Doranz B, Grossman M, Wilson JM. Adenovirus-mediated transfer of the CFTR gene to lung of nonhuman primates: biological efficacy study. Hum Gene Ther.1993;4:759-69.
- Engelhardt JF, Ye X, Doranz B,

Wilson JM. Ablation of E2A in recombinant adenoviruses improves transgene persistence and decreases inflammatory response in mouse liver. Proc Natl Acad Sci U S A. 1994;91:6196-6200.
- Flugelman MY, Jaklitsch MT, Newman KD, Casscells W,Bratthauer GL, Dichek DA. Low-level in vivo gene transfer into the arterial wall through a perforated balloon catheter. Circulation. 1992;3:1110-7.
- Garver RI Jr, Chytil A, Courtney M, Crystal RG. Clonal gene therapy: transplanted mouse fibroblast clones express human ±1- antitrypsin gene in vivo. Science. 1987;237:762-4.
- Gerard RD, Herz J. Adenovirus-mediated low density lipoprotein receptor gene transfer accelerates cholesterol clearance in normal mice. Proc Natl Acad Sci U S A. 1993;90:2812-6.
- Graham FL, Prevec L. Adenovirus-based expression vectorsand recombinant vaccines. In: Ellis RW, ed. Vaccines: New Approaches to Immunological Problems. Boston, Mass: Butterworth-Heinemann; 1992:363-390.
- Grossman M, Raper SE, Kozarsky K, Stein EA, Engelhardt JF, Muller D, Lupien PJ, Wilson JM. Successful ex vivo gene therapy directed to liver in a patient with familial hypercholesterolaemia. Nat Genet. 1994;6:335-41.
- Guzman RJ, Lemarchand P, Crystal RG, Epstein SE, Finkel T. Efficient and selective adenovirus-mediated gene transfer into vascular neointima.Circulation. 1993;88:2838-48. Hagiwara
- N., Irisawa H., Kameyama M. (1988) Contribution of two types of calcium currents to the pacemaker potentials of rabbit sinoatrial node cells. J. Physiol. (Lond.) 395:233-253.
- Hagiwara N., Irisawa H., Kasanuki H., Hosoda S. (1992) Background current in sinoatrial node cells of the rabbitheart.J.Physiol.(Lond.)448:53-72.
- Henning RJ, Abu-Ali H, Balis JU, Morgan MB, Willing AE, Sanberg PR. Human umbilical cord blood mononuclear cells for the treatment of acute myocardial infarction. Cell Transplant. 2004;13(7-8):729-39.
- Henry T.D., Annex B.H., Azrin M.A., et al.(1999) Double blind, placebo controlled trial of recombinant human vascular endothelial growth factor. The VIVA Trial [abstract] J ACoII Cardiol 33:384A.
- Herreros J, Prosper F, Perez A, Gavira JJ, Garcia-Velloso MJ, Barba J, Sanchez PL, Canizo C, Rabago G, Marti-Climent JM, HernandezM,Lopez-HolgadoN,Gonzalez-SantosJM, Martin-LuengoC,AlegriaE.Autologous intramyocardial injection of cultured skeletal mus cle-derived stem cells in patients with non-acute myocardial infarction. Eur Heart J 2003; 24:2012-20.
- Hock RA, Miller AD. Retrovirus-mediated transfer and expression of drug resistant genes in human haematopoietic progenitorcells.Nature.1986;320:275-7.
- Hu CH, Wu GF, Wang XO et al. Transplanted human umbilical cord blood mononuclear cells improve left ventricular function through angiogenesis in myocardial infarction. Chin Med J (Engl). 2006;119(18):1499-506.
- J, Guetta E, Feinberg MS et al. Human umbilical cord blood-derived CD133+ cells enhance function and repair of the infarcted myocardium. Stem Cells. 2006;24(3):772-80.
- Kornowski R., Fuchs S., Vodovotz Y., et al.(1999) Successful gene transfer in a porcine ischemia model using the Biosense(tm) guided transendocardial injection catheter

[abstract] J Am Coll Cardiol 33:355A.
- Lee SW, Trapnell BC, Rade JJ, Virmani R, Dichek DA. In vivo adenoviral vector-mediated gene transfer into balloon-injured rat carotid arteries. Circ Res. 1993;73:797-807.
- .Lemarchand P, Jones M, Yamada I, Crystal RG. In vivo gene transfer and expression in normal uninjured blood vessels using replication-deficient recombinant adenovirus vectors. Circ Res. 1993;72:1132-8.
- Levi M., Coronel R.(1997) Gene therapy in the cardiovascular system. Cardiovasc Res 35:389–90. Li J.,Qu J., Nathan R.D. (1997) Ionic basis of ryanodine's negative chronotropic effect on pacemaker cells isolated from the sinoatrial node. Am. J. Physiol273:H2481-H2489
- Losordo D.W., Vale P.R., Symes J.F., et al.(1998) Gene therapy for myocardial angiogenesis: initial clinical results with direct myocardial injection of phVEGF165 as sole therapy for myocardial ischemia
- Macris M.P., Igo S.R.(1999) Minimally invasive access of the normal pericardium: initial clinical experience with a noveldevice.ClinCardiol22:I36–39.
- Ma N. Ladilov Y, Kaminski A, Piechaczek C. Stamm C. Umbilical cord blood cell transplantation for myocardial regeneration. Transplant proc. 2005;38(3):771-3.12Leor
- Ma N, Stamm C, Kaminski A, Li W, et al. Human cord blood cells induce angiogenesis following myocardial infarction in NOD/scid-mice. Cardiovascular Research. 2005;66(1):45-54.
- March K.L., Woody M., Mehdi K., et al(1999) Efficient in vivo catheter-based pericardial gene transfer mediated by adenoviral vectors. Clin Cardiol 22:I23–I2
Melillo G., Scoccianti M., Kovesdi I., et al.(1997) Gene therapy for collateral vessel development. Cardiovasc Res 35:480–489.
- Miller DG, Adam MA, Miller AD. Gene transfer by retrovirus vectors occurs only in cells that are actively replicating at the time of infection. Mol Cell Biol. 1990;10:4239-42
- Muller DWM, Gordon D, San H, Yang ZY, Pompili VJ, Nabel GJ, Nabel EG. Catheter-mediated pulmonary vascular gene transfer and express. Circ Res.1994;75:1039-49.
- Nabel EG, Plautz G, Boyce FM, Stanley JC, Nabel GJ. Recombinant gene expression in vivo within endothelial cells of the arterial wall. Science.1989;244:1342-4.
- N, Copin H, Barnoux M, Ie Bert M, Samuel JL, Rappaport L,Menasche P. Can cellular transplantation improve function in doxorubicin-induced heart failure? Circulation 1998; 98(suppl 11):11-151-11-156.
- Nishiyama N, Miyoshi S, Hida N, et al. The significant cardiomyogenic potential of human umbilical cord blood-derived mesenchymal stem cells in vitro. Stem Cells. 2007;25(8):2017-24.
- Noma A., Irisawa H. (1975) Effects of Na+ and K+ on the resting membrane potential of the rabbit sinoatrial node cell.Jpn.J.Physiol25:287-302.
- Ohno T, Gordon D, San H, Pompili VJ, Imperiale MJ, Nabel GJ, Nabel EG. Gene therapy for vascular smooth muscle cell proliferation after arterial injury. Science. 1994;265:781-784.
- Ono K., Ito H. (1995) Role of rapidly activating delayed rectifier K+ current in sinoatrial node pacemaker activity. Am. J.Physiol269:H453-H462.
- Ratko T.A., Cummings J.P., Blebea J.,Matuszewski K.A. (2003) Clinical gene therapy for nonmalignant disease. Am. J. Med 115(7):560-569.
- Rivard A., Silver M., Chen D., et al.(1999) Rescue of diabetes-related impairment of angiogenesis by intramuscular gene therapy with adeno-VEGF. Am J Pathol 154:355–63.
- Roe TY, Reynolds TC, Yu G, Brown PO. Integration of murine leukemia virus DNA depends on mitosis. EMBO J. 1993;12:2099-2108.
- Scorsin M, Hagege AA, Dolizy I, Marotte F, Mirochnik Simon RH, Engelhardt JF, Yang Y, Zepeda M, Weber-Pendleton S, Grossman M, Wilson JM. Adenovirus-mediated transfer of the CFTR gene to lung of nonhuman primates: toxicity study. Hum Gene Ther. 1993;4:771-780.
- Simons M.Ware J.A. (2003) Therapeutic angiogenesis in cardiovascular disease. Nature reviews. Drug Discov 2(11):863-871.
- Strauer B.E., Brehm M., Zeus T., et al. (2002) Repair of infracted myocardium by autologous intracoronary monomuclear bone marrow cell transplantation in humans.Circulation 106:1913-18.
- Tal I., Schaper W.(1997) Angiogenesis by gene therapy: a new horizon for myocardial revascularization? Cardiovasc Res 35:490–7.
- Teirstein P.S., Massullo V., Jani S., et al.(1999) Two-year follow-up after catheter-based radiotherapy to inhibit coronary restenosis. Circulation 99:243–47.
- Tripathy SK, Goldwasser E, Lu MM, Barr E, Leiden JM. Stable delivery of physiological levels of recombinant erythropoietin to the systemic circulation by intramuscular injection of replication-defective adenovirus. Proc Natl Acad SciUA1994;91:11557-11561.
- Verrier R.L., Waxman S., Lovett E.G., Moreno R.(1998) Transatrial access to the normal pericardial space: a novel approach for diagnostic sampling, pericardiocentesis, and therapeutic management
- Wilson JM, Birinyi LK, Salomon RN, Libby P, Callow AD, Mulligan RC. Implantation of vascular grafts lined with genetically modified endothelial cells. Science. 1989;244:1344-6.
- Wilson JM, Jefferson DM, Chowdhury JR, Novikoff PM, Johnston DE, Mulligan RC. Retrovirus-mediated transduction of adult hepatocytes. Proc Natl Acad Sci U S A. 1988;85:3014-18.
- Wollert KC, Meyer GP, Lotz J, Ringes-Lichtenberg S, Lippolt P,Breidenbach C, Fichtner S, Korte T, Hornig B, Messinger D, Arseniev L, Hertenstein B, Ganser A, Drexler H. Intracor-onary autologous bone-marrow cell transfer after myocardial infarction: the BOOST randomi sed controlled clinical trial. Lancet 2004; 364:141-8.
- Yamada Y, Yokoyama S, Fukuda N, et al. A novel approach for myocardial regeneration with educated cord blood cells cocultured with cells from brown adipose tissue. Biochem Biophys Res Commun. 2007;353(1):182-
- Zabner J, Petersen DM, Puga AP, Graham SM, Couture LA, Keyes LD, et al. Safety and efficacy of repetitive adenovirus-mediated transfer of CFTR cDNA to airway epithelia of primates and cotton rats. Nat Genet. 1994;6:75-83.

CHAPTER

Management of Heart Failure with Implantation of Newer Devices

Several new devices for the treatment of heart failure (HF) patients have been introduced and are increasingly used in clinical practice or are under clinical evaluation in either observational and/or randomized clinical trials. These devices include cardiac contractility modulation, spinal cord stimulation, carotid sinus nerve stimulation, cervical vagal stimulation, intracardiac atrioventricular nodal vagal stimulation, and implantable hemodynamic monitoring devices. This task force believes that an overview on these technologies is important. Special focus is given to patients with HF New York Heart Association Classes III and IV and narrow QRS complex, who represent the largest group in HF compared with patients with wide QRS complex. An overview on potential device options in addition to optimal medical therapy will be helpful for all physicians treating HF patients.

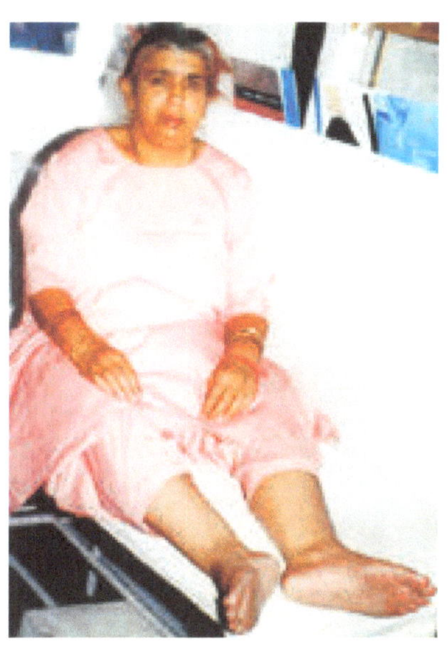

Fig. 17.1 Rough, dry hair, skin, facial puffiness, edema of whole body and cardiomegaly in a middle aged lady with hypothyroidism and heart failure.

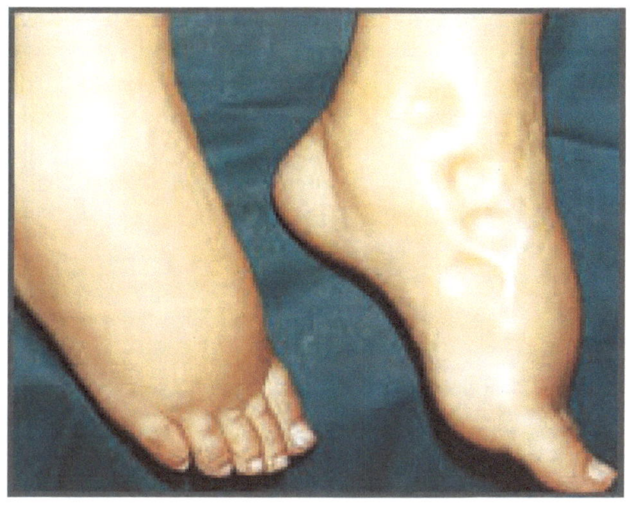

Fig. 17.2 Pitting Edema - Bilateral, dependent pitting edema occurs with heart failure.

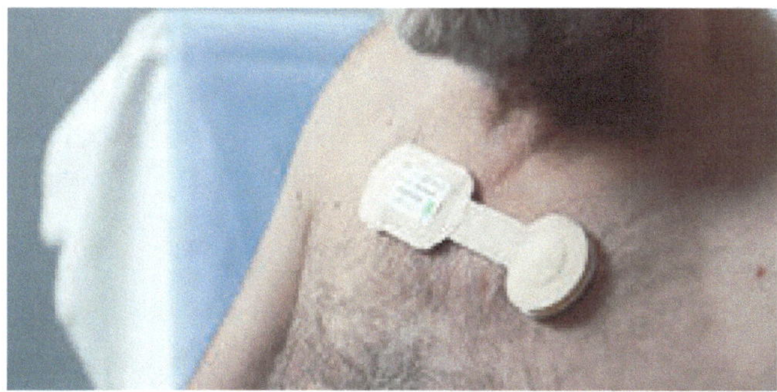

Fig 17.3 Low cost wireless ECG cardiac monitor can save lives and cut healthcare costs developed by British medical services startup Isansys – and based on the class-leading performance of Nordic nRF24AP2 ANT chips – the LifeTouch HRV011 cardiac monitor supports low cost yet continuous, clinical-grade ECG monitoring for the first time and can thus be used to detect post cardiac arrest and other problems when they are usually straight-forward to treat, avoiding life-threatening and costly emergency room re-admissions.

The Committee for scientific documents of the European Heart Rhythm Association felt, that several new devices for the treatment of heart failure (HF) patients have been introduced and are increasingly used in clinical practice or are under clinical evaluation in either observational and/or randomized clinical trials. So far, most of these technologies, if not all, have not been addressed in guidelines or position papers. Recently, several expert consensus documents and guidelines on device therapy in HF have been published followed by the publication of the 2012 EHRA/HRS consensus statement and new 2013 ESC Guidelines on cardiac pacing and cardiac resynchronization therapy in 2013. Therefore, this position paper does not include any recommendation on cardiac resynchronization therapy (CRT) in heart failure.

Recommendations should represent evidence-based medicine. However, except for cardiac contractility modulation (CCM), no data based on randomized trials are available, and for none of the new devices clinical outcome data, in particular mortality data, are available.

Nevertheless, this task force believes that an overview on these new technologies is important and necessary. Special focus is given to patients with HF New York Heart Association (NYHA) Classes III and IV and narrow QRS complex, who represent the largest group in HF compared with patients with wide QRS complex. Therefore, the task force believes that an overview on potential device options in addition to optimal medical therapy (OMT) would be helpful for all physicians treating HF patients.

CARDIAC CONTRACTILITY MODULATION

Resynchronization Therapy Device

Cardiac contractility modulation signals are non-excitatory signals which, when applied during the absolute refractory period, enhance the strength of left ventricular (LV) contraction and improve exercise tolerance as well as QoL in patients with heart failure. As the signals influence cell function without any affecting activation sequence, the effects are independent of QRS duration and should be additive to those of CRT.

Concept of Cardiac Contractility Modulation

Cardiac contractility modulation signals are electrical impulses delivered during the absolute refractory period. Cardiac contractility modulation signals used in clinical practice are delivered ~30 ms after detection of the QRS complex onset and consist of two biphasic ±7 V pulses spanning a total duration of >20 ms. These signals do not elicit a new action potential or contraction, as is the case with extra- or post-extrasystolic contractions. Moreover, they do not affect the sequence of electrical or mechanical activation, nor do they recruit additional contractile elements. On this basis, CCM signals are referred to as 'non-excitatory'.

If your heart is not beating efficiently and you meet the eligibility criteria, you may be eligible for a cardiac resynchronization therapy (CRT) heart device.

A CRT device sends small, undetectable electrical impulses to both lower chambers of the heart to help them beat together in a more synchronized pattern. This improves the heart's ability to pump blood and oxygen to the body.

The heart device itself is actually a tiny computer, plus a battery, contained in a small titanium metal case that is about the size of a pocket watch. It weighs about 3 ounces.

In addition to the heart device, insulated wires called leads are implanted for two purposes: to carry information signals from your heart to the heart device, and to carry electrical impulses to your heart.

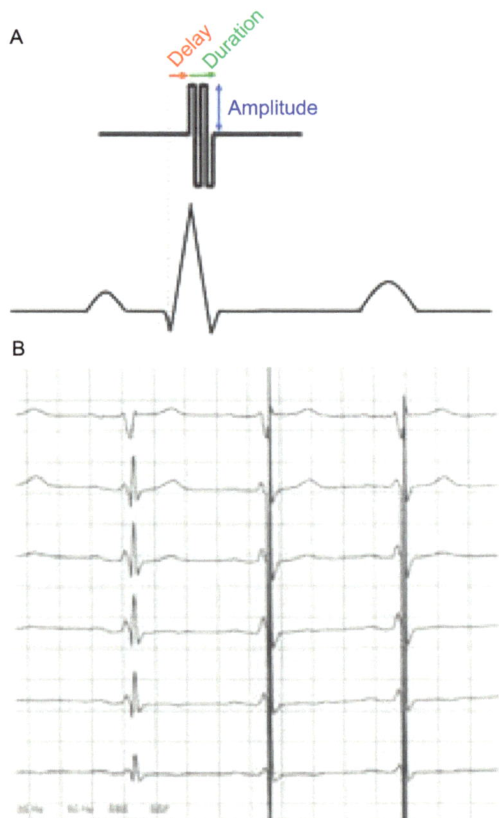

Fig. 17.4(A)Top and middle: Cardiac contractility modulation (CCM) signals are biphasic pulses, delivered after a defined delay from detection of local electrical activation. (B) Body surface electrocardiogram (leads V1–V6) showing one beat prior to initiating CCM signals and the first two beats of CCM signal application. Please note the stimulation artefact in Beats 2 and 3 reflect CCM signals.

The third part of your implantable device system is a programmer, an external computer located in your doctor's office or clinic that is used to program the heart device and retrieve information from your heart device that will assist your doctor in your heart failure treatment.

There are two types of implantable heart failure heart devices: a CRT pacemaker and a combination CRT pacemaker with defibrillation therapy. Both of these devices help to coordinate the heart's pumping action and improve blood flow. They can also speed up a heart that is beating too slowly.

The CRT pacemaker with defibrillation therapy (CRT-D) also offers the ability to detect and treat dangerously fast heart rhythms, which some individuals with a damaged heart muscle may be at risk for developing. Your doctor will determine which CRT device is appropriate for your medical condition.

Cardiac resynchronization therapy improves symptoms, quality of life (QoL), exercise tolerance, and reduces hospitalizations in patients with advanced HF and prolonged electrical activation (i.e. increased QRS duration). The results of a recent study showed that patients with mechanical dyssynchrony detected by tissue Doppler imaging but a normal QRS duration did not benefit from CRT. While the results of outcome trials of CRT in patients with a normal QRS duration are negative including Echo-CRT, a QRS $\geq$ 120 ms remains as one of the criterion for selecting patients for CRT. Patients with a QRS duration >120 ms represent 31% of HF patients in a recent trial. The indications for CRT have been summarized in a recent update of ESC guidelines on devices in heart failure.

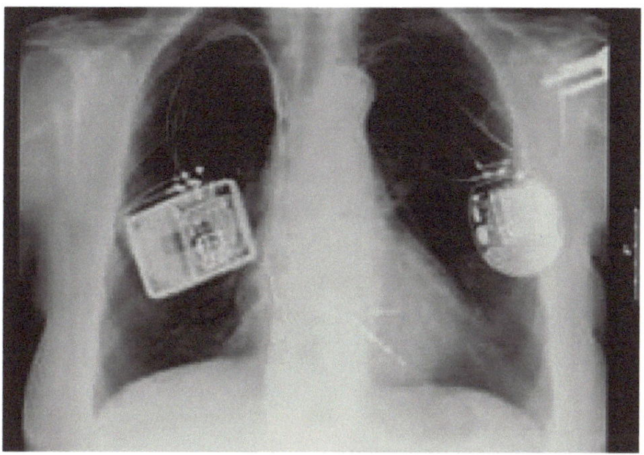

Fig.17.5 Chest X-ray showing an implanted CCM system (CCM, right side) and an one-chamber ICD device (left side). The CCM system consists of a can and three pace-sense electrodes. Two of them are fixed to the mid-septum and the third one to the right atrium.

Although CRT is indicated in patients with a prolonged QRS duration, up to 60% of patients with HF have a normal QRS duration. According to European registries published recently, even in the broad QRS population, those cared in hospital cardiology setting and meeting the current indications to CRT therapy were 6%, and among them approximately one-third only were actually implanted with a CRT device. Therefore, although the last ESC guidelines on HF extended the indications to CRT in chronic heart failure, a substantial proportion of patients remain either not eligible for CRT or simply do not respond. At a time when pharmacological therapy for HF has made only little advances, it is appropriate to explore whether new device-based therapies have anything else to offer to patients with heart failure.

The CCM system consists of a can and three pace-sense electrodes. Two of them are fixed to the mid-septum and the third one to the right atrium. The impact of a HF therapy on myocardial energetics is an important factor to consider in long-term safety and efficacy. Therefore, the acute effects of CCM on myocardial energetics were investigated in a clinical study in which myocardial oxygen uptake (MVO_2) and LV dP/dt_{max} were measured in nine patients exposed to acute CCM signals. In this study, acute CCM was associated with an increase in dP/dt_{max} from ~630 to ~800 mmHg/s (an ~20% increase). Despite an acute increase in contractility, there was no detectible increase in myocardial oxygen consumption. These data were compared with those of Nelson et al., who had also measured MVO_2 and dP/dt_{max} during temporary RV and biventricular pacing (BIV) pacing. In this study, contractility was increased first by applying CRT and then dobutamine to achieve a comparable increase in dP/dt_{max}. As expected from its effects on calcium cycling, dobutamine increased both dP/dt_{max} and MVO_2. In contrast, CCM increased dP/dt_{max} but not MVO_2. Thus, like CRT, the acute, modest increase in contractility achieved by CCM does not increase energy demands. In addition to acute haemodynamic effects noted above, improvement in global ventricular function has also been reported during chronic CCM signal application. In one study, 30 patients with ejection fraction (EF) < 35% and NYHA III symptoms despite OMT underwent three-dimensional echocardiography at baseline and 3 months after CCM treatment. Left ventricular ejection fraction (LVEF) increased by 4.8 ± 3.6% and LV end-systolic volumes decreased by 11.5 ± 10.5%, respectively. These findings indicate that LV reverse remodelling could be achieved by CCM in the background of optimum medical therapy.

Combining Cardiac Contractility Modulation with Cardiac Resynchronization Therapy

As discussed above, CCM signals applied in the acute setting to HF patients simultaneously receiving CRT provide additive effects on LV contractility indexed by dP/dt_{max}. In view of the fact that symptoms persist in more >30% of patients with prolonged QRS duration receiving CRT, it can be postulated that addition of CCM treatment may provide an option for these patients. The initial experience of combining CCM in a CRT non-responders has been published.

Table 17.1 New therapeutic devices in heart failure

	Characteristics	*Effects and status of trials*
Cardiac contractility modulation (CCM)	of proteins and genes involved in Ca handling • CCM signals are non-excitatory signals delivered to the LV ~30 ms after QRS onset • Effects are independent of QRS duration and additive to those of CRT • CCM signals acutely affect calcium handling but also expression	• Enhances the strength of LV contraction • Decreases LV volumes and increases EF • Improves exercise tolerance and quality of life • RCTs: FIX-HF-4, FIX-HF-5
Spinal cord stimulation	• Stimulation of afferent spinal nerve fibres • Increase of central vagal tone and decrease of sympathetic tone via central reflex activation	• Improves cardiac output, reduces peripheral resistance • Increases cardiac work efficiency, decreases myocardial oxygen demand • Reduces risk of ischaemic ventricular arrhythmia • SCS-HEART (ongoing non-RCT) • DEFEAT-HF (ongoing RCT)
Carotid sinus nerve stimulation	• Stimulation of afferent fibres coupled to arterial baroreceptors • Increase of central vagal tone and decrease of sympathetic tone via central reflex activation	• Improves systolic and diastolic LV function • Slight decrease of heart rate and blood pressure • XR-1 Heart Failure Study; HOPE4HF study (ongoing RCTs)
Cervical vagal nerve stimulation	• Stimulation of cervical pre-ganglionic parasympathetic fibres • Direct activation of overall cardiac vagal tone	• Antiarrhythmic, rate slowing, antifibrotic, anti-inflammatory, and reverse remodelling effects • Decreases LV volumes and increases EF • Improves exercise tolerance and quality of life • CardioFit study (non-RCT) • INNOVATE-HF (ongoing RCT)
Intracardiac AV-nodal vagal stimulation	• Stimulation of post-ganglionic cardiac parasympathetic nerves selectively innervating AV node	• Dynamic ventricular rate control during AF • AV nodal selective • May avoid inappropriate shock delivery in patients with AF and ICD/CRT-D • AVNS study (ongoing non-RCT)

Table 17.2 Implantable haemodynamic monitoring devices

Device	*Characteristics*	*Clinical outcome*
RV-pressure monitoring	Monitors: • Systolic and diastolic RV pressure • RV d*P*/d*t* • Pulmonary artery diastolic pressure • Heart rate • Patient activity • Core body temperature	• Non-significant reduction of all CHF-related events (COMPASS-HF)
LA-pressure monitoring (Heart-POD)	Monitors: • LA pressure • Intracardiac electrogram • Body temperature	• Reduces death and CHF events • Adequate adjustment of drug-therapy results in improvement of NYHA class and LVEF (HOMEOSTASIS study)
Pulmonary artery pressure (CardioMEMS)	• Monitors PAP	• Reduces significantly rate and duration of CHF-related hospitalization (CHAMPION study)

It was demonstrated that the implantation procedure is technically feasible, that the OPTIMIZER and CRT defibrillator (CRT-D) devices can coexist without interference and that acute haemodynamic and clinical improvements can be observed. These preliminary results, however, have to be confirmed in a prospective study that is underway to systematically investigate the effects of CCM in CRT non-responders.

Clinical Perspectives

Two large-scale studies have validated the safety and suggested the effectiveness of CCM therapy. Results of these trials show that CCM improves exercise tolerance as indexed by peak VO_2. Other indices of exercise tolerance (e.g. 6 min hall walk) and QoL (NYHA class and MLWHFQ) have also been shown to improve. Data from both clinical trials suggest that mortality rates are unaffected by CCM therapy. However, the aim of these studies was to demonstrate an absence of increase in mortality as a safety end-point and was not powered to show a mortality benefit. The level of recommendation would be substantially higher if a gain in mortality can be demonstrated. In this respect, a specific subgroup of HF patients (EF ≥ 25%) is more likely to respond favourably. Moreover, more research is probably required to determine the optimal pacing configuration (single or biphasic stimuli, optimal delay from the pacing spike, optimal duration of each phase, and optimal amplitude of the signal), the optimal daily duration of application, the optimal localization of the pacing sites, and the optimal number of pacing sites to gain the maximal benefit from this therapy. The potential interest of CCM in early stages of HF has not been investigated.

Required Technical Improvement

Some technical limitations should be solved in the future: (i) with the last version of the device, CCM cannot be delivered in patients with AF or frequent ectopy, as it is designed to inhibit CCM delivery on arrhythmias and relies on detection of a P-wave. A future device is supposed to incorporate an algorithm that does not rely on P-wave detection and therefore could be used in patients with AF. (ii) The development of a device combining CCM with implantable cardioverter defibrillator (ICD) functions would be desirable in this population of HF patients. Future studies will be required to define whether CCM is additive to CRT pacemaker or CRT-D in patients with wide QRS. This would be facilitated by the development of a single device that incorporates pacing, antitachycardia therapies, and CCM. (iii) A simple peri-implantation method to guide lead positioning would be desirable, beyond the invasive LV dP/dt_{max} measurement.

NEUROMODULATION

Heart failure is associated with significant perturbances of the autonomic balance with predominant sympathetic activation over the parasympathetic system. Several indirect markers of cardiac vagal tone like heart rate variability, heart rate turbulence, baroreflex sensitivity are suppressed in CHF which in turn is predictive for a worse outcome of CHF. Likewise, an increase of cardiac vagal tone by pharmacological β-receptor blockade has substantially improved functional status and survival of HF patients. Cardiac vagal tone is controlled by pre-ganglionic parasympathetic cardiac neurons mainly residing in the nucleus ambiguus and the dorsal motor nucleus of the brainstem. Of note, parasympathetic cardiac efferent neurons in the nucleus ambiguus are intrinsically electrically silent,thus needing presynaptic input to generate and modulate parasympathetic efferent activity and tone. Such input is likely provided by sensory afferent fibres from arterial baroreceptors or respiratory sensory neurons, but spinal cord afferent fibres

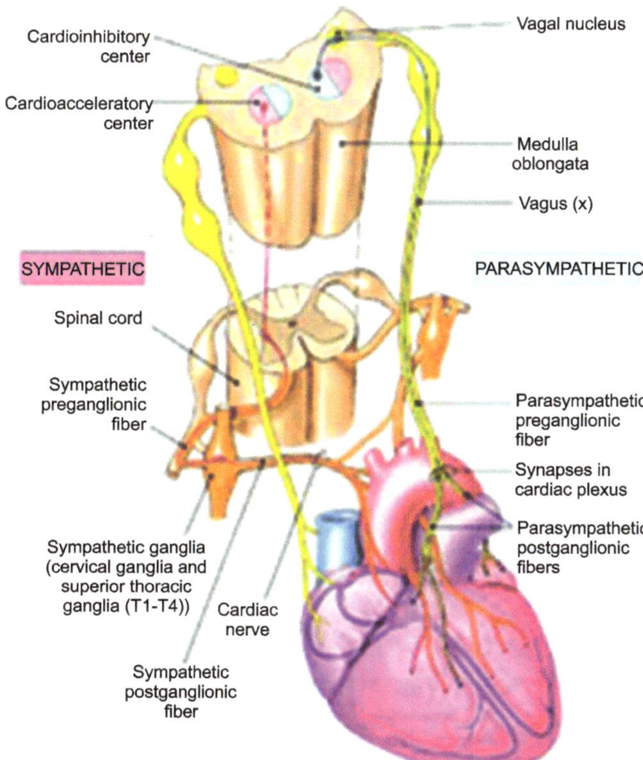

Fig.17.6 Parasympathetic and sympathetic innervations of the heart. Functional anatomy: efferent pre-ganglionic vagal nerve (parasympathetic) fibres course from the brain stem towards the heart and connect with post-ganglionic cells in circumscript epicardial ganglionic plexus. Sympathetic pre-ganglionic fibres (orange colour) switch to post-ganglionic fibres inside the stellate ganglion. Major afferent inputs to the central autonomic centres are the carotid sinus nerves and spinal cord afferents.

may also connect to the brainstem and modulate cardiac vagal tone Thus, attempts to therapeutically increase the cardiac parasympathetic tone by electrical neural stimulation may operate at any part of this integrative circuit. This has led to four neurostimulation approaches, two of which are focusing on reflex activation of the parasympathetic tone and sympathetic inhibition via afferent fibre stimulation [spinal cord stimulation (SCS), carotid sinus nerve stimulation], while two are concentrating on efferent parasympathetic stimulation (cervical vagal and intracardiac vagal stimulation)

Spinal Cord Stimulation

Preliminary work suggests some benefits from neuromodulation with SCS in HF patients. Spinal cord stimulation has been used for over 40 years in the management of chronic intractable pain. According to the American Association of Neurosurgical Surgeons , as many as 50,000 neurostimulators are implanted worldwide every year. Among multiple indications, the benefits have been confirmed in patients with refractory angina associated with end-stage CAD and in the absence of CAD (syndrome X) Positive effects have also been demonstrated in the peripheral vascular beds: patients with severe pain due to distal atherosclerosis, in Raynaud's disease, and at the level of cerebral vasculature.

Mechanisms of Action

Spinal cord stimulation compared positively with surgical and laser endo-myocardial revascularization in patients with severe refractory angina associated with severe CAD without any increase in adverse ischaemic events. This suggests that the improvement in symptoms and the clinical condition of these patients was mediated only partially through the 'gate-control' mechanisms described by Melzack and Wall in 1965. The involved mechanisms remain incompletely understood and appear to be far more complex than just the suppression of the nociceptive influx associated with myocardial ischaemia:SCS seems to affect the balance between oxygen demand and supply. Since there is little evidence that SCS improves the coronary blood flow in ischaemic patients, other factors acting in the balance between oxygen requirements and supplies have to play an important role. Spinal cord stimulation applied at the low cervical (C7–C8) and/or high thoracic (T1–T6) level exerts effects through reflex activation of the vagus nerve and sympathetic.

Overall, the cumulated effects on both the sympathetic and the parasympathetic system seems to be a re-equilibrium of the balance in favour of the latter. Other positive effects via the cytokines and the NO/NOS system have been identified and there may even be some direct protective mechanisms on the myocardium during ischaemia.

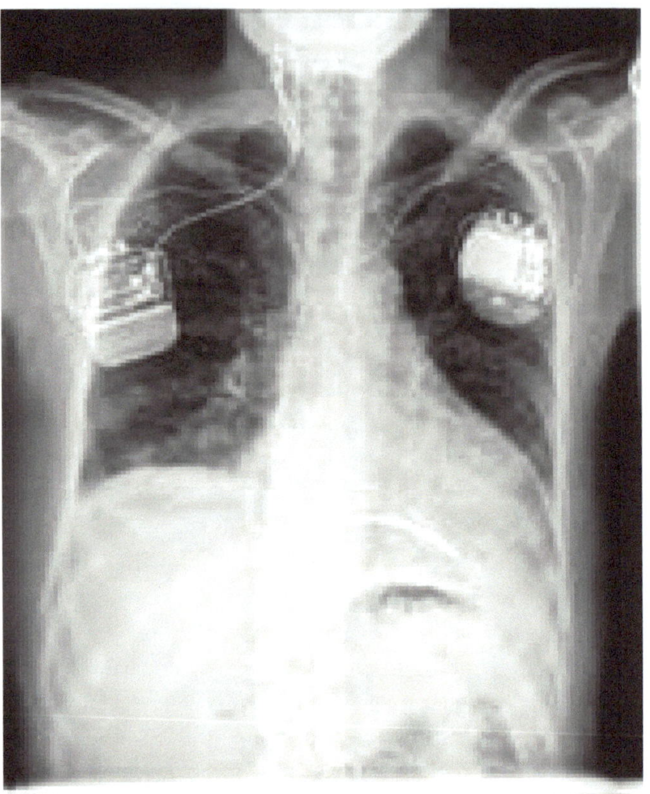

Fig. 17.7 CardioFit: CardioFit is an implantable electrical stimulation device designed to restore balance in the autonomic nervous system and improve heart function in patients with HF.

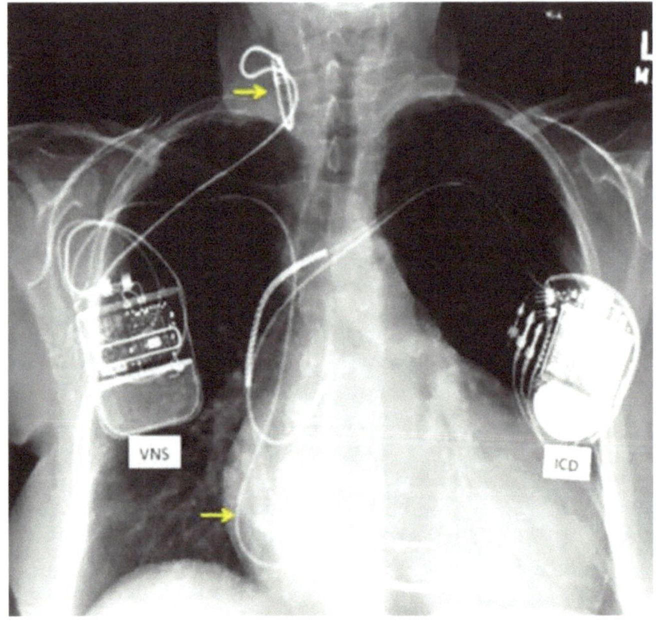

Fig. 17.8 X-ray of a patient with a vagal nerve stimulator with a previously implanted implantable cardioverter defibrillator. The arrows show a lead attached to the vagus nerve on the right side and an additional right ventricular sensing lead connected to the vagal nerve stimulator device.

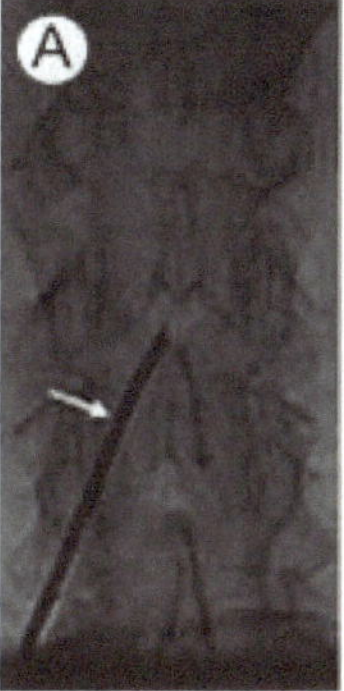

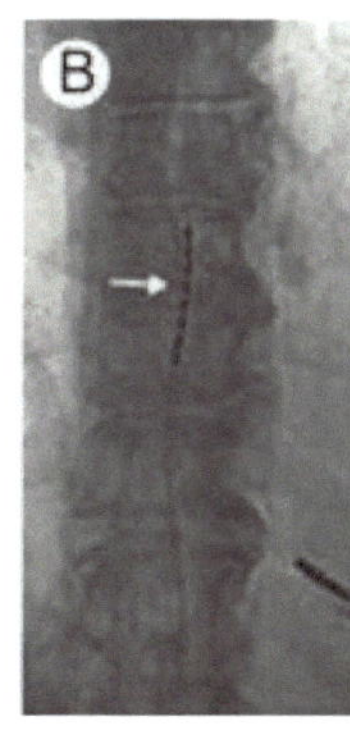

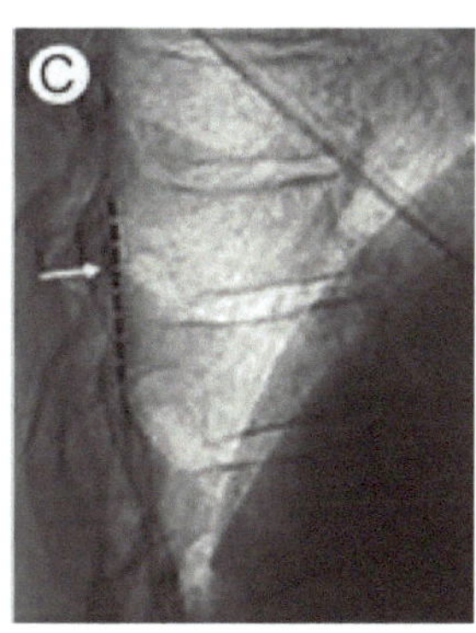

Fig17.9 Spinal cord stimulation: single-lead placement. A. Introducer (arrow) is directed into the epidural space. (B and C) anteroposterior and lateral views demonstrate the lead in the posterior epidural space in the mid-thoracic region at approximately T1 (arrows).

Clinical Perspectives

Spinal cord stimulation, via complex mechanisms, appears promising in pre-clinical experiments to improve the systolic function of the LV and to decrease the ventricular arrhythmias associated with this condition. According to Clinicaltrials.org, there are at the present time two ongoing clinical studies that are directly addressing the role—and possible benefits—of SCS in severely afflicted HF patients. SCS-HEART is a non-randomized feasibility study that aims to determine the safety of SCS in 20 patients with a LVEF between 20 and 35%, in NYHA functional class III, and who already have an ICD implanted. Results should be available in the second part of 2014. On the other hand, DEFEAT-HF (sponsored by Medtronic) is a single blind randomized study involving similar patients but that will compare SCS 'ON' vs. 'OFF' in 250 recipients. Results are also expected for the end of 2014. Until these studies are completed, it remains impossible to recommend this therapy in HF patients outside of the current recognized indications.

Table 17.3 Major findings reported with SCS

Spinal cord stimulation has been shown to have positive impact on cardiac ischaemia due to CAD:
1. The mechanisms involved go beyond suppression of the nociceptive stimuli. 2. SCS has limited impact on coronary blood flow, therefore the mechanisms must lie somewhere else. 3. SCS has a profound positive impact on the cardiac sympathetic/para-symapathetic balance. 4. SCS also affects positively the NO/NOS and cytokines system at the myocardial level.
Spinal cord stimulation has shown some effects on LV function and ventricular arrhythmias:
1. One preliminary report on four HF patients who improved clinically with SCS. 2. SCS was associated with smaller deterioration of LVEF due to adenosine administration in patients with multivessel CAD. 3. SCS was associated with better invasive haemodynamic evaluation in patients with normal LV function. 4. SCS was associated with reduced risk of ventricular arrhythmias and LV function improvement in animal models of HF.

Carotid Sinus Nerve Stimulation

Baroreceptors are embedded into the wall of arterial vessels and can be preferentially found in the aortic arch at the origins of the brachiocephalic or left subclavian artery, in the brachiocephalic artery at its bifurcation into the right subclavian and right common carotid artery, in the carotid sinuses, along both common carotid arteries, and in both common carotid arteries at the origin of the superior thyroid artery. They respond to changes in arterial pressure and mediate their signals via afferent rapid conducting (2.5–60 m/s) myelinated A fibres and slow conducting (< 2.5 m/s) non-myelinated C fibres to the brainstemwhere they connect to efferent vagal neurons. A-type receptors respond to normal arterial pressures and are regularly discharging at high frequency (>100 Hz) synchronously to the pulsatile pressure wave. By contrast, C-type baroreceptor respond to higher threshold values of the mean arterial pressure with irregular firing at lower frequency of 20–30 Hz. Increases of arterial blood pressure elicit a reflectory activation of efferent vagal fibres resulting in a decrease of the sinus heart rate. The baroreflex activation is considered as powerful contributor to the baseline parasympathetic tone.

Mechanisms of Action

Electrical stimulation of the baroreceptor fibres (carotid sinus nerve fibres) elicits a graded response decrease of heart rate and arterial pressure via parasympathetic efferent activation and sympathetic withdrawal and has recently been clinically introduced for treatment of resistant arterial hypertension. The potential of electrical carotid sinus nerve stimulation to shift the autonomic balance towards a higher parasympathetic tone has also been investigated in HF models. In fact, chronic low-intensity carotid sinus stimulation, which lowers blood pressure by only 10–15 mmHg and which does not critically decrease heart rate was able to improve survival in dogs with pacing-induced HF. In addition, LV systolic and diastolic function improved due to reverse LV geometric and interstitial remodelling. In parallel, the downregulation of β1 receptor density in CHF was almost normalized to control levels and serum catecholamine levels declined which may be taken as evidence for a direct or reflectory decrease of the systemic sympathetic tone in these models. (Fig. 17.10)

Clinical Data

The Rheos system was the first baroreceptor stimulation system by CVRx implanted in hypertensive patients. The Rheos system was so far evaluated in three multicentre clinical studies in patients with resistant hypertension: the DEBuT-HT/ DEBuT-HET in Europe and the Rheos Feasibility Trial and Rheos Pivotal Trial which mostly included patients in the USA. The Rheos pivotal trial is in long-term follow-up by now. The randomized part of the trial with a 12-month blinded follow-up was published in 2011: 265 patients with resistant hypertension received the device and were either randomized to immediate BAT or delayed BAT following the 6-month visit. Three of the five pre-specified co-primary endpoints were met: long-term sustained response to baroreceptor activation therapy, with 88% responders after 12 months of follow-up, incidence of short-term AEs (6-month follow-up), and long-term AEs (12-month follow-up). The study did not meet the endpoints for acute responders (54 vs. 46% responders after 6-month follow-up) and procedural safety (event-free rate 74.8%). A majority of these events were related to the carotid sinus lead placement and involved transient or permanent nerve injury that occurred during the implant. The majority (76%) of procedure-related AEs resolved completely.

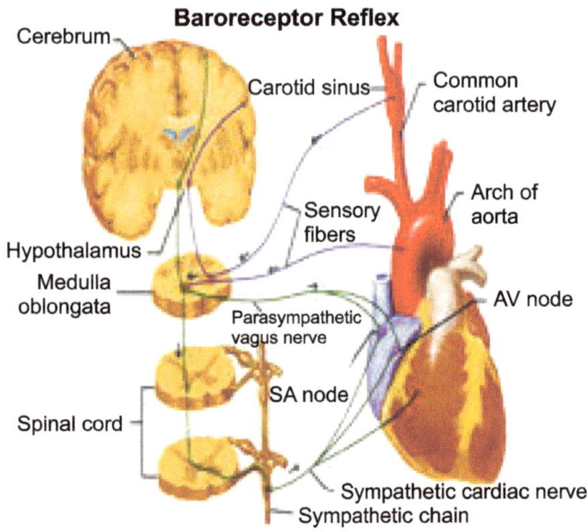

Fig.17.10 Baroreceptor reflexes. Congestive heart failure is a syndrome that is usually initiated by a reduction in pump function of the heart, i.e. a decrease in cardiac output. Initially, a reduction in cardiac output leads to unloading of baroreceptor reflex that, in turn, increases heart rate through vago-sympathetic mechanisms and total peripheral resistance via an increase in sympathetic outflow to vascular beds. During human HF, this baroreflex is profoundly suppressed and worsens with deterioration of CHF. Thus, electrical stimulation of afferent carotid sinus nerves, which connect baroreceptors to the brainstem may evolve as tool for increasing cardiac vagal tone during HF.

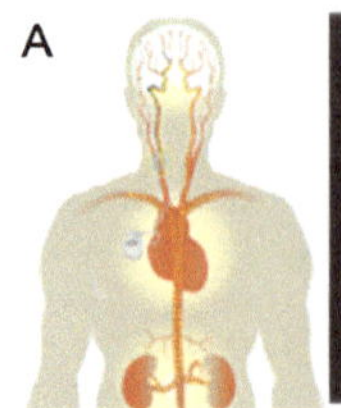

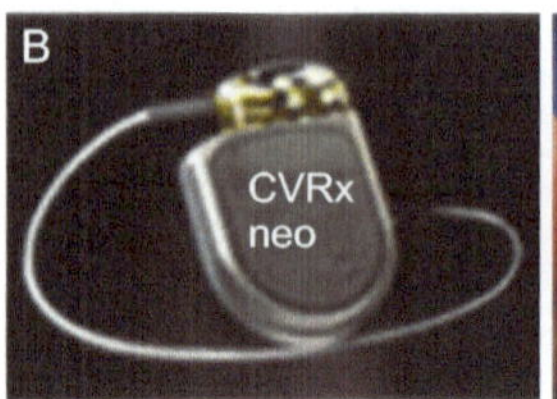

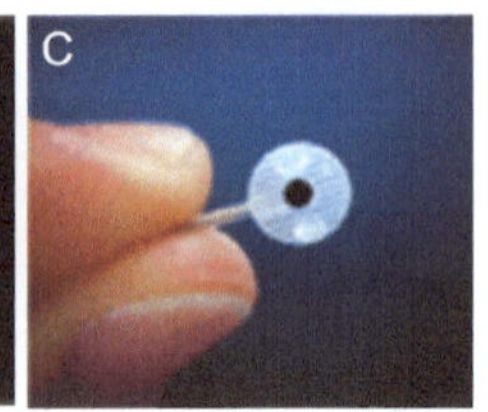

Fig.17.11(A) Shows the principle of carotid sinus nerve stimulation. The device is implanted via the right side and is connected to a patch electrode fixed on the right-sided carotid sinus. (B) Shows an example of a carotid sinus nerve stimulator. The device carries one electrode connected to the patch electrode. (C) Demonstrates a patch electrode which will be fixed to the carotid sinus nerve.

To date, there exist no randomized clinical data evaluating the effectiveness of BAT in patients with systolic HF. In addition to experimental data, several sub-studies and single-centre data indicated beneficial physiological effects of BAT beyond just blood pressure reduction.

Cervical Vagal Nerve Stimulation

The efferent cardiac parasympathetic signalling chain comprises pre-ganglionic parasympathetic neurons originating in the brainstem, which course inside the vagal nerve and connect via nicotinergic acetylcholine receptors to post-ganglionic neurons, which are aggregated in circumscript cardiac ganglionic plexus inside the heart. Post-ganglionic fibres then innervate the cardiac target cells via muscarinergic acetylcholine receptors. During CHF, the density of cardiac muscarinergic receptors is increased, which is most probably due to an adaptive upregulation secondary to a decreased efferent vagal input. However, the post-ganglionic vagal nerve transmission seems to be intact in HF: selective electrical stimulation of post-ganglionic vagal nerve fibres to the sinus node leads to a larger decrease of the sinus rate in HF dogs than in controls, which would be in line with an increased number of muscarinergic receptors in HF. By contrast, electrical stimulation of presynaptic cervical vagal fibres led to a smaller decrease of the sinus rate in CHF animals as compared with control animals. Thus, pre- to post-ganglionic parasympathetic efferent neurotransmission via nicotinergic acetylcholine receptors seems to be impaired during CHF.Importantly, these nicotinergic receptors are agonist dependent and chronic exposure to a nicotinic agonist during HF has been shown to re-establish efferent parasympathetic neural control of the sinus node.These experiments form a pathophysiological rationale to apply electrical pre-ganglionic cervical vagal nerve stimulation to re-establish the diminished cardiac vagal tone in CHF. ((Figs 17.12–17.13)

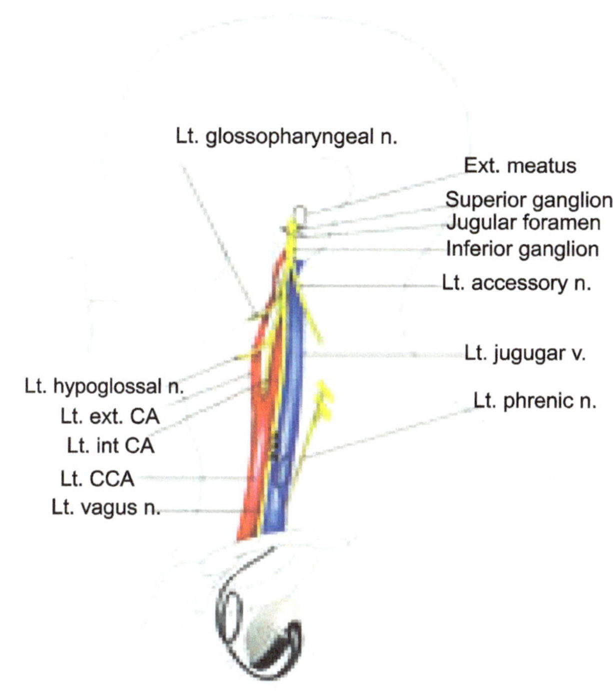

Fig. 17.12 anatomical relationship between vagus nerve and surrounding structures and location of VNS

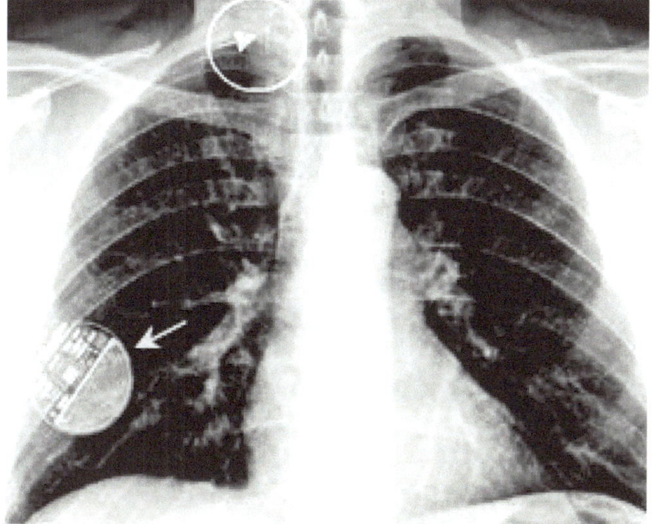

Fig.17.13 Plain thoracic x-rays displaying the vagus nerve stimulator (VNS) implanted on the right side in a patient. Encircled upper arrow points to the VNS around the right vagus nerve trunk. VNS generator is positioned at the right paraaxillary region (arrow)

Mechanisms of Action

Several studies in various chronic HF animal models have shown a reduction of the progression of HF and a survival benefit with cervical vagal nerve stimulation. Major contributing mechanisms are detailed as follows:

Antiarrhythmic effects: Vagal nerve stimulation increases the ventricular refractory period in humans, leads to a prolongation of the epicardial action potential duration, and decreases ventricular vulnerability to ventricular fibrillation. These electrophysiological effects may contribute to its potent antifibrillatory effects as demonstrated during cervical vagal nerve stimulation experiments in post-infarction animal models. In addition, vagal nerve stimulation in HF reduces the loss of Cx43, which may prevent proarrhythmic conduction delays and dispersion of action potential duration.

Rate slowing effects: Vagal nerve stimulation exerts profound negative chronotropic and dromotropic effects. Since an increased heart rate is associated with adverse prognosis in CHF, a reduction of heart rate both in SR and AF might contribute beneficial therapeutic effects in CHF.

Antifibrotic effects: In a coronary microembolization-induced HF model, chronic cervical vagal nerve stimulation has been shown to decrease ventricular replacement fibrosis and to blunt the development of CHF-associated cellular hypertrophy of remaining myocytes.

Anti-inflammatory effects: Vagal nerve stimulation has potent anti-inflammatory effects. Recently, vagal nerve stimulation was shown to blunt HF-associated increases of tumour necrosis factor-α, interleukin-6, and C-reactive protein in two animal models of HF.

Reverse remodelling: Vagal nerve stimulation decreases ventricular end-systolic and end-diastolic diameters and improves LVEF. Chronic vagal stimulation has also been shown to reduce NT-proBNP levels in a dog HF model and biventricular weight in a rat HF model.

Clinical Data

The first multicentre, open-label phase II, two-staged study (8-patient feasibility phase plus 24-patient safety and tolerability phase) enroled 32 NYHA Class II–IV patients (age 56 + 11 years, LVEF 23 + 8%). Right cervical vagal nerve stimulation (VNS) with an implantable system started 2–4 weeks after implant, slowly raising intensity; patients were followed 3 and 6 months thereafter with optional 1-year follow-up. Overall, 26 serious AEs occurred in 13 of 32 patients (40.6%), including three deaths and two clearly device-related AEs (post-operative pulmonary oedema, need of surgical revision). Expected non-serious device-related AEs (cough, dysphonia, and stimulation-related pain) occurred early but were reduced and disappeared after stimulation intensity adjustment. There were significant improvements (P = 0.001) in NYHA class QoL, 6 min walk test (from 411 + 76 to 471 + 111 m), LVEF (from 22 + 7 to 29 + 8%), and LV systolic volumes (P = 0.02). These improvements were maintained at 1 year.

Several scientific articles have summarized the use of cervical vagal nerve stimulator (CVS) in patients with CHF. Naturally, the data provided in those articles are limited, due to the small patient cohort and the non-randomized nature of first in man and safety and feasibility studies; however important considerations can be drawn from them:

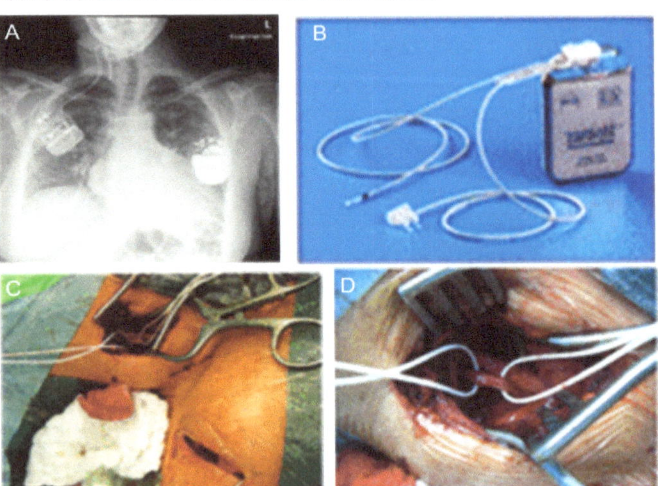

Fig.17.14 (A) Chest X-ray of an implanted cervical vagal nerve stimulator in a patient with severely reduced LV systolic function. The device has been implanted via the right side and consists of a ventricular sensing lead and a cervical vagal nerve electrode. On the left side an ICD had been previously implanted. (B) Example of a cervical vagal stimulator. The device carries two electrodes: one conventional RV screw-in pace/sense electrode monitors the heart rate during vagal nerve stimulation, while the other cuff electrode is wrapped around the cervical vagal nerve. (C) Local implanta-tion site of the CVS: there are two incisions, one for exposure of the cervical vagal nerve and a second one for implanting the RV electrode. The vagal electrode is tunnelled subcutaneously to the impulse generator, which is implanted below the collarbone. (D) Exposed cervical vagal nerve.

- Patients with mild-to-moderate HF can tolerate the higher current amplitudes and other parameters used in chronic vagal stimulation vs. the parameters used for treatment of epilepsy.
- Vagal stimulation may generate side effects like hoarseness, voice alteration, and increased cough. The majority of side effects are related to the underlying disease or a multitude of co-morbidities.
- In patients with both CVS and ICD, no interferences from vagal stimulation were recognized by the ICD nor were detectable on the intracardiac electrogram of the device.
- CVS increased parasympathetic tone of subjects with HF (as measured by heart rate variability on 24 h Holter recordings; and as inferred by reduction of resting heart rate).
- Vagal stimulation improved subjective, as well as objective clinically relevant parameters of functional class, quality of life, sub-maximal exercise capacity, and cardiac structure and function in a first clinical study.

UNRESOLVED ISSUES

Atrial Proarrhythmia

At the atrial level, an increased vagal tone substantially shortens the atrial refractory period and increases the heterogeneity of refractory periods in the atria. Whether this might promote the occurrence of AF especially in HF patients with a diseased atrial substrate is unknown.

Experimental evidence in healthy dogs, however, suggests that the occurrence of AF during cervical vagal nerve stimulation depends on the intensity of vagal stimulation with no AF occurrence at lower level stimulation. Data on the occurrence of AF during vagal stimulation in HF patients need to be gathered prospectively. (Fig. 17.14)

Selectivity of Neural Stimulation

The cervical vagal nerve contains efferent and afferent fibres coursing not only to the thoracic but also to or from the abdominal viscera. So far, the issue of concomitant stimulation of efferent parasympathetic fibres to the gastrointestinal tract has not yet been thoroughly investigated. Such inadvertent stimulation might increase gastric acid secretion or increase intestinal motility. Likewise, afferent electrical stimulation or block of the vagal nerve below the diaphragm has been shown to decrease food intake and to reduce weight gain. Since these fibres potentially course through the cervical vagal nerve inadvertent stimulation or block of these fibres may occur during vagal nerve stimulation for HF possibly inducing weight loss masking as cardiac cachexia.

Intracardiac Atrioventricular Nodal Vagal Stimulation

Thirty to forty percent of patients with CHF eventually will develop AF. Rapid ventricular rates during AF may further deteriorate HF or decrease the degree of LV resynchronization in patients with cardiac resynchronization devices and may ultimately lead to inappropriate shock delivery in up to 5% of ICD recipients. Long-term selective atrioventricular (AV) nodal vagal stimulation for ventricular rate control has been developed as potential adjunctive treatment modality for these patients. (Figs. 17.15–17.18)

Mechanisms and Experimental Models

Post-ganglionic cardiac vagal fibres, which preferentially supply the AV node reside in an inferior right ganglionated plexus (IRGP) at the postero-inferior interatrial septum.This makes them amenable to stimulation from the endocardial surface,

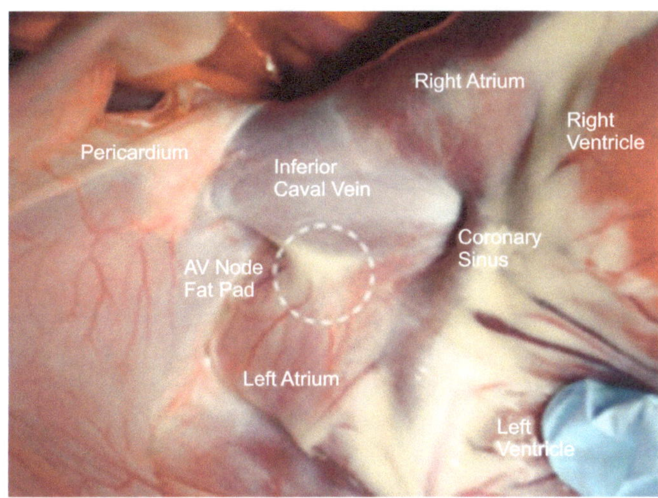

Fig. 17.15 Anatomical location of the atrioventricular node Fat Pad.The diagram uses as a background a real anatomical epicardial image of heart. The heart has been lifted up toward the head to show the anatomical position of the epicardial AV node fat pad (dashed circle).

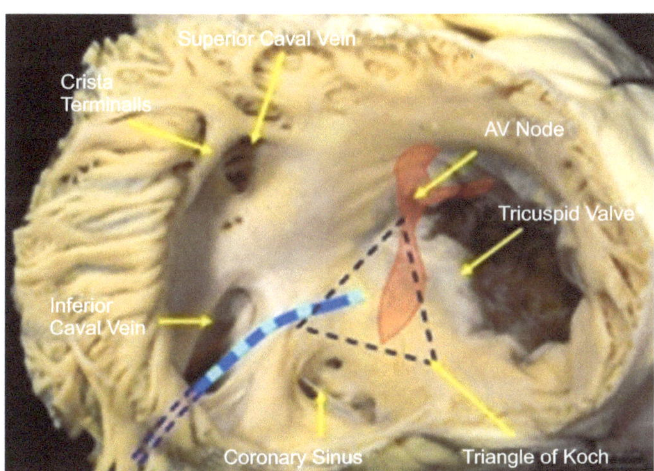

Fig.17.16 Vagal stimulation site for endocardial approach in the human heart. A schematic diagram showing the site at the posterior right atrium at which optimal AV conduction delay could be achieved by electrical postganglionic vagal stimulation delivered with an endocardial catheter inserted through the inferior caval vein. Anatomical image of endocardial view of human right atrium provided by Prof. R.H.Anderson.)

thus resulting in a graded response negative dromotropic effect. Chronic stimulation of the IRGP in animal models provides reliable and well-tolerated ventricular rate control in dogs and has been shown to be haemodynamically superior to His bundle ablation and RV pacing probably because ventricular conduction over the His–Purkinje system is maintained.

Technology and Implant Technique

The IRGP is located at the epicardial surface of the heart between the ostium of the coronary sinus and the entrance of the inferior vena cava. For chronic electrostimulation of this plexus, atrial pacing leads of current technology can be screwed into the IRGP from the right atrial endocardial site at the postero-inferior interatrial septum either by using specifically shaped guiding catheters or manually shaped conventional mandrins.

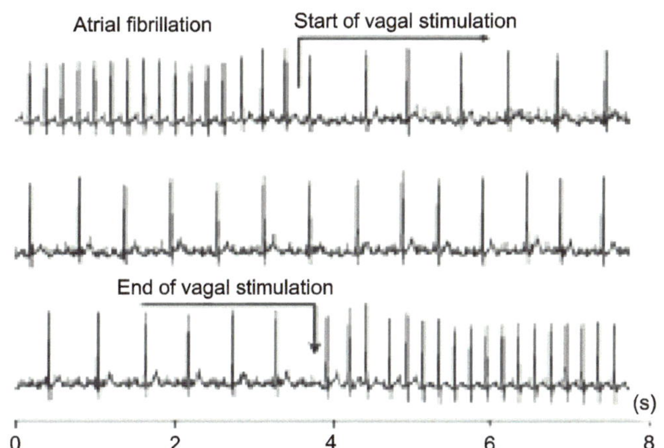

Fig.17.17 Surface ECG recordings from A chronic dog implanted with an AV node vagal stimulation device.The top trace shows at the beginning a rapid ventricular rate (>240 bpm) during AF without vagal stimulation. The arrow indicates the start of vagal stimulation and the immediate resultant slowing of the ventricular rate. The middle trace shows the maintenance of slow ventricular rate (105 bpm) during continuous vagal stimulation. The bottom trace shows the prompt restoration of the initial (fast) ventricular rate after vagal stimulation was terminated (arrow).

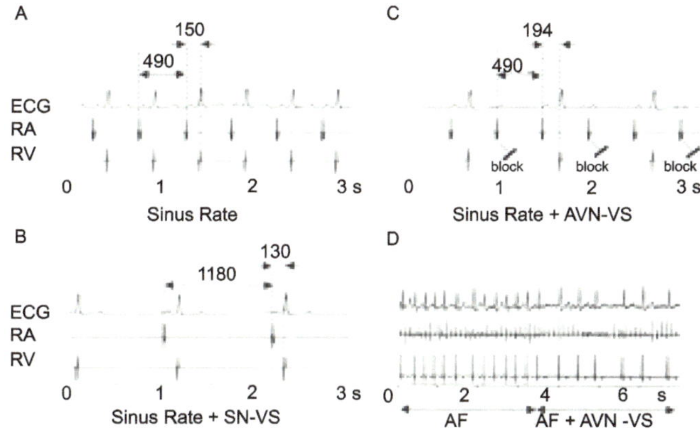

Fig. 17.18 Effects of subthreshold epicardial stimulation of the fat pads. (A) control sinus rate. Numbers refer to the sinus cycle length and the AV conduction time, respectively. (B) stimulation of the SN fat pad. Note the strong chronotropic effect and the associated shortening of the control AV conduction time. (C) stimulation of the AVN fat pad. There was no change in the control sinus cycle length, whereas AV conduction was strongly depressed and 2:1 Wenckebach periodicity was observed. (D) atrial fibrillation (AF) alone (left), followed by AF in combination with AVN fat-pad stimulation (right). Note the slowing of the ventricular rate during vagal stimulation. ECG, electrocardiogram; RA, right atrium; VS, vagal stimulation.

Clinical Data

Recently, the feasibility of such an approach was shown in a series of chronic human implants in HF patients with AF. A prospective multicentre study (AVNS: AV node stimulation study, which investigates whether short-term probatory AV nodal vagal stimulation may avoid inappropriate shock delivery in patients with resynchronization defibrillators is ongoing.

Electrical Determinants of Neurostimulation

Electrical stimulation of parasympathetic pre- or post-ganglionic efferent fibres obeys the same fundamental laws as myocardial electrostimulation with the exception that the chronaxie time of 180 μs is shorter. In contrast to the myocardial action potential, the action potential of neurons is very short lasting only 10–20 ms. Thus, transmitter release and physiological effects may be elicited by electrical stimulation at higher frequencies, which typically is set to 20–50 Hz during cervical vagal stimulation for seizures or depression, 100 Hz for carotid sinus stimulation, or 4–20 Hz for cervical vagal stimulation in HF.For post-ganglionic efferent parasympathetic stimulation the frequency-response curve is bell-shaped with an optimum at 40 Hz. Since most stimulated nerve structures contain afferent and efferent autonomic fibres with varying fibre diameter and conduction velocities,efforts have been undertaken to preferentially stimulate efferent fibres. For example, cervical vagal nerve stimulation for treatment of HF aims to stimulate efferent parasympathetic B fibres coursing towards the heart but tries to avoid afferent A and C fibre excitation. This can be achieved by hyperpolarizing the nerve fibres at the anode thus preventing excitation and simultaneously depolarizing fibres at the cathode. Since larger afferent A fibres (diameter 5–20 μm) are more sensitive to hyperpolarization than smaller efferent B fibres (1–3 μm) inside the vagal nerve preferential efferent stimulation can be accomplished. Besides electrode configuration, the applied stimulus strength also affects differential recruitment of A–C fibres and changes the frequency dependence of afferent neural stimulation. Finally, the application of biphasic impulses may bare the benefit of decharging the membrane with the second phase of the impulse thus preventing damage to the neurocytes.

Implantable Haemodynamic Monitoring Devices

Clinical management to prevent acute decompensated heart failure (ADHF) and/or hospitalization in ambulatory HF patients remains challenging. There is an urgent need to develop strategies to reduce hospitalizations and re-admission rates for HF. Frequent monitoring of physiological data is imperative in the management of HF. The development of wireless and remote technology makes it possible to frequently monitor and transfer data via telemonitoring. The concept of telemonitoring involves patient-activated automatic devices which provide physiological parameters such as weight, blood pressure, heart rate, rhythm, and activity logs. Results of studies using telemonitoring have been contradictory. A meta-analysis demonstrated that telemonitoring may provide better outcomes compared with usual care, with a reduction in mortality and HF hospitalizations. Recently, the value of telemonitoring has been challenged by two randomized clinical trials. The results of the Telemedical Interventional Monitoring in Heart Failure (TIM-HF) trial showed no significant difference in all-cause mortality (primary endpoint) or in the composite of cardiovascular death or HF hospitalization. The study of Chaudhry et al demonstrated that telemonitoring failed to reduce HF hospital admissions, duration of hospital stay, or the frequency of admissions. One explanation might be the insensitivity of daily weight monitoring to predict HF hospitalization, which is >20%. Another strategy is the use of cardiac implantable devices (defibrillators and CRT) to stratify the risk of ADHF based on a single parameter as thoracic impedanceor heart rate variability, or a combination of parameters. These parameters, single or combined, have a sensitivity of 60–70%, a positive predictive value up to 7.8%, and false-positive alarms ranging from 1.8 to 2.7 per patient-year of monitoring. Although these parameters enable physicians to identify patients at increased risk of ADHF, they do not impact patient outcomes and are not sufficiently accurate to adjust treatment. A new approach to monitor the status of ambulatory HF patients and preventing potential hospitalizations may involve implantable devices providing real-time haemodynamic data to the clinician. Device companies began to develop new implantable devices designed to collect haemodynamic data. These investigational devices include RV, left atrial pressure (LAP), and pulmonary artery pressure (PAP) sensors. (Figs. 17.19–17.20)

Right Ventricular Pressure Monitoring

The device, implantation, and monitored data. The Chronicle (model 9520, Medtronic Inc.) is an implantable haemodynamic monitor. The system consists of a specialized transvenous lead that has a sensor incorporated near the tip to measure intracardiac pressure and a programmable device similar in size and shape to a pacemaker. Details of the components have been previously described. The device is able to monitor and telemeter systolic and diastolic RV pressure, RV dP/dt (positive and negative), to estimate pulmonary artery diastolic pressure, to monitor heart rate and patient's activity, and to measure core body temperature. In addition, continuous remote monitoring of data is available. The implantation procedure is similar to that of a single-lead pacemaker. The device is positioned subcutaneously in the pectoral area and the lead is placed transvenously in the RV outflow tract or septum. The patient is furnished with a small external device, which aids in correcting for barometric pressure.

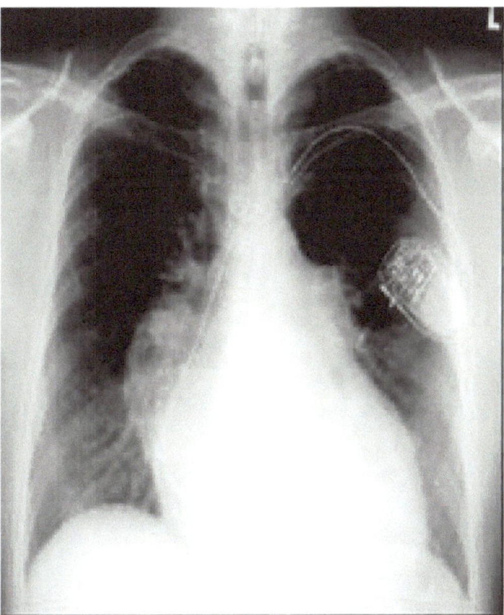

Fig.17.19The implant procedure of the Chronicle implantable haemodynamic monitoring is similar to that of a cardiac pacemaker, whereby the device is positioned subcutaneously in the pectoral area with the lead positioned transvenously in the right ventricular outflow tract. Average implant time is >1 h.

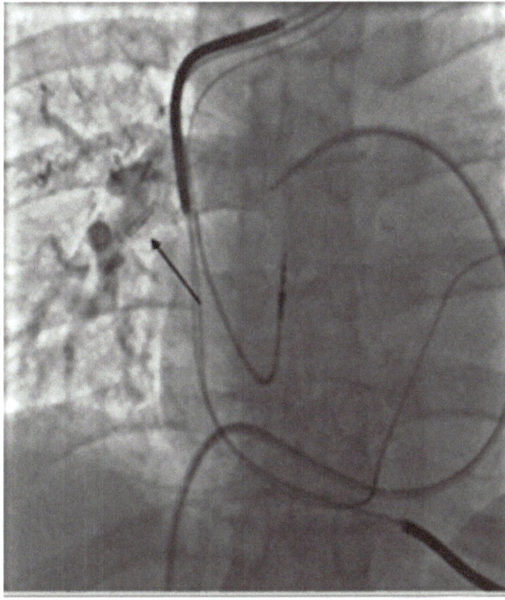

Fig. 17.20 Heart failure sensor implanted through right heart catheterization in the right pulmonary artery (arrow), although left is the preferred location. Flow is noted around the sensor on venogram

The monitor capabilities includes pressure sensing circuitry and a memory to store continuous pressure trends, as well as specific triggered events such as bradyarrhythmias, tachyarrhythmias, or patient-activated episodes. The device continuously measures and stores RV systolic, diastolic, and pulse pressure, estimated pulmonary arterial diastolic pressure (ePAD), RV dP/dt, pre-ejection interval, and systolic time interval. The ePAD is defined as the RV pressure at the time of pulmonary valve opening or maximal RV dP/dt and has been shown to correlate with PA diastolic pressures (r = 0.87 at baseline and 1 year), thus reflecting LV filling pressure. In addition, heart rate, patient activity levels, and central venous temperature are also monitored and stored.

Clinical Perspectives

In March 2007, FDA's Circulatory System Devices Panel voted against the approval of Chronicle implantable haemodynamic monitor because its use was not proved to significantly improve clinical outcomes in the COMPASS-HF randomized, controlled trial. The following step has been the planning of a trial designed to test the potential usefulness of combining the haemodynamic monitoring capabilities of an implantable monitoring device with an ICD in patients at risk of sudden cardiac death. Indeed, a new trial, REDUCEhf, was designed to enrol 850 patients (then increased to 1300) with indication for an ICD (NYHA functional class II or III with reduced LVEF) to test the hypothesis that the use of RV pressure-guided patient management would reduce HF-related events (hospitalization and emergency department or urgent clinic visit requiring parenteral therapy). Because of technical complications, REDUCEhf was prematurely ended after enrolment of 400 patients. Data analysis showed no benefit from haemodynamic monitoring and a lower than expected event rate. Demonstrating the efficacy of HF disease management programmes using RV pressure monitoring was particularly difficult and many issues appear to condition the ability to demonstrate a substantial clinical benefit. These factors include the degree of HF severity in the tested population, the quality of comparative usual care (with a potential low-external validity if the trial is managed by highly specialized centres), the choice of the primary endpoint (the need for medical visits may actually increase during continuous monitoring in view of earlier detection of worsening HF, but this may imply avoidance of subsequent hospitalizations), as well as the specific characteristics of the disease management programme adopted. Moreover, it is possible that a substantial improvement in patient care will require to couple the information provided by an implantable haemodynamic sensor to an effect or capable of promptly instituting an appropriate therapy, thus 'closing the loop' and limiting the need for interventions of healthcare providers.

Left Atrial Pressure Monitoring

Patients admitted for decompensated HF usually have elevated LAP causing pulmonary congestion and oedema. The rise in LAP is usually gradual and precedes the onset of symptoms. Therefore, monitoring of LAP has the potential to forecast and abort HF decompensation by adjusting drug therapy. (Figs. 17.20–17.22)

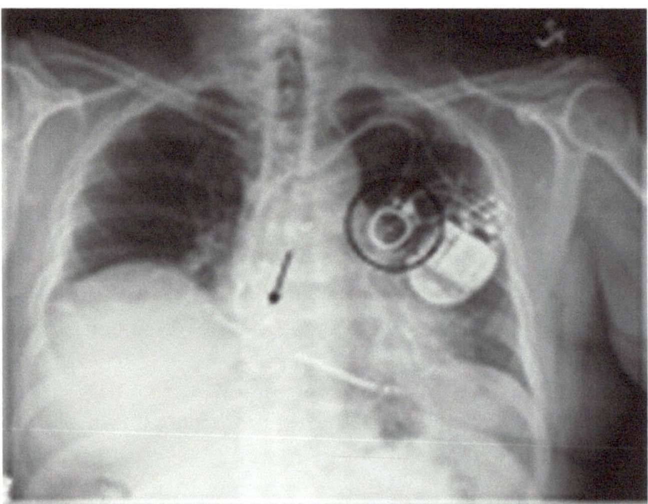

Fig. 17.21 Heartpod (left atrial pressure sensor, arrow) in the trans-septal location attached to the coil antenna (circle) implanted in the subpectoral area. This patient also has a dual-chamber defibrillator for primary prevention with right atrial and right ventricular leads.

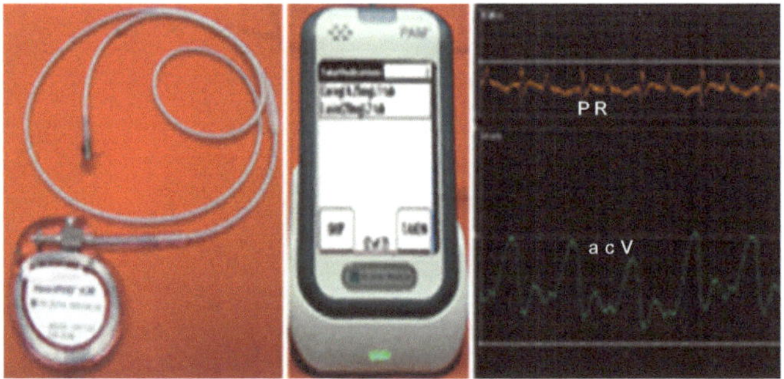

Fig.17.22Left: A standalone HeartPOD device with the communicator module connected to the sensor lead.Middle: the PAM that powers the HeartPOD by telemetry, records data, and provides therapeutic advice to the patient. Right: electrograms and LAP waveforms recorded by the HeartPOD (reproduced with kind permission by St Jude Medical).

The device

The HeartPOD (St Jude Medical) comprises an implantable sensor lead that measures pressure, intracardiac electrograms, and temperature, coupled to a coil antenna positioned in the subcutaneous tissue . Folding proximal and distal nitinol anchors fix the sensor lead onto the interatrial septum. The device is either standalone or coupled to a CRT-D unit. A handheld patient advisory module (PAM) powers the implanted device (which has no battery) by radiofrequency wireless transmission. The PAM also measures the atmospheric pressure, that is then subtracted from the pressure measured in the implant to obtain LAP. During interrogation, physiological waveforms of LAP and intracardiac electrograms are captured in the memory of the PAM for periods of up to 20 s. The PAM has the capacity to store ~3 months of data with six daily interrogations.

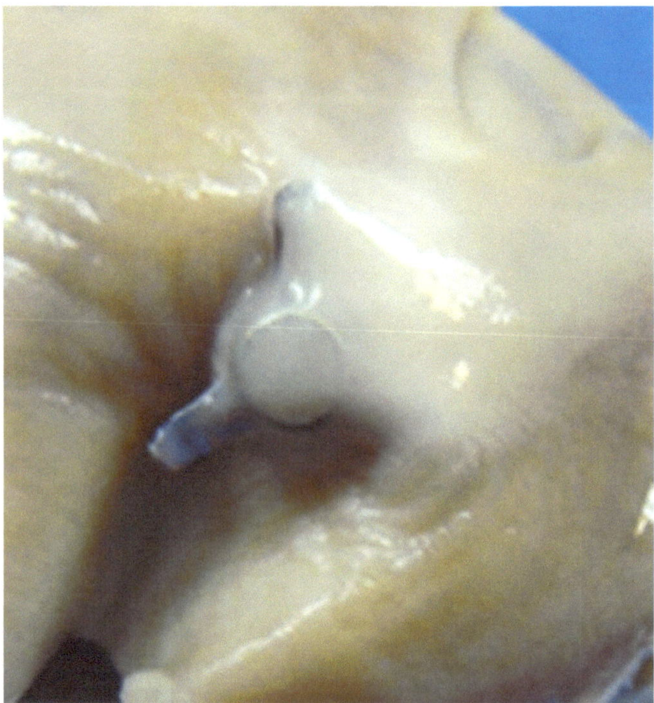

Fig.17.23Autopsy in a patient after 37 months of implantation of a HeartPOD showing endothelialisation of the pressure sensor (reproduced with kind permission by St Jude Medical).

Clinical perspectives

Self-titration of HF therapy by patients based upon LAP readings (similar to diabetics adjusting insulin levels with glycaemia) is a paradigm shift in HF management. This strategy of course requires patient participation and compliance, and may not be suitable for many individuals. Patients with diastolic HF are a therapeutic challenge, in whom volume overload may rapidly cause pulmonary congestion. Analysis of the LAPTOP-HF data in this subset of patient will clarify whether titration of diuretics based upon LAP readings improves outcome. LAP data may be of use to optimize AV delays in CRT-HeartPOD devices (as the left atrial A-wave is recorded), but has not as yet been tested.

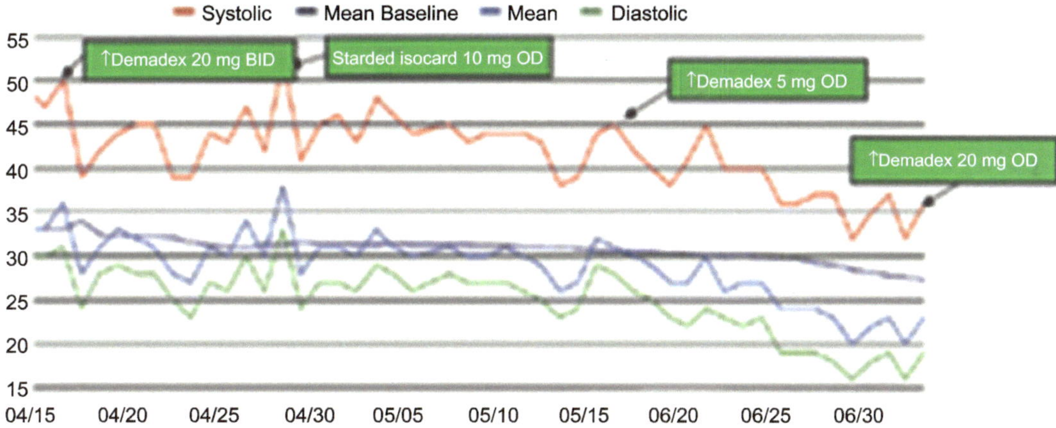

Fig. 17.24 Pressure-guided sensor has been used in a patient with heart failure. The patient had a history of NYHA class III ischaemic cardiomyopathy, cardiac resynchronization therapy combined with a defibrillator, atrial fibrillation, and renal insufficiency. At device implantation, the patient was on low-dose angiotensin-converting enzyme inhibitor, diuretic, and β-blocker. Vasodilating therapy and diuretic doses were titrated to maintain pre-specified target pressures.

In conclusion, preliminary data relating to the HeartPOD show good mid-term device function and hold promise for improving patient self-management in HF. These data however need to be confirmed by the ongoing randomized LAPTOP-HF trial. Device implantation requires special training, and techniques are still evolving. The presence of a lead allows extraction (contrary to PAP monitor), but further experience is required to better evaluate procedural complications. (Figs. 17.23—17.24)

PULMONARY ARTERY PRESSURE MONITORING

The device

The CardioMEMS heart failure sensor (CardioMEMSInc.) consists of a coil and a pressure-sensitive capacitor housed in a hermetically sealed silica capsule covered in medical-grade silicone. Two wired nitinol loops at the ends of the capsule serve as anchors to prevent distal migration of the sensor. The coil and capacitor form an electrical circuit that resonates at a specific frequency. The coil allows for electromagnetic coupling to the sensor by an external antenna, which is held against the patient's body. The antenna powers the implanted device, continuously measures its resonant frequency, which is then converted to a pressure waveform. The interrogating device measures the atmospheric pressure, which is subtracted from the pressure measured by the implanted sensor. The CardioMEMS sensor is designed to measure PAP.

Sensor delivery system and implantation

The CardioMEMS sensor is supplied pre-loaded and attached to a tether wire at the end of the delivery catheter. The sensor is implanted by using a venous femoral approach. First, a Swan–Ganz catheter is advanced into the deployment site in the pulmonary artery. After identification of the target artery, a guidewire (0.018–0.025 inch) is placed through the Swan–Ganz catheter to allow the sensor delivery catheter system to be advanced. The delivery catheter is advanced over the wire and released in the target vessel. After removal of the delivery catheter, the Swan–Ganz catheter is replaced into the pulmonary artery proximal to the sensor. Subsequently, the implanted sensor is calibrated using PAPs acquired from the Swan–Ganz catheter. (Figs. 17.25—17.26)

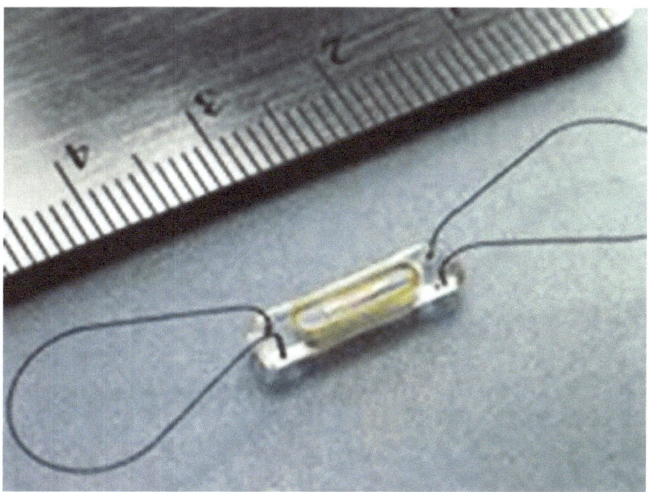

Fig.17.25 The CardioMEMS sensor consists of a coil and a pressure-sensitive capacitor housed in a hermetically sealed silica capsule covered in medical-grade silicone. Two wired nitinol loops at the ends of the capsule serve as anchors to prevent distal migration of the sensor

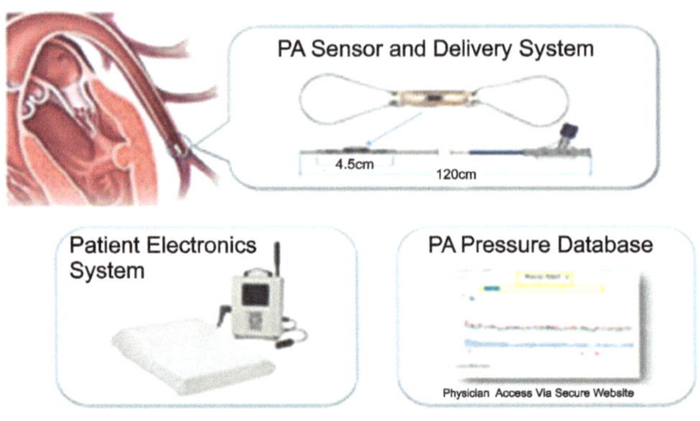

Fig. 17.26 FDA approves first implantable wireless device with remote monitoring to measure pulmonary artery pressure in certain heart failure patients.

Clinical perspectives

In November 2011, FDA's Circulatory System Devices Panel voted against the approval of the CardioMEMS implantable haemodynamic monitor because its use was not proved to significantly improve clinical outcomes in the randomized, single-blind CHAMPION trial. The greatest concern is the trial's design, which made it impossible to distinguish any treatment effect from the device itself in the single-blind trial. Physicians knew which patients had the device and specific treatment recommendations were made in the treatment group and not in the control group. Ambulatory HF patients are at high risk for hospital admission. There is an urgent need to develop strategies to reduce hospitalizations and re-admission rates for HF. New technologies for invasive haemodynamic monitoring have been developed as an adjunct to clinical follow-up. The results of studies with implantable haemodynamic monitoring devices show great promise as adjunctive tools in the management of HF patients. The technology of haemodynamic monitoring is not incorporated in current defibrillators or devices with CRT. Future studies have to evaluate whether a role exists for combining impedance measurements by current cardiac devices with haemodynamic sensors.

Bibliography and Acknowledgement

Abraham WT, *et al.* Cardiac resynchronization in chronic heart failure. N Engl J Med 2002; **346**:1845–53.

Abraham WT, *et al.* Subgroup analysis of a randomized controlled trial evaluating the safety and efficacy of cardiac contractility modulation in advanced heart failure. J Card Fail 2011; **17**:710–7.

Abraham WT, et al Wireless pulmonary artery haemodynamic monitoring in chronic heart failure: a randomised controlled trial. Lancet 2011; **377**:658–66.

Adamson PB, *et al.* Continuous hemodynamic monitoring in patients with mild to moderate heart failure: results of The Reducing Decompensation Events Utilizing Intracardiac Pressures in Patients with Chronic Heart Failure (REDUCEhf) trial. Congest Heart Fail 2011; **17**:248–54.

Andresen MC, *et al.* Nucleus tractussolitarius—gateway to neural circulatory control. Annu Rev Physiol1994; **56**:93–116.

Ardell JL, *et al.* Dorsal spinal cord stimulation obtunds the capacity of intrathoracic extracardiac neurons to transduce myocardial ischemia. Am J Physiol Regul Integr Comp Physiol 2009; **297**:R470–77.

Armour JA, *et al.* Long-term modulation of the intrinsic cardiac nervous system by spinal cord neurons in normal and ischaemic hearts. Auton Neurosci 2002; **95**:71–9.

Bedder MD, *et al.* Spinal cord stimulation surgical technique for the non-surgically trained. Neuromodulation2009; **12**:1–19.

Beshai JF, *et al.* Cardiac–resynchronization therapy in heart failure with narrow QRS complexes. N Engl J Med2007.

Bibevski S, *et al.* Ganglionic mechanisms contribute to diminished vagal control in heart failure. Circulation1999; **99**:2958–63.

Bibevski S, *et al.* Prevention of diminished parasympathetic control of the heart in experimental heart failure.Am J Physiol Heart Circ Physiol 2004; **287**:H1780–5.

Binkley PF, *et al.* A polymorphism of the endothelial nitric oxide synthase promoter is associated with an increase in autonomic imbalance in patients with congestive heart failure. Am Heart J 2005; **149**:342–8.

Binkley PF, *et al.* Parasympathetic withdrawal is an integral component of autonomic imbalance in congestive heart failure: demonstration in human subjects and verification in a paced canine model of ventricular failure. J Am Coll Cardiol 1991; **18**:464–72.

Bisognano JD, *et al.* Baroreflex activation therapy lowers blood pressure in patients with resistant hypertension: results from the double-blind, randomized, placebo-controlled Rheos pivotal trial. J Am Coll Cardiol2011; **58**:765–73.

Blank M, *et al.* Initial interactions in electromagnetic field-induced biosynthesis. J Cell Physiol 2004; **199**:359–63.

Borggrefe MM, *et al.* Randomized, double blind study of non-excitatory, cardiac contractility modulation electrical impulses for symptomatic heart failure. Eur Heart J 2008; **29**:1019–28.

Bourge RC, *et al.* Randomized controlled trial of an implantable continuous hemodynamic monitor in patients with advanced heart failure: the COMPASS-HF study. J Am Coll Cardiol 2008; **51**:1073–9.

Brandt MC, *et al.* Baroreflex activation as a novel therapeutic strategy for diastolic heart failure. Clin Res Cardiol 2011; **100**:249–51.

Brignole M, *et al.* ESC guidelines on cardiac pacing and cardiac resynchronization therapy: the task force on cardiac pacing and resynchronization therapy of the European Society of Cardiology (ESC). Developed in collaboration with the European Heart Rhythm Association (EHRA). Europace 2013; **15**:1070–118.

Bristow MR, *et al.* Cardiac–resynchronization therapy with or without an implantable defibrillator in advanced chronic heart failure. N Engl J Med 2004; **350**:2140–50.

Bristow MR, *et al.* Decreased catecholamine sensitivity and beta-adrenergic-receptor density in failing human hearts. N Engl J Med 1982; **307**:205–11.

Brodison A, *et al.* Spinal-cord stimulation in management of angina. Lancet 1999; **354**:1748–9.

Brook AL, *et al.* Spinal cord stimulation: a basic approach. Tech Vasc Interv Radiol 2009; **12**:64–70.

Brunner-La Rocca HP, *et al.* Effect of cardiac sympathetic nervous activity on mode of death in congestive heart failure. Eur Heart J 2001; **22**:1136–43.

Burkhoff D, *et al.* Nonexcitatory electrical signals for enhancing ventricular contractility: rationale and initial investigations of an experimental treatment for heart failure. Am J Physiol Heart Circ Physiol 2005; **288**:H2550–6.

Burkhoff D, *et al.* 'Responder analysis' for assessing effectiveness of heart failure therapies based on measures of exercise tolerance. J Card Fail 2009; **15**:108–15.

Butter C, *et al.* Cardiac contractility modulation electrical signals improve myocardial gene expression in patients with heart failure. J Am Coll Cardiol 2008; **51**:1784–9.

Butter C, *et al.* Enhanced inotropic state of the failing left ventricle by cardiac contractility modulation electrical signals is not associated with increased myocardial oxygen consumption. J Card Fail 2007; **13**:137–42.

Cameron T. Safety and efficacy of spinal cord stimulation for the treatment of chronic pain: a 20-year literature review. J Neurosurg 2004; **100**:254–67.

Cardinal R, *et al.* Spinal cord activation differentially modulates ischaemic electrical responses to different stressors in canine ventricles. Auton Neurosci 2004; **111**:37–47.

Cardinal R, *et al.* Spinal cord stimulation suppresses bradycardias and atrial tachyarrhythmias induced by mediastinal nerve stimulation in dogs. Am J Physiol Regul Integr Comp Physiol 2006; **291**:R1369–75.

Castro PF, *et al.* A wireless pressure sensor for monitoring pulmonary artery pressure in advanced heart failure: initial experience. J Heart Lung Transplant 2007; **26**:85–8.

Chandler MJ, *et al.* A mechanism of cardiac pain suppression by spinal cord stimulation: implications for patients with angina pectoris. Eur Heart J 1993; **14**:96–105.

Creager MA, *et al.* Arterial baroreflex regulation of blood pressure in patients with congestive heart failure. J Am Coll Cardiol 1994; **23**:401–5.

Cygankiewicz I, *et al*; MuerteSubita en InsuficienciaCardiaca Investigators. Heart rate turbulence predicts all-cause mortality and sudden death in congestive heart failure patients. Heart Rhythm 2008; **5**:1095–102.

Czachurski J, *et al.* Localization of neurons with baroreceptor input in the medial solitary nucleus by means of intracellular application of horseradish peroxidase in the cat. Neurosci Lett 1982; **28**:133–7.

Daubert JC, *et al.* EHRA/HRS expert consensus statement on cardiac resynchronization therapy in heart failure: implant and follow–up recommendations and management. Europace 2012; **14**:1236–86.

de Jongste MJ, *et al.* Stimulation characteristics, complications, and efficacy of spinal cord stimulation systems in patients with refractory angina: a prospective feasibility study. Pacing Clin Electrophysiol 1994; **17**:1751–60.

de Vries J, *et al.* An open label, single-centre, randomized trial of spinal cord stimulation vs. percutaneous myocardial laser revascularization in patients with refractory angina pectoris: the spirit trial. Eur Heart J2006; **27**:1631–2. author reply 1632.

Dickstein K, et al ; ESC Committee for Practice Guidelines. 2010 Focused Update of ESC Guidelines on device therapy in heart failure: an update of the 2008 ESC Guidelines for the diagnosis and treatment of acute and chronic heart failure and the 2007 ESC Guidelines for cardiac and resynchronization therapy. Developed with the special contribution of the Heart Failure Association and the European Heart Rhythm Association. Europace 2010; **12**:1526–36.

Diedrichs H, *et al.* [Increased myocardial blood flow after spinal cord stimulation in patients with refractory angina pectoris]. Med Klin (Munich) 2003; **98**:146–50.

Diedrichs H, *et al.* Symptomatic relief precedes improvement of myocardial blood flow in patients under spinal cord stimulation. Curr Control Trials Cardiovasc Med 2005; **6**:7.

Eckberg DL, *et al.* Defective cardiac parasympathetic control in patients with heart failure. N Engl J Med1971; **285**:877–83.

Ekre O, *et al.* Feasibility of spinal cord stimulation in angina pectoris in patients with chronic pacemaker treatment for cardiac arrhythmias. Pacing Clin Electrophysiol 2003; **26**:2134–41.

Eliasson T, *et al.* Myocardial turnover of endogenous opioids and calcitonin-gene-related peptide in the human heart and the effects of spinal cord stimulation on pacing-induced angina pectoris. Cardiology 1998; **89**:170–7.

Eliasson T, *et al.* Spinal cord stimulation in angina pectoris with normal coronary arteriograms. Coron Artery Dis 1993; **4**:819–27.

Enggaard TP, *et al.* Spinal cord stimulation for refractory angina in patients implanted with cardioverter defibrillators: five case reports. Europace 2010; **12**:1336–7.

Fan W, *et al.* Graded and dynamic reflex summation of myelinated and unmyelinated rat aortic baroreceptors.Am J Physiol 1999; **277**:R748–56.

Ferrero P, *et al.* Spinal cord stimulation affects T-wave alternans in patients with ischaemic cardiomyopathy: a pilot study. Europace 2008; **10**:506–8.

Foody JM, *et al.* Beta-blocker therapy in heart failure: scientific review. JAMA 2002; **287**:883–9.

Foreman RD, *et al.* Modulation of intrinsic cardiac neurons by spinal cord stimulation: Implications for its therapeutic use in angina pectoris. Cardiovasc Res 2000; **47**:367–75.

Georgakopoulos D, *et al.* Chronic baroreflex activation: a potential therapeutic approach to heart failure with preserved ejection fraction. J Card Fail 2011; **17**:167–78.

Gersbach PA, *et al.* Spinal cord stimulation treatment for angina pectoris: more than a placebo? Ann Thorac Surg 2001; **72**:S1100–04.

Gibbons DD, *et al.* Neuromodulation targets intrinsic cardiac neurons to attenuate neuronally mediated atrial arrhythmias. Am J Physiol Regul Integr Comp Physiol 2012; **302**:R357–64.

Hautvast RW, *et al.* Effect of spinal cord stimulation on heart rate variability and myocardial ischemia in patients with chronic intractable angina pectoris—a prospective ambulatory electrocardiographic study. Clin Cardiol1998; **21**:33–8.

Hautvast RW, *et al.* Spinal cord stimulation in chronic intractable angina pectoris: a randomized, controlled efficacy study. Am Heart J 1998; **136**:1114–20.

Hegarty D. Spinal cord stimulation: the clinical application of new technology. Anesthesiol Res Pract2012; **2012**:375691.

Henderson JM, *et al.* Nans training requirements for spinal cord stimulation devices: selection, implantation, and follow-up. Neuromodulation 2009; **12**:171–4.

Heusser K, *et al.* Chronic baroreflex activation: a potential therapeutic approach to heart failure with preserved ejection fraction carotid baroreceptor stimulation, sympathetic activity, baroreflex function, and blood pressure in hypertensive patients. Hypertension 2010; **55**:619–26.

Hosobuchi Y. Electrical stimulation of the cervical spinal cord increases cerebral blood flow in humans. Appl Neurophysiol 1985; ; **48**:372–6.

Illig KA, *et al.* An implantable carotid sinus stimulator for drug-resistant hypertension: surgical technique and short-term outcome from the multicenter phase II Rheos feasibility trial. J Vasc Surg 2006; **44**:1213–8.

Imai M, *et al.* Therapy with cardiac contractility modulation electrical signals improves left ventricular function and remodeling in dogs with chronic heart failure. J Am Coll Cardiol 2007; **49**:2120–8.

Issa ZF, *et al.* Thoracic spinal cord stimulation reduces the risk of ischemic ventricular arrhythmias in a postinfarction heart failure canine model. Circulation 2005; **111**:3217–20.

Jacques F, *et al.* Spinal cord stimulation causes potentiation of right vagus nerve effects on atrial chronotropic function and repolarization in canines. J Cardiovasc Electrophysiol 2011; **22**:440–7.

Jesus S, *et al.* Initial experience with spinal cord stimulation (SCS) for the treatment of advanced heart failure.J Card Fail 2010; **16**:S67.

Kadish A, *et al.* A randomized controlled trial evaluating the safety and efficacy of cardiac contractility modulation in advanced heart failure. Am Heart J 2011; **161**:329–37.

Kirchheim HR. Systemic arterial baroreceptor reflexes. Physiol Rev 1976; **56**:100–77.

Klomp HM, *et al.* Systematic review and meta-analysis of controlled trials assessing spinal cord stimulation for inoperable critical leg ischaemia (Br J Surg 2004; 91:948–955). Br J Surg 2005; **92**:120. author reply 120–1.

Kollai M, *et al.* Relation between baroreflex sensitivity and cardiac vagal tone in humans. Am J Physiol1994; **266**:H21–7.

Kosharskyy B, *et al.* Feasibility of spinal cord stimulation in a patient with a cardiac pacemaker. Pain Physician2006; **9**:249–51.

Kujacic V, *et al.* Assessment of the influence of spinal cord stimulation on left ventricular function in patients with severe angina pectoris: an echocardiographic study. Eur Heart J 1993; **14**:1238–44.

Lanza GA, *et al.* Effect of spinal cord stimulation on spontaneous and stress-induced angina and 'ischemia-like' ST-segment depression in patients with cardiac syndrome X. Eur Heart J 2005; **26**:983–9.

La Rovere MT, et al; ATRAMI (Autonomic Tone and Reflexes After Myocardial Infarction) Investigators.Baroreflex sensitivity and heart-rate variability in prediction of total cardiac mortality after myocardial infarction.Lancet 1998; **351**:478–84.

Latif OA, *et al.* Spinal cord stimulation for chronic intractable angina pectoris: a unified theory on its mechanism. Clin Cardiol 2001; **24**:533–41.

Lawo T, *et al.* Electrical signals applied during the absolute refractory period: an investigational treatment for advanced heart failure in patients with normal QRS duration. J Am Coll Cardiol 2005; **46**:2229–36.

Liu Y, *et al.* Thoracic spinal cord stimulation improves cardiac contractile function and myocardial oxygen consumption in a porcine model of ischemic heart failure. J Cardiovasc Electrophysiol 2011.

Li W, *et al.* Inflammatory cytokines and nitric oxide in heart failure and potential modulation by vagus nerve stimulation. Heart Fail Rev 2011; **16**:137–45.

Long DM, *et al.* Electrical stimulation of the spinal cord and peripheral nerves for pain control. A 10-year experience. Appl Neurophysiol 1981; **44**:207–17.

Lopshire JC, *et al.* Spinal cord stimulation improves ventricular function and reduces ventricular arrhythmias in a canine postinfarction heart failure model. Circulation 2009; **120**:286–94.

Lund LH, *et al.* Prevalence, correlates, and prognostic significance of QRS prolongation in heart failure with reduced and preserved ejection fraction. Eur Heart J 2013; **34**:529–39.

Maggioni AP, *et al.* EURObservational Research Programme: the Heart Failure Pilot Survey (ESC–HF Pilot). Eur J Heart Fail 2010; **12**:1076–84.

Mannheimer C, *et al.* The problem of chronic refractory angina; report from the esc joint study group on the treatment of refractory angina. Eur Heart J 2002; **23**:355–70.

Marin-Neto JA, *et al.* Abnormal baroreflex control of heart rate in decompensated congestive heart failure and reversal after compensation. Am J Cardiol 1991; **67**:604–10.

Markos F, *et al.* Nitric oxide facilitates vagal control of heart rate via actions in the cardiac parasympathetic ganglia of the anaesthetised dog. Exp Physiol 2002; **87**:49–52.

McMurray JJ, *et al.* ESC guidelines for the diagnosis and treatment of acute and chronic heart failure 2012: The Task Force for the Diagnosis and Treatment of Acute and Chronic Heart Failure 2010 of the European Society of Cardiology. Developed in collaboration with the Heart Failure Association (HFA) of the ESC. Eur Heart J2012; **33**:1787–847.

McNab D, *et al.* An open label, single-centre, randomized trial of spinal cord stimulation vs. percutaneous myocardial laser revascularization in patients with refractory angina pectoris: the spirit trial. Eur Heart J2006; **27**:1048–53.

Mekhail NA, *et al.* Retrospective review of 707 cases of spinal cord stimulation: indications and complications.Pain Pract 2011; **11**:148–53.

Melzack R, *et al.* Pain mechanisms: a new theory. Science 1965; **150**:971–9.

Mendelowitz D. Firing properties of identified parasympathetic cardiac neurons in the nucleus ambiguus. Am J Physiol 1996; **271**:H2609–14.

Merchant FM, *et al.* Implantable sensors for heart failure. Circ Arrhythm Electrophysiol 2010; **3**:657–67.

Mohri S, *et al.* Cardiac contractility modulation by electric currents applied during the refractory period. Am J Physiol Heart Circ Physiol 2002; **282**:H1642–7.

Molon G, *et al.* ICD and neuromodulation devices: is peaceful coexistence possible? Pacing Clin Electrophysiol 2011; **34**:690–3.

Morita H, *et al.* Cardiac contractility modulation with nonexcitatory electric signals improves left ventricular function in dogs with chronic heart failure. J Card Fail 2003; **9**:69–75.

Nägele H, *et al.* Cardiac contractility modulation in non-responders to cardiac resynchronization therapy.Europace 2008; **10**:1375–80.

Neelagaru SB, *et al.* Nonexcitatory, cardiac contractility modulation electrical impulses: feasibility study for advanced heart failure in patients with normal QRS duration. Heart Rhythm 2006; **3**:1140–7.

Nelson GS, *et al.* Left ventricular or biventricular pacing improves cardiac function at diminished energy cost in patients with dilated cardiomyopathy and left bundle-branch block [In Process Citation]. Circulation (Online)2000; **102**:3053–9.

Olgin JE, *et al.* Effects of thoracic spinal cord stimulation on cardiac autonomic regulation of the sinus and atrioventricular nodes. J Cardiovasc Electrophysiol 2002; **13**:475–81.

Olshansky B, *et al.* Parasympathetic nervous system and heart failure: pathophysiology and potential implications for therapy. Circulation 2008; **118**:863–71.

Ooi YC, *et al.* Simultaneous use of neurostimulators in patients with a pre-existing cardiovascular implantable electronic device. Neuromodulation 2011; **14**:20–5. discussion 25–26.

Pappone C, *et al.* Cardiac contractility modulation by electric currents applied during the refractory period in patients with heart failure secondary to ischemic or idiopathic dilated cardiomyopathy. Am J Cardiol 2002; **90**:1307–13.

Pappone C, *et al.* Electrical modulation of cardiac contractility: clinical aspects in congestive heart failure.Heart Fail Rev 2001; **6**:55–60.

Pappone C, *et al.* First human chronic experience with cardiac contractility modulation by nonexcitatory electrical currents for treating systolic heart failure: mid-term safety and efficacy results from a multicenter study. J Cardiovasc Electrophysiol 2004; **15**:418–27.

Reig E, *et al.* Spinal cord stimulation: a 20-year retrospective analysis in 260 patients. Neuromodulation2009; **12**:232–9.

Ritzema J, *et al.* Direct left atrial pressure monitoring in ambulatory heart failure patients: initial experience with a new permanent implantable device. Circulation 2007; **116**:2952–9.

Ritzema J, *et al.* Physician-directed patient self-management of left atrial pressure in advanced chronic heart failure. Circulation 2010; **121**:1086–95.

Romano M, *et al.* Efficacy and safety of permanent cardiac DDD pacing with contemporaneous double spinal cord stimulation. Pacing Clin Electrophysiol 1998; **21**:465–7.

Rydlewska A, *et al.* Changes in autonomic balance in patients with decompensated chronic heart failure. Clin Auton Res 2011; **21**:47–54.

Sabbah HN, *et al.* Cardiac contractilty modulation with the impulse dynamics signal: studies in dogs with chronic heart failure. Heart Fail Rev 2001; **6**:45–53.

Sabbah HN, *et al.* Chronic electrical stimulation of the carotid sinus baroreflex improves left ventricular function and promotes reversal of ventricular remodeling in dogs with advanced heart failure. Circ Heart Fail2011; **4**:65–70.

Schau T, *et al.* Long-term outcome of cardiac contractility modulation in patients with severe congestive heart failure. Europace 2011; **13**:1436–44.

Scheffers IJM, *et al.* Novel baroreflex activation therapy in resistant hypertension: results of a European multi-center feasibility study. J Am Coll Cardiol 2010; **56**:1254–8.

Schimpf R, *et al.* Potential device interaction of a dual chamber implantable cardioverter defibrillator in a patient with continuous spinal cord stimulation. Europace 2003; **5**:397–402.

Schwartz PJ, *et al.* Sympathetic-parasympathetic interaction in health and disease: abnormalities and relevance in heart failure. Heart Fail Rev 2011; **16**:101–7.

Shenkman HJ, *et al.* Congestive heart failure and QRS duration: establishing prognosis study. Chest2002; **122**:528–34.

Sibell DM, *et al.* Successful use of spinal cord stimulation in the treatment of severe Raynaud's disease of the hands. Anesthesiology 2005; **102**:225–7.

Southerland EM, *et al.* Preemptive, but not reactive, spinal cord stimulation mitigates transient ischemia-induced myocardial infarction via cardiac adrenergic neurons. Am J Physiol Heart Circ Physiol 2007; **292**:H311–7.

Stix G, *et al.* Chronic electrical stimulation during the absolute refractory period of the myocardium improves severe heart failure. Eur Heart J 2004; **25**:650–5.

Tordoir JH, *et al.* An implantable carotid sinus baroreflex activating system: surgical technique and short-term outcome from a multi-center feasibility trial for the treatment of resistant hypertension. Eur J Vasc Endovasc Surg2007; **33**:414–21.

Troughton RW, *et al.* Direct left atrial pressure monitoring in severe heart failure: long-term sensor performance. J Cardiovasc Transplant Res 2011; **4**:3–13.

Ubbink DT, *et al.* Spinal cord stimulation for non-reconstructable chronic critical leg ischaemia. Cochrane Database Syst Rev 2005:CD004001.

Vanoli E, *et al.* Vagal stimulation and prevention of sudden death in conscious dogs with a healed myocardial infarction. Circ Res 1991; **68**:1471–81.

Vatner DE, *et al.* Physiological and biochemical evidence for coordinate increases in muscarinic receptors and Gi during pacing-induced heart failure. Circulation 1996; **94**:102–7.

Verdejo HE, *et al.* Comparison of a radiofrequency-based wireless pressure sensor to swan-ganz catheter and echocardiography for ambulatory assessment of pulmonary artery pressure in heart failure. J Am Coll Cardiol2007; **50**:2375–82.

Visocchi M, *et al.* Spinal cord stimulation and cerebral hemodynamics: updated mechanism and therapeutic implications. Stereotact Funct Neurosurg 2011; **89**:263–74.

Wang J, *et al.* Synaptic and neurotransmitter activation of cardiac vagal neurons in the nucleus ambiguus. Ann N Y Acad Sci 2001; **940**:237–46.

Wang M, *et al.* Long-term baroreflex activation therapy increases the threshold for the induction of lethal ventricular arrhythmias in dogs with chronic advanced heart failure. Circulation 2008; **118**:S_721.

Whellan DJ, *et al.* Review of advanced heart failure device diagnostics examined in clinical trials and the potential benefit from monitoring capabilities. Prog Cardiovasc Dis 2011; **54**:107–14.

Wu M, *et al.* Putative mechanisms behind effects of spinal cord stimulation on vascular diseases: a review of experimental studies. Auton Neurosci 2008; **138**:9–23.

Wustmann K, *et al.* Effects of chronic baroreceptor stimulation on the autonomic cardiovascular regulation in patients with drug-resistant arterial hypertension. Hypertension 2009; **54**:530–6.

Yu CM, *et al.* Impact of cardiac contractility modulation on left ventricular global and regional function and remodeling. JACC Cardiovasc Imaging 2009; **2**:1341–9.

Yu CM, *et al.* Intrathoracic impedance monitoring in patients with heart failure: correlation with fluid status and feasibility of early warning preceding hospitalization. Circulation 2005; **112**:841–8.

Zucker IH, *et al.* Chronic baroreceptor activation enhances survival in dogs with pacing-induced heart failure.Hypertension 2007; **50**:904–10.

CHAPTER

Recent Advances in Drug Therapy In Cardiovascular Diseases

1.New Pharmacological Agents for Arrhythmias

Despite advances in catheter ablation techniques and device-based therapies for cardiac arrhythmias, antiarrhythmic drugs remain essential components of any comprehensive therapeutic strategy. Antiarrhythmic drug therapy, however, has been limited by both incomplete efficacy and a substantial potential for cardiac and extracardiac toxicity. As a result, only a few new antiarrhythmic agents have successfully completed clinical development programs and reached routine clinical usage over the past 20 years.Antiarrhythmic drugs may be indicated for ventricular tachycardia, sudden death prevention, or specific types of supraventricular arrhythmia. Implantable cardioverter-defibrillator (ICD) therapy has evolved as the primary treatment for most life-threatening ventricular arrhythmias, and antiarrhythmic drugs for these rhythms are currently mostly used either as acute interventions or as adjuncts to chronic ICD therapyAnother approach has been to seek agents that synergistically affect multiple channels simultaneously, resulting in a net beneficial effect while minimizing toxicity. Other nontraditional targets for drug therapy that do not directly involve ion channels have also emerged as our understanding of the mechanisms of arrhythmias has improved. As a result, several new compounds are now at or near completion of phase 3 clinical trials, and other promising agents are in earlier phases of clinical testing.

Agents Similar to Amiodarone

Amiodarone is generally accepted to be a valuable antiarrhythmic drug, but it accumulates in tissues during long-term therapy, which may result in significant toxicity in several organ systems. Several compounds that were designed to be similar in structure and electrophysiological effects to amiodarone have completed or are now in clinical trials

Dronedarone

Dronedarone is, like amiodarone, a benzofuranyl compound with iodine removed and a methane sulfonyl group added . Removing iodine from the molecule was intended to eliminate or reduce iodine-related organ toxicity. The side chain modification decreased lipophilicity, resulting in a shorter elimination half-life with less potential for tissue accumulation. The basic and clinical pharmacology of dronedarone has been recently reviewed. Dronedarone retains many of amiodarone's electrophysiological effects.

It is a multichannel blocker with effects on the rapid and slow components of the delayed rectifier current (IKr and IKs), L-type calcium currents, (ICa-L), the inward sodium current (INa), and the inward rectifier potassium current (IK1). Dronedarone also inhibits the acetylcholine receptor-dependent K+ current (IKAch) and the pacemaker current (If) and is a noncompetitive α- and β-adrenergic antagonist. Dronedarone reduces sinus rate and prolongs AV nodal conduction and refractoriness. Effects on the QT and QTc intervals have been variable when studied in different species. In several animal models of ischemia or reperfusion-induced arrhythmias, dronedarone effectively prevents spontaneous and inducedventricularfibrillation.

The pharmacokinetic properties

The pharmacokinetic properties of dronedarone are complex. Dronedarone is well absorbed after oral ingestion but undergoes extensive first-pass metabolism mediated by CYP3A4, resulting in a net bioavailability of only 15% when taken with meals. Several metabolic pathways are active, including N-debutylation, oxidative N-deamination, and direct oxidation.The steady-state elimination half-life for dronedarone is estimated to be 13 to 24 hours. The N-debutyl derivative (SQ35021A) is electrophysiologically active but less potent than the parent compound. In the large clinical trials, using 400 mg twice daily, the trough plasma concentration at steady state has been 60 to 150 ng/mL. Potent CYP3A4 inhibitors (eg, ketoconazole, erythromycin, etc) can markedly increase dronedarone plasma concentrations. Less potent CYP3A4 inhibitors (eg, diltiazem, verapamil, moderate amounts of grapefruit juice, etc) produce lesser effects. Potent CYP3A4 inducers (eg, rifampin, phenytoin, St John's wort, etc) should not be used with dronedarone. Dronedarone inhibits both CYP3A4 and CYP2D6. Interactions with CYP3A4 substrates (eg, many statins and calcium antagonists) are possible and should be considered. Dronedarone does not inhibit CYP2C9 or CYP2C19, and interactions with warfarin have not been reported. Dronedarone increases serum digoxin levels by inhibiting P-glycoprotein-mediated renal excretion. Dronedarone also inhibits renal organic cation transport, and this effect may cause serum creatinine levels to rise without decreasing glomerular filtration as measured by inulin clearance.8 Dronedarone should not be used in patients with severe hepatic dysfunction. Dosage reduction is not required in patients with renal insufficiency. The dronedarone dose was 400 mg twice daily. It seems likely that dronedarone will provide a valuable addition to our therapeutic options in patients with atrial fibrillation. Dronedarone was released in the United States for use in patients with atrial fibrillation in July 2009. It has moderate efficacy and, at least during intermediate term therapy, little serious toxicity. Although it may not be as potent as amiodarone, the impressive hospitalization and mortality data from ATHENA suggest that a safe and moderately effective drug can favorably affect important patient outcomes.

Budiodarone

Unlike dronedarone, budiodarone (AT1-2042), another compound that structurally resembles amiodarone, retains 2 iodine atoms in its molecular structure (Figure 1). A sec-butyl acetate side chain has been added at position 2 of the benzofuranyl ring. This ester modification changes the compound's metabolic pathways such that budiodarone undergoes rapid degradation by plasma and tissue esterases, not by CYP3A-mediated oxidation, to an inactive compound. During in vitro studies, budiodarone has shown electrophysiological properties similar to amiodaroneOnly limited clinical data on budiodarone are available. One study assessed twice-daily placebo or doses of 200, 400, 600, and 800 mg during sequential 2-week periods in a very small group of patients with paroxysmal atrial fibrillation and implanted pacemakers. Atrial fibrillation burden (defined as percent time in atrial fibrillation) was calculated during each period. Budiodarone reduced total atrial fibrillation burden by reducing the duration but not the number of atrial fibrillation episodes. Preliminary data from a similar but a larger phase 2 trial compared placebo and budiodarone (200, 400, and 600 mg twice daily) in 72 patients with pacemakers and paroxysmal atrial fibrillation. There were 54.4% and 75% reductions in AF burden in the 400 mg and 600 mg groups. Some patients manifested a rise in thyroid-stimulating hormone, but clinical symptoms of thyroid disease did not appear. There are as yet no published data on long-term exposure to budiodarone, so its potential for chronic toxicity is unknown.

Celivarone

Celivarone (SSR149744C) is another noniodinated benzofuran derivative with electrophysiological effects similar to amiodarone.18 Few clinical data have been published in manuscript form, but a phase 2 trial tested celivarone's efficacy at 300- or 600-mg daily doses for conversion of atrial fibrillation and flutter (CORYFEE, NCT00232310) and a dose ranging study compared celivarone at 50, 100, 200, or 300 mg once daily with amiodarone for maintenance of sinus rhythm (MAIA, NCT00233441) have been completed but not yet published. A preliminary report from the dose-ranging study showed the lowest rate of atrial fibrillation recurrence at the 50 mg dose with no enhanced efficacy at the higher doses.In another study in patients with ICDs, 2 doses of celivarone (100 and 300 mg daily) were compared with placebo over 6 months of therapy.20 A 46% reduction in the number of sustained ventricular arrhythmia episodes requiring ICD therapy was noted in the 300 mg daily group, but this reduction did not achieve statistical significance (P=0.172). Additional trials in patients with ventricular arrhythmias and ICDs are plannedVernakalant Vernakalant is an atrial-selective, multiple ion channel blocker that is in the advanced stages of investigation for the treatment of atrial fibrillation.

Both intravenous and oral forms of vernakalant have undergone clinical trials. The intravenous form has been recommended for approval by the Cardiorenal Advisory Committee of the Food and Drug Administration, but a formal letter of approval has not been issued. Vernakalant is an atrial repolarization-delaying agent with its major target IKur. Vernakalant also blocks Ito and INa, although there is little effect on IKr or IKs.22 As IKur is present in higher density in the atria, vernakalant is relatively atrial selective. The INa inhibition is rate- and voltage-dependent. Vernakalant has, therefore, a much greater effect in fibrillating atria than in the ventricle and is less likely to be proarrhythmic. Vernakalant is hepatically metabolized by CYP2D6. It is not clear what effect abnormal liver function has on the metabolism of the drug. In a study of intravenous vernakalant, coadministration of CYP2D6 inhibitors did not appear to decrease clearance, and little difference was seen in maximum plasma concentrations between CYP2D6 poor and extensive metabolizers. Differences in renal function, age, sex, race, blood pressure, and heart failure status have not been shown to affect the pharmacokinetics of vernakalant. Vernakalant demonstrates 2-compartment elimination pharmacokinetics, and its half-life after intravenous administration is 2 to 5 hours. The oral bioavailability of vernakalant is approximately 20%.

During oral therapy in the dose range of 300 to 600 mg twice daily, steady-state concentrations are achieved in 4 days. It remains to be seen whether CYP2D6 poor and extensive metabolizers will require different doses during chronic oral therapy.In summary, intravenous vernakalant for cardioversion of recent onset AF is moderately effective for rapid termination of atrial fibrillation with durable maintenance of sinus rhythm up to 24 hours. The side effect profile shows relatively modest potential for toxicity. Age, sex, ethnicity, and concomitant illnesses do not appear to alter efficacy. Of course, drugs used only for the acute conversion of atrial fibrillation must also be compared with electrical cardioversion as well as other agents. Oral vernakalant may prove useful for maintenance of sinus rhythm, but phase 3 trials have yet to be completed. If these trials show efficacy, vernakalant probably will be more widely used in conversion attempts as a step to long-term therapy. There are no clinical data on the effects of vernakalant in ventricular arrhythmias, and its mechanisms of action suggest it would not be useful.

Ranolazine

Ranolazine is currently approved for the treatment of chronic angina pectoris. Ranolazine reduces myocardial ischemia by its effects on the late inward Na+ current (INaL). During myocardial ischemia and heart failure, INaL is augmented. This results in increased sodium entry and, via sodium-calcium exchange, increased cytosolic calcium concentrations. These changes produce action potential prolongation and increased susceptibility to early afterdepolarizations. Ranolazine is an inactivated sodium channel blocker.At concentrations near its therapeutic range for angina (2 to 6 μmol/L, IC50 ≈6 μmol/L), ranolazine inhibits INaL. In the same concentration range, ranolazine inhibits peak INa in the atrium but not the ventricle This effect results in reduced atrial excitability and a rate-dependent increase in postrepolarization atrial refractoriness. Ranolazine also inhibits IKr but with a higher IC50 ≈12 μmol/L. In experiments using an isolated canine ventricular wedge preparation, ranolazine results in either no change or a decrease in transmural ventricular dispersion of refractoriness and does not produce early afterdepolarizations, triggered activity, or polymorphic ventricular tachycardia. In other experiments, ranolazine has been shown to suppress excitability and triggered activity in an isolated canine pulmonary vein sleeve preparation, terminate acetylcholine- and isoproterenol-induced atrial fibrillation, and prevent its reinitiation.Ranolazine has variable systemic availability after oral administration due to its extensive first-pass metabolism in the gut and liver. Metabolism is mainly via CYP3A4 and, to a lesser extent, CYP2D6. The terminal elimination half-life is 7 hours. The recommended dosage in patients with angina is 500 to 1000 mg twice daily. Ranolazine should not be used as concurrent therapy with strong CYP3A4 inhibitors (eg, ketoconazole), and dose reduction is recommended with moderate CYP3A4 inhibitors

(eg, diltiazem) or P-glycoprotein inhibitors. Ranolazine is a weak inhibitor of CYP3A4 and a moderate inhibitor of CYP2D6 and P-glycoprotein. One form of the long-QT syndrome (LQT3) is caused by mutations in the SCN5A sodium channel that lead to enhanced and sustained activity of late INa. Moss et al41 administered intravenous ranolazine to 5 patients with LQT3. During the infusion, ranolazine shortened QTcf by 26 3 ms. Diastolic function on echocardiography was also improved. Ranolazine may also prove useful in another form of the long-QT syndrome. The Timothy syndrome (LQT8) is a multisystem disorder characterized by facial dysmorphism, syndactyly, QT prolongation, and premature sudden death. The syndrome is caused by a missense mutation in Cav1.2, the gene that encodes the α-subunit of the L-type calcium channel, resulting in a gain in function of the L-type calcium current. In an animal model of the Timothy syndrome, ranolazine suppressed polymorphic ventricular tachycardia induced by the calcium channel agonist Bay K8644.40 Clinical data on the chronic treatment of arrhythmias in LQT3 and Timothy syndrome patients are not available.
At present, the only approved indication for ranolazine is the treatment of angina. It remains to be proven whether it will also be useful as an antiarrhythmic agent.

Ivabradine

Ivabradine selectively inhibits the spontaneous pacemaker activity of the sinus node by blocking the If current.43 This reduces the heart rate without altering myocardial contractility or other hemodynamics.44 Ivabradine has been approved for use as an antianginal in Europe.45 It has also been used off-label in Europe as a treatment for inappropriate sinus tachycardia. It has not yet been approved for any use in the United States. The blockage of the If current is dose-dependent and heart rate-dependent. There is a greater efficiency in blocking If at faster heart rates, limiting the risks of symptomatic bradycardia.46 Electrophysiological studies of ivabradine in humans have shown little effect on the conduction system or on atrial and ventricular refractoriness. Some remodeling of the sinus node appears to occur in response to ivabradine, but no rebound tachycardia has been seen after discontinuing the drug.
Ivabradine is 80% hepatically metabolized by the CYP3A4 enzyme and cannot be used concomitantly with drugs that inhibit this enzyme, such as azoles and macrolide antibiotics.49 There does not appear to be a difference in heart rate response between patients who are CYP3A4 rapid metabolizers and those who are slow metabolizers. It is 20% renally cleared. The oral bioavailability is approximately 40% and it takes 60 to 90 minutes to reach maximal plasma concentrations. The half-life is approximately 2 hours.

A previous study compared ivabradine with atenolol for treatment of patients with stable angina and found that ivabradine was as effective as atenolol. It is on this basis that it was approved for use in Europe. Composite data from phase 2 and phase 3 trials suggest that most side effects are dose-related. Ion channels in the retina that generate the Ih current are also affected by ivabradine. This is the mechanism for ivabradine's major side effect, visual luminous phenomena, also known as phosphenes (14.5%). Phosphenes usually resolve with continued treatment and are a rare cause of drug discontinuation. Severe bradycardia is seen in 3.3% of patients. Other less common side effects include palpitations, nausea, headaches, vertigo, muscle cramps, hypereosinophilia, and hyperuricemia. Little trial data exists regarding the treatment of atrial tachyarrhythmias with ivabradine. The mechanism of action suggests that ivabradine may benefit patients with inappropriate sinus tachycardia. In Europe, where the drug is being marketed, it is used off-label in the treatment of inappropriate sinus tachycardia. Further data will be needed as to its effectiveness in treating this condition.

Adenosine A1 Receptor Agonists Adenosine is frequently used for termination of supraventricular tachycardias (SVT). Adenosine terminates SVT in patient with AV nodal or AV reentry by stimulating the A1 adenosine receptor to produce transient AV block. However, adenosine induces atrial fibrillation in up to 15% of patients by decreasing the refractory period of the atrium.In addition, adenosine also stimulates the A2A, A2B, and A3 adenosine receptor subtypes, which contribute to its adverse effect profile. Stimulation of these receptors leads to a variety of systemic side effects, including flushing (18%), dyspnea (12%), and chest pain (7%). Efforts have been made to identify A1 receptor-selective agonists for both the termination of SVT and rate control for atrial fibrillation. Several are under investigation currently, including tecadenoson, selodenoson, and PJ-875. Tecadenoson is the furthest along in the development process. A phase 3 trial has been completed evaluating tecadenoson for the termination of SVT, and preclinical data are promising for rate control of atrial fibrillation. Selodenoson and PJ-875 are both in the early stages of evaluation for treatment of atrial fibrillation.

Preclinical trials indicate that tecadenoson is a potent and selective agonist of the A1 receptor. Studies in animal models showed that it caused significant prolongation of AV nodal conduction and refractoriness without causing hypotension or negative inotropic effects. In addition, those effects were dose-dependent and persistent with chronic administration of the drug. A phase 1 dose-escalation trial in 32 patients showed a dose-dependent prolongation of the AH interval.60 There was no effect on the HV interval. The peak effect on AH interval was at 1 minute, and resolution occurred at 20 minutes. Four patients had significant heart block and 3 patients had atrial fibrillation (2 after atrial pacing). Two patients had neurological effects. There is incomplete published information regarding the pharmacokinetics tecadenoson. It appears to follow a 2-compartment model and has a longer half-life than adenosine (20 to 30 minutes).

In summary, the available data regarding adenosine A1 receptor agonists, particularly tecadenoson, is promising for the conversion of SVT and for short-term rate-control of atrial fibrillation. The rate of conversion for SVT is similar to that of adenosine, but the systemic side effects are milder. In addition, although adenosine A1 receptor stimulation is the presumed mechanism for the induction of atrial fibrillation, tecadenoson appears less likely to cause atrial fibrillation, perhaps because the maximal action potential shortening seen with a bolus of adenosine is not observed with longer-acting agents. Future Targets for Antiarrhythmic Drugs Additional approaches to antiarrhythmic therapy continue to be explored,

It is probable that novel agents directed at these targets will enter clinical trials in the next several years. If these efforts prove successful, drug therapy may reemerge as an equal partner to ablation and device approaches in the treatment of patients with arrhythmias.

Table.18.1 Future Targets for Novel Antiarrhythmic Drugs

- Specific acetylcholine-regulated K+ current inhibition
- Abnormal calcium handling
- Gap junction modification
- Na+/Ca+ exchanger inhibition
- Stretch-induced or ischemia-induced ATP-sensitive K + current inhibitors
- Gene and cellular therapy

11 Treatment of stable ischaemic heart disease: the old and the new

Coronary artery disease (CAD) is one of the main causes of morbidity and mortality in the world.1 Coronary artery disease is a condition characterized by a clinical continuum consisting of stable ischaemic heart disease (SIHD) ranging from asymptomatic patients with subclinical or non-obstructive CAD to those who have obstructive CAD without obvious angina (often referred to as 'silent myocardial ischaemia') with or without previous myocardial infarction (MI), passing through the classical group suffering from chronic stable angina and finally to patients with rapid deterioration or progressive angina that culminate in acute coronary syndrome (ACS). In a nutshell, SIHD can be defined as documentation of ischaemic heart disease in the absence of recent acute events; typically the interval of time free from acute events is considered to be 12 months

The pathophysiology of cardiac ischaemia

The pathophysiology of cardiac ischaemia involves the presence of fibrotic and often calcific atherosclerosis (with a low tendency to rupture) which limits blood flow within a coronary artery causing a discrepancy between the demand and supply of oxygen to the myocardium. This occurs in particular at the increase in heart rate and wall stress of the left ventricle; less frequent alternative mechanisms of ischaemia are plaque spasm and microvascular dysfunction

Chronic angina therapy includes drugs that slow the progression of the disease and reduce cardiovascular events (ASA, statins) and drugs that improve symptoms and therefore the quality of life. With regard to the latter, there is clear scientific evidence of the effectiveness in reducing angina, while the data related to the reduction of 'hard' clinical endpoints (mortality, need for revascularization interventions, and MI) are much less solid. For this reason, the definition of optimal medical therapy in SIHD is not of univocal interpretation and presents substantial differences even among the clinical researches that have studied this pathology. In this work, we will analyse the state of the art in the pharmacological treatment of stable CAD.

Beta-blockers

Beta-adrenergic antagonists, or beta-blockers (BBs), are the most commonly used drugs for the treatment of angina. The BBs exert their anti-angina action by blocking the β1 adrenergic receptor and thereby reducing heart rate, myocardial contractility, left ventricular wall tension, and blood pressure. By reducing the heart rate, the duration of diastole increases, thus improving coronary perfusion.3 The above mechanisms improve the balance between oxygen supply and demand and increase the threshold of appearance of angina .Beta-blockers improve prognosis, in addition to anti-angina symptoms, in patients with a history of MI or left ventricular dysfunction 85. The American and European guidelines for the management of SIHD, published respectively in 2012 and 2013, recognize the importance of this class of drugs and recommend their use on the front line for the treatment of angina, even in patients without history of MI or left ventricular dysfunction. However, in this latter population, there is no clear evidence of a prognostic benefit. Historical randomized studies on BB in stable angina showed no improvement in survival: Pepine et al.9 analysed the issue in the ASIST study, a multicentre, randomized placebo-controlled trial involving patients with asymptomatic or minimally symptomatic ischaemia. Atenolol significantly reduced the primary composite endpoint (death, tachycardia/ventricular fibrillation resuscitation, hospitalization for unstable angina, non-fatal MI, and angina worsening). It should be noted that this result was mainly driven by the reduction in angina frequency, with no difference in mortality. In the TIBET trial, conducted by Dargie et al., subjects with SIHD were randomized to atenolol, nifedipine or a combination of the two drugs. There were no significant differences in mortality or other end points (non-fatal MI,need for surgical revascularization, or coronary angioplasty) among the three treatment regimens. Rehnqvist et al. conducted the APSIS study in which, in patients with SIHD, the effects of metoprolol vs. verapamil were compared regarding mortality: no differences were found in cardiovascular mortality and for all causes.

A meta-analysis performed by Shu et al. on BB in patients with SIHD found no mortality benefit in patients with or without previous MI. Furthermore, an observational analysis from the REACH registry did not document a survival benefit of BB in patients with SIHD and without previous MI.In contrast, BB therapy was associated with adverse effects and a non-significant increase in hospitalization rates.

Again in contrast to previously reported historical data, analyses performed by Bangalore et al.14 using data from the REACH register and CHARISMA (Clopidogrel for High Atherothrombotic Risk and Ischaemic Stabilization, Management, and Avoidance) showed no difference in mortality with BB therapy in patients with previous history of MI. This temporal discrepancy in results with an apparent lack of benefit in more recent studies could be explained by the overall improvements in the treatment of ACS, with aggressive reperfusion, secondary prevention (concomitant use of drugs such as aspirin, enzyme inhibitors of angiotensin conversion and statins), and lifestyle interventions. This accounts for the position of the 2013 European Society of Cardiology (ESC) guidelines that exclude BBs from treatments that improve prognosis in SIHD patients.

Nitrates

Organic nitrates are among the oldest drugs used in the treatment of angina. Nitrates increase the distribution of nitric oxide to vascular smooth muscle, resulting in decreased calcium entry into cells and increased levels of cyclic guanosine monophosphate, thus causing vasodilation. Nitrates mainly cause veno-dilatation, leading to a decrease in preload and a decrease in systolic and diastolic pressure of the left ventricle, thus reducing the stress of the left ventricular wall and myocardial oxygen consumption. Furthermore, nitrates cause coronary vasodilation, leading to redistribution of blood flow to the ischaemic myocardium 91. Like calcium channel blockers (CAs) and BBs, nitrates are quite effective in improving angina symptoms. However, their most noteworthy limitation with frequent use is the development of tachyphylaxis. This limitation has been addressed with the development of pharmaceutical preparations and dosage regimens that allow nitrate-free intervals of 8–10 h every day. There are several nitrate preparations for the treatment of angina. Quick-acting preparations such as sublingual nitrates or sprays are used for immediate relief from angina symptoms. Instead, long-term preparations such as isosorbide mononitrate or isosorbide dinitrate are frequently used for angina prophylaxis. Guidelines recommend the use of long-acting nitrates as second-line agents after BBs or when BBs are contraindicated. Although previous studies have clearly shown the role of nitrates in improving exercise capacity and reducing angina episodes, high-quality studies that examine the impact of nitroglycerine on 'hard' clinical endpoints are lacking. In fact, nitrates are thought to have a minimal impact on long-term prognosis, based on the GISSI-3 and ISIS-4 trials conducted in patients with MI. These studies did not show a mortality benefit from chronic nitrate administration. Currently, nitrates are therefore recommended for the management of the angina crisis and to reduce the frequency of episodes, by virtue of a low cost and the absence of serious side effects. The most frequent adverse reaction is indeed the headache

Calcium channel blockers

Calcium channel blockers (CAs) work by blocking the L-type calcium receptor which leads to decreased calcium influx into the cell. The dihydopyridine CAs, traditionally represented by nifedipine, act mainly on the systemic and coronary vascularization to produce vasodilation with a consequent decrease in afterload. The peripheral effects (vasodilation) of the dihydropyridine group are more evident than the cardiac effects (negative chronotrope and negative dromotrope). In contrast, drugs of the non-dihydropyridine group, which includes diltiazem and verapamil, produce a more pronounced negative inotropic and negative chronotropic effect and less intense systemic vasodilation In terms of anti-angina efficacy, numerous studies over the last few decades have clearly identified calcium channel blockers (dihydropyridines and others) as an effective therapy for reducing angina symptoms. Calcium channel blockers are currently recommended in angina as second-line therapy after BBs, along with nitrates. In particular, CAs remain the therapy of choice for patients with coronary vasospasm or Prinzmetal angina.In the age of statins, the number of high-quality studies examining the role of CA on long-term prognosis is verylow.The randomized ACTION study examined the use of long-acting nifedipine in patients with known CAD by comparing it with placebo.20 The study dispelled concerns about the increased mortality from reflex tachycardia associated with long-term use of dihydropyridine agents. No reduction in mortality with the use of nifedipine was also observed. Importantly, 80% of patients in both arms of the study took BBs and 50% nitrates, which could explain the lack of benefit with nifedipine.

Subsequently, a meta-analysis from Bangalore et al. examining 15 trials (including the ACTION) compared dihydropyridine agents and non-dihydropyridine agents. This meta-analysis also did not show a mortality benefit with chronic CA, while documenting a good safety of this class of drugs.

.Trimetazidine

It increases cellular tolerance to ischaemia by inhibiting the metabolism of fatty acids and secondly, by stimulating glucose metabolism. A meta-analysis of 23 studies showed that trimetazidine is effective in reducing the occurrence of stress-induced ischaemia at electrocardiogram.Trimetazidine is recommended as a second-line agent by European guidelines, while it is not recommended in the USA.

Nicorandil

It exerts its anti-angina effect by vasodilation: the drug stimulates the potassium channels. This drug, like trimetazidine, is recognized by European guidelines.

The newer Drugs

Ranolazine

Ranolazine is a new anti-angina agent belonging to the class of metabolic modulators. The mechanism of action with which it acts in angina is not entirely clear: the hypothesis foresees that ranolazine blocks the delayed sodium current in the ischaemic myocardium, leading to the decrease of intracellular calcium and, finally, to the reduction of oxygen demand. This drug does not affect heart rate or blood pressure The efficacy of ranolazine as anti-angina has been evaluated in multiple randomized clinical trials as monotherapy and in combination with other drugs. The guidelines suggest it if the symptoms are not well-controlled with BB, calcium channel blockers, or nitrates or if hypotension and bradycardia limit the use of these drugs (Class IIa indication of European and American guidelines).

The relatively high cost and the absence of generic formulations have so far limited its adoption in a widespread manner in clinical practice. The propensity of ranolazine to prolong QTc, although without an increase in malignant arrhythmias or arrhythmic deaths, combined with pharmacological interactions contributed to limiting its adoption.Several studies have confirmed the effectiveness of ranolazine in reducing angina symptoms and angina-free exercise time. The MARISA trial (Monotherapy Assessment of Ranolazine in Stable Angina) evaluated the efficacy of ranolazine in patients with stress angina treated with nitrates, calcium antagonists, and BBs. In patients treated, during stress test, there was a significant increase in the duration of the effort and an increase in the time to onset of angina and of the ST-segment subsidence.TheCARISAtrial (Combination Assessment of Ranolazine in Stable Angina) evaluated whether ranolazine was able to improve the total exercise time of patients with symptoms of chronic angina, and manifestation of angina and ischaemia after reduced workloads, despite the assumption of standard dosages of atenolol (50 mg), amlodipine (5 mg), or diltiazem (180 mg). The study, carried out with 12-week follow-up, involved 823 adults with chronic symptomatic angina, who were randomized to receive placebo or two different dosages of ranolazine (750 mg or 1000 mg × 2/day). In patients treated with the two dosages of ranolazine, the duration of exercise increased by 115.6 s from baseline to 91.7 s in patients in the placebo group (P = 0.01). Ranolazine also reduced angina episodes and the use of nitroglycerine. In a post hoc analysis, the group treated with ranolazine 750 and 1000 mg showed a reduction in glycosylated haemoglobin of 0.48% (P = 0.008) and of 0.70% (P = 0.0002), respectively, over placebo. Finally, in the ERICA trial (Efficacy of Ranolazine in Chronic Angina), the efficacy of ranolazine in the chronic treatment of patients with SIHD and at least three angina attacks/ week was evaluated. In the treated group a reduction in the frequency of angina attacks and a reduction in the use of sublingual nitrates was highlighted.However, data on the reduction of mortality with ranolazine have not yet emerged. The MERLIN-TIMI study examined the role of ranolazine in ACS patients. No improvement in the composite endpoint of cardiovascular death, non-fatal MI, or recurrent ischaemia was demonstrated.Wilson et al. performed a subgroup analysis in patients with a history of SIHD and demonstrated a reduction in the primary endpoint (mainly driven by lower recurrent ischaemia) but no change in mortality or MI.

In the recent multicentre randomized trial, the RIVER-PCI, conducted in patients treated by percutaneous coronary intervention (PCI) but incomplete revascularization, ranolazine did not benefit in reducing the risk of the combined endpoint of revascularization for ischaemia or admission for angina

Ivabradine

Ivabradine is the only drug belonging to the class of sinus node inhibitors that has been approved for clinical use. It acts through the inhibition of the late Na current (also known as If), which controls the spontaneous diastolic depolarization of the sinus node cells. The BEAUTIFUL trial evaluated the efficacy of ivabradine in reducing cardiovascular mortality and morbidity in patients with CAD and left ventricular systolic dysfunction. Between 2004 and 2006, 10 917 patients with CAD and left ventricular ejection fraction <40% were enrolled. Ivabradine had no effect on the primary composite endpoint [hazard ratio (HR) 1.0; P = 0.94].31 However, in the subgroup of patients with resting heart rate >70 b.p.m., ivabradine significantly reduced the incidence of secondary endpoints of admission for fatal and non-fatal AMI [HR 0.64; 95% confidence interval (CI) 0.49–0.84; P = 0.001] and coronary revascularization (HR 0.7; 95% CI 0.52–0.93; P = 0.016). The most important results were obtained in the subgroup of patients presenting with limiting stress angina (13.8% of patients enrolled in the study). In this group, ivabradine significantly reduced (−24%) the primary endpoint of cardiovascular death, hospitalizations for fatal and non-fatal MI or heart failure (HR 0.76; 95% CI 0.58–1.00; P = 0.05) and 42% hospitalizations for AMI (HR 0.58; 95% CI 0.37–0.92; P = 0.05).These positive data have not been confirmed by the recent randomized SIGNIFY study (Study Assessing the Morbidity-Mortality Benefits of the If Inhibitor in Patients with Coronary Artery Disease), conducted in patients with stable CAD and resting HR

>70 b.p.m. in the absence of left ventricular dysfunction (FE > 40%). This trial enrolled 19 102 patients and the primary endpoint was a composite of death from cardiovascular causes and MI. Ivabradine did not reduce the primary endpoint during a median follow-up of 27.8 months. The drug led to a significant improvement in angina in CCS > II patients, at the price of an increased incidence of the primary endpoint in this subgroup.32 Ivabradine is not approved in the USA foranginatreatment.

Non-anti-anginadrugs

In addition to symptom control therapies, prognosis-improving drugs such as antithrombotics and statins play a central role in SIHD. Indeed, the SIHD population presents a high risk of cardiovascular events, particularly if a previous MI or a revascularization for ACS is present in the history.

Antiplatelettherapy

It is a cornerstone in patients with CAD and is historically represented by aspirin.34 Recently, the opportunity of a dual antiplatelet therapy in patients with post-infarct SIHD was evaluated in the PEGASUS trial: in selected (low haemorrhagic risk) patients the addition of ticagrelor 60 mg b.i.d. at 1–3 years after the acute event, it has allowed to save in 10 000 patients 42 cardiovascular events/year at the price of 31 TIMI majorhaemorrhages/year

In the COMPASS study, three antithrombotic regimens were compared in coronary heart disease patients (previous MI, angina, previous percutaneous, or surgical coronary revascularization): rivaroxaban 2.5 mg b.i.d. plus ASA, rivaroxoban 5 mg bid, ASA alone: a significant reduction in the combined primary endpoint (cardiovascular death, MI, and stroke) was observed in the ASA + rivaroxaban group: 347 (4%) out of 8313 vs. 460 (6%) out 8261 (HR 0.74, 95% CI 0.65–0.86, $P < 0.0001$)36; at the same time, an increase in bleeding was observed with this latter treatment compared to ASA alone, however with a clear clinical benefit in favour of dual therapy and a reduction in mortality. The reduction of systemic inflammation using an antiinterleukin 1β monoclonal antibody has been shown to significantly reduce events; canakinumab was tested vs. placebo in the CANTOS trial in post-MI patients and with C-reactive protein >2 mg/dL and led to a reduction in MACE: HR 0.85 (0.76–0.96) in a 5-year follow-up. Among the other pharmacological and non-pharmacological interventions capable of modifying the prognosis, the inhibitors of the renin–angiotensin system, the control of diabetes, the cessation of smoking, the control of weight, and the reduction of cholesterol by statins are to be mentioned. With regard to the latter aspect, the recent Fourier study showed an important reduction in cardiovascular events in patients with a history of previous MI, previous stroke, or peripheral arterial disease using Evolocumab, a PCSK9 inhibitor; the drug was compared with placebo in patients already on high-dose statin treatment, thus demonstrating the benefit of achieving particularly low LDL cholesterol.

Hyper-uricaemia

It has been associated with a worse prognosis in patients with heart failure; some evidence seems to suggest a negative impact also in ischaemic heart disease, through a mechanism of increased oxidative stress and consequent endothelial dysfunction; to support this, some studies have shown that allopurinol can reduce angina symptoms and increase blood supply to the heart muscle.

Therapeutic angiogenesis using vascular endothelial growth factors, although promising, is still premature for a clinical setting.40 Important studies on the use of stem cells are underway, however, it is not yet clear which cells are most suitable for the treatment of patients with angina, as well as the best method of administration. Attention is currently focusing on autologous CD34 + cells, which appear to be quite promising

Conclusions

The medical treatment of chronic ischaemic heart disease is often underutilized, despite the good efficacy, and solid scientific proof, in reducing symptoms. However, the lack of clarity of the guidelines, combined with the difficulty in managing association therapies, still lead a large part of patients with SHID to undergo PCI before having optimized anti-angina therapy. The most recently introduced drugs, ranolazine and ivabradine, have not been shown to modify the patients' prognosis and their adoption in clinical practice has been anything but disruptive, however, they are an important resource in hypotensive and bradycardic patients. Future scenarios will probably see the arrival of cellular therapies and the use of angiogenic factors that will change the scenario in patients suffering from refractory angina and not candidate for revascularization. However, the road to their concrete adoption is still very long. Undoubtedly, a central role in the prognosis of patients with SIHD can be played by measures that slow the progression of atherosclerotic disease and reduce the risk of acute ischaemic events.

111.New drug targets for hypertension

Hypertension is a major contributing factor for cardiovascular disease (CVD) and renal diseases, that can increase the risks of comorbidities such as myocardial infarction, stroke and heart failure (HFStudies have revealed that risk factors such as obesity and genetic factors can influence the occurrence and development of hypertension In addition, complicated regulatory networks, including the renin-angiotensin-aldosterone system (RAAS), the nervous system and arterial remodeling also affect the progression of hypertension. Because blood pressure (BP) is difficult to control, the priority is finding drug targets to effectively control and manage BP in the hypertensive population. Below is the description of the classical and new drug targets used in hypertension therapy

Classical targets in hypertension

Renin-angiotensin-aldosterone system (RAAS) plays an important role in human body. The imbalance of RAAS could result in the occurrence of the hypertension directly. Briefly, Renin (or angiotensinogenase) secreted by kidney catalyzes its substrate angiotensin which is the other component in RAAS system synthesized by liver, contributing to form angiotensin II accompanying with the effect of the angiotensin-converting enzyme (ACE). Meanwhile, aldosterone secreted by adrenal gland could maintain sodium potassium homeostasis by increasing sodium reabsorption with mineralocorticoid receptor (MR). Hence, the component of RAAS system can serve as therapeutic targets to regulate blood pressure and many pharmacological antihypertensive drugs Classical antihypertensive drugs include renin inhibitor, ACE inhibitors, angiotensin II receptor blockers (blocking the activity of Ang1–7/Mas and Ang II-Ang type 1 receptor (AT1R)/Ang type 2 receptor (AT2R)), β-adrenoreceptor blockers (blocking the secretion of renin), aldosterone-related blocker (blocking the activity of the synthesis of aldosterone and receptor).

AngII-AT1R/AT2R axis

Ang II mainly works by activating AT1Rs and AT2Rs. AT1Rs mediate vascular smooth muscle contraction, aldosterone secretion, dipsogenic responses, renal sodium reabsorption and pressor and tachycardiac responses . Conversely, AT2Rs generally induce the opposite effects, including vasodilation, natriuresis, cellular differentiation and growth inhibition [24]. Therefore, AT2R agonists could serve as a potential therapeutic drug for the treatment of hypertension. Compound 21 (C-21) is a highly selective nonpeptide AT2R agonist which is the first reported AT2R agonist.C-21-induced AT2R activation evoked a bradykinin-nitric oxide (NO)-cyclic guanosine 3,5-monophosphate (cGMP) signaling cascade that stimulated the downstream signaling mediators Src kinase and extracellular signal-related kinase, leading to the internalization/inactivation of the major renal proximal tubule (RPT) Na+ transporters Na +/H+ exchanger 3 (NHE3) and Na+/K+ ATPase (NKA) and resulting in natriuresis. Prior studies found that Ang II can increase sodium retention and BP in rats, however, the injection of C-21 prevented Ang II-mediated sodium retention and BP elevation. The activation of chronic AT2R initiates and sustains receptor translocation to RPT apical plasma membranes. It also promotes the internalization/ inactivation of NHE3 and NKA and prevents Na+ retention, which results in a negative cumulative Na+ balance and lowers BP in models of experimental Ang II-induced hypertension. The results indicated that C-21 is a potential drug candidate for the treatment of hypertension and Na+ retaining states in humans. In addition, in the clipped kidneys of two-kidney, one-clip hypertensive rats model, C-21 significantly reduced TNF-α, IL-6 and TGF-β1 levels and increased nitric oxide (NO) and cGMP levels in the kidneys . These results suggest that AT2R is a new target for the treatment of hypertension and AT2R agonists may act as novel anti-hypertensive drugs in the future

ACE2/Ang1–7/Mas receptor axis

In addition to the classic ACE-Ang II-ATR1 axis, the RAAS system also features the ACE2/Ang1–7/Mas axis. In contrast to the ACE-Ang II-ATR1 axis, the ACE2/Ang1–7/Mas axis inhibits ventricular remodeling and lowers BP by inducing systemic and regional vasodilation, promoting diuresis and natriuresis and inhibiting the proliferation and migration of smooth muscle cells, cardiomyocytes, fibroblasts and glomerular and adjacent tubular cells]. ACE2 is similar to ACE structurally. It can generate Ang1–9 by cleaving Ang I and Ang1–7 can be generated from Ang1–9 through the action of ACE. It can also directly cleave Ang II into Ang1–7 [69]. Ang1–7 participates in vasodilation, natriuresis and BP reduction by binding to the MAS receptor. Therefore, drugs targeting ACE2 or MAS may be useful in the treatment of hypertension. AVE 0991, a MAS receptor agonist , can reduce mean arterial BP (MABP) in rats with hypertension induced by deoxycorticosterone acetate (DOCA). When combined with renin inhibitors, the anti-hypertensive effect is stronger [70]. Moreover, AVE 0991 can reduce BP and cardiac inflammatory cell infiltration and collagen fiber deposition in renovascular hypertensive rats and it plays a role in reducing BP-induced cardiac remodeling and improving baroreflex sensitivity .A study involving 161 patients with essential hypertension and 47 age- and sex-matched normotensive healthy subjects revealed that plasma ACE2 levels were significantly elevated in patients with hypertension, compared with healthy individuals. Additionally, the concentration of ACE2 in serum was positively correlated with left atrial diameter, left ventricular end-diastolic diameter and left ventricular mass in patients with hypertension. In addition, a prospective controlled study found that the expression of ACE2 was increased in patients with acute ST-elevation myocardial infarction and ACE2 activity in plasma was closely related to the infarct area, left ventricular systolic dysfunction and the occurrence of left ventricular remodeling These results suggest that ACE2 may participate in the development of hypertension and cardiovascular disease. Human and murine recombinant ACE2 are pharmacological tools for strenthening the activity of ACE2. A study illustrated that compared with the results in the control group, mice with Ang II-induced hypertension that were injected with murine recombinant ACE2 exhibited lower BP pressure [74]. Previous research indicated that in mice infused with Ang II (1.5 mg/kg/day) for 4 days, Ang II levels and nicotinamide adenine dinucleotide phosphate oxidase activity were higher in ACE2-knockout mice than in wild-type mice. Meanwhile, pro-inflammatory cytokine and fibrosis-associated gene levels were also higher in ACE2-knockout mice than in wild-type mice. Then, the mice were treated with recombinant human ACE2 (2 mg/kg/day, intraperitoneal), and the results confirmed that recombinant human ACE2 prevents Ang II-induced hypertension, renal oxidative stress and tubulointerstitial fibrosis . These results suggest that BP can be reduced by enhancing ACE2 activity.In prior studies, the ACE2 activator XNT (1-[(2-dimethylamino)ethylamino]-4-(hydroxymethyl)-7-[(4- methylphenyl)sulfonyloxy]-9H-xanthene-9-one) was found to lower BP in SHRs and Wistar-Kyoto (WKY) rats, as well as improving the heart function of SHRs and reverse myocardial, peripheral vascular and renal fibrosis . In addition, XNT reduced BP in Ang II-induced hypertensive, wild-type and ACE2-knockout mice . All of these studies indicate that the development of drugs targeting the ACE2/Ang1–7/Mas receptor axis will be of great significance for the treatment of hypertension and the reduction of heart and kidney fibrosis.

ACE2inCOVID-19

Recently, it is a widespread idea that ACE2, an important component in RAAS system is the cell membrane receptor of SARS-Cov-2, the causative virus of the COVID-19 pandemic, which emerged from Wuhan, China in 2019 [28]. The entry of SARS-CoV-2 into host cell is mediated by a spike protein which is a special region in SARS-Cov-2. The binding of spike protein with ACE2 and its “accomplice” protein TMPRSS2 leads SARS-Cov-2 to host cell, increasing the secretion of inflammatory cytokine and causing the consequent inflammation storm in lung. Recent studies showed that SARS-CoV-2 can directly infect engineered human blood vessel organoids and human kidney organoids, which can be inhibited by human recombinant soluble ACE2 (hrsACE2). Moreover, research showed that circulating Ang II levels were markedly elevated compared with healthy control [28], and overexpression of the Fc domain of spike protein elevated ANG II levels which indicated that imbalance of ACE2 and ANG II existed in the RAAS.Based on that, many classical antihypertensive drugs including angiotensin-converting enzyme inhibitors (ACEIs) and angiotensin II receptor blockers (ARBs) were applied to treat the COVID-19 patients due to the ability of blocking ACE2 and down-regulating the ANG II. Among the COVID-19 patients with severe symptoms, most of them have pre-existing comorbidity such as hypertension and so on. In one study, among the patients with severe symptoms of COVID-19, 58% of them had hypertension, 25% of them had heart disease and 44% of them had arrhythmia. Hence, it is useful and necessary to treat the patients with antihypertensive agents. A retrospective, single-center study showed that ARBs/ACEIs group had significantly lower concentrations of Hs-CRP and procalcitonin compared with non- ARBs/ACEIs group, and a lower proportion of critical patients and a lower death rate were observed in ARBs/ACEIs group than non-ARBs/ ACEIs group, whereas it failed to reach statistical significance [34]. These results revealed that ACE2 played an important role in the development and treatment of COVID-19 besides hypertension

.

Aldosterone

The aldosterone synthetase CYP11B2 can catalyze the synthesis of aldosterone . CYP11B2 is a key enzyme involved in the final stages of the biosynthesis of aldosterone. Therefore, inhibition of the expression of CYP11B2 is a potential treatment strategy for diseases such as hypertension, congestive HF and myocardial fibrosis . Ménard et al. revealed that the aldosterone synthase inhibitor FAD286A dose-dependently reduced the urine aldosterone concentration in spontaneously hypertensive rats (SHRs) and increased plasma renin concentrations. Furthermore, this drug reversed hypokalemia induced by treatment with the diuretic furosemide. In addition, in uninephrectomized rats treated with Ang II and high-salt diet, FAD286 reduced BP and plasma aldosterone levels. The compound also decreased hypertrophy and interstitial fibrosis of the kidneys and heart and exerted protective effects against end-organ damage LCI699 was the first aldosterone synthase inhibitor to be used orally in humans . Studies revealed that in transgenic rats harboring the renin and angiotensinogen genes, LCI699 reduced the aldosterone levels in plasma and urine in a dose-dependent manner. LCI699 also reduced heart and kidney dysfunction and prolonged the lifespan of rats. In addition, a randomized double-blind experiment involving 99 healthy subjects revealed that compared with the control group, the levels of aldosterone in plasma and urine were decreased by 49 ± 3 and 39 ± 6% respectively in the 0.5 mg LCI699 group together with increased urinary sodium excretion and plasma renin activity .These results suggest that the inhibition of aldosterone synthase is an effective strategy for treating diseases associated with excess aldosterone. The CLCI699A2201 study designed to investigate the role of LCI699 in patients with essential hypertension indicated that compared with the placebo group, all doses of LCI699 (0.25 mg once daily, 0.5 mg once daily, 1.0 mg once daily and 0.5 mg twice daily) reduced systolic BP (SBP) in the clinic. In addition, a study of 14 patients with increased primary aldosterone revealed that subjects taking LCI699 had lower plasma aldosterone concentrations and higher 11-deoxycorticosterone and potassium ion concentrations. Most importantly, LCI699 reduced 24-h dynamic SBP by 4.1 mmHg [43]. These results suggest that aldosterone synthase inhibitors can be used to treat hypertension. Because aldosterone synthase (CYP11B2) and cortisol synthase (CYP11B1) have high homology, aldosterone synthase can affect the synthesis of cortisol. In the aforementioned CLCI699A2201 study, LCI699 suppressed adrenocorticotropic hormone-induced cortisol secretion in approximately 20% of the subjects. Amar et al. also revealed that plasma cortisol response to corticotropin was reduced in patients with increased primary aldosterone who took LCI699. These results suggest that LCI699 could inhibit cortisol synthesis in addition to inhibiting aldosterone synthesis . Therefore, it is necessary to explore the maximum tolerated dose (MTD) of LCI699 that does not seriously affect cortisol synthesis. One study,explored the MTD of LCI699 in patients with hypertension, indicated that LCI699 can lower BP and increase plasma aldosterone levels in line with previous results. Furthermore, the MTD was obtained using a threshold of an ACTH-stimulated cortisol response of <400 nmol/L in no more than 20% of patients and no clinical symptoms of adrenal insufficiency. It was estimated that the MTD was 1.30 mg once daily with a 90% confidence interval (CI) of 0.88–181 mg once daily. Because the selectivity of LCI699 is not strong, researchers have recently applied a ligand-based approach to synthesize a series of novel pyridyl- or isoquinolinyl-substituted indolines and indoles. Compared with LCI699, these compounds are more selective for CYP11B2 than for CYP11B1 . The novel aldosterone synthase inhibitor BI 689648 [6-(5-methoxymethyl-pyridin-3-yl)-3,4-dihydro-2H-[1,8]naphthyridine-1-carboxylic acid amide] was recently discovered. Results revealed that compared with FAD286 and LCI699, BI 689648 has higher selectivity for aldosterone synthase than cortisol synthetase in vitro. Similarly, BI 689648 was found to be more selective than FAD286 and LCI699 in rhesus monkeys [46]. Whether these new aldosterone synthase inhibitors can selectively inhibit aldosterone synthesis also requires animal experiments and clinical trials.

Aldosterone receptor (AR)

Aldosterone is a mineralocorticoid secreted by the globular zone of the adrenal cortex that can promote the reabsorption of sodium and chloride ions and increase the excretion of potassium and hydrogen ions in the renal tubules. Aldosterone exerts its effects by binding with the mineralocorticoid receptor (MR). MR activation in the kidneys promotes the development of hypertension by increasing the expression of potassium channels, thereby promoting the reabsorption of water and sodium and causing the loss of potassium in tissues. In addition, the activation of MR in extrarenal tissues such as the heart and blood vessels increases NADPH oxidase levels and the production of reactive oxygen species and promotes the development of hypertension and CVD. Mineralocorticoid receptor antagonists (MRAs) antagonize the action of aldosterone on MR [10]. The two types of MRAs are classic steroids and new nonsteroidal compounds. Steroidal compounds such as spironolactone and eplerenone inhibit the effects of aldosterone by competitively binding its ligand-binding domain on MR and preventing MR from forming its active structure. Spironolactone was the first reported MRA . Studies have revealed that in patients with resistant hypertension with and without primary aldosteronism, the combination of low-dose spironolactone, an angiotensin (Ang)-converting enzyme (ACE) inhibitor or Ang receptor blocker, and diuretics can reduce BP in patients with resistant hypertension. Chapman et al. also reported similar results. Their study found that spironolactone can effectively lower BP in patients with uncontrolled hypertension. In addition, , Pitt et al. demonstrated that the combination of spironolactone with standard therapy can substantially reduce the risks of morbidity and death in patients with severe HF. The aforementioned results illustrated that spironolactone played an important role in the prevention and treatment of resistant hypertension. However, spironolactone non-selectively binds to MR,and it can also antagonize the androgen receptor, thereby causing a variety of sexual adverse events inboth men and women . Subsequently, eplerenone, a more selective MRA, was developed. This drug appears to have weaker anti-androgenic effects than spironolactone Finerenone is an analog ofdihydronaphthyridine compound. Dihydropyridines have anti-MRA activity and function as Ca2+ channel blockers. Previous studies found that finerenone has stronger cardiorenal protective effects than eplerenone inhypertension-inducedHFrats.

Meanwhile,hypertension-induced cardiac hypertrophy mouse, finerenone exerted a stronger inhibitory effect on myocardial hypertrophy than eplerenone. Dihydropyridine calcium channel blockers can function as MRAs and inhibit aldosterone-induced MR activation . The drug was proven to be a potent and highly selective nonsteroidal MRAA mineralocorticoid receptor antagonist tolerance study (ARTS) was designed to assess the safety and tolerability of finerenone in patients with HF and reduced left ventricular ejection fraction associated with mild or moderate chronic kidney disease (CKD). The study illustrated that finerenone has the same effect with spironolactone in reducing ventricular remodeling. In addition, finerenone can reduce the occurrence of hyperkalemia and renal impairment . Currently, two Phase IIB clinical studies of finerenone are ongoing. Two studies aimed to assess the effect of drug in patients with worsening chronic HF and type 2 diabetes mellitus and CKD (ARTS-HF; The aforementioned results demonstrated that anti-hypertensive drugs targeting AR have good clinical effects, but these drugs are limited by shortcomings such as drug resistance and side effects. It is necessary to develop new anti-hypertensive drugs targeting AR

New targets in hypertension

Aminopeptidase of the brain renin-Ang system (RAS) In recent years, studies have uncovered that excessive activation of the brain RAS plays an important role in the occurrence and maintenance of hypertension in various experimental and genetic hypertension animal . The activation of RAS in the brain can improve sympathetic tone and consequently increase vascular resistance and the release of arginine vasopressin which lead to elevated BP level . The main biologically active substances are Ang II and Ang III. Aminopeptidase A (APA) is a membrane-bound zinc metalloprotease. It is responsible for the N-terminal cleavage of Ang II and it can convert Ang II to Ang III . One study, demonstrated that Ang III generated by APA is one of the main effector peptides of the brain RAS, exerting tonic stimulatory control over BP in conscious hypertensive rats. Therefore, APA can be considered a candidate target for hypertension treatment. EC33 [(S)-3-amino-4-mercaptobutyl sulfonic acid] [84] is a specific APA inhibitor. RB150 [4,40-dithio[bis(3-aminobutyl sulfonic acid)] is a systemically active prodrug of EC33. RB150 inhibited the biological effects of APA. Yannick et al. [86] revealed that compared with the effects of oral saline, administration of RB150 orally (100 mg/kg) in SHRs significantly inhibited brain APA activity by 31%. RB150 treatment reduced the increase in APA activity in SHRs by 58% compared with normotensive WKY rats. Additionally, oral RB150 (15–150mg/kg) dose-dependently decreased MABP in conscious SHRs, and the ED50 was 30.5 mg/kg. The maximal decrease in MABP (37.2 ± 8.0 mmHg) was observed at a dose of 150 mg/kg. The hypotensive effect peaked at 5–7 h after administration. In addition, concomitant oral administration of RB150 (100 mg/kg) with the systemic RAS blocker enalapril (1 mg/kg) significantly reduced BP in conscious SHRs within 2 h, and the maximum decrease in MABP was observed 6 h after administration. These results suggest that RB150 may be the prototype of a new class of centrally active anti-hypertensive agents, and it can be used in combination with classic systemic RAS blockers to improve BP control. Subsequently, phase I clinical trials were conducted to evaluate the safety, pharmacokinetics and pharmacodynamic effects of RB150 in humans. The study included 56 healthy male volunteers, and the results demonstrated that RB150 was well tolerated and safe among healthy volunteers. Azizi et al. conducted a pilot multicenter, double-blind, randomized,placebo-controlled, crossover pharmaco dynamic study to evaluate the effects of RB150 on BP and hormones in patients with hypertension in phase II clinical trial. The study included 34 hypertensive patients who were randomly assigned to receive either RB150 and then placebo for 4 weeks each or vice versa after a 2-week run-in period. After 4 weeks, daytime ambulatory SBP had decreased by 2.7 mmHg and office SBP was decreased by 4.7 mmHg in the RB150 group versus placebo group. These results suggested that RB150 can reduce daytime SBP in patients with hypertension without significant effects on systemic RAS activity. In another multicenter, open-label, phase II study, 256 overweight or obese hypertensive patients were recruited, and 54% of the participants were of Black or Hispanic. After 8 weeks of oral administration, RB150 lowered systolic automated office BP (AOBP) by 9.5 mmHg and diastolic AOBP by 4.2 mmHg. Meanwhile, the BP-lowering effects differed among the races. Systolic AOBP was decreased by 10.5 mmHg in Black participants, versus 8.9 mmHg in other participants . The results of this study confirmed that RB150 has a hypotensive effect in the diverse high-risk population. Vasoactive intestinal peptide (VIP) receptor VIP is a neuropeptide that exerts positive inotropic, chronotropic and vasodilatory effects by activating the G protein-coupled receptors VPAC1 and VPA 2 [90]. VIP is associated with several CVDs and cardiopulmonary diseases, making it a key treatment target for both systemic and pulmonary hypertension as well as HF. Vasomera (PB1046) was developed by fusing an analog of VIP with an elastin-like polypeptide. This drug exerts its effects through selectively binding VPAC2, thereby avoiding the gastrointestinal side effects associated with VPAC1 activation. In addition, PB1046 has a longer half-life than native VIP. At present, two phase I randomized, double-blind, placebo-controlled studies evaluating the safety, tolerability, pharmacokinetics and pharmacodynamics of PB1046 in patients with essential hypertension have been completed (NCT 01873885, NCT 01523067), but the results have not beenpublished..

IntestinalNHE3

The imbalance of sodium intake and excretion plays an important role in the pathogenesis of hypertension and its complications, such as HF and CKD. NHE3 expressed on enterocytes throughout the intestinal lumen plays a dominant role in intestinal sodium absorption

Therefore, inhibition of NHE3 has been considered a potential strategy for controlling hypertension and its complications. Studies indicated that oral administration of the NHE3 inhibitor tenapanor reduced the uptake of sodium in rats. In salt-fed nephrectomized rats with induced hypervolemia combined with cardiac hypertrophy and arterial stiffening, tenapanor reduced the extracellular fluid volume, left ventricular hypertrophy, albuminuria and BP. In addition, compared with enalapril alone, combined treatment with tenapanor improved cardiac diastolic dysfunction and arterial pulse wave velocity .

SAR21803(SAR)

It is an orally nonabsorbable specific NHE3 inhibitor. Linz et al. reported that in senescent lean hypertensive rats developed by feeding lean SHRs drinking water containing 0.7% NaCl, SAR (1 mg/kg per day in chow) increased fecal sodium excretion and reduced urine sodium excretion. At the same time, the drug increased feces water content and reduced SBP. In addition, the hypotensive effect of SAR can be significantly enhanced when combined with the ACE inhibitor ramipril. In hypertensive, obese and hyperinsulinemic rats (obese SHRs, not loaded with NaCl), SAR exerted a similar anti-hypertensive effect. In addition to its anti-hypertensive effect, Labonté et al. demonstrated that tenapanor can protect against vascular calcification in CKD rats by decreasing serum creatinine and phosphorus levels

Endothelinreceptor(ETR)

Endothelin-1 (ET-1) is an endothelium-derived contractile factor released by vascular endothelial cells. To date, it is the most potent vasoconstrictor and an important factor for maintaining vascular tension.ET-1 can bind with its specific receptors ETRs including ETAR and ETBR which are G-protein coupled receptors. The binding of ET-1 to ETAR can promote vasoconstriction, cell proliferation, tissue fibrosis and vascular endothelial injury, which are involved in the pathogenesis of hypertension . The binding of ET-1 to ETBR can activate endothelial cells to produce NO, thereby relaxing vascular smooth muscle and inhibiting vasoconstriction and cell proliferation.Therefore, inhibition of ETAR may be a strategy for the treatment of hypertension.At present, a variety of ETR antagonists (ETRAs) have been developed, and they can be divided into three categories according to their function: selective ETAR antagonists such as darusentan and ambrisentan; nonselective ETRAs such as bosentan and macitentan; and selective ETBR antagonists . The first anti-hypertensive ETRA used in clinical trial was bosentan. Studies have illustrated that bosentan at 0.5 or 2.0 g/day in patients with essential hypertension significantly decreased BP after 4 weeks, and its anti-hypertensive effect was comparable to that of enalapril.

Darusentan is a selective ETAR antagonist. A multicenter, randomized, double-blind, parallel-group, dose-response study found that darusentan dose-dependently reduced BP in patients with essential hypertension.Macitentan is a novel dual ETAR/ETBR antagonist. Another study found that in Dahl salt-sensitive hypertensive and pulmonary hypertensive bleomycin-treated rats, macitentan more strongly reduced mean arterial pressure and mean pulmonary artery pressure than bosentan.In addition, in a randomized, double-blind study involving 27 patients with hypertension and CKD, the ETRA sitaxentan restored a normal circadian rhythm of BP . A meta-analysis of 18 studies including 4898 patients evaluating the effectiveness and safety of ETRAs in this population concluded that ETRAs significantly reduced 24-h ambulatory and sitting BP. At the office, the mean decreases in systolic and diastolic BP (DBP) were 6.12 and 3.81 mmHg, respectively, and 24-h ambulatory SBP and DPB were reduced by 7.65 and 5.92 mmHg, respectively . These results illustrated that ETRAs have beneficial effects on elevated BP. Aprocitentan is a dual ETAR/ETBR antagonist. Recently, a randomized, double-blind, parallel study was conducted in patients with essential hypertension to evaluate the anti-hypertensive effect of aprocitentan. The study included 490 patients who were administered 5, 10, 25, or 50 mg of aprocitentan, placebo or 20 mg of lisinopril as a positive control once daily for 8 weeks.The results indicated that aprocitentan at doses of 10, 25 and 50 mg lowered placebo-corrected SBP/DBP in the clinic by 7.05/4.93, 9.90/6.99 and

7.58/4.95 mmHg, respectively.In addition, placebo-corrected 24-h SBP was reduced by 3.99, 4.83 and 3.67 mmHg, respectively, by these doses, whereas 24-h DBP was reduced by 4.04, 5.89 and 4.45 mmHg, respectively. Compared with lisinopril group, the *aprocitentan* 25 mg group exhibited reductions of SBP and DBP of 4.84 and 3.81 mmHg, respectively. Conversely, there was no significant difference in the incidence of side effects between the aprocitentan and placebo groups.At present, research on aprocitentan in combination with other drugs in the treatment of resistant hypertension.

The results of these studies suggest that targeting ETRs may have therapeutic effects for the treatment of hypertension. Drugs targeting the NO pathway NO is a vasodilation factor that plays an important role in BP regulation. NO is synthesized from L-arginine by at least three different forms of NO synthase (NOS): neuronal NO synthase, endothelial NO synthase and inducible NOS. Asymmetric and symmetric dimethylarginine (ADMA and SDMA, respectively) are endogenous NOS inhibitors that can inhibit the production of NO . Moreover, a recent study showed that another NO synthase inhibitor NG-nitro-L-arginine methyl ester hydrochloride (L-NAME) could induce hypertension and elicit macrophage infiltration and inflammation. The detrimental effect L-NAME-induced was reversed by metallothionein, a heavy metal-binding scavenger which indicated that NO synthase has served as a novel target .The vascular endothelium is stimulated by shear force and other factors to induce the production and release of NO into surrounding tissues and cells, thereby reducing BP by inhibiting the vascular tone and the proliferation of smooth muscle cells. These results suggest that increasing NO levels in the body may reduce BP. Therefore, NOS substrates and drugs that reduce ADMA and ADMA levels and NO donors may be useful for reducing BP. Sphingosine-1-phosphate, the bioactive lipid mediator is a potent activator of endothelial nitric oxide synthase through G protein-coupled receptors.The autocrine/paracrine activation of Sphingosine-1-phosphate receptors (SIPR) plays an important role in the regulation of BP level. Recent studies showed that S1PR1signaling is a keypathway in BP homeostasis, genetically ablation of BP increases BP level in both physiological and pathological conditions. Moreover, an FDA-approved drug FTY702 which acts as antagonist of S1PR1 could increase BP and exacerbate hypertension in ANG II mouse model, indicating that S1PR1 may serve as a novel therapeutic target for the treatment of hypertension. One study found that the oral administration of NOS substrates such as L-arginine or its precursor L-citrulline can lower BP in hypertensive rats. In hypertensive uremic rats, oral administration of 0.1% L-arginine lowered BP by increasing plasma NO2/NO3 levels and decreasing ET-1 levels in the aorta and kidneys. Additionally, L-arginine can alleviate kidney injury. Treatment with 0.25% L-citrulline for 8 weeks significantly reduced BP in SHRs.Additionally,L-citrullinetreatment dramatically altered L-arginine and ADMA levels in the kidneys of rats, thereby increasing the L-arginine/ADMA ratio. This result illustrated that NO bioavailability was restored and oxidative stress was reduced in SHR kidneys. In addition, similar results were reported in clinical trials .A clinical trial found that the administration of 12 g of L-arginine daily for 4 weeks significantly reduced both SBP and DBP in patients with hypertension. These results indicated that NOS substrates have protective effects on the kidneys in addition to the anti-hypertensive effects.Drugs that reduce ADMA and SDMA levels such as resveratrol, melatonin, and N-acetylcysteine (NAC) can also play an important role in regulating BP. Hsu et al. reported that in dexamethasone (DEX)-or2,3,7,8-tetrachlorodibenzo-p-dioxin-exposed female rats, the administration of resveratrol reduced BP by decreasing ADMA and SDMA levels and increasing NO levels in plasma in offspring rats. In maternal rats with hypertension induced by fructose diet combined with high-salt diet feeding, oral melatonin reduced plasma AMDA and SDMA levels and protected adult offspring against programmed hypertension.

In offspring rats exposed prenatally to DEX and fed a high-fat diet postnatally, NAC administration reduced the levels of ADMA and restored the L-arginine/ADMA ratio in plasma, thereby preventing programmed hypertension . In addition, studies indicated that NO donors such as sodium nitrate and pentaerythritol tetranitrate can also lower BP. In SHRS, plasma L-arginine and ADMA levels were decreased by treatment with 1 mmol/kg/day sodium nitrate and BP pressure was also significantly decreased. Meanwhile, maternal pentaerythritol tetranitrate treatment led to a persistent BP reduction in female offspring .In the future, more drugs associated with the NO pathway could be developed to reduce hypertension.

Vaccines

In the long history of immunotherapy, vaccines targeting the RAS for the treatment of hypertension have been reported since the 1950s .Ang I and Ang II vaccines, as well as those targeting Ang receptors, can successfully lower BP in rat and mouse. An Ang I vaccine consisting of an AI analog conjugated with a tetanus toxoid carrier protein and adjuvanted with aluminum hydroxide reduced BP in Sprague-Dawley rats .An Ang II-derived peptide was conjugated to the virus-like particle (VLP) Qb (AngQb). In SHR immunized with 400 mg of AngQb, the average SBP was reduced by up to 21 mmHg compared with the findings in rats administered Qb alone, and total Ang II levels (antibody-bound and free) were increased by 9-fold compared with those in the VLP controls. Then a placebo-controlled, randomized phase I trial of 12 healthy volunteers was conducted. The results indicated that Ang II-specific antibody levels were elevated in all participants, giving a 100% responder rate, and AngQb was well tolerated. The ATRQβ-001 vaccine is another peptide (ATR-001) derived from human AT1R conjugated with Qβ bacteriophage VLPs. ATRQβ-001 lowered BP by up to 35 mmHg in mice with Ang II-induced hypertension (143 ± 4 mmHg versus 178 ± 6 mmHg; P = 0.005) and by up to 19 mmHg in SHRs (173 ± 2 mmHg versus 192 ± 3 mmHg; P = 0.003), and the vaccine protected against end-organ damage caused by hypertension In addition, other studies demonstrated that in streptozotocin-induced diabetic nephropathy rats, in addition to lowering BP, ATRQβ-001 ameliorated streptozotocin-induced diabetic renal injury [104]. Some clinical trials of vaccines have also been conducted. The Ang I vaccine PMD3117 significantly increased the titers of anti-Ang I antibody in both phase I and phase II clinical trials, but it had no obvious anti-hypertensive effect. Therefore, further studies will be required to explore whether higher titers can lead to a decrease in BP. A multicenter, double-blind, randomized, placebo-controlled clinical trial of the Ang II vaccine AngQb-Cyt006 included 72 patients with mild-to-moderate hypertension. The subjects received subcutaneous injections of either 100 or 300 μg of the conjugate (CYT006-AngQb) or placebo at weeks 0, 4 and 12. SBP and DBP were reduced by 9.0 and 4.0 mmHg, respectively, in patients in the 300 μg vaccine dose group versus the baseline levels .This study confirmed that a vaccine can have a hypotensive effect in humans for the first time. In the future, the antihypertensive effect of vaccines must be verified in a broader population with hypertension.

Gastrointestinalmicrobiota

A large number of microbes are present in the human intestine, and these microorganisms play an important role in human health. The abundance, diversity, and uniformity of the intestinal flora are important indicators reflecting its composition. In 2005, Eckburg et al.used metagenomics to divide intestinal microorganisms into six categories: Firmicutes, Bacteroidetes, Proteobacteria, Actinobacteria, Verrucomicrobia and Fusobacteria. Bacteroidetes and Firmicutes are the dominant flora, and the ratio of Firmicutes to Bacteroidetes (F/B ratio) can reflect the degree of intestinal flora disorder. Dysbiosis of the gastrointestinal microbiota is closely related to the progression of hypertension, and the metabolites of the gastrointestinal microbiota play an important role in BP regulation .Mell et al. were the first group to present differences between the cecal microbial components of Dahl salt-sensitive and Dahl salt-resistant rats. In the same year, Yang et al. also found that compared with normotensive WKY rats, there were significant decreases in the abundance, diversity and evenness of microbial and an increase in the F/B ratio in SHR rats that were accompanied by declines in acetate- and butyrate-producing bacteria. Similar results were also found in chronic Ang II infusion rat.These results demonstrated that at the animal level, hypertension is correlated to disorders of the intestinal flora.

Recently, a study conducted in China performed comprehensive metagenomic and metabolomic analyses in a cohort of 41 healthy controls, 56 patients with pre-hypertension, and 99 individuals with primary hypertension. The results found that compared with healthy control group, microbial abundance and diversity were dramatically reduced in the pre-hypertension and hypertension groups. In addition, the counts of bacteria related to health status were reduced, whereas those of bacteria such as Prevotella and Klebsiella spp. were increased. Furthermore, by transplanting the stools of patients with hypertension into germ-free mice, BP was increased, indicating that increases in BP are transferrable through the microbiota. This study illustrated that the intestinal flora can directly regulate BP in the host. The aforementioned results indicate that changes in the composition of the gut microbiota play an important role in the progression of hypertension. It was found that after changes in the bacterial composition observed in animals and humans of hypertension, the level of bacterial metabolic end-products in the bloodstream was also changed . One of the main functions of the human intestinal microbiota is to ferment indigestible dietary fiber in the large intestine. The products of this fermentation process are short-chain fatty acids (SCFAs), including acetate, propionate, and butyrate. SCFAs are either absorbed by the gastrointestinal tract or excreted in feces. SCFAs mainly regulate BP by activating Olfr78 and Gpr41, both of which are G protein-coupled receptors, in vascular or renal tissues. Olfr78 is expressed in the renal juxtaglomerular apparatus, and it mediates renin secretion in response to SCFAs. Olfr78-knockout mice had lower plasma renin levels and baseline blood pressure levels than wild-type mice . There are also studies revealing that an acute SCFA bolus decreases BP in anesthetized mice, and this effect is mediated primarily via Gpr41. Therefore, Olfr78 is currently considered primarily responsible for raising BP, whereas Gpr41 is primarily responsible for lowering BP. The opposite effect of these receptors may be to regulate BP in the normal range when SCFA levels change. It has been demonstrated that the number of SCFAs produced by the intestinal microbiota is reduced in SHRs . In addition, a study demonstrated that compared with Dahl salt-sensitive rats fed a normal salt diet, Dahl salt-sensitive rats fed a high-salt diet exhibited increased levels of acetate, propionate, and isobutyrate in the stool, whereas butyrate levels did not increase significantly

A clinical trial illustratethat high intake of fruit and vegetables,which are considered as sources of SCFAs, can reduce BP, and they are associated with a lower incidence of cardiovascular mortality.

These results were inconsistent, and thus, more studies are needed to clarify the mechanism by which SCFAs influence the development of hypertension. A large number of studies have confirmed that regulating the intestinal microbiota may be an effective strategy for treating hypertension. Lactobacilli comprise a subdominant component of the human intestinal microbiota. Lactobacilli can enhance the release of anti-inflammatory factors. They can also reduce paracellular permeability and prevent the invasion of pathogenic bacteria. A randomized, placebo-controlled study indicated that Lactobacillus helveticus LBK-16H-fermented milk, which contains bioactive peptides, has a BP-lowering effect in hypertensive subjects. Ahren et al. reported that in rats with hypertension induced by NG-nitro-L-arginine methyl ester, blueberries fermented with the tannase-producing bacterium L. plantarum DSM 15313 can lower BP in rats and exert anti-hypertensive effect and reduce the risk of CVD. In another study, oral administration of recombinant L. plantarum NC8 (RLP) can express ACE inhibitory peptides and significantly reduce SBP in SHRs. Furthermore, the administration of RLP led to increased levels of NO and decreased levels of ET and Ang II in the plasma, heart and kidneys . Aoyagi et al. found that elderly people who drink fermented milk products containing L. casei strain Shirota at least three times a week had a significantly lower risk of hypertension. All the results indicate that lactobacilli can play a protective role against the development of hypertension, and probiotic intervention may be a potentially effective method for treating hypertension by restoring the intestinal microbial inhabitants. In the future, it will be necessary to further explore the mechanism of the interaction between the gastrointestinal microbiota and the host. We need to investigate the effects of different types of probiotics and explore the potential molecular mechanisms responsible for improved BP to elucidate the beneficial effect of probiotics on hypertension.

Leptin

Obesity lead to many adverse metabolic and

cardiovascular outcomes. Among this, obesity hypertension (HTN) has gained widespread interest. Obesity is the most common cause of primary HTN and is directly proportional to increases BMI. Although the pathophysiology of obesity HTN has not yet been fully elucidated, leptin, derived from obese gene, is increasingly implicated in obesity HTN. The relationship of leptin and hypertension is mutual. On the one hand, leptin increases arterial BP by activating aldosterone synthase (CYP11B2), which augments aldosterone secretion from the zona glomerulosa. On the other hand, leptin-induced cardiac contractile response was abrogated by hypertension. In addition, a theory named selective leptin resistance has emerged. Selective leptin occurs in obese humans and then contribute to the sympathetic overactivity and hypertension. Study has showed that leptin administration resulted in dose-dependent suppression of weight and appetite in lean mice. Besides, ablation of leptin receptors in the subfornical organ resulted in a drop in BP level . However, leptin -induced aldosterone levels failed to increase and BP reduction by adrenergic blockade was less marked in female rat which suggested that leptin failed to show the specificity of therapeutic target . Whether the selective leptin antagonists have the property of antihypertensive drugs remains unclear. Sodium-glucose cotransporter 2 (SGLT2) The SGLTs are one classes of carrier protein which mediate the reabsorption of the filtered glucose. About 90% of the filtered glucose is reabsorbed in the early proximal tubule via the action of SGLT2 expressed in kidney. Inhibition of SGLT2 decreases glucose reabsorption and modestly lowers blood glucose levels. However, the ability to lower blood glucose is limited by the filtered load of glucose and the osmotic diuresis . A meta-analysis of 45 placebo-controlled studies showed that SGLT2 inhibitor contributed to the mean reduction in systolic blood pressure (SBP) of −3.77 mmHg . In addition, SGLT2 inhibitors seem to reduce nighttime BP compared with daytime . The mechanisms of SGLT2 inhibitors lowering BP level may be via natriuresis and osmotic diuresis, but it is not clarified fully. The first FDA-approved drug of SGLT2 inhibitor class was canagliflozin . A multicenter double-blind, placebo-controlled dose-ranging study of 451 individuals randomized to escalating doses of canagliflozin (50 to 300 mg daily) added to metformin, sitagliptin, or placebo found a reduction in SBP ranging from − 0.9 mmHg with 50 mg once daily to −4.9 mmHg with 300 mg once daily, compared to −1.3 mmHg with placebo and − 0.8 mmHg with sitagliptin . Dapagliflozin was also a class of SGLT2 inhibitor. A randomized, placebo-controlled clinical trial showed that 10 mg dapagliflozin decreased the SBP by 4.3 mm. The effect could be explained by the synergy with β-blockers and calcium channel blockers. Furthermore, other SGLT2 inhibitors have been approved in some countries of the world, like empagliflozin, ipragliflozin, luseogliflozin and tofogliflozin.

Other factors in hypertension

Chemerin

Chemerin, a new relatively adipokine, can drive pathological changes in BP levels. The effect of chemerin in BP levels was mediated by the contraction of isolated arteries and the effect of established vasoconstrictors such as ET-1. Although as concrete molecule the mechanisms which chemerin modify and participate in hypertension is not clarified fully, it plays an important role in the component of blood vessel. In endothelial cells, chemerin increases reactive oxygen species (ROS) and may lead to decreased nitric oxide (NO) production Chemerin is a mitogen in vascular smooth muscle cells and elevates blood pressure . Moreover, chemerin promotes angiogenesis in the microvasculature . However, the specific drugs targeting chemerin need further investigation.

Autophagy

Autophagy maintains endothelial cell function and the integrity of blood vessels, plays a protective role in the development of pulmonary hypertension and atherosclerosis. In the past, blood pressure overload-induced cardiac dysfunction suppressed the process of autophagyA genome-wide association study showed that a common variant in the damage-regulated autophagy modulator locus was associated with hypertension whereas increased autophagy may account for the pulmonary arterial hypertension-induced ventricular

Table18. 2. New drug target for hypertension.

Target	Drug	Mode of action	Status
Aminopeptidase A	Firibastat (RB150)	APA inhibitor	Phase I/II
Vasoactive intestinal peptide	Vasomera (PB1046)	VIP receptor agonists	Phase I
Na+/H+ exchanger 3	Tenapanor	NHE3 inhibitor	
	SAR218034	NHE3 inhibitor	
Endothelin-1	Bosentan	Nonselective ETR antagonists	Approved
	Macitentan	Dual ETAR/ETBR antagonist	Approved
	Darusentan	Selective ETR antagonists	Approved
	Aprocitentan	Dual ETAR/ETBR antagonist	Approved
Nitric oxide	NG-nitro-L-arginine methyl ester hydrochloride	NO synthase inhibitor	Preclinical
	L-arginine or L-citrulline	NO synthase	Preclinical
	Pentaerythritol tetranitrate	NO	Preclinical
Sphingosine-1-phosphate	FTY702	S1PR1 antagonist	Approved
Ang I and Ang II	CYT006-AngQβ	ANGII antibody	Phase II
	PMD3117	ANGI antibody	Phase I/II
	ATRQβ-001	ANGII type 1 receptor antibody	Preclinical
Sodium-glucose cotransporter 2	Canagliflozin	SGLT2 inhibitor	Approved
	Dapagliflozin	SGLT2 inhibitor	Approved

APA, Aminopeptidase A; VIP, Vasoactive intestinal peptide; NHE3, Na+/H+ exchanger 3; ETR, endothelin receptor; NO, Nitric oxide; S1PR1, Sphingosine-1-phosphate; SGLT2, Sodium-glucose cotransporter 2.

hypertrophy and diastolic heart failure , which was a contradictory result of autophagy in hypertension. To date, the role of autophagy in vascular biology and blood pressure regulation remains unknown.

Acetylation

Acetylation and deacetylation of functional proteins are essential for hypertension. In spontaneously hypertensive rat, inhibition of histone deacetylases could suppress cardiac hypertrophy and fibrosis by elevating histone 3 acetylation on promoters of MR target genes . In addition, inhibition of lysine deacetylases also increased the acetylation of MR and attenuated hypertension. Depletion of SIRT3 causes hyperacetylation of mitochondrial SOD2 and overproduction of oxidative stress, which results in endothelial dysfunction, vascular inflammation and hypertension in mice Many research fellows have realized that monotherapy in the treatment of hypertension may represent ineffectiveness due to the additional effects and adverse effects on BP control. In addition to the new targets mentioned above (Table 1), the investigation of new mechanisms and new drug targets in antihypertensive was challengeable. Thus, many companies in the market have focused on developing fixed-dose combinations (FDCs) of two or more agents [99]. In the past, ACE inhibitors can be combined with ARBs and dihydropyridine calcium-channel blockers can be combined with all other first-line antihypertensive drugsMost late-stage antihypertensive drugs consist of dual or triple combinations, and they refer to dual or triple targets. For example, phase III trials are under way for candesartan cilexetil/nifedipine and fimasartan/amlodipine, both of which are FDCs of an ARB and a calcium channel blocker (CCB). Valsartan/ amlodipine/rosuvastatin is in phase III trials while valsartan/amlodipine/atorvastatin is in phase I trials. Similar trials were also under investigation.

1V. Trends in Antidiabetic Drug Discovery

The complexity of T2DM has prompted a significant interest in developing new pharmaceutical therapies to control diabetes. A broad range of drug therapies has been approved by the United States Food and Drug Administration (FDA) that address different biological systems and mechanisms implicated in the disease (Gourgari et al., 2017). In this rapidly developing area of pharmacology, hundreds of compounds with antihyperglycemic activity have been discovered in nature or synthesized in recent years, many of which are currently undergoing clinical trials (Artasensi et al., 2020). Furthermore, there are several agents in different stages of clinical development that target both established pathways and novel mechanisms of actions for antidiabetic drugs. Excellent reviews have been published that focus on specific aspects of diabetes drug discovery, for example on FDA-approved antihyperglycemic agents (Gourgari et al., 2017; Artasensi et al., 2020), specific delivery systems to improve drug efficacy (Veiseh et al., 2015), and on targeting particular pathways that are being investigated in clinical development. However, the landscape of approved agents for the treatment of diabetes is dynamic, with both drug approvals and discontinuations taking place (Scheen et al., 2017; Chikara et al., 2018). Hence, an updated comprehensive analysis is needed to examine the current state of diabetes drug discovery and search for new diabetology approaches.

The main aim of this writing is to shed light on the current trends of FDA-approved antidiabetic pharmaceuticals and all the drugs to treat diabetes in clinical development from 2015 to 2020. It will also discuss the mechanisms of action of the main classes of antihyperglycemic compounds and present new and promising, but not yet approved, therapeutic approaches for treating T2DM. The FDA has approved 59 unique antihyperglycemic drugs since human insulin (Humulin) approval in 1982.The approved drugs include 36 new molecular entities (NMEs) as monotherapies and 23 unique drug combinations of two or more antihyperglycemic agents. Most recently approved NMEs trends in antidiabeticdrug discovery approval.Thus, approximately half of the clinical agents target already established pathways, i.e., molecular targets that have been validated through the FDA approval of an agent targeting that pathway for the treatment of diabetes. However, a surprising number of the drugs in clinical trials have novel molecular targets, as monotherapies or combinations, that have not yet been validated through the approval of an agent by the FDA. A large proportion of clinical development is dedicated to new avenues for treating diabetes. Notably, at least six of these agents are in phase III trials, which indicates that potential first-in-class drugs for diabetes management may be approved soon.

Established Drug Classes for the Treatment of Diabetes

1 . Types of Insulin

Different types of insulin comprise a considerable portion of FDA-approved drugs for diabetes treatment with at least 14 unique analogues and combination regimens. Insulin is perhaps one of the most studied proteins and has been an integral part of T2DM treatment. Recombinant insulin analogues have been developed that act in several different ways. Rapid-acting insulin analogues supply a bolus insulin level needed at mealtimes (prandial insulin) and include insulin lispro, aspart, and glulisine. Longer-acting insulins released slowly over a more extended period supply the basal insulin level needed throughout the day and night (basal insulin) and include detemir, glargine, and the ultra-long-acting degludec. Such a spectrum of insulin analogues enables combinations of different insulin forms, providing an effective basal-bolus therapy that more closely reflects physiological insulin secretion (Petersen and Shulman, 2018). In addition to insulin plus insulin combination regimens, insulin plus glucagon-like peptide-1 (GLP1) receptor agonist combinations have also been approved. Furthermore, basal insulin therapy combinations with other drugs or adjunctive therapies are also prescribed (Chaudhury et al., 2017). Even though insulin has been an important discovery for the treatment of diabetes, it is rarely used as a first-line treatment choice (van den Boom et al., 2020). Insulin administration comes with risks of developing severe hypoglycemia, cancer, and cardiovascular complications, and most often occurs when patients develop insulin tolerance and the dose administered has to be increased (Lebovitz,(Lebovitz, 2011).

2 Sulfonylureas (SU0

Until the approval of metformin, sulfonylureas (SU) were the only approved insulin competitors and were extensively used to treat T2DM. While currently, only three SU drugs are available for the prescription (glyburide, glipizide, and glimepiride). There have been at least four additional unique chemical SU compounds previously approved that are now discontinued (refer to Supplementary Table S2 for a full description of previously approved and now discontinued drugs for the T2DM treatment). Two SU and metformin combination regimens have been FDA-approved that are currently marketed: glyburide/metformin, glipizide/metformin. Combinations of glimepiride and metformin do exist, e.g., Amaryl M and Glimetal Lex, but are not approved by the FDA or the European Medicines Agency (Kim et al., 2014; AdisInsight, 2021). However, in the FDA approval of Amaryl (Glimepiride, 2021) it is stated that the two drugs can be taken together if monotherapies of each fail to work. The first SU compounds were discovered in the 1940s and entered the pharmaceutical market in the mid-1950s. The evolution of insulin therapies went in parallel with the search for alternative approaches. Among the first such attempts, compounds from the SU class were most interesting. Sulfonylureas mimic the effect of ATP in pancreatic beta cells and act as insulin-secreting agents (Tian et al., 1998; Al-Omary, 2017). SU molecules interact with the sulfonylurea receptors (SURs) on the surface of beta cells, which leads to inhibition of ATP-dependent inward-rectifier potassium ion channels (Ashcroft, 1996; Szewczyk, 1997; Liu et al., 2016). As a result, the intracellular concentration of potassium cations increases, leading to plasma membrane depolarization. These conditions stimulate the opening of voltage-gated calcium channels, and an increased concentration of cytosolic calcium cations leads to a surge in insulin secretion (Sulis et al., 2019). SU drugs have been extensively prescribed to treat T2DM for more than 50 years. SUs are well-tolerated, and their popularity could be attributed to their low cost and the possibility of use as a monotherapy or in combination with metformin (Sola et al., 2015). SUs do not only interact with SURs in pancreatic beta cells, but also in smooth muscle cells and cardiac myocytes. This may explain why SU agents have been linked to a greater prevalence of hypoglycemia and cardiovascular risk (Rao et al., 2008; Schramm et al., 2011). However, most reports support the cardiovascular safety of SUs (Pop and Lingvay, 2017).

3 Biguanides

The approval of the biguanide metformin in 1995 significantly changed T2DM therapy and is the only FDA-approved antihyperglycemic agent in this drug class. Metformin selectively inhibits the mitochondrial isoform of glycerophosphate dehydrogenase, indirectly activates adenosine monophosphate-activated protein kinase (AMPK), and reduces cytosolic dihydroxyacetone phosphate while raising cytosolic NADH/NAD ratio (Musi et al., 2002; Wang et al., 2019). This results in decreased plasma glucose and lactate levels, reduced liver gluconeogenesis, hepatic glucose secretion, and endogenous glucose production (Foretz et al., 2014; Rena et al., 2017; Wang et al., 2019). Moreover, metformin can increase insulin sensitivity in muscle tissues. Currently, metformin is the only antihyperglycemic drug recommended by the American Diabetes Association and the European Association for the Study of Diabetes as initial oral therapy for patients with T2DM (Hostalek et al., 2015).

4 Alpha-Glucosidase Inhibitors

The first alpha-glucosidase inhibitor (AGI), acarbose, was approved by the FDA as an antihyperglycemic agent in 1995 and the second AGI, miglitol, followed in 1996. These are the only two AGIs approved for the United States market, although another AGI, voglibose, was approved by the Pharmaceuticals and Medical Devices Agency in Japan (Oki et al., 1999).

In clinical development, the chewable tablet BTI-320 (PAZ320) recently completed a proof-of-concept study that showed low dose BTI-320 attenuated postprandial rise in blood glucose and reduced body weight modestly in pre-diabetic subjects.

It is currently in the product pipeline at Boston Therapeutics, and due to the ease of administration and high levels of tolerance, it can be used as an adjunct to lifestyle modification for diabetes prevention(Trasketal.,2013).

Alpha-glucosidase is a widely expressed enzyme that cleaves glucosidic bonds. Inhibition of alpha-glycosidase prevents the digestion of complex carbohydrates to monosaccharides in the small intestine (Bischoff, 1994; Zhang et al.,2016).

Thus, these agents act as pseudo-carbohydrates (substrate analogues), where they inhibit digestive enzymes and prevent oligo- and polysaccharides from being catabolized to monomers (Goto et al., 1995; Taira et al., 2000). This leads to less sugar being absorbed, resulting in lower postprandial glucose levels and reducing hyperglycemia (Lebovitz, 2011). AGIs have been shown to have similar efficacy as metformin, so they are often prescribed as a first-line treatment or combined with other antidiabetics. However, typical side effects of AGIs are flatulence, abdominal bloating and discomfort, and diarrhea. At the same time, a recent meta-analysis found that the use of AGI leads to an increase in liver transaminases, indicative of hepatotoxicity (Zhang et al., 2016)

5.Thiazolidinediones

Thiazolidinediones (TZDs) act as insulin sensitizers which activate peroxisome proliferator-activated receptors (PPARs), a broad family of nuclear receptors. The first TZD drug, troglitazone, was approved by the FDA in 1997; however, it was discontinued in 1999 due to severe hepatotoxicity. Currently, there are two marketed TZDs, rosiglitazone and pioglitazone, which were FDA-approved in 1999. TZD use has previously been limited due to concerns with safety issues and side effects. In addition, there was some controversy over cardiovascular toxicity with rosiglitazone and an increase in bladder cancer with pioglitazone.

However, recent studies show no longer significant issues (see Lebovitz (2019) for review). Furthermore, the beneficial effects of TZDs on the cardiovascular risk factors associated with insulin resistance have been well documented. TZD drugs can be effective as a monotherapy or in a combination regimen. One combination regimen that consists of pioglitazone and metformin is currently marketed. Four TZD monotherapies and one combination with a dipeptidyl peptidase-4 (DPP4) inhibitor are in trials in clinical development. The most clinically advanced is lobeglitazone, which has already been approved in South Korea and is currently in phase III trials for additional combination treatments.TZD molecules can interact with PPAR-α and PPAR-γ isoforms expressed primarily on fatty tissues and skeletal muscle. This leads to activating these receptors and stimulating complexation with another essential constituent–the retinoid X receptor. The triple complex can bind specifically to DNA by peroxisome proliferative response elements (PPRE)and act as a target gene promoter, thus stimulating gene expression (Yau et al., 2013). This therapeutic method leads to increased adiponectin levels, decreased gluconeogenesis, and increased glucose uptake in the muscle and fat. Adiponectin is a hormone secreted in adipose tissue that regulates glucose concentration by improving insulin sensitivity (Yu et al., 2002).

In general, prescription rates for SU and TZD drugs are experiencing a gradual decline (Kohro et al., 2013; Eibich et al., 2017; Wilkinson et al., 2018; Giorda et al., 2020). From 2000 to 2006, there was a rapid surge in TZD prescriptions (45%); however, most likely due to reports of safety issues, TZD use decreased (Wilkinson et al., 2018; Secrest et al., 2020). Currently, a guideline recommends a series of intensification steps to a baseline of initial metformin monotherapy in case of intolerance to metformin (Irons and Minze, 2014; American Diabetes Association, 2019). However, each country may manage the situation differently due to income levels, medicine development degrees, and population differences in physiology (Singla et al., 2019).

6. Incretin-Dependent Therapies (GLP1 Receptor Agonists and DPP4 Inhibitors)

In 2005 and 2006, the first incretin dependent T2DM therapies were approved, and they have become increasingly popular as monotherapies and in combination regimens since then. Incretin-depending treatments include glucagon-like peptide-1 (GLP1) mimetics which act as GLP1 receptor agonists and DPP4 inhibitors. Six injectable GLP1 receptor agonists were approved, including exenatide, liraglutide, dulaglutide, albiglutide, lixisenatide, and semaglutide. They differ in their lifetime in the bloodstream and in their ability to treat hyperglycemia (Yamamoto-Honda et al., 2018). Incretin therapies account for 30% of antidiabetic drugs in clinical development, with GLP1R agonists comprising the most significant proportion (20%). The clinical outcome of GLP1R agonists is robust, with 21 agents in clinical trials and the majority of them in phase I and II trials. Fifteen of these receptor agonists target just GLP1R, four agents also target the glucagon receptor (GCGR), one drug targets GLP1R plus GCGR plus the gastric inhibitory polypeptide receptor (GIPR), and one drug targets GLP1R and GIPR. The only GLP1R agonist in phase III trials is efpeglenatide from Hanmi Pharm; it demonstrated a dose-proportional pharmacokinetic profile, with an extended half-life and slow absorption in patients with T2DM (Sharma et al., 2018; Del Prato et al., 2020; Yoon et al., 2020). There are currently four DPP4 inhibitors that have been FDA-approved: sitagliptin, saxagliptin, linagliptin, and alogliptin. However, at least seven additional DPP4 inhibitors have obtained approval from other regulating agencies and are currently registered in phase III and IV trials. It is not clear whether all these agents will seek FDA marketing approval or not. Also, there are ten DPP4 inhibitors in clinical development–two additional phase III drugs and one agent in phase II trials. The introduction of DPP4 inhibitors as antihyperglycemic agents brought significant changes in T2DM prescription trends. In Japan, for example, they were the most frequently prescribed drugs in the elderly in 2013 (49.1%) (Yamamoto-Honda et al., 2018). GLP1 is one of the most crucial hormones in glucose metabolism and is released into the bloodstream by special L-cells in the ileum and colon. It is one of two significant incretins (intestinal secretion of insulin) hormones which stimulate insulin secretion and suppress glucagon synthesis (Meier et al., 2003; Andersen et al., 2018; Mathiesen et al., 2019). They act on the pancreas within 2–4 min and are rapidly inactivated afterwards. DPP4 selectively cleaves N-terminal dipeptides from proteins containing proline or alanine in the penultimate positionand GLP1 is its substrate (Röhrborn et al., 2015). Usually, this cleavage does not have any adverse effects on the glucose level–on the contrary–this inactivation is necessary. Nevertheless, in T2DM, the production of incretins is reduced, and their effects are weakened. Furthermore, the inactivation occurs so rapidly that there is not enough time for incretins to perform their physiological functions (Drucker and Nauck, 2006; Nauck and Meier, 2018). Therefore, this inactivation of incretins by DPP4, which is usually necessary, leads to hyperglycemia in T2DM patients. To overcome this, two possible mechanisms have been implemented: to create artificial long-acting GLP1 mimetics and to prevent the enzyme from cleaving its substrates. Both GLP1 receptor agonists and DPP4 inhibitors share some remarkable effects regarding beta-cell physiology in that they can improve beta-cell functioning and reduce apoptosis (Lee and Jun, 2014; Bugliani et al., 2018; Wang, et al., 2018; Jiang et al., 2020). However, this advantage may have a simultaneous drawback; with an increase in the survival of beta cells due to the reduced apoptosis, the potential risk of cancer increases. It is also worth mentioning that liraglutide and semiglutide, GLP1 receptor agonists, act as cardiovascular protectors (Marso et al., 2016; Bethel et al., 2018; Davies et al., 2018; Sharma et al., 2018; Husain et al., 2019; Husain et al., 2020). Moreover, the usage of GLP1 receptor agonists is associated with weight loss. At the same time, while DPP4 inhibitors do not influence weight gain, it is controversial whether or not they increase the risk of heart failure (Khalse and Bhargava, 2018; Sano, 2019).

7.Meglitinides

Two meglitinides have been FDA-approved: nateglinide in 2009 and repaglinide in 2013. Currently, there are no meglitinides in clinical trials. Meglitinides share a similar mechanism of action to sulfonylurea agents in that they increase insulin secretion in the pancreas. They bind to SURs in pancreatic beta cells but at a binding site different than SUs and induce the same reaction cascade that leads to insulin secretion (O'Brien et al., 2018). In contrast to SUs, meglitinides, nateglinide in particular, exhibit glucose-sensitive action whereby their potency increases at higher glucose concentrations (Hu et al., 2000). Meglitinides are short-acting and associated with lower hypoglycemia risks, weight gain, and chronic hyperinsulinemia than sulfonylurea drugs (Guardado-Mendoza et al., 2013). Other studies have since demonstrated that meglitinides could be associated with increased risk of hypoglycemia in diabetic patients with advanced chronic kidney disease (Wu et al., 2017).

8.Sodium-GlucoseCotransporter Type2 Inhibitors

The most modern and promising drug class is SGLT2 inhibitors. The first SGLT2 inhibitors, canagliflozin, and dapagliflozin were approved in 2013, followed by additional monotherapy agents including empagliflozin in 2014 and ertugliflozin in 2017. Additionally, SGLT2 inhibitors are popular in combination regimens with metformin and DPP4 inhibitors and combinations of all three and TZD drugs. SGLT2 inhibitors are the second largest group of antidiabetic agents in clinical trials (12%) after incretin therapies. Three of the twelve drugs in phase II, III, and IV clinical trials have been previously approved by other regulating agencies. Five other

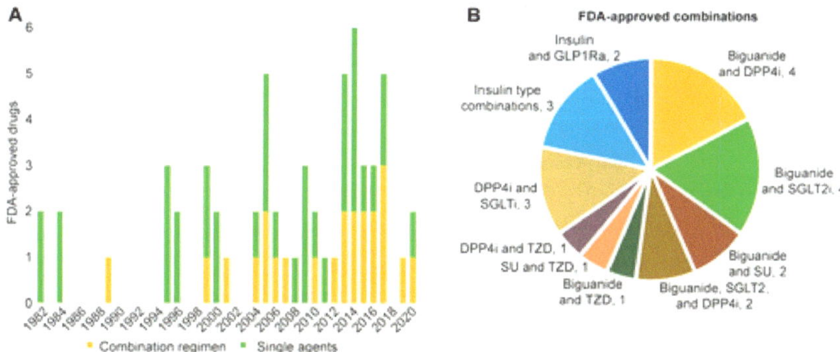

FIG.18.1 FDA-approved monotherapies and combination regimens. (A) The current 59 FDA-approved anti-diabetic agents. The data includes the year of first approval for new molecular entities and unique combinations. Single agents are indicated in green while combination regimens are in yellow. (B) FDA-approved unique combinations. Data compiled and verified using the United States Drugs@FDA resource. DPP4i, Dipeptidyl peptidase 4 (DPP4) inhibitor; GLP-1Ra, Glucagon-like peptide-1 (GLP-1) receptor agonist; SGLT2i, Sodium-glucose co-transporter-2 (SGLT2) inhibitor; SU, Sulfonylureas; TZD, Thiazolinediones.

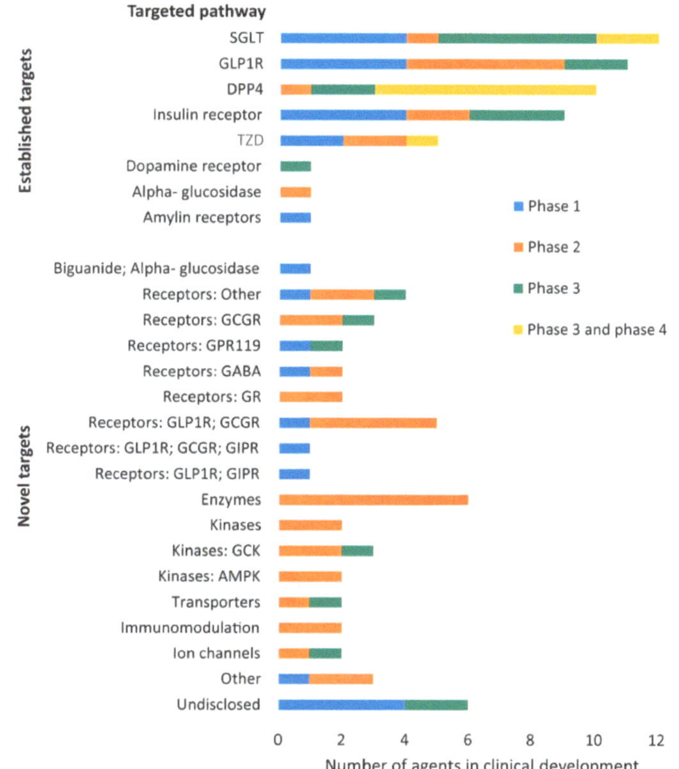

FIG 18.2 The molecular targets of the 99 anti-diabetic agents in clinical trials. The phase status is the highest clinical phase each agent has achieved. A surprising number clinical agents–nearly half–target novel molecular targets or combination regimens. Novel targets or pathways are those that have not yet been validated through approval of an FDA-approved drug for treatment of diabetes. Approximately half of the agents target already established pathways, i.e., molecular targets that have been validated through the FDA-approval of an agent targeting that pathway for the treatment of diabetes. Six of the agents had an undisclosed mechanism of action. DPP4, Dipeptidyl peptidase 4; GLP-1R, Glucagon-like peptide-1 (GLP-1) receptor; SGLT2, Sodium-glucose co-transporter-2; TZD, Thiazolinediones; GCGR, Glucagon receptor; GPR119, Glucose-dependent insulinotropic receptor (G-Protein coupled receptor 119); GR, Glucocorticoid receptor; GIPR, Gastric Inhibitory Polypeptide Receptor; GCK, glucokinase; AMPK, 5'-AMP-activated protein kinase.

agents are in phase III trials, indicating that new SGLT2 inhibitors may be approved soon. Even though SGLT inhibitors reduce renal glucose reabsorption levels, which leads to glucose excretion (glucosuria) and weight loss (Taylor, et al., 2015; Lupsa and Inzucchi, 2018; Brown et al., 2019), they also appear to have good pharmacokinetic properties and are well tolerated (Ito et al., 2016). Moreover, this drug class has been shown to improve cardiovascular conditions in both diabetic and non-diabetic populations (Martens et al., 2017).Therefore SGLT-2 inhibitors have become the preferred glucose-lowering drugs to treat patients with T2DM at high risk of cardiovascular events, although it is also associated with urogenital infections (Wu et al., 2016; Kramer, et al., 2018). As a result, prescription rates for newer therapies, such as DPP4 and SGLT2 inhibitors, have grown. In the United Kingdom, in 2017, new prescription rates for DPP4 and SGLT2 inhibitors accounted for 42 and 22%, respectively (Eibich et al., 2017).

Table18.3 Examples of oral hypoglycemic agents with their mechanism of action.

	Mechanism of action	Examples	Approximate A1C reduction (%)	Impact on CV events	Adverse effects
Biguanides	Activates AMPK	Metformin	1–2	Reduction in MI, all-cause mortality	diarrhea, nausea, lactic acidosis
Sulfonylureas	Increase insulin secretion via ATP-sensitive K channel on beta cells	Glimepiride, Glipizide, Glyburide	1–2	No effect; risk of hypoglycemia	hypoglycemia, weight gain
DPP-IV inhibitors	Prevents degradation of GLP-1	Saxagliptin, Sitagliptin, Vildagliptin	0.5–0.8	Increased heart failure hospitalization for saxagliptin	Nausea (generally resolves)
Thiazolidinediones	Bind PPAR gamma, decrease insulin resistance and increase glucose utilization	Rosiglitazone, Pioglitazone	0.5–1.4	Increased risk of heart failure; pioglitazone may be associated with reduced MACE	Peripheral edema, HF, weight gain, fractures
SGLT-2 Inhibitors	Block glucose resorption in proximal renal tubule	Canagliflozin, Empagliflozin, Dapagliflozin, Ertugliflozin	0.5–0.8	Reduction in HF hospitalization, CV mortality	GU infections, increased lower extremity amputation with canagliflozin (0.6% v 0.3% in placebo)
GLP-1 Agonists	Activated glucagon-like-peptide 1 receptor, increasing insulin secretion, decreasing glucagon selection	Liraglutide, Semaglutide, Exenatide	0.4–0.9	Reduction in CV mortality, all-cause mortality, MI/stroke	GI side effects. Higher rates of retinopathy with semaglutide

AMPK, 5' adenosine monophosphate-activated protein kinase; MI, myocardial infarction; CV, cardiovascular; MACE, major adverse cardiovascular event; ATP, adenosine triphosphate; K, potassium, DPP-IV, dipeptidyl peptidase 4; GLP-1, glucagon like peptide 1; PPAR, peroxisome proliferator-activated receptor; HF, heart failure; SGLT-2, sodium-glucose cotransporter 2; GU, genitourinary; GI, gastrointestinal.

Table 18.4 Examples of oral hypoglycemic agents with their mechanism of action.

Class	*Example*	*Mechanism*	*Side effects*
Biguanides	Metformin	↓Hepatic glucose production ↑Peripheral insulin sensitivity	Hypoglycemia Lactic acidosis GI symptoms
Sulfonylurea derivatives	Tolbutamide	↑Insulin release by depolarizing pancreatic β-cell	Hypoglycemia
GLP1 agonists DPP4 inhibitors	Liraglutide, Linagliptin	↑Insulin release by depolarizing pancreatic β-cell ↓Hepatic glucose release by ↓glucagon delay gastric emptying	Hypoglycemia (if combined with insulin or sulfonylurea) GI symptoms Upper RTI
SGLT2 inhibitors	Dapagliflozin	↓Glucose resorption in renal tubule	Diabetic Ketoacidosis Dehydration Hypoglycemia (if combined with insulin or sulfonylurea)
Thiazolidinedione	Pioglitazone	↑Peripheral insulin sensitivity (via PPARγ)	Hypoglycemia (if combined with insulin or sulfonylurea) Fluid retention
Others	Acarbose	↓Glucose absorption in small intestine (↓Conversion of polysaccharides into monosaccharides)	Treatment of any hypoglycemia requires glucose and not other sugars or carbohydrates

DPP4, dipeptidyl peptidase-4; GI, gastrointestinal; GLP1, glucagon-like peptide-1; PPARγ, peroxisome proliferator-activated receptor gamma; RTI, respiratory tract infection; SGLT2, sodium/glucose cotransporter2.

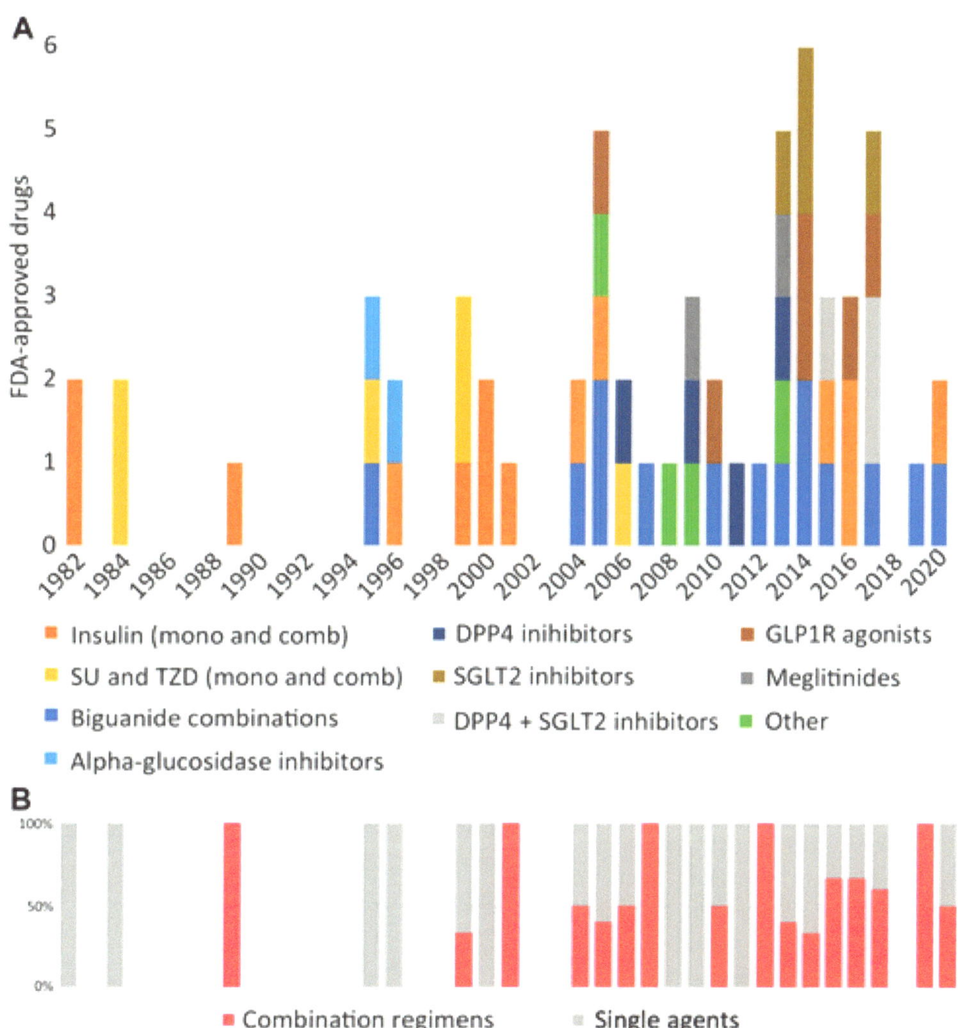

Fig.18.3 FDA-approved drug classes per year. (A) Timeline of the major classes of antihypertensive drugs that have approved including monotherapies (mono) and combinations (comb). DPP4, Dipeptidyl peptidase 4; GLP-1R, Glucagon-like peptide-1 (GLP-1) receptor; SGLT2, Sodium-glucose co-transporter-2; SU, Sulfonylureas; TZD, Thiazolinediones. (B) The proportion of combination regimens in comparison to monotherapies.

9 Drug Combinations

The different types of approved oral combinations have steadily increased, along with the proportion of combinations being approved in comparison to monotherapies. Nearly 40% of the approved antidiabetic drugs are combination regimens. FDA-approved combinations of antihyperglycemic drugs can be divided into two generations. First-generation combinations were mixtures of different insulin isoforms, where they differed in the method of preparation, natural source, duration of action, or concentrations. By 2004, the increase in the proportion of drug combinations began in earnest as second-generation antihyperglycemic combinations evolved. They consisted mainly of drugs that require oral administration, and in most cases, one of the components was metformin. To date, there are 23 unique antihyperglycemic drug combinations. The first triple combination regimen was approved in 2019, consisting of metformin, saxagliptin, and dapagliflozin. Another triple combination approval for metformin, linagliptin, and empagliflozin followed in 2020. This trend expounds on the idea that it is necessary to use all known approaches for the comprehensive treatment of T2DM.Analysis shows that most combinations that have been created are based on metformin. It also correlates well with global prescribing trends. Currently, metformin is the most optimal drug for monotherapy. Its prescription trends have dramatically increased over the past years, which cannot be said about other options for the initial therapy of T2DM. For instance, in the United Kingdom prescriptions for SUs and insulin declined by almost tenfold between 2000–2017 (Wilkinson et al., 2018; Ramzan et al., 2019). The 1998 United Kingdom Prospective Diabetes Study (UKPDS) shifted the trend toward using metformin instead of using SUs. Moreover, the introduction of long-acting insulins benefited patients with T2DM in the last stages of progression, often being the very last frontier to achieve glycemic control and help prevent chronic implications (Eibich et al., 2017).

NovelDrugTargets

More than 40% of the agents identified in clinical trials target novel therapeutic molecules or combinations of targets . Receptors and enzymes and the largest classes of novel targets, followed by transporters and ion channels.

1.Receptors

Glucose protein-coupled receptor 119 (GPR119) plays a critical role in glucose homeostasis and is expressed in pancreatic β-cells and enteroendocrine cells (Fredriksson et al., 2003; Neelamkavil et al., 2018). Previous studies have shown that agonism of GPR112 stimulates insulin and incretin secretion (Semple et al., 2008; Kang, 2013; Ritter et al., 2016). Thus, the mechanism of action resembles the incretin effect in glucose metabolism. Furthermore, animal studies suggest that agonism of GPR119 has favorable outcomes regarding weight gain and food intake (Overton et al., 2008). However, due to the chemistry of GPR119 agonists thus far, unintended side effects may occur and may have been a contributing factor in the discontinuation of previous clinical agents (Ritter et al., 2016). The second-generation GPR119 agonist DA-1241 is currently in phase I trials and will hopefully provide diabetic patients with significant glucose-lowering benefits and better safety profiles (Kang, 2013; Ritter et al., 2016).The gastric inhibitory polypeptide (GIP) is an incretin hormone that works similarly to GLP1 in stimulating pancreatic β cells for insulin secretion in a glucose-dependent manner. Tirzepatide is currently active in clinical trials (Phase III), which acts as a dual agonist. Binding to both the GLP1 receptor and GIP receptor, a study with GIP showed decreased body weight and hemoglobin A1c (Mathiesen et al., 2019).

Thyroid hormone receptors (THR) have typically been targeted in the treatment of metabolic disorders, but they have also been shown to be attractive targets in the treatment of diabetes (Saponaro et al., 2020). THR agonism studies in mice resulted in increased energy expenditure, increased insulin sensitivity, and lowered glucose concentrations. These effects may be because THR is highly expressed in the liver, skeletal muscles, and kidneys (Lin and Sun, 2011; Zambad et al., 2011). There is one thyroid hormone receptor agonist (TRC150094), which is a functional analogue of iodothyronines. It is currently active in phase III clinical trials to evaluate the safety in lowering cardiovascular risk in patients with diabetes

2. Enzymes–General

Diacylglycerol acyltransferase (DGAT) is a crucial enzyme in triacylglycerol (TAG) synthesis, which catalyzes the final dedicated step of TAG synthesis. DGAT deficient mice showed a significant reduction in the postprandial increase of plasma TAG and were resistant to diet-induced obesity due to increased energy expenditure. Even more, the DGAT1 knockout mice had enhanced insulin sensitivity. However, increased activity of DGAT in T2DM patients can cause beta-cell dysfunction. Therefore, selective DGAT inhibitors have been designed to manage metabolic diseases such as obesity and T2DM due to their ability to prevent abnormal TAG levels and beta-cell damage. Currently, at least one promising agent (IONIS DGAT2Rx) from this drug group has completed phase II clinical trials. Being a hepatoprotectant, it is not a classic hyperglycemic drug, but it indirectly affects glycemia by increasing insulin sensitivity and protecting islet β-cells (Zhu et al., 2019; Hong et al., 2020).

The kallikrein-kinin system may also provide an exciting approach for diabetes treatment. It has been shown that bradykinin (BK) resulted in increased glucose uptake and insulin sensitivity through the bradykinin type 2 receptor (BK2R) signaling (Lau et al., 2020). In addition, studies on diabetic mice models treated with human tissue kallikrein 1 gene resulted in lowered glucose concentration, controlled hypoglycemia, and reversed insulin resistance (Kolodka et al., 2014). This therapeutic strategy is being investigated with DM-199,, a recombinant human tissue kallikrein-1 protein currently in phase II trials to treat diabetes.Fructose-1,6-bisphosphatase-1 (FBP1), an enzyme involved in gluconeogenesis, is another constituent in glucose homeostasis (Zhao et al., 2018). An unmet issue in T2DM pathology is the endogenous glucose production in the liver, which may be mediated by inhibiting FBP1. While metformin can indirectly mediate this activity (Hunter et al., 2018), the investigative agent VK 0612 directly inhibits FBP1 and has completed phase II clinical trials.

Methionine aminopeptidase 2 (MetAP2) is an enzyme that cleaves off methionine from the N-terminus of new proteins. It has been shown that MetAP2 has a crucial role in angiogenesis, which is why MetAp2 inhibitors have been used in cancer treatment (Chun et al., 2005; Morgen et al., 2016). However, recent studies have shown that inhibition of MetAP2 is a strong candidate for treating obesity and diabetes (Joharapurkar et al., 2014). Inhibition of MetAP2 induced clinically meaningful reductions in blood glucose and increased weight loss (Siddik et al., 2019; Wentworth et al., 2020). The clinical agent ZGN-1061 is a MetAP2 inhibitor with promising results with improved glucose control and lowered weight in preclinical studies and a recently completed phase II clinical trial (Burkey et al., 2018; Wentworth et al., 2020).

Angiopoietin-related protein 3 (ANGPTL3) is another protein involved in angiogenesis and hence cancer; however, it also has essential functions in glucose metabolism. Its principal function is inhibiting lipoprotein lipase and controlling triglyceride levels in plasma (Lupo and Ferri, 2018; Ahmad et al., 2019; Lang and Frishman, 2019). How exactly ANGPTL3 functions in glucose metabolism is unclear. However, it is speculated that it lowers insulin sensitivity and increases insulin resistance by increasing free fatty acids (Christopoulou et al., 2019). Thus, inhibition of ANGPTL3 is a promising strategy and a potential drug target for T2DM and other metabolic disorders. ISIS-703802, a designed ANGPTL3 inhibitor, recently completed phase II trials in subjects with hypertriglyceridemia, T2DM, and non-alcoholic fatty liver disease (Jiang et al., 2019).

2.1 Enzymes–Kinases

Glucokinase is a crucial enzyme that maintains normal glucose homeostasis and has a glucostatic effect in the blood because it initiates gluconeogenesis. Activating glucokinase by small molecule therapeutics may increase insulin secretion from the pancreas, promote glycogen synthesis in the liver, and thus reduce hepatic glucose output (Toulis et al., 2020). Therefore, a promising strategy for antihyperglycemic drugs is through glucokinase activators (GKA). Research and development began in the early 1990s, and preclinical animal studies showed that GKAs effectively normalize blood glucose levels; however, the activation leads to severe hyperlipidemia, vascular hypertension, and other negative consequences (Matschinsky, 2013). Hence many GKAs have entered trials (e.g., Piragliatin, ARRY-403, AZD1656, PSN010), although they have subsequently discontinued clinical progression. However, there has been renewed interest due to the development of several next-generation GKAs: dorzagliatin, a novel, dual-acting agent that targets both pancreatic and hepatic glucokinases, and TTP399, a hepatoselective compound (Toulis et al., 2020). Dorzaliatin is currently in phase III trials, and TTP339 and SY004, another new GKA, are in phase II trials.AMP-activated protein kinase (AMPK) is an enzyme for energy regulation. When energy levels are low, it promotes glucose update in skeletal muscles and reduces gluconeogenesis. It was found that a healthy lifestyle that includes calorie restriction, exercise, and hormones that encourage longevity like leptin and adiponectin activate AMPK. In addition, some antihyperglycemic drugs, such as metformin or canagliflozin, can indirectly activate AMPK via regulating cation transporters (Coughlan et al., 2014; Steinberg and Carling, 2019). Currently, direct activators of AMPK have been designed, and several are registered in trials: PXL770 and PBI-4050 have recently completed phase II studies.

Fructokinase (FK) is an enzyme in the liver, intestine, and kidney cortex that converts fructose into fructose-1-phosphate. Since fructokinase lacks a negative feedback system, its activation leads to the depletion of phosphates, thus leading to activation of AMP deaminase and the formation of uric acid, which causes inflammation in the cells. This inflammation happens in pancreatic islets and can lead to insulin resistance (Khitan and Kim, 2013). Thus, inhibition of this pathway could be an exciting approach in the treatment of hyperglycemia. The fructokinase inhibitor, PF-06835919, is currently in phase II clinical trials.Tolimidone (MLR-1023) has completed phase II in patients with uncontrolled T2DM and is currently active in phase II with patients treated with metformin. It is a potent Lyn protein tyrosine kinase stimulant (Ochman et al., 2012; Saporito et al., 2012). Lyn tyrosine kinase is vital for insulin sensitivity and glucose metabolism. It phosphorylates insulin receptor substrates which attenuate insulin receptor signaling (Lee et al., 2020; Lipinski and Reaume, 2020). It was shown to lower blood glucose similarly to metformin in preclinical studies without a hypoglycemic episode. In addition, tolimidone is insulin-dependent and was shown to increase insulin sensitivity (Ochman et al., 2012).

Transporters

Another attractive agent is MSDC-0602K which acts as a mitochondrial membrane transport protein modulator that increases insulin sensitivity. Impaired mitochondrial function has been previously connected with the development of diabetes and its complications (Sivitz and Yorek, 2010). MSDC-0602K is the second generation of insulin sensitizers expected to have fewer side effects than the first-generation compounds. It is planned to start phase III clinical trials in 2022 (Harrison et al., 2020).

Targets Not Currently Active in Clinical Development

11-beta-hydroxysteroid dehydrogenase 1 (EC 1.1.1.146) converts cortisone to cortisol, thus indirectly increasing glucose output in the liver via the ability of cortisol to activate corticoid receptors and transcription of phosphoenolpyruvate kinase. It was estimated that 11β-HSD1 activity increases in patients with T2DM, and hence why synthesizing potent inhibitors has looked promising. Several agents (e.g., Poxel, CNX-010, SAR-184841) have reached preclinical studies or early research phases, but there were no recent reports of further development. At least one 11β-HSD1 inhibitor, INCB13739, has completed phase II in clinical trials as an antihyperglycemic agent, but neither statements of development nor discontinuation were identified (Paranjeet et al., 2018; Shukla et al., 2019).Increased cannabinoid-1 (CB1) receptor activity can cause obesity and obesity-related T2DM; peripheral effects of CB1 antagonism are decreased bodyweight, improved glucose tolerance, increased adiponectin, and decreased insulin resistance. All of these consequences are favorable in regards to the treatment of hyperglycemia. However, CB1 antagonism in the central nervous system increases anxiety and depression (Lu et al., 2016). The first cannabinoid-1 receptor antagonist, rimonabant, initially approved in Europe for T2DM treatment, was subsequently withdrawn due to the risk of severe mood disorders (Williams et al., 2020). Another antagonist, Tetrahydrocannabivarin-9, has completed phase II in clinical trials but has not clinically progressed .

Major advancements within diabetes research have been made since the ground-breaking discovery of insulin in the early 1920s (Quianzon and Cheikh, 2012). Today's antihyperglycemic drugs target a variety of pathological mechanisms implicated in T2DM, ranging from insulin secretion (e.g., SUs), peripheral glucose uptake (e.g., biguanides) and glucose reabsorption (e.g., SGLT2 inhibitors) (Chaudhury et al., 2017). Although insulin analogues remain a reliable approach to treat late stage T2DM, insulin therapy is no longer used in the initial stages of the disease. Over the past decades, the number of approved insulin analogues on the pharmaceutical market has remained relatively constant. However, the FDA recently withdrew approval of two insulin combinations (Ryzodeg was discontinued in 2018, and Novolog Mix 50/50 in 2019); while novel combinations containing insulins and GLP1R agonists have been approved, such as Xultophy (insulin degludec/ liraglutide) and Soliqua (insulin glargine/lixisenatide). Since 1995, metformin has become the leading antihyperglycemic agent in the initial stages of T2DM and in combination with other drugs in the later stages (13 out of 24 drug combinations approved by the FDA contain metformin). Recent approvals have been made for triple drug combinations containing metformin and other modern antihyperglycemic drugs, including four unique formulae with SGLT2is and two metformin/ SGLT2i/DPP4is.

In conclusion, there has been major progress in T2DM pharmacological therapy during the last decade. The rapid pace in which diabetology is developing makes it challenging to keep up with the interesting and innovative therapeutic approaches currently used. Therefore, we considered it necessary to compile up to date antihyperglycemic drugs approved by the FDA and explore recent data on new potential antidiabetic agents. Our review provides key points regarding each significant class of antihyperglycemic drugs, gives insight into which treatment options have been successful, and the novel mechanisms currently explored in clinical development.

V. Novel Antiplatelet Therapies for Atherothrombotic Diseases

Antiplatelet therapies are an essential tool to reduce the risk of developing clinically apparent atherothrombotic disease and are a mainstay in the therapy of patients who have established cardiovascular, cerebrovascular, and peripheral artery disease. Strategies to intensify antiplatelet regimens are limited by concomitant increases in clinically significant bleeding. The development of novel antiplatelet therapies targeting additional receptor and signaling pathways, with a focus on maintaining antiplatelet efficacy while preserving hemostasis, holds tremendous potential to improve outcomes among patients with atherothrombotic diseases. Atherosclerosis is a pan-vascular arterial disease process involving the coronary, cerebral, and peripheral arteries and remains the leading cause of mortality in the urbanized areas.1 The common pathophysiologic pathway of atherosclerosis ends in narrowing or obliteration of the arterial lumen through erosion or rupture of lipid-laden and highly inflammatory plaques, with subsequent thrombosis. The clinical manifestations correspond directly to the organ system affected, although atherosclerosis in 1 vascular bed is predictive of disease in other territories. Antiplatelet therapy remains a cornerstone in the management of patients with atherothrombotic diseases. The use of single or dual antiplatelet therapy (DAPT) regimens has been effective in reducing cardiovascular events among patients with stable coronary artery disease (CAD), acute coronary syndrome (ACS), peripheral artery disease (PAD), and cerebrovascular disease. During the past several years, oral and intravenous antiplatelet therapies have been developed with escalating potency to reduce further clinical atherothrombotic events among at-risk patients However, adoption of these agents has occurred with a concomitant increase in clinically significant bleeding. Consequently, there has been an interest in additional strategies to improve net clinical outcomes, such as the development of tools to predict individual bleeding and ischemic risk, minimizing antiplatelet exposure among patients with low ischemic or high bleeding risk, and improving percutaneousstent technologiesto mitigate late thrombotic risks. Additionally, there are now focused and innovative efforts to develop novel pharmacotherapies which target receptors and pathways in the thrombotic process while preserving the normal hemostatic function of platelets. Here, we review current state-of-the-art and novel antiplatelet strategies to treat atherothrombotic diseases.

Established Antiplatelet Therapies

Aspirin

Aspirin nonselectively and irreversibly acetylates a serine residue on the COX (cyclooxygenase) enzymes, suppressing the production of prostaglandins and TxA2 (thromboxane A2), a potent platelet activator. Aspirin is a foundation in antiplatelet regimens, both as a single agent, and in combination with other antiplatelet or antithrombotic agents, particularly for the secondary prevention of cardiovascular events. The landmark Antithrombotic Trialists' Collaboration meta-analysis of 287 studies including 212 000 patients demonstrated the efficacy of aspirin in reducing nonfatal myocardial infarction (MI), stroke, and cardiovascular death among patients with ACS (new or old), stroke, or who were at increased risk for vascular events.2 Based on this evidence, aspirin is commonly used for secondary prevention in patients with CAD, cerebrovascular accident, and PAD. The role of aspirin for primary prevention of cardiovascular disease remains controversial and a topic of ongoing clinical investigation. A recent study randomized 19 114 patients in Australia and the United States who were ≥70 years of age (or ≥65 years among blacks and Hispanics in the United States) without cardiovascular disease to receive 100 mg of enteric-coated aspirin or placebo.3 After a median of 4.7 years of follow-up, there was no improvement in the rates of cardiovascular disease between groups but a significantly higher risk of hemorrhage among those randomized to aspirin.A separate study randomized 15 480 patients with diabetes mellitus but without clinically apparent cardiovascular disease to receive enteric coated aspirin at a dose of 100 mg daily or placebo.4 After a mean follow-up of 7.4 years, there was a 12% reduction in serious vascular events, although a 29% increase in major bleeding rates among aspirin-treated patients. Finally, a recent study of 12 546 patients across 7 countries with a moderate estimated risk of first cardiovascular event randomized to enteric-coated aspirin 100 mg daily or placebo followed for a median of 60 months found no difference in rates of cardiovascular events but a >2-fold increase in gastrointestinal bleeding events.5 Thus, the potential role of aspirin in primary prevention seems confined to high-risk primary prevention (based on older studies) or patients with diabetes mellitus at low bleeding risk but at high ischemic risk.

P2Y12 Receptor Antagonists

The P2Y12 receptor is a G-protein coupled receptor which binds ADP, stored in platelet dense granules until platelet activation. ADP binding to the P2Y12 receptor inhibits adenylate cyclase–mediated signaling and the formation of cyclic AMP, which consequently enhances sustained platelet aggregation through intracellular signal activation and conformational changes of the GP (glycoprotein) IIb/IIIa receptor. These conformational changes in the GP IIb/IIIa receptor augment its affinity for its major ligand, soluble fibrinogen. This sequence may be interrupted by various P2Y12 receptor antagonists.

Clopidogrel

Clopidogrel is an oral, irreversible, competitive, thienopyridine P2Y12 receptor antagonist, which has been widely studied and shown to reduce cardiovascular events among patients with atherosclerotic disease. Among high-risk patients with ischemic stroke, MI, or established PAD, clopidogrel monotherapy was associated with a 7.9% relative risk reduction in MI, ischemic stroke, vascular death, or rehospitalization compared with aspirin.6 Among patients with ACS, the addition of clopidogrel to aspirin reduces ischemic events by 20% in the first 30 days and results in similar reductions between 30 days and 12 months of treatment.7 Additionally, a subgroup analysis of the CHARISMA trial (Clopidogrel for High Atherothrombotic Risk and Ischemic Stabilization, Management, and Avoidance) suggested that patients with a history of MI, ischemic stroke, or symptomatic PAD, may benefit from escalation on antiplatelet therapy with the addition of clopidogrel to aspirin for the reduction for cardiovascular death, MI, or stroke.8,9 Current practice patterns suggest a high utilization of DAPT even beyond 12 months, particularly among patients with CAD. Among patients with ACS in Europe and Asia, a recent study demonstrated that 57% of patients were receiving DAPT beyond 12 months. In another registry cohort of patients from the United States, France, Germany, Italy, and Greece, 43% of patients with ACS and 57% of patients who underwent elective percutaneous coronary intervention (PCI) received DAPT at the end of 2 years of follow-up.The role of clopidogrel in the treatment of stroke and transient ischemic attack (TIA) has been recently investigated. The CHANCE trial (Clopidogrel in High-Risk Patients With Acute Nondisabling Cerebrovascular Events) was a randomized, double-blind, placebo-controlled trial that randomly assigned patients with small ischemic strokes or high-risk TIA to a combination of clopidogrel and aspirin or aspirin alone for 90 days.12 The study, conducted in a Chinese population, demonstrated a reduction in stroke with combination therapy (8.2% versus 11.7%; hazard ratio [HR], 0.68; 95% CI, 0.57–0.81; p<0.001), without an increased risk of moderate or severe hemorrhage. Recently, the POINT trial (Platelet-Oriented Inhibition in New TIA and Minor Ischemic Stroke) tested this hypothesis in an international population and confirmed a reduction in major ischemic strokes (5.0% versus 6.5%; HR, 0.75; 95% CI, 0.59–0.95; p=0.02), but demonstrated an increase in major hemorrhage with combination therapy (0.9% versus 0.4%; HR, 2.32; 95% CI, 1.10–4.87; p=0.02).

Recent investigations have sought to determine whether a pharmacogenetic-guided strategy to the use of clopidogrel as anti-platelet therapy may be beneficial. Clopidogrel is a prodrug that is extensively metabolized by the liver, mediated by the cytochrome P450 system. Clopidogrel is first metabolized to the 2-oxo-clopidogrel intermediate metabolite, with subsequent metabolism yielding a thiol derivative which is the active metabolite. This pathway is mediated by CYP3A4, CYP2C19, CYPA12, and CYP2B6.14 Ex vivo platelet aggregation studies have demonstrated differences in antiplatelet effects of clopidogrel according to the CYP2C19 genotype. Specifically, the CYP2C19*1 allele yields fully functional metabolism, whereas the CYP2C19*2 and CYP2C19*3 alleles yield reduced metabolism and antiplatelet therapy. The association between CYP2C19 genotype and clinical outcomes among patients receiving clopidogrel therapy is not well established. A recent multisite investigation of 1815 patients sought to determine whether genotype-guided antiplatelet therapy improved outcomes among patients undergoing PCI.15 In this study, 31.5% of patients had a loss of function allele. Among those with a loss of function allele who received clopidogrel versus alternative antiplatelet therapy, there was a 2-fold risk of cardiovascular events, whereas there was no significant difference in major adverse cardiovascular events rates among those with a loss of function allele treated with an alternate antiplatelet agent and those without a loss of function allele treated with clopidogrel. This strategy has yet to be established as beneficial in a randomized trial setting Overall, the primary role of clopidogrel in CAD remains as an adjunct to aspirin in DAPT regimens after PCI and for treatment of ACS with or without PCI.18 The addition of clopidogrel to aspirin may be reasonable for treatment of patients with a small stroke or TIA within 24 hours for 21 days and for patients with recent stroke or TIA within 30 days attributable to severe stenosis of a major intracranial artery for a duration of 90 days. Additionally, clopidogrel in addition to aspirin may be reasonable in select patients with symptomatic PAD after lower extremity revascularization to prevent limb-related events.

Prasugrel

Prasugrel is an oral, irreversible, competitive, thienopyridine P2Y12 receptor antagonist. Prasugrel is approved only for patients with CAD who present with ACS and undergo PCI, based on results of the TRITON-TIMI 38 study (Trial of Assess Improvement in Therapeutic Outcomes by Optimizing Platelet Inhibition With Prasugrel-Thrombolysis in Myocardial Infarction 38).23 In this randomized study of 13 608 patients, prasugrel in addition to aspirin, lead to a 19% risk reduction of cardiovascular (CV) death, MI, or stroke compared with the combination of clopidogrel and aspirin. Subgroup analyses additionally revealed a lack of net clinical benefit and higher rates of major bleeding among patients age ≥75 years and with body weight <60 kg. Prasugrel is also contraindicated in patients with prior TIA or stroke.The TRITON-TIMI 38 trial did not assess the role of prasugrel in medical management of ACS. However, the TRILOGY ACS study (Targeted Platelet Inhibition to Clarify the Optimal Strategy to Medically Manage Acute Coronary Syndromes) did not demonstrate improvement in the composite outcome of death, MI, or stroke among either patients under the age of 75 years or the entire study population when treated with prasugrel compared with clopidogrel for the medical management of ACS.However, there was a significant benefit with prasugrel over clopidogrel in TRILOGY ACS in those patients who had undergone coronary angiography, perhaps representing those patients who had true ACS versus troponin elevation because of other causes. Current guidelines suggest that prasugrel in place of clopidogrel is a reasonable option for antiplatelet therapy in addition to aspirin for patients with ACS treated with PCI.

Ticagrelor

Ticagrelor is an oral, direct acting, noncompetitive, reversible cyclopentyl triazolopyrimidine P2Y12 receptor antagonist. Compared with the thienopyridines, ticagrelor does not require hepatic metabolism for activation, is more rapidly acting, and more potent.The landmark PLATO (Study of Platelet Inhibition and Patient Outcomes) randomized 18 624 patients presenting with ACS to ticagrelor or clopidogrel in addition to aspirin.26 The study demonstrated a 16% risk reduction for the composite end point of CV mortality, MI, or stroke (9.8% versus 11.7%; HR, 0.84; 95% CI, 0.77–0.92; p<0.001), as well as a significant reduction in all-cause mortality (4.5% versus 5.9%; p<0.001) with ticagrelor. Ticagrelor was associated with higher rates of major noncoronary artery bypass grafting related bleeding and higher rates of intracranial hemorrhage.A strategy of long term DAPT with ticagrelor and aspirin was evaluated among patients with a history of MI in the PEGASUS-TIMI 54 study (Prevention of Cardiovascular Events in Patients With Prior Heart Attack Using Ticagrelor Compared to Placebo on a Background of Aspirin–Thrombolysis in Myocardial Infarction 54).27 This study randomized 21 162 patients with a history of MI 1 to 3 years before enrollment to receive ticagrelor 90 mg twice daily, ticagrelor 60 mg twice daily, or placebo, in addition to low-dose aspirin. After 33 months of follow-up, there was a 16% risk reduction in the composite outcome of CV death, MI, or stroke in the group that received 60 mg of ticagrelor twice daily (7.77% versus 9.04%; HR, 0.84; 95% CI, 0.74–0.95; p=0.004), with an increase in major bleeding compared with the placebo-controlled study arm. A PEGASUS-TIMI 54 substudy of patients with PAD demonstrated a 4.1% absolute reduction in major adverse cardiovascular events

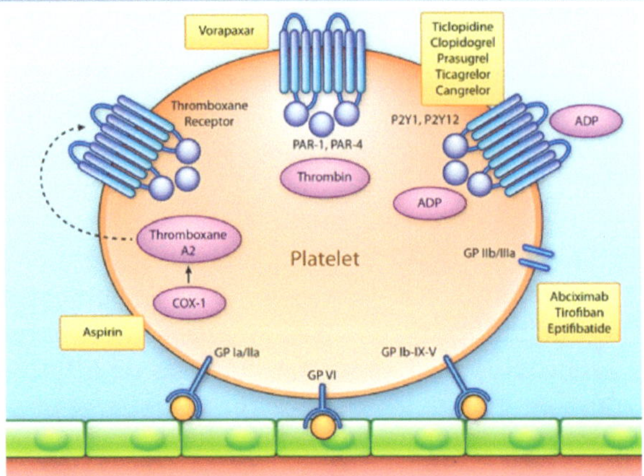

Fig.18.4 Commonly used and approved antiplatelet drugs and their targets. Platelet activation and aggregation occur through a complex interplay involving several platelet receptors and their ligands. Platelet adhesion initially occurs through interactions between GP (glycoprotein) Ib and von Willebrand factor, and GP VI and subendothelial collagen. Platelet activation additionally occurs through interactions of soluble agonists, such as TXA2 (thromboxane A2), and ADP which binds the P2Y12 receptor, promoting platelet aggregation. Intracellular signaling leads to conformation changes and activation of the GP IIb/IIIa receptor, enhancing its affinity for its major ligand, fibrinogen, which allows linking of platelets. The drugs depicted interrupt these pathways to provide antiplatelet activity. COX indicates cyclooxygenase; and PAR, protease activating receptor.

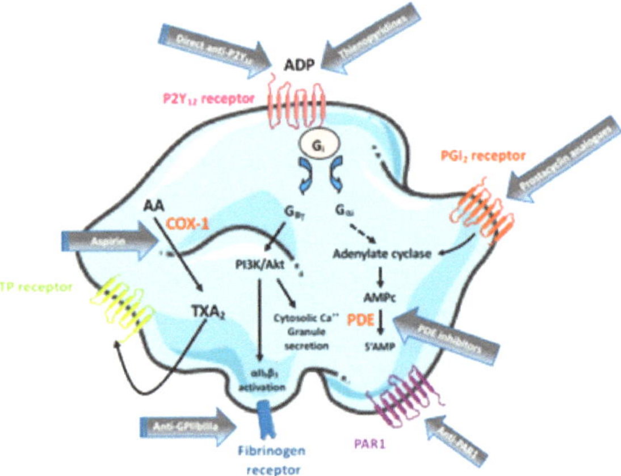

Fig.18.5 Targetsof the commercialized antiplatelet agents. Arachidonic acid (AA) is produced by membrane phospholipids upon the action of phospholipase A2. It is metabolized in cyclic endoperoxydes by the cycloxygenase-1 (COX-1) enzyme, then in thromboxane A2 (TXA2) by the thromboxane synthase. TXA2 activates the Thromboxane Prostanoid (TP) receptor in return. ADP, by activating P2Y12 receptor, induces an inhibition of adenylate cyclase which downregulates cAMP (a powerful platelet inhibitor) synthesis. It also stimulates the phosphoinositide 3-kinase (PI3K) via Gβγ protein complex resulting in Akt stimulation, which activates a number of downstream substrate proteins thereby increasing the cytosolic Ca2+ levels and inducing granule secretion. Inversely, prostacyclin (PGI2) binds to its receptor on platelet surface and increases cAMP intraplatelet level. cAMP is metabolized by phosphodiesterases (PDE) in 5'AMP. Blocking ADP binding site with a P2Y12 receptor antagonist (including thienopyridines and direct anti-P2Y12), stimulating PGI2 receptor or inhibiting PDE maintains cAMP intraplatelet concentration at a high level thus keeping platelets in a resting state. Following coagulation activation, thrombin is generated and cleaves its receptor on platelet surface, i.e., the protease-activated receptor 1 (PAR1), resulting in its activation. TP, P2Y12, or PAR1 activation leads to a conformational change of the glycoprotein (GP)IIbIIIa (also called the integrin αIIbβ3) on platelet surface which links fibrinogen resulting in platelet aggregation. This figure does not aim to represent platelet physiology with the different signaling pathways. It rather illustrates in a very simple manner the targets of the currently available antiplatelet drugs.

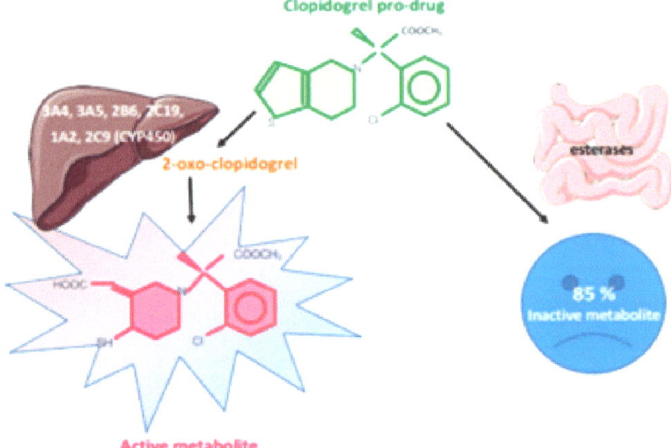

Fig.18.6 Clopidogrel metabolism pathways. Clopidogrel is a pro-drug. Eighty-five percent of the administered dose is metabolized into an inactive metabolite by intestinal esterases. The remaining 15% undergoes two sequential oxidative reactions involving several CYP enzymes leading, respectively, to 2-oxo-clopidogrel then to the active metabolite.

The subgroup with diabetes mellitus also showed significant relative and absolute benefits with ticagrelor, including lower CV mortality.The role of ticagrelor monotherapy among patients with PAD was assessed in the EUCLID study (Examining Use of Ticagrelor in Peripheral Artery Disease), which did not demonstrate a significant improvement in the composite primary outcome of CV death, MI, or ischemic stroke compared with clopidogrel.30 Ticagrelor monotherapy for nonsevere ischemic stroke or high-risk TIA was assessed in the international SOCRATES study (Acute Stroke or Transient Ischaemic Attack Treated With Aspirin or Ticagrelor and Patient Outcomes) and did not demonstrate a significant reduction in time to occurrence of stroke, MI, or death within 90 days compared with aspirin. Combination therapy with ticagrelor and aspirin for acute ischemic stroke or TIA is being evaluated in the THALES trial (Acute Stroke or Transient Ischaemic Attack Treated With Ticagrelor and Aspirin for Prevention of Stroke or Death; Unique identifier: NCT03354429). The role of ticagrelor monotherapy compared with aspirin after PCI with a drug-eluting stent is being evaluated in the TWILIGHT (Ticagrelor with Aspirin or Along in High-Risk Patients After Coronary Intervention) and TICO (Ticagrelor Monotherapy After 3 Months in the Patients Treated With New Generation Sirolimus Stent for Acute Coronary Syndrome.There has additionally been interest in leveraging potential off-target effects of ticagrelor and other antiplatelet agents. However, a recent study of the effects of ticagrelor, prasugrel, and clopidogrel on endothelial function and vascular biomarkers found no difference in the reactive hyperemia index or biomarker levels in a population of post-ACS patients treated with the various agents.33 Additionally, the study found no evidence that ticagrelor increases plasma adenosine levels compared with other antiplatelet agents, although this has been previously implicated as a mechanism to explain ticagrelor related side effects, including bradycardia and dyspnea.

Overall, current evidence supports ticagrelor as a first line agent for ACS with or without PCI in addition to aspirin, and for long term therapy among patients with a history of MI, assuming they are at low bleeding risk. The role of ticagrelor as an adjunct to aspirin in patients with stroke or PAD is uncertain, and the role of ticagrelor monotherapy in patients with CAD remains under investigation.

Cangrelor

Cangrelor is an intravenous, reversible, nonthienopyridine, ATP analog, P2Y12 receptor antagonist. Cangrelor has a rapid onset of action, with demonstrable platelet inhibition within 2 minutes, rapid reversibility with an elimination half-life of 3 to 6 minutes, and return of normal platelet function in 1 hour. Cangrelor was initially studied in the CHAMPION (Clopidogrel Versus Standard Therapy to Achieve Optimal Management of Platelet Inhibition) PCI and CHAMPION PLATFORM studies which suggested the possibility of a reduction in stent thrombosis without an excess of severe bleeding in patients treated with cangrelor. Subsequently, the pivotal CHAMPIONPHOENIX study prospectively evaluated the efficacy and safety of cangrelor versus clopidogrel pretreatment among patients undergoing urgent or elective PCI.36 The primary efficacy end point, a composite of all-cause mortality, MI, ischemia-driven revascularization, or stent thrombosis 48 hours after randomization was significantly reduced in the cangrelor-treated study arm (4.7% versus 5.9%; adjusted odds ratio, 0.78; 95% CI, 0.66–0.93; p=0.005), with no significant difference in the primary safety end point. A pooled analysis of patient-level data from the 3 trials of cangrelor additionally supported this finding and demonstrated that cangrelor was associated with a 19% reduction in odds for the composite outcome of death, MI, ischemia-driven revascularization, or stent thrombosis at 48 hours. Cangrelor use was also independently associated with a 38% reduction in odds for stent thrombosis (0.8% versus 1.4%; odds ratio, 0.62; 95% CI, 0.43–0.90; p=0.01).Real-world experience with cangrelor has supported a potential role among patients with cardiogenic shock, who are uniquely at risk for gut malabsorption and likely to benefit from direct acting, intravenous agents. However, these benefits must be balanced with the increased risk of bleeding among critically ill patients. Strategies to avoid potentiating bleeding risk in patients with and without cardiogenic shock, such as avoiding the concomitant use of glycoprotein IIb/IIIa inhibitors, are critical.Presently, no randomized clinical trial evidence among patients with cardiogenic shock is available. Cangrelor had additionally been used off-label as a bridging therapy before cardiac surgery after discontinuation of thienopyridines, offering the potential advantage of rapid reversal of antiplatelet action with discontinuation 1 hour before surgery.40 Additional evidence suggests that the benefits of cangrelor are maintained across several high-risk subgroups, including those with a history of stroke ≥1 year from the time of PCI, older patients, and in those on a background of anticoagulant therapy with heparin, without concomitant increases in the rates of major bleeding

Table18.5. FDA-approved antiplatelet agents

Drug*	Mechanism of action	Route of administration	Frequency	Side effects	Limitations
Aspirin	Irreversible acetylation of Ser529 of cyclooxygenase 1	Oral	Daily	• Bleeding • Gastrointestinal toxicity: heartburn, indigestion, nausea, vomiting and gastric ulceration	• Weak antiplatelet agent
Ticlopidine (Ticlid; Roche)	The active metabolite irreversibly inhibits $P2Y_{12}$ receptors	Oral	Twice daily	• Bleeding • Gastrointestinal toxicity: heartburn, indigestion, nausea and vomiting • Rash • Neutropaenia • Thrombotic thrombocytopaenic purpura (rare)	• More side effects than clopidogrel
Clopidogrel (Plavix; Bristol–Myers Squibb/ Sanofi–Aventis)	The active metabolite irreversibly inhibits $P2Y_{12}$ receptors	Oral	Daily	• Bleeding • Rash • Neutropaenia • Thrombotic thrombocytopaenic purpura (rare)	• Patient-to-patient variability in response
Prasugrel (Effient; Lilly/ Daiichi Sankyo)	The active metabolite irreversibly inhibits $P2Y_{12}$ receptors	Oral	Daily	• Bleeding	• More haemorrhagic side effects and greater cost than clopidogrel • Contraindicated in patients with a history of stroke or transient ischaemic attacks • Not recommended in patients >75 years old unless they are at high risk of cardiovascular events
Abciximab (ReoPro; Lilly)	Integrin αIIbβ3 antagonist	Intravenous	Once	• Bleeding • Thrombocytopaenia EDTA-induced pseudo-thrombocytopaenia	• Requires intravenous administration
Eptifibatide (Integrilin; Millennium Pharmaceuticals/ Shering–Plough)	Integrin αIIbβ3 antagonist	Intravenous	Once	• Bleeding • Thrombocytopaenia EDTA-induced pseudothrombocyto-paenia	• Requires intravenous administration
Tirofiban (Aggrastat; Merck)	Integrin αIIbβ3 antagonist	Intravenous	Once	• Bleeding • Thrombocytopaenia EDTA-induced pseudo-thrombocytopaenia	• Requires intravenous administration
Dipyridamole (Boehringer Ingelheim)	Antiplatelet and vasodilatory effects through inhibition of cyclic nucleotide phosphodiesterase- and of adenosine uptake	Oral	Two or three times daily	• Headache • Dizziness • Hypotension and blood pressure lability • Flushing • Gastrointestinal toxicity: nausea, vomiting, diarrhoea and abdominal pain • Rash	• Benefit is most evident in combination with low-dose aspirin
Cilostazol (Pletal; Otsuka)	Antiplatelet and vasodilatory effects through inhibition of cyclic nucleotide phosphodiesterase 3	Oral	Twice daily	• Bleeding • Headache • Diarrhoea • Palpitations • Dizziness • Rash • Pancytopaenia	• Side effects lead to discontinuation of the drug in ~15% of patients

EDTA, ethylenediaminetetra-acetic acid; FDA, US Food and Drug Administration; ND, not determined; $P2Y_{12}$, P2Y purinoceptor 12; *For chemical structu
Supplementary information S1 (figure).

PAR-1 Antagonists

The PAR (protease-activated receptor)-1 is the site of action of thrombin, which is highly active at sites of clotting. Vorapaxar is a competitive PAR-1 antagonist, which was studied among patients with a history of atherothrombotic events (MI, PAD, or stroke) in the TRA 2P TIMI 50 study (Thrombin Receptor Antagonist in Secondary Prevention of Atherothrombotic Ischemic Events– Thrombolysis in Myocardial Infraction 50).45 The majority of patients enrolled in the study were on background antiplatelet therapy with aspirin, and a significant proportion was additionally being treated with a thienopyridine or dipyramidole. The trial was stopped early in patients with a history of stroke because of evidence of increased rates of intracranial hemorrhage. However, compared with patients receiving placebo, there was a reduction in the composite end point of cardiovascular death, MI, or stroke at 3 years with vorapaxar (9.3% versus 10.5%; HR, 0.87; 95% CI, 0.80–0.94; P<0.001), primarily driven by a reduction in MI. This came at the expense of increased moderate or severe bleeding (4.2% versus 2.5%; HR, 1.66; 95% CI, 1.43–1.93; P<0.001) and an increase in the rate of intracranial hemorrhage in the vorapaxar group (1.0% versus 0.5% in the placebo group; P<0.001). Vorapaxar is contraindicated in patients with a history of stroke, TIA, or intracerebral hemorrhage.In a substudy of patients with symptomatic lower extremity PAD, vorapaxar was associated with a reduction in acute limb ischemia (2.3% versus 3.9%; HR, 0.58; 95% CI, 0.39–0.86; p=0.006) and reduction in peripheral artery revascularization (18.4% versus 22.2%; HR, 0.84; 95% CI, 0.73–0.97; p=0.017).47 However, in this cohort, bleeding occurred more frequently with vorapaxar (7.4% versus 4.5%; HR, 1.62; 95% CI, 1.21–2.18; p=0.001), and there was no reduction in the composite primary end point of cardiovascular death, MI, or stroke

Experimental Therapies

Current approaches to improving antiplatelet efficacy have relied on pharmacotherapies with increasing potency. However, in virtually all cases, increasing potency is linked to a concomitant increase in bleeding. This observation has led to a paradigm shift as new targets, and novel approaches for antiplatelet therapies are being developed. Instead of simply developing more potent therapies, preclinical and early clinical studies have supported the notion that thrombosis pathways may be targeted while preserving hemostasis and may, therefore, maintain efficacy while improving safety compared with currently available therapies

Developing thrombi are now known to consist of 2 distinct regions. The platelet response at the site of arterial injury comprises a core of fully activated platelets located close to the lesion and is highly dependent on soluble agonists such as thrombin. Separately, a propagating thrombus is composed primarily of platelets in lower activation states, and their recruitment is minimally sensitive to standard antiplatelet drugs. This distinction between the hemostatic response, which relies on the thrombus core, and the thrombotic response that regulates the growth of a propagating outer shell of thrombus has provided a conceptual framework for developing novel therapies.

Phosphatidylinositol 3 Kinase B

PI3KB (phosphatidylinositol 3 kinase B) is a lipid kinase with important functions in signaling pathways downstream of platelet receptor activation and for mediating platelet activation at sites of thrombus propagation. AZD6482 is a novel PI3KB inhibitor that has undergone preclinical and early clinical (phase I) study to determine its general safety and tolerability. In animal studies using a canine model, AZD6482 produced antithrombotic effects without any increase in bleeding time or blood loss. These effects extended to healthy human volunteers, and the drug demonstrated moderate platelet inhibition at levels between aspirin and clopidogrel. The beta isoform-selective PI3K inhibitor, TGX221, was shown to decrease cyclic flow reductions in a preclinical carotid artery stenosis model, without bleeding sequelae. Recent evidence suggests that P13KB also has a critical role in maintaining the integrity of a formed thrombus in an environment of elevated shear stress, and thus, inhibition of this pathway may theoretically increase the risk of thrombus embolization, although the clinical impact of this finding is yet uncertain and requires additional study

Protein Disulfide-Isomerase

PDI (protein disulfide-isomerase) exist in platelet granules and the platelet surface where they are involved in thrombosis through their action on several intravascular targets. PDI inhibitors in preclinical studies have been shown to reduce platelet aggregation and reduce thrombus formation under flow conditions, and have been shown to protect mice from carotid artery occlusion.54 The PDI inhibitor isoquercetin underwent phase I clinical study and was shown to diminish platelet-dependent thrombin generation by blocking generation of platelet factor Va. Isoquercetin is currently in phase II/III clinical study to evaluate its potential role in preventing venous thrombosis in patients with pancreatic, nonsmall cell lung, or colorectal cancer .The primary end point of the phase III portion of the study is the cumulative incidence of venous thromboembolic disease. A clinical role for isoquercetin and other PDI inhibitors in preventing arterial thrombosis in humans has not yet been established. Additional PDI inhibitors which have been shown to inhibit platelet aggregation and are not cytotoxic include rutinoside and the more potent, small molecule inhibitor ML359

Novel GP IIb/IIIa Receptor Antagonism

GP IIb/IIIa is a highly abundant platelet receptor and is the binding site for fibrinogen. GP IIb/IIIa has an essential role in platelet adhesion and aggregation. Current therapies targeting GP IIb/IIIa receptors are highly potent with a bleeding risk that limits their clinical utility for long-term therapy. However, it is now recognized that GP IIb/IIIa exists in both low- and high-affinity states. On platelet activation, signaling from within the platelet induces conformational changes of the receptor (inside-out signaling), allowing it to bind its primary ligand, soluble fibrinogen. Once a ligand binds to the GP IIb/IIIa receptor, so-called outside-in signaling is thought to mediate intracellular events which allow thrombus propagation and are distinct from those which allow hemostasis. Current GP IIb/IIIa inhibitors, which are ligand mimetic agents, may paradoxically potentiate platelet activation through this mechanismscFv (single-chain variable fragments) have been developed which target the GP IIb/IIIa receptor specifically in its high-affinity configuration. This strategy can block fibrinogen from binding to the receptor without potentiating outside-in signaling. In murine models and ex vivo primate models, these agents demonstrated potency similar to ligand mimetic agents without increases in bleeding. In addition, intracellular inhibitors of GP IIb/IIIa have been developed which disrupt integrin activation and switching to the high-affinity state or which can specifically inhibit outside-in signaling

Separately, the drugs RUC-1 and RUC-4, identified through high throughput screens for small molecule inhibitors of fibrinogen binding, are specific for the alpha IIb subunit of the GP IIb/IIIa receptor. These agents maintain the receptor in a low-affinity state, unable to bind its major ligand fibrinogen. Studies of RUC-4 have demonstrated that it does not induce conformational changes or platelet activation through outside-in signaling. Unlike a strategy of using scFvs, RUC-4 affects all platelets because its binding is not dependent on the receptor being in an active state, and evidence on its safety profile, particularly with respect to bleeding risk, is lacking at this time.These agents represent a renewed interest in the potential of GP IIb/IIIa antagonists to provide therapeutic antiplatelet benefits with an improved safety profile

PAR-4 Antagonists

Despite the efficacy of PAR-1 antagonists, their clinical utilization has been limited because of concerns for significant bleeding. Additional PAR-1 specific antagonists, including SCH 79797 and F 16618, remain under development.

However, thrombin activates platelets through its action on both PAR-1 and PAR-4. There has been growing interest in the role of PAR-4 receptor as a target for platelet antagonism. PAR-4 expression is highly dynamic and is altered by numerous thrombotic and inflammatory stimuli. The PAR-4 specific antagonist BMS-986120 completed a phase I clinical trial where it was demonstrated to provide selective and reversible PAR-4 antagonism and platelet aggregation. Ex vivo total thrombus area was significantly reduced, driven by reductions in platelet-rich thrombus deposits.64 Additionally, the drug was shown to have no effect on thrombus formation at low shear conditions and did not demonstrate an increase in coagulation time.

An additional PAR-4 specific antagonist, BMS-986141, was also developed with greater potency than BMS-986120. BMS-986141 was studied for reduction of stroke recurrence in a phase II clinical study among patients with history of stroke or TIA already on aspirin. An additional class of PAR-1 inhibitors, called paramodulins, have been developed which target the cytoplasmic face of PAR-1 without modifying the ligand binding site. This distinction may allow paramodulins to maintain the cytoprotective effects of PAR-1 signaling.65,66 This is a significant distinction from orthosteric antagonists, such as vorapaxar or atopaxar, which inhibit all signaling downstream of the PAR-1 receptor.

GP VI Mediated Adhesion Pathways

GP VI mediates platelet activation through binding of subendothelial collagen. Collagen binding promotes crosslinking of GP VI receptors, which facilitates platelet aggregation and activation through release of platelet agonists, such as ADP and TxA2, and activation of the GP IIB/IIIa receptor. Additionally, both experimental blockade and genetic deficiency of GP VI lead to reduced thrombus formation without major bleeding complications.70 For these reasons, GP VI is a site of significant interest as an antiplatelet target.

Revacept is a fusion protein comprising the extracellular domain of GP VI and a human Fc immunoglobulin region. It can bind immobilized collagen and prevent platelet adhesion and activation. A phase I clinical study of Revacept demonstrated dose-dependent inhibition of collagen-induced platelet activation without an increase in bleeding time.71 Studies in animal models suggest that Revacept may reduce thrombus formation and improve vascular endothelial function.72 In mouse cerebral infarct models, the addition of Revacept to varying doses of recombinant tissue plasminogen activator improved efficacy compared with r-tPA (recombinant tissue-type plasminogen activator) alone, without an increase in intracranial bleeding.73 It has also been suggested that Revacept may have a role as part of DAPT regimens, in addition to aspirin or P2Y12 receptor antagonist and has been shown to improve platelet inhibition as an adjunct to aspirin or ticagrelor. Phase II clinical studies of Revacept in patients with stable CAD ACT017 is an additional GP VI inhibitor currently under investigation. ACT017 is a humanized Fab fragment with high specificity and affinity for GP VI. It has undergone a dose escalation study and was shown to be effective in inhibiting collagen-induced platelet aggregation ex vivo after injection into a macaque. Additionally, there was no evidence of thrombocytopenia or excess bleeding with its use. The GP Ia/IIa receptor for collagen also remains another target of interest for antiplatelet therapies. Inhibitors of GP Ia/IIa may reduce thrombus formation after arterial injury in preclinical models

GP Ib/IX/V inhibition

The GP Ib/IX/V receptor binds to von Willebrand factor (vWF) during injury and under conditions of high shear stress, allowing early platelet adhesion to the subendothelium. The GP Ib/IX/V receptor and vWF have been proposed as additional antiplatelet targets, although antibodies developed against vWF have demonstrated unacceptably high rates of bleeding, leading to their discontinuation. ARC1779 is an intravenous oligonucleic acid aptamer that binds vWF and had entered phase II/III clinical study in patients undergoing carotid endarterectomy, but the study was halted because of lack of funding. Available data suggested that the drug reduced carotid embolic events but was associated with an excess of bleeding. The single-domain antibody caplacizumab, which also binds vWF, was studied in a phase I/II clinical trial among patient with stable angina and shown to improve peripheral endothelial function. The drug was also studied as an adjunct to DAPT in patients with ACS but was found to have prohibitive bleeding risk. However, caplacizumab has emerged as a potential treatment for patients with thrombotic thrombocytopenic purpura, where it has demonstrated significant reduction in thrombotic complications and is now poised for phase III study.The snake venom derivative anfibatide is a direct anti-GP Ib antagonist that also inhibits vWF. Anfibatide has been shown to inhibit platelet adhesion and aggregation in preclinical models and was protective of ischemic stroke and reperfusion injury in mice.A phase II clinical trial to assess the safety and efficacy of anfibatide in patients with ST-segment–elevation myocardial infarction before PCI is also underway . Additional preclinical agents, directly targeting GP Ib or the vWF binding domain, are under development at this time.

Novel P2Y12 and P2Y1 Inhibition

Novel, direct, P2Y12 inhibitors remain under development at this time, including the highly potent inhibitors ACT-246475, AZD1283, and SAR2164 ACT-246475 was associated with less bleeding, higher selectivity, and equivalent antithrombotic efficacy to ticagrelor in rat models and is now undergoing phase II study. The P2Y1 receptor initiates ADP induced platelet aggregation and shape change, whereas P2Y12 activation is responsible for amplification and stabilization. The potential of P2Y1 inhibition as an antiplatelet strategy to reduce bleeding risk has been recently explored. The compound BMS-884775 demonstrated similar efficacy with less bleeding compared with prasugrel in a rabbit model. In a preclinical study, the P2Y1 receptor antagonist MRS2500 was shown to prevent carotid artery thrombosis in cynomolgus monkeys.The potential of combined P2Y1 and P2Y12 receptor inhibition is also of interest and led to the development of the compound diadenosine tetraphosphate and additional derivative compounds.86 Of these, GLS-409 has shown significant potential in preclinical studies, where it has been shown to be highly potent, and to improve coronary blood flow recovery in a canine model of unstable angina, with minimal increase in bleeding time.

12-Lipoxygenase Inhibitors

12-LOX (platelet 12-lipoxygenase) is an oxygenase predominantly expressed in human platelets. 12-LOX utilizes arachidonic acid as a substrate to form bioactive metabolites that have been shown to play a role in platelet activation and granule secretion.89 For this reason, there is an interest in the utility of specific 12-LOX inhibitors as antiplatelet therapy. A recent study of the first inhibitor of 12-LOX, ML355, demonstrated dose-dependent inhibition of human platelet aggregation.89 Ex vivo flow chamber assays confirmed attenuation of platelet adhesion and thrombus formation at arterial shear over collagen in whole blood, with effects comparable to aspirin. Additionally, in a mouse model, oral ML355 treatment impaired thrombus growth in an arteriole thrombus model, with minimal bleeding.

Conclusions

Antiplatelet therapies remain an essential tool to reduce the risk of developing clinically apparent atherothrombotic disease and are a mainstay in the therapy of patients who have established cardiovascular, cerebrovascular, or peripheral artery disease. Strategies to intensify antiplatelet regimens should be complemented by approaches that focus on targeting thrombosis while preserving hemostasis. Several novel antiplatelet therapies which are being developed target a wide range of receptors and signaling pathways that have been unexplored and hold tremendous potential to improve patient outcomes by maintaining antiplatelet efficacy and preserving hemostasis Figure Figure2.2. Additional study in human subjects and with randomized trials will clearly be required before such agents can be widely disseminated, but their therapeutic promise gives reason for optimism and excitement in the treatment of atherothrombotic diseases.

V1. Recent Advances in Anticoagulant Treatment of Immune Thrombosis:

For more than 10 years, direct oral anticoagulants (DOACs) have been increasingly prescribed for the prevention and treatment of thrombotic events However, their use in immunothrombotic disorders, namely heparin-induced thrombocytopenia (HIT) and antiphospholipid syndrome (APS), is still under investigation. The prothrombotic state resulting from the autoimmune mechanism, multicellular activation, and platelet count decrease, constitutes similarities between HIT and APS. Moreover, they both share the complexity of the biological diagnosis. Current treatment of HIT firstly relies on parenteral non-heparin therapies, but DOACs have been included in American and French guidelines for a few years, providing the advantage of limiting the need for treatment monitoring. In APS, vitamin K antagonists are conversely the main treatment (+/− anti-platelet agents), and the use of DOACs is either subject to precautionary recommendations or is not recommended in severe APS. While some randomized controlled trials have been conducted regarding the use of DOACs in APS, only retrospective studies have examined HIT. In addition, vaccine-induced immune thrombotic thrombocytopenia (VITT) is now a part of immunothrombotic disorders, and guidelines have been created concerning an anticoagulant strategy in this case. This literature review aims to summarize available data on HIT, APS, and VITT treatments and define the use of DOACs in therapeutic strategies.

Since 2008, direct oral anticoagulants (DOACs) have been increasingly prescribed for the treatment and prevention of thromboembolic events. Their efficacy and safety are well documented for the prevention of thromboembolism events in the case of non-valvular atrial fibrillation and for the treatment and prevention of venous thromboembolism (VTE) and pulmonary embolism (PE) but their efficacy for immunothromboembolic disorders requires further investigation, particularly in antiphospholipid syndrome (APS) and heparin-induced thrombocytopenia (HIT). DOACs have also been recently proposed for the treatment of vaccine-induced immune thrombotic thrombocytopenia (VITT), which rarely appears after administering adenovirus-vector-based vaccines against the severe acute respiratory syndrome CoronaVirus-19 (SARS-CoV-2). DOACs provide advantages, including oral administration, rapid onset of anticoagulant effects, fixed doses for each indication, fewer drug interactions, and no routine laboratory monitoring. They are thus easier to manage than vitamin K antagonists (VKA) and parenteral anticoagulant drugs; however, they display a long half-life and have limited use in patients with renal or hepatic dysfunction or with altered gut absorption. In this review we aim to

Table 18.6 **Comparison of HIT and APS.**

	HIT	APS
Clinical expression	Thrombosis Thrombocytopenia +++	Thrombosis and/or obstetrical events Thrombocytopenia
Main immunoglobulin isotype	IgG1 and IgG3 (IgM)	IgG2 IgM
Antibody targets	PF4/H complexes	β2GPI-CL PS/PT
Cellular activation	Multicellular activation via FcγRII (on platelets +++, endothelial cells, monocytes, neutrophils)	Multicellular activation via activation cascades of intracellular kinases
	TF expression and secretion of procoagulant microparticles	
Mechanism of platelet activation and thrombocytopenia	Strong platelet activation FcγRII +++	Weak platelet activation F(ab')2 ++ (FcγRII)
Recommended laboratory tests	Detection of anti-PF4/H antibodies Platelet functional assays	Detection of anti-CL, anti-β2GPI, or LAC activity; twice, 12 weeks apart.
Standard care	Non-heparin treatment (argatroban, danaparoid, bivalirudin, fondaparinux) Contraindication of VKA until platelet count = 150 G/L	VKA +/- low-dose aspirin LMWH
DOAC use	Recommended in stable patients Rivaroxaban +++	Still debated Contraindicated in triple-positive patients Not recommended in patients with arterial thrombosis
DOAC RCT	None	Cohen H. et al., 2016 [6]

APS: antiphospholipid syndrome; CL: cardiolipin; β2GPI: β2 glycoprotein I; DOAC: direct oral anticoagulant; HIT: heparin-induced thrombocytopenia; Ig: Immunoglobulin; LAC: Lupus anticoagulant; LMWH: low molecular weight heparin; PF4/H: platelet factor 4/heparin; PS/PT: phosphatidylserine/prothrombin; RCT: randomized controlled trial; TF: tissue factor; VKA: vitamin K antagonist.

to summarize available data regarding the use of DOACs in immunothrombotic diseases with a focus on HIT, APS, and VITT.

Differences and Similarities between HIT andAPS

HIT and APS are two immunothrombotic disorders with challenging anticoagulation strategies. Both are responsible for venous and/ or arterial thrombosis affecting large vessels and microcirculation, and APS is sometimes accompanied by obstetrical morbidity, mainly recurrent fetal loss . The prevalence of HIT is estimated at 20,000 cases/year in the USA (1/1500 to 1/5000 hospitalizations) , while the incidence of APS is estimated at 40–50cases/100,000persons

In APS, the immune reaction is mediated by antiphospholipids (aPL) antibodies directed against cardiolipin, β2-glycoprotein I (β2GPI), and/ or phosphatidylserine/prothrombin (PS/PT) complexes. These antibodies have the potential to prolong coagulation time in laboratory tests, which is called lupus anticoagulant (LAC) activity. Cardiolipin is an anionic phospholipid (PL) of the mitochondrial membrane also present in plasma, while β2GPI (also called apolipoprotein H) is a five "sushi domains" glycoprotein synthesized by the liver, with a high affinity for negatively charged molecules such as cardiolipin. The conformation of platelet factor4 (PF4) is modified when bound to heparin, whereby β2GPI changes its 3D conformation secondary to cardiolipin bonding via its domain 5, from a close (O shape) to an open conformation (J and S shape), leading to the exposure of pathogenic antibodies binding-sites on domain 1. These antibodies induce a dimerization of the glycoprotein, which further increases β2GPI affinity for negatively charged PL, triggering various membrane receptors (Apolipoprotein E Receptor 2, GPIb, Toll-like receptors, GPVI) and intracellular signaling pathways, thereby resulting in the activation of many kinases Diagnosing these two pathologies requires further expertise than a single detection of immunoglobulins (Ig). Indeed, HIT antibodies must be able to activate platelets as evidenced by platelet functional assays (namely serotonin-release assay (SRA), heparin-induced platelet aggregation (HIPA), or light transmission aggregometry) while in APS, aPL must persist for at least 12 weeks to be considered as a diagnostic criterion

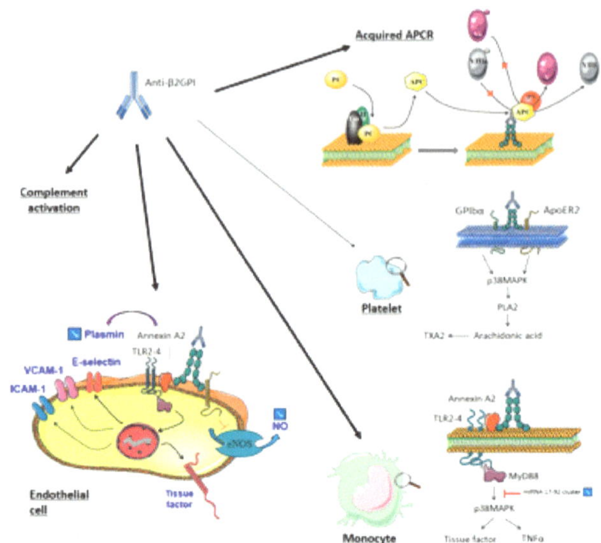

Fig.18.7 Mechanism of action of anti-β2GPI antibodies in APS. Adapted from Masliah-Planchon J. et al., Rev. Med. Int., 2012 [14]. Anti-β2GPI antibodies bind to negative phospholipids of endothelial cells, monocytes, and, to a lesser extent, platelets. By interacting with membrane receptors (GPIbα, ApoER2, TLR, and annexin A2), they trigger the activation of many intracellular kinases, thereby modulating the expression of procoagulant and anticoagulant molecules. In addition, this binding to membrane phospholipids induces acquired APCR by preventing the formation of coagulation factor complexes on the cell surface which reduces inhibition of factor Va and VIIIa by protein C/ protein S complex. These antibodies are also involved in complement activation. APCR: activated protein C resistance; ApoER2: apolipoprotein E receptor 2; GP: glycoprotein; ICAM1: intracellular adhesion molecule; MAPK: mitogen-activated protein kinases; miRNA: microRNA; PC: protein C; PS: protein S; PLA2: phospholipase A2; TLR: toll-like receptor; TM: thrombomodulin; TXA2: thromboxane A2; VCAM: vascular cell adhesion molecule.

The link between Ig emergence and thromboembolic events regards a multicellular activation. In HIT, anti-PF4/heparin (PF4/H) antibodies activate platelets upon binding with FcγRIIA receptors, thereby triggering the secretion of granules and production of membrane microparticles, ultimately resulting in thrombocytopenia In APS, a mild thrombocytopenia (platelet count between 30 and 100 G/L) is observed in 22% of cases , which appears secondary to antibodies directed against platelet membrane glycoprotein (GP) IbIX and GPIIbIIIa. Pardos-Gea J et al. recently have associated thrombocytopenia with poor long-term prognoses, where thrombocytopenic patients have a higher risk of death secondary to thrombosis (15% vs. 1%) . Moreover, the onset or worsening of thrombocytopenia may be a sign of thrombosis or a catastrophic APS. A recent study also showed that anti-prothrombin (aPT) antibodies inducing LAC activity are able to trigger platelet activation mediated by FcγRII . In APS and HIT, monocytes and endothelial cells are also activated, leading to tissue factor expression and coagulation activation, thereby increasing thrombin generation and the release of procoagulant microparticles. Moreover, neutrophil adhesion to endothelial cells is enhanced, resulting in neutrophils extracellular traps (NETs) formation. Another molecular aspect in APS pathophysiology is the modulation of microRNA (miRNA) levels, which results in the increase of tissue factor expression in monocytes and in the development of a pro-inflammatory response whereby miRNA effects pro and anti-inflammatory cytokines levels .

HIT and APS, therefore, represent procoagulant disorders that may be life-threatening and that require rapid management, including primary or secondary prevention of thrombosis. In HIT, 20% to50% of patients who develop thrombocytopenia sufferfromnewor progressive thromboembolic complications .

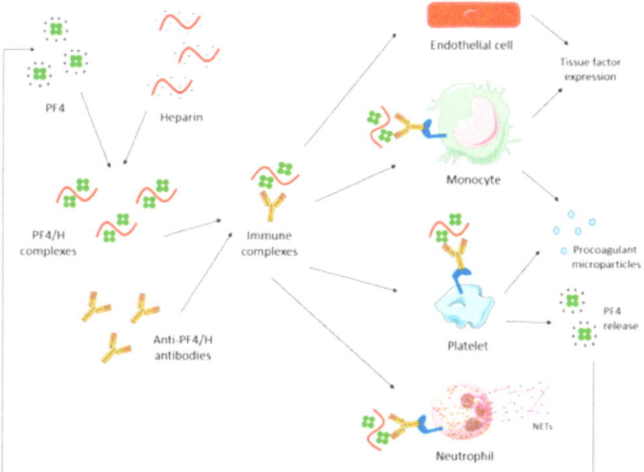

Fig.18.8 HIT pathophysiology. Antibodies directed against PF4/H complexes induce a multicellular activation, leading to the production of procoagulant microparticles from platelets and monocytes, the tissue factor expression by endothelial cells and monocytes, and the production of NETs by neutrophils. NETs: Neutrophil extracellular traps; PF4: platelet factor 4; PF4/H: PF4/heparin.

HIT: Diagnosis and Standard of Care

Diagnosing HIT is of crucial importance and remains challenging. HIT diagnosis is based on clinical and biological features, and the risk of developing HIT is high (>1%) in cases of unfractionated heparin (UFH) treatment in medical, surgical, obstetrical, or circulatory assistance contexts.

HIT should be suspected whenever the platelet count drops by 50% or when new thrombosis occurs in a patient 5 to 14 days after beginning heparin therapy. The 4Ts score represents a reliable prediction tool that considers the degree of platelet count decrease, the time to onset of platelets decrease, the occurrence of thrombosis while receiving heparin treatment, and the presence of other causes of thrombocytopenia . When the 4Ts score is 3 or less, the probability of HIT is low, and heparin treatment can be continued; with a score of 4 or 5, the probability of HIT is intermediate, while a 4T score ≥6 highly favors HIT When the HIT probability is intermediate to high, an anti-PF4/H antibodies enzyme-linked immunosorbent assay (ELISA) must be performed as soon as possible, which conveys an accurate negative predictive value (varying between 96.5% and 98.9%, depending on the kit used) and can quickly rule out HIT diagnosis When ELISA is positive, functional platelet assays should be performed in order to confirm the capacity of anti-PF4/H antibodies to activate platelets from healthy donors in the presence of heparin, thereby confirming the HIT diagnosis . SRA is a common functional assay and is considered the gold standard for HIT diagnosis. This assay measures serotonin release from platelets previously incubated with radioactive serotonin in the presence of low or high heparin concentration or in the absence of heparin . Other tests are available, including light transmission aggregometry, HIPA , and flow cytometry-based assays. Functional assays confirm HIT diagnoses when platelet activation is observed only in the presence of a low concentration of heparin, thereby indicating that the platelets' activation by HIT antibodies depends on heparin.As soon as HIT is clinically suspected, with at least an intermediate probability 4Ts score, heparin treatment must immediately be ceased and replaced by a non-heparin agent where the latter should have a rapid onset of anticoagulant effect. Until recently, the only therapeutic options for these patients were parenteral anticoagulant drugs, including argatroban, bivalirudin, danaparoid, and fondaparinux.

The French Working Group on Perioperative Haemostasis (GIHP) recommends argatroban as a first-line treatment except for patients with severe hepatic impairment.

Danaparoid is a mixture of heparan, dermatan, and chondroitin sulfates which potentiates the anticoagulant activity of antithrombin, thereby inhibiting the activated factor Xa and thrombin to a much lesser extent. Danaparoid has a long half-life (≈25 h) and can be safely used in patients with non-severe renal insufficiency.The GIHP does not recommend prophylactic doses of danaparoid for the treatment of acute HIT; instead, curative IV doses should be prescribed, and treatment efficacy should be monitored using specific anti-Xa activity not represent safe alternative drugs as long as the hypercoagulable state persists .Fondaparinux represents an attractive alternative treatment of HIT and is a subcutaneous factor Xa inhibitor prescribed off-label in HIT patients. It does not require any systematic laboratory monitoring, and the bridging to VKA is simple since fondaparinux does not affect global hemostasis assays, particularly the prothrombin time and the international normalized ratio (INR) values. Fondaparinux is also renally cleared, which means that kidney function should be considered in treated patients VKA should not be used in acute HIT, and their

Table 18.7 **Estimating the pre-test probability of heparin induced thrombocytopenia: the "4 T's"**

Category	2 points	1 point	0 point
Thrombocytopenia	>50% fall, or nadir of 20–100×10^9/l	30–50% fall, or nadir of 10–19×10^9/l	30% fall or nadir <10×10^9/l
Timing of platelet count fall	Days 5 to 10, or ⩽1 day if heparin exposure within past 30 days	>Day 10 or unclear (but its with HIT), or ⩽1 day if heparin exposure within past 30–100 days	⩽1 day (no recent heparin)
Thrombosis or other sequelae	Proven thrombosis, skin necrosis, or, after heparin bolus, acute systemic reaction	Progressive, recurrent, or silent thrombosis; erythematous skin lesions	None
Other cause for thrombocytopenia	None evident	Possible	Deinit e

*Points assigned in each of four categories are totalled, and the pre-test probability of HIT by total points is as follows: 6 to 8=high, 4 to 5=intermediate; 0 to 3=low. Adapted with permission from Warkentin *et al. Hematology/the education program of the American Society of Hematology*. Copyright 2003, American Society of Hematology.

introduction must be delayed until normal platelet count recovery. In addition, switching to VKA in an acute HIT setting exposes the patient to a risk of warfarin-induced skin necrosis and gangrene due to the depletion of protein C and protein S . Warkentin and Kelton showed a comparable rate of thrombosis if heparin is immediately switched to VKA or is ceased without any alternative anticoagulant therapy (10/21 vs. 20/36 HIT patients).

HIT: Update on DOACs Use

Rivaroxaban was the most studied DOACs in HIT. In 2016, Linkins, LA. et al. evaluated the efficacy and safety of rivaroxaban in HIT patients in a multicenter, single-arm, prospective cohort study, where 5 out of 12 HIT-positive patients received rivaroxaban 15 mg bidaily (bid), 3 of which were thrombocytopenic at treatment initiation. The other 7 patients received a short course of danaparoid or fondaparinux before being switched to rivaroxaban, and 4 out of these 7 patients were still thrombocytopenic when rivaroxaban was initiated. Platelet recovery occurred in a median time of 7 days in 9 of the 10 initially thrombocytopenic patients. The rivaroxaban dosage was reduced to 20 mg daily upon platelet recovery in patients with isolated HIT or after 21 days in those with HITT. One patient had symptomatic recurrent VTE during the 30-day follow-up (extension of apheresis catheter-related thrombosis that may have preceded rivaroxaban introduction). Another patient underwent bilateral lower limb arterial thrombosis, which was not resolved by an anticoagulation switch and increased platelet count. Finally, one gastrointestinal bleeding event occurred in a patient suffering from gastric cancer.

APS: Diagnosis and Standard of Care

Diagnosing APS requires the association of at least one clinical and one biological criterion. According to the Sydney classification , clinical criteria for APS are defined as follows: ≥1 episode of venous, arterial, or microvascular thromboembolism in any tissue or organ; ≥1 unexplained fetal loss beyond the 10th week of gestation; ≥1 premature birth before the 34th week of gestation due to eclampsia, pre-eclampsia, or placental insufficiency; or ≥3 unexplained consecutive spontaneous fetal losses before the 10th week of gestation. The biological criteria include the presence of a LAC activity, the detection of IgG or IgM anticardiolipin (aCL) antibody in medium or high titer (i.e., >40 GPL or MPL), or IgG or IgM anti-β2GPI antibody with a titer > 99th percentile. The laboratory criteria should be persistent and remain positive on 2 or more occasions at least 12 weeks apart. No more than 5 years should separate the positive aPL test and the clinical manifestations

The accidental discovery of an isolated high-risk aPL profile (thus with no history of thrombosis or obstetrical complication) justifies initiating low-dose aspirin therapy as a primary prophylaxis to reduce the risk of a first thrombotic event In APS patients who underwent a first VTE, VKA are the first choice for secondary thromboprophylaxis with a recommended target INR of 2-3 (higher treatment intensity has shown no benefit ; however, aPL antibodies can interfere with some prothrombin time reagents, thereby complicating the reliable measurement of INR and consequently the VKAdosage adjustment, and human recombinantthromboplastins should not be used in this case . LAC may also interfere with the INR measured with point-of-care devices, whose use is thus not advised in APS patients with LAC.In cases of arterial thrombosis, VKA remains the first-line therapy with a recommended target INR of 2–3 or 3–4 alone or combined with low-dose aspirin while considering the individual risk of bleeding and recurrent thrombosis.

DOACs' Therapeutic Use in APS

Multiple studies evaluating the efficacy and safety of DOACs for secondary thromboprophylaxis in APS have been published (Table 3), but a high level of incertitude persists regarding their benefit-risk balance in this context. Study populations are often heterogeneous (excluding arterial thrombosis, mixing different biological profiles etc.), as well as the primary endpoints (arterial or venous events, bleedings, all events together).

Like in HIT, most published studies have focused on rivaroxaban with some conflicting results. In RAPS trial [6], patients were treated with rivaroxaban (n = 57) or warfarin (n = 59), and no thrombotic or bleeding events were observed during the 6-month follow-up. In contrast, TRAPS study [7] was prematurely stopped due to the large number of undesirable events (composite primary endpoint: thromboembolism, major bleeding, and vascular death) in the rivaroxaban group compared to the warfarin group (Hazard Ratio = 6.7 [CI95%: 1.50–30.5]).

Finally, the European Alliance of Associations for Rheumatology agrees that DOACs should not be used as secondary thromboprophylaxis in triple-positive patients or patients with first arterial thrombosis, but it concedes that DOACs could be considered in patients unable to achieve target INR despite strict adherence to VKA or those with contraindications to VKA. Like VKA, DOACs are contraindicated or strongly not recommended during pregnancy or breastfeeding; therefore, they should not be prescribed for patients with obstetric APS

In conclusion, the role of DOACs in antithrombotic therapeutic strategies has continuously been grown over recent decades; however, further studies are needed to expand our knowledge on DOACs' use in immune thrombosis.

V11. New anticoagulants: Moving beyond the direct oral anticoagulants

Although anticoagulants have been in use for more than 80 years, heparin and vitamin K antagonists were the sole available options until recently. Although these agents revolutionized the prevention and treatment of thrombotic diseases, their use has been hampered by the necessity for coagulation monitoring and by bleeding complications resulting in part from their multiple sites of action. Owing to advances in basic science, animal models, and epidemiology, the arsenal of available anticoagulants has expanded in the past two decades. This evolution has yielded many novel compounds that target single coagulation enzymes. Initially, thrombin and factor Xa were targeted because of their critical roles in coagulation. However, attention has now shifted to compounds that target upstream reactions, particularly those catalyzed by factors XIIa and XIa, which are part of the contact system. This shift is predicated on epidemiological and experimental evidence suggesting that these factors are more important for thrombosis than for hemostasis. With the goal of developing a new class of anticoagulants associated with a lower risk of bleeding than currently available agents, dozens of drugs targeting the contact system are now in development. This section focuses on the rationale, development, and testing of these new agents with a concentration on those that have reached or completed phase 2 evaluation for at least one indication.

The pace of development of new anticoagulants has accelerated. Heparin and vitamin K antagonists (VKAs) were the only anticoagulants available for most of the 20th century . These drugs, which were the mainstay of anticoagulant therapy for more than 50 years, demonstrated the efficacy of anticoagulation for prevention and treatment of thrombosis. Whereas heparin and VKAs have multiple targets in the coagulation pathway, the more recent generation of drugs is aimed at single targets. Thus, thrombin and factor (F) Xa became the targets of anticoagulants introduced at the turn of the century.Hirudin, bivalirudin, and argatroban were developed because of their specificity for thrombin. In parallel, further refinement of low molecular weight heparin (LMWH), which favors FXa over thrombin, led to the development of fondaparinux, which only inhibits FXa. These second and third generation parenteral anticoagulants provided proof of concept that sole inhibition of thrombin or FXa is effective and safe.Replacement of VKAs remained elusive until advances in structure-based drug design and high throughput screening enabled the development of direct oral anticoagulants (DOACs), small molecules that inhibit the active site of thrombin or FXa.After the initial disappointment with ximelagatran, an oral thrombin that was withdrawn because of the potential for hepatic injury, additional DOACs soon entered the market. These include dabigatran, which inhibits thrombin, and apixaban, betrixaban, edoxaban, and rivaroxaban, which inhibit FXa.5 When evaluated in phase 3 trials that included more than 100 000 patients, the DOACs were at least as effective as VKAs for stroke prevention in atrial fibrillation (AF) or for treatment of venous thromboembolism (VTE) and were associated with less bleeding, particularly less intracranial hemorrhage. With similar efficacy, better safety, and the convenience of fixed dose administration without the need for routine coagulation monitoring, guidelines now give preference to the DOACs over VKAs for many indications.Nonetheless, like with all anticoagulants, bleeding remains the major side effect of the DOACs. This is problematic because the fear of bleeding likely contributes to the underuse of oral anticoagulant prophylaxis in eligible patients with AF and the inappropriate overuse of low-dose DOAC regimens. Furthermore, the DOACs are contraindicated in patients with end stage renal disease (ESRD) and in patients with mechanical heart valves. Therefore, there remains a need for anticoagulants with a reduced incidence of bleeding complications, little or no renal clearance, and with the capacity to attenuate clotting triggered by medical devices such as mechanical heart valves or central venous catheters. To achieve this goal, attention has moved further up the coagulation pathway. Thus, FXI and FXII have garnered interest as novel targets. Focusing on these advances, this review (a) outlines our current understanding of the role of the contact system in thrombosis, (b) identifies FXI and FXII inhibitors under investigation, (c) describes the pharmacological properties of these new agents, (d) identifies potential indications for FXI and FXII inhibitors, (e) describes the clinical trial data available to-date with these agents and the ongoing studies, and (f) provides perspective on the opportunities and challenges for this new class of anticoagulants.

Contribution Of The Contact SystemTo Thrombosis

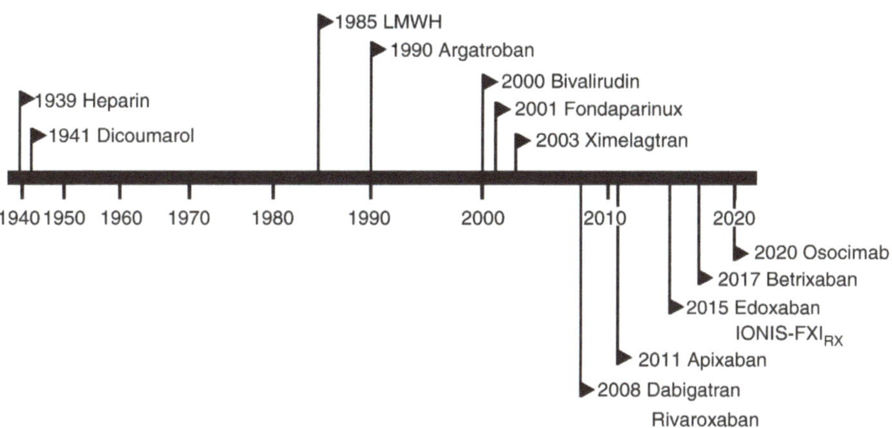

Fig.18.9 Timeline of major landmarks in the development of anticoagulants. The year of approval of drugs for therapeutic use or of completion of phase 2 trials with newer agents is shown

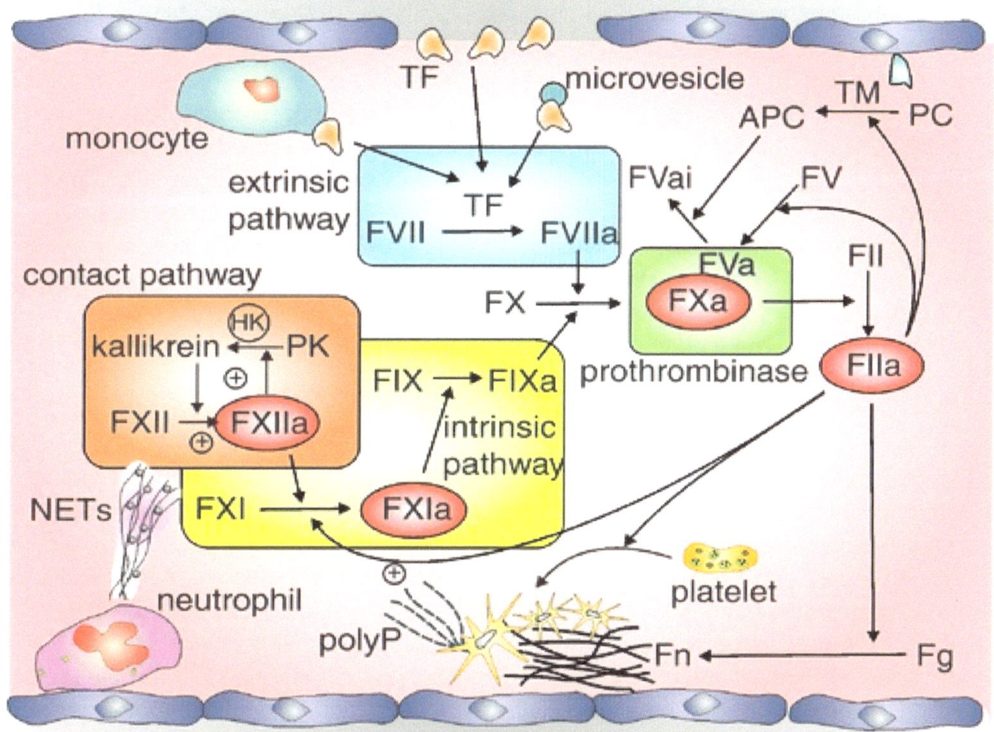

Fig.18.10 Role of the contact system in hemostasis. The extrinsic pathway is initiated when tissue factor (TF) is exposed on subendothelium, leukocytes, or circulating microvesicles. TF promotes activation of factor (F) VII to FVIIa. The TF-FVIIa complex activates FX to FXa, which assembles into the prothrombinase complex along with cofactor FVa on negatively charged membrane surfaces. The prothrombinase complex converts prothrombin (FII) to thrombin (FIIa). The intrinsic pathway is initiated by activation of the contact pathway, whereby FXII and prekallikrein (PK) engage in reciprocal activation by their activated forms, FXIIa and kallikrein, respectively. FXIIa activates FXI to FXIa, which activates FIX and subsequently FX. Platelets and neutrophils release procoagulant molecules upon stimulation, including polyphosphate (polyP) and neutrophil extracellular traps (NETs), respectively. These polyanions contribute to coagulation by potentiating upstream reactions (shown by ⊕), namely the contact system and thrombin-mediated activation of FXI. Ultimately, thrombin cleaves fibrinogen (Fg) to generate fibrin (Fn), which polymerizes into long strands that bind platelets and other cells. Coagulation is downregulated by activation of protein C (PC) by thrombin in the presence of thrombomodulin (TM). Activated PC (APC) attenuates coagulation by degrading FVa into an inactive form (FVai)

The contact system is composed of FXII, prekallikrein (PK), and high molecular weight kininogen . FXI also is considered part of the system because it binds HK, is activated by activated FXII (FXIIa), and activates FIX. Therefore, FXI provides a direct link between the contact system and the intrinsic pathway.The contact system requires an autoactivation step for initiation. FXII autoactivates in the presence of polyanions. FXIIa then activates PK bound to HK, generating kallikrein (Ka). Ka reciprocally activates FXII, completing a cyclic amplification loop. FXIIa activates FXI, thereby leading to activation of the intrinsic pathway. Upstream connection with the distal coagulation pathway was provided by the demonstration that thrombin back-activates FXI. This observation served as an impetus to re-examine the role of FXI in coagulation, and prompted a revision of the basic cascade model of clotting that was established in the 1960s Still missing, however, was knowledge of the contribution of the contact system to thrombosis. This information came from three sources: basic science, epidemiological studies, and the findings from animal models of thrombosis.

NEWANTICOAGULANTS

With evidence of its contribution to thrombosis and the paucity of bleeding complications, the contact system has emerged as a target for development of new anticoagulants. The first consideration is whether FXII or FXI represent a better target. The epidemiological data linking coagulation factor levels with the risk of thrombosis are stronger for FXI than for FXII. Conversely, FXII may be a safer target than FXI because of the lack of a bleeding diathesis with FXII deficiency. The difference in the risk of bleeding likely reflects the fact that FXI has a direct role in the intrinsic pathway because of its back-activation by thrombin, whereas FXII only contributes to the intrinsic pathway when it undergoes autoactivation upon exposure to contact activators. With pros and cons for either target, FXII and FXI have both received attention as targets for development of new anticoagulants. Agents directed against these factors include inhibitors of biosynthesis, antibodies, small molecules, and derivatives of naturally occurring inhibitors. A major accomplishment of the new generation anticoagulants is specificity. Most of the agents under investigation are targeted to single molecules. This limits non-specific effects and may eventually reveal which target is most appropriate for each indication. Currently, there are more agents in development that target FXI than FXII .This imbalance likely reflects uncertainty about the role of FXII in thrombosis and the concern that feedback-activation of FXI by thrombin may bypass the effect of FXII inhibitors. ASOs directed against FXI have been shown to be effective in numerous animal models, including models in mice, rabbits, and baboons. An ASO directed against FXI (Ionis 416858) effectively reduces plasma FXI levels in humans.31 Several monoclonal antibodies directed against FXI are under investigation. Antibodies O1A6 and 14E11 interfere with FXI activation by FXIIa and are effective in mouse and nonhuman primate models of thrombosis. Other antibodies, such as DEF and osocimab (BAY1213790), are directed against FXIa and inhibit its activity.Perhaps of greatest interest are the small molecule inhibitors of FXI, which are directed at the active site or exosites. Notably, BMS-262084, BMS-654457, and ONO-8610539 are parenteral agents directed against the active site of FXIa that have been shown to attenuate thrombosis in animal models. Orally available FXIa inhibitors include JNJ-70033093 (BMS-986177), BAY 2433334, and ONO-5450598. Naturally occurring inhibitors of FXIa include derivatives from nematodes (acaNAP10), snakes (fasxiator), bats (desmolaris), and ticks (boophilin).A smaller arsenal of agents is directed against FXII, and includes monoclonal antibodies (15H8, DO6, CSL312), small molecules (FXII304), an ASO, and naturally occurring inhibitors such as infestin-4 and Ixodes ricinus contact phase inhibitor (Ir-CPI), which also inhibits FXIa

PHARMACOLOGICAL PROPERTIES OF FXI AND FXII INHIBITORS

The pharmacological properties of FXI and FXII inhibitors vary, which may limit their indications First, ASOs, antibodies, and naturally occurring inhibitors require parenteral delivery by subcutaneous or intravenous injection, whereas small molecules can be delivered orally or parenterally. Second, ASOs have a slow onset of action requiring about 4 weeks to achieve therapeutic levels, thus disqualifying them for use in acute settings. In contrast, antibodies and small molecules have a rapid onset of action, which enables their use in both acute and chronic settings. Third, ASOs and antibodies have long half-lives, which may enable once-monthly administration but could necessitate development of reversal strategies. The need for specific reversal agents may be less with oral small molecules, which are expected to have half-lives of <24 hours and are likely to be administered once or twice daily, much like DOACs.

Potential Clinical Indications

Thrombosis is responsible for one in four deaths worldwide and the burden of disease is likely to

Tab 18.8 Relative advantages and disadvantages of factor (F) XII or FXI as targets for new anticoagulants.

	FXII	FXI
Epidemiological data	Weak	Strong
Risk of bleeding	None	Low
Level of evidence for role in thrombosis	Preclinical	Phase 2
Potential for bypassing inhibition	Thrombin-mediated back activation of FXI could bypass FXII inhibition	None
Potential for off-target effects	May modulate inlammation b y inhibiting bradykinin generation	Low

increase with the aging of the population. Anticoagulants are a mainstay for the prevention and treatment of thrombosis, which creates a global need for effective and safe agents. However, recent advances have addressed many of the unmet needs. Thus, DOACs have replaced VKAs for stroke prevention in most patients with AF and for VTE treatment. In addition, dual-pathway inhibition with low-dose rivaroxaban plus aspirin has been shown to reduce major adverse cardiovascular and limb events to a greater extent than aspirin alone in patients with coronary artery disease (CAD) or peripheral artery disease (PAD), thereby creating another niche for DOACs. Although DOACs are more expensive than VKAs and reimbursement can be problematic in some jurisdictions, the cost of the DOACs is likely to decrease with the introduction of generics. Therefore, it is on this background that the development of new anticoagulants needs to be considered. Despite the many advantages of the DOACs over VKAs, there still are problems. These include more bleeding from some anatomical sites with DOACs than with VKAs, and uncertain efficacy of DOACs in some patient populations and lack of efficacy in others. For example, gastrointestinal and genitourinary bleeding is more common with some DOACs than with VKAs.Furthermore, even though the risk of major bleeding is lower with DOACs than with VKAs, bleeding remains the major side effect. The fear of bleeding leads to the underuse of DOACs in some patients with AF and inappropriate use of low-dose DOAC regimens .

The risk of bleeding with DOACs and VKAs is higher in patients with renal impairment than in those with normal renal function. In contrast to VKAs, the DOACs are cleared through the kidneys, which poses a risk of drug accumulation and bleeding in patients with severe renal dysfunction. Although dosing information for apixaban and rivaroxaban is provided for patients with ESRD on hemodialysis in the United States label, it is based only on pharmacokinetic data derived from a small cohort of subjects. A retrospective study using claims-data reported less major bleeding with apixaban than with warfarin in AF patients on hemodialysis, but no reduction in the risk of intracranial or gastrointestinal bleeding with apixaban. Furthermore, the risk of stroke was only lower with apixaban than with warfarin in patients given the higher dose ofapixaban regimen. Without more robust efficacy and safety information, therefore, many clinicians are reluctant to use DOACs for stroke prevention in AF patients with ESRD.

Special populations in which DOACs are contraindicated include patients with mechanical heart valves and those with antiphospholipid syndrome (APS) who are triple-positive for lupus anticoagulant and anticardiolipin and anti-β2-glycoprotein I antibodies. The black box warning against the use of DOACs in patients with mechanical heart valves stems from a study comparing dabigatran with warfarin for this indication that showed a trend for more thromboembolic and bleeding events with dabigatran. Likewise, the recommendation against the use of DOACs in APS arose from studies indicating higher rates of recurrent thrombosis with rivaroxaban than with VKAs in such patients.46, 47Consequently, VKAs remain the only available oral anticoagulants for patients with mechanical heart valves and APS. Therefore, there exists a need for safer anticoagulants, particularly agents with minimal renal clearance and the capacity to attenuate clotting induced by medical devices, such as central venous catheters, heart valves, cardiac assist devices, and extracorporeal circuits.

Clinical evaluation of new anticoagulants often starts in patients undergoing joint replacement surgery because such patients are at high risk of postoperative venous thromboembolism, particularly asymptomatic deep vein thrombosis (DVT), which can be detected on routine venography. Consequently, the dose response for efficacy can readily be determined by quantifying the rate of DVT relative to that of a comparator such as LMWH or a DOAC. Once effective doses are identified, they can then be evaluated in other indications. In addition to medical device–associated clotting, such indications might include secondary stroke prevention in patients with non-cardioembolic stroke, prevention of major adverse cardiac or limb events in patients with CAD or PAD, and vascular protection in patients with ESRD from which half of the deaths are cardiovascular in origin.

CLINICAL TRIALS WITH FXI AND FXII INHIBITORS

Agents that inhibit contact factors are at various stages of development and testing in humans. None has reached phase 3 evaluation; completed and ongoing phase 2 studies with each agent will briefly be described . There are more studies with FXI inhibitors than with inhibitors of FXII.

Antisense oligonucleotides

The drug that has progressed furthest is IONIS-FXIRx (IONIS416858), an ASO directed against FXI. In a phase 1 study in healthy volunteers, subcutaneous IONIS-FXIRx reduced FXI levels in a concentration-dependent manner.49 Maximum reductions occurred after 3 to 4 weeks of treatment and restoration of FXI to baseline levels was delayed for several weeks after treatment stopped. In a phase 2 study, this ASO was compared with enoxaparin for postoperative thromboprophylaxis in 300 patients undergoing elective knee arthroplasty. Patients received subcutaneous injections of IONIS-FXIRx at doses of 200 or 300 mg starting 35 days prior to surgery. These doses were chosen because in the phase 1 study, they were shown to reduce FXI levels by about 60% and 80%, respectively. Venography performed 8 to 12 days after surgery demonstrated a comparable 30% and 27% incidence of VTE with enoxaparin and the 200 mg dose of IONIS-FXIRx, respectively. In contrast, the incidence of VTE was significantly reduced to 4% with the 300 mg dose of IONIS-FXIRx. The incidence of major or clinically relevant nonmajor bleeding was 3% with both doses of IONIS-FXIRx and 8% with enoxaparin; differences that were not statistically significant. The major side effect of IONIS-FXIRx is injection site reactions, which do not appear to be serious.

Osocimab (BAY 1213790)

A fully human immunoglobulin G (IgG)1 monoclonal antibody generated using phage display, osocimab binds the catalytic domain of FXIa and blocks its activity. When given as a single intravenous bolus to healthy volunteers, osocimab prolonged the aPTT in a concentration-dependent manner and had no effect on the bleeding time.52 The half-life tended to increase with higher doses to around 30 to 44 days.In a phase 2 noninferiority study osocimab was compared with enoxaparin and apixaban for thromboprophylaxis in patients undergoing elective knee arthroplasty (NCT03276143).53 A total of 813 patients were randomized to single intravenous osocimab postoperative doses of 0.3, 0.6, 1.2, or 1.8 mg/kg; single preoperative osocimab doses of 0.3 or 1.8 mg/kg; or 40 mg of subcutaneous enoxaparin once daily or 2.5 mg of oral apixaban twice daily until venography. VTE (detected by bilateral venography and symptomatic events) at 10 to 13 days postoperatively occurred in 23.7% of patients receiving 0.3 mg/kg, 15.7% receiving 0.6 mg/kg, 16.5% receiving 1.2 mg/kg, and 17.9% receiving 1.8 mg/kg of osocimab postoperatively; 29.9% receiving 0.3 mg/kg and 11.3% receiving 1.8 mg/kg osocimab preoperatively; and 26.3% receiving enoxaparin and 14.5% receiving apixaban. Major or clinically relevant nonmajor bleeding was observed in up to 4.7% of those receiving osocimab, 5.9% receiving enoxaparin, and 2% receiving apixaban; all bleeding events were limited to the surgical site and there was no intracranial bleeding or bleeding into another critical site. Given postoperatively, the 0.6, 1.2, and 1.8 mg/kg doses of osocimab met the criteria for noninferiority compared with enoxaparin at the prespecified noninferiority margin of 5%. Although the preoperative 1.8 mg/kg dose of osocimab met the criteria for superiority compared with enoxaparin, the 4.7% rate of major clinically relevant bleeding identified the 0.6 and

1.2 mg/kg doses as those most promising for future investigation. Pilot studies evaluating single intravenous and multiple subcutaneous doses of osocimab in patients with ESRD undergoing hemodialysis are underway (NCT03787368).

Abelacimab (MAA868)

Abelacimab is a fully human IgG1 antibody that binds to the catalytic domain of FXI with high affinity and locks it in the zymogen conformation.54 Once bound to FXI, abelacimab inhibits its activation by FXIIa and thrombin; abelacimab also inhibits FXIa. In a phase 1 study single subcutaneous abelacimab doses ranging from 5 to 240 mg were compared with placebo in healthy volunteers with normal body weight and in otherwise healthy obese subjects.54 Abelacimab was well tolerated with no bleeding events, hypersensitivity reactions, or injection site reactions. There was a dose-dependent increase in exposure with median time to maximum concentration ranging from 7 to 21 days and mean terminal elimination half-life ranging from 20 to 28 days. Abelacimab prolonged the aPTT in a dose-dependent manner up to a dose of 150 mg. There was no further prolongation of the aPTT with higher doses but the duration of aPTT prolongation was longer.

Abelacimab is being compared with placebo in a pilot study in patients with AF who are at low risk of thromboembolism (NCT04213807). Patients receive once monthly subcutaneous injections of abelacimab at three different dose levels or placebo for 3 months. The primary outcome is the extent of FXIa inhibition at trough antibody concentrations. In a phase 2 study, abelacimab is being compared with enoxaparin for postoperative thromboprophylaxis in 600 patients undergoing elective knee arthroplasty. Patients will be randomized to single intravenous doses of abelacimab in one of three different doses or to subcutaneous enoxaparin. The results of this study will inform dose selection for other indications.

Garadacimab (CSL312)

An affinity matured variant of 3F7, a fully humanized monoclonal antibody against FXIIa, garadacimab was scheduled to undergo phase 2 evaluation in cancer patients who are receiving systemic chemotherapy via a percutaneously inserted central catheter (PICC; NCT04281524). A single intravenous infusion of garadacimab (in one of four different doses) was to be compared with placebo in such patients with the primary efficacy outcome being the incidence of symptomatic and asymptomatic PICC-associated thrombosis detected up to 30 days after PICC insertion. This study was withdrawn based on a company business decision. However, garadacimab is being compared with placebo in patients with coronavirus disease 2019 pneumonia with the primary outcome being the need for intubation or death (NCT04409509).

Xisomab (AB203)

A humanized version of 14E11, an antibody that binds to the apple 2 domain of FXI, xisomab inhibits FXIIa-mediated but not thrombin-mediated FXI activation. Although it binds to FXI, xisomab has no effect on FXIa activity. Therefore, xisomab functions as FXIIa inhibitor. In a phase 1 study, xisomab prolonged the aPTT in a dose-dependent manner.32, 55 It has a short half-life with low doses, which likely reflects its rapid binding to FXI. Once FXI is saturated, the half-life of xisomab increases likely reflecting slower clearance of the antibody-FXI complex. A phase 2 trial is comparing the safety and efficacy of xisomab and heparin in patients with ESRD undergoing hemodialysis (NCT03612856).

JNJ70033093 (BMS-986177)

A potent and selective small molecule inhibitor of FXIa, JNJ70033093 binds reversibly to the active site of FXIa and inhibits its activity. Phase 1 evaluation has been conducted in healthy volunteers, in healthy Japanese subjects, and in patients with ESRD or with hepatic dysfunction. Two phase 2 trials are underway. One study is comparing JNJ70033093 with enoxaparin for postoperative thromboprophylaxis in up to 1200 patients undergoing elective knee arthroplasty (NCT03891524). Twice daily doses of JNJ70033093 ranging from 25 to 200 mg and once daily doses of 25, 50, or 100 mg are being evaluated. The second phase 2 study is comparing JNJ70033093 with placebo for secondary stroke prevention in up to 2250 patients with non-cardioembolic stroke or transient ischemic attack (NCT03766581). All patients receive aspirin plus clopidogrel for 21 days followed by aspirin alone thereafter. The primary endpoint is the 90-day rate of recurrent overt stroke or covert stroke detected by repeat magnetic resonance imaging (MRI) of the brain.

BAY 2433334

Like JNJ70033093, BAY 2433334 is an active site directed, small molecule inhibitor of FXIa. Three phase 2 trials with BAY 2433334 are under way as part of the PACIFIC (Phase 2 Program of Anticoagulation via Inhibition of FXIa by the Oral Compound BAY 2433334) program. PACIFIC-AF will compare once daily doses of BAY 2433334 (either 20 or 50 mg) with apixaban in 750 patients with non-valvular AF (NCT04218266). Treatments will be given for 12 weeks and the primary endpoint will be safety as evidenced by the composite of major and clinically relevant nonmajor bleeding.PACIFIC-STROKE will compare BAY 2433334 at once daily doses of 10, 20, or 50 mg with placebo on top of antiplatelet therapy in 1800 patients with non-cardioembolic stroke (NCT04304508). Treatments will be given for up to 54 weeks and the choice of antiplatelet therapy will be at the discretion of the investigators. The primary efficacy endpoint is the composite of symptomatic recurrent ischemic stroke and covert brain infarcts detected on repeat MRI brain imaging, whereas the principal safety endpoint is the composite of major and clinically relevant nonmajor bleeding.

PACIFIC-AMI will compare BAY 2433334 at once daily doses of 10, 20, or 50 mg with placebo on top of dual antiplatelet therapy for prevention of major adverse cardiac events in 1600 patients with acute myocardial infarction (MI; NCT04304534). Treatments will be given for a minimum of 26 weeks and a maximum of 52 weeks. The primary efficacy endpoint is the composite of cardiovascular death, MI, stroke, or stent thrombosis, whereas the principal safety endpoint is the composite of major and clinically relevant nonmajor bleeding.

Animal models

Mice deficient in FXII or FXI have normal bleeding after tail tip amputation, but exhibit attenuated clot formation at sites of arterial or venous injury.10 Similarly, antibodies directed against FXII or FXI abrogate thrombosis in these models.11 In nonhuman primate models, antibodies directed against FXI reduce fibrin and platelet deposition on vascular grafts, whereas those directed against FXII are less effective.10 Likewise, knockdown of FXI levels with an antisense oligonucleotide (ASO) reduces arterio-venous shunt thrombosis in baboons and knockdown of FXII or FXI attenuates central vein catheter thrombosis in rabbits.24, 25 Thus, animal studies have been instrumental in demonstrating a potential contribution of the contact system to thrombosis.

MAXIMIZING SAFETY OF NEW ANTICOAGULANTS

Inherent in the quest for new anticoagulants is minimizing the risk of bleeding while on therapy. The challenge in differentiating hemostasis from thrombosis is that they reflect different outcomes originating from the same processes. Thus, it is difficult to attenuate coagulation without impairing hemostasis. Nonetheless, selective inhibition of FXa or thrombin brought us one step forward. Thus, compared with VKAs, which reduce the functional levels of multiple clotting factors, the DOACs are associated with a 50% reduction in the risk of intracranial bleeding.26 Even with the DOACs, however, the annual rate of major bleeding in elderly patients with AF is approximately 3% and the annual rate of major plus clinically relevant nonmajor bleeding can be up to 10% to 12%. Therefore, there remains room for improvement.

CONCLUSIONS AND FUTURE DIRECTIONS

Recent years have witnessed great strides in the expansion of our repertoire of anticoagulants and indications for their use. After a 60-year hiatus during which VKAs were the only available oral anticoagulants, the DOACs have taken over. From the first investigations into the role of the contact system in thrombosis, it has taken <20 years to advance agents targeting factor XI into clinical trials to prevent thrombosis in humans.56 Consequently, the bar is set at a new high for the next generation of anticoagulants and the question is whether FXI or FXII inhibitors can fill this space.The results from the phase 2 studies with IONIS-FXIRx and osocimab provide proof of concept for FXI as a target. Tissue factor is likely to be a major driver of postoperative thrombosis. The efficacy of FXI inhibition in this setting suggests that feedback-activation of FXI by thrombin is important for thrombus growth and stabilization. If these initial successes are indicative, upstream inhibition of FXI may prove to be at least as effective as downstream inhibition at the level of FXa alone or combined inhibition of FXa and thrombin. Whether the benefit-risk profiles of FXI inhibitors exceed those of the DOACs remain to be established. Head-to-head trials comparing FXI inhibitors with DOACs will require large numbers of patients to determine whether FXI inhibitors are at least as effective as DOACs but associated with less bleeding. Even if there is less bleeding with the new agents, the benefit will need to be substantial to induce payers to provide a premium to achieve that result. The easiest studies will be those evaluating FXI inhibitors for indications for which the DOACs have yet to be tested, such as secondary stroke prevention, or for which the DOACs have failed, such as prevention of clotting on medical devices. Although most of the current attention is focused on FXI inhibitors, by inhibiting the root cause of clotting on medical devices and extracorporeal circuits, FXII inhibitors may be better than FXI inhibitors for this indication. With a plethora of new agents under investigation and a wide array of phase 2 trials ongoing, the clinical potential of FXI and FXII inhibitors should become clearer over the next few years.

Bibliography and Acknowledgement

- A Randomized Trial Assessing the Effects of Inclisiran on Clinical Outcomes Among People With Cardiovascular Disease (ORION-4). ClinicalTrials.gov Identifier: NCT03705234.
- Adams D, Bridges CR, Casey DE, et al. ACCF/AHA focused update of the guideline for the management of patients with unstable angina/non-ST-elevation myocardial infarction (updating the 2007 guideline and replacing the 2011 focused update): a report of the American College of Cardiology Foundation/
- American Heart Association Task Force on Practice Guidelines. Circulation.2012;126:875–910.
- Alehagen U, Alexander J, Aaseth J (2016) Supplementation with selenium and coenzyme Q10 reduces cardiovascular mortality in elderly with low selenium status. A secondary analysis of a randomised clinical trial. PLoS One 11:e0157541
- Alexanian I, Parissis J, Farmakis D, Pantziou C, Ikonomidis I, Paraskevaidis I, Ioannidou S, Sideris A, Kremastinos D, Lekakis J, Filippatos G (2014) Selenium contributes to myocardial injury and cardiac remodeling in heart failure. Int J Cardiol 176:272–27
- Arai H, Yamashita S, Yokote K, Araki E, Suganami H, Ishibashi S; K-877 Study Group. Efficacy and Safety of Pemafibrate Versus Fenofibrate in Patients with High Triglyceride and Low HDL Cholesterol Levels: A Multicenter, Placebo-Controlled, Double-Blind, Randomized Trial. J Atheroscler Thromb. 2018;25:521-38.
- Arnaud L., Mathian A., Ruffatti A., Erkan D., Tektonidou M., Cervera R., Forastiero R., Pengo V., Lambert M., Martinez-Zamora M.A., et al. Efficacy of aspirin for the primary prevention of thrombosis in patients with antiphospholipid antibodies: An international and collaborative meta-analysis. Autoimmun. Rev. 2014;13:281–291.
- Arya A, Silberbauer J, Teichman SL, Milner P, Sulke N, Camm AJ. A preliminary assessment of the effects of ATI-2042 in subjects with paroxysmal atrial fibrillation usingimplantedpacemaker methodology. Europace. 2009;
- Ballantyne CM, Laufs U, Ray KK, Leiter LA, Bays HE, Goldberg AC, Stroes ES, MacDougall D, Zhao X, Catapano AL. Bempedoic acid plus ezetimibe fixed-dose combination in patients with hypercholesterolemia and high CVD risk treated with maximally tolerated statin therapy. Eur J Prev Cardiol. 2020;27:593-603.
- Banach M, Duell PB, Gotto AM Jr, Laufs U, Leiter LA, Mancini GBJ, Ray KK, Flaim J, Ye Z, Catapano AL. Association of Bempedoic Acid administration with atherogenic lipids levels in phase 3 randomized clinical trials of patients with hypercholesterolemia. JAMA Cardiol. 2020;5:1-12.
- Barlow A., Barlow B., Reinaker T., Harris J. Potential Role of Direct Oral Anticoagulants in the Management of Heparin-induced Thrombocytopenia. Pharmacotherapy. 2019;39:837–853. doi: 10.1002/phar.2298.
- Barrowcliffe TW. Low molecular weight heparins. Br J Haematol. 1995;90:1–7. doi: 10.1111/j.1365-2141.1995.tb03373.x.
- Bays HE, Banach M, Catapano AL, Duell PB, Gotto AM Jr, Laufs U, Leiter LA, Mancini GBJ, Ray KK, Bloedon LT, Sasiela WJ, Ye Z, Ballantyne CM. Bempedoic acid safety analysis: Pooled data from phase 3 clinical trials. J Clin Lipidol. 2020;14:649-59.
- Carr JA, Silverman N. The heparin-protamine interaction. A review. J Cardiovasc Surg (Torino) 1999;40:659–666
- Clinical Investigator's Brochure: SR33589B Dronedarone. Bridgewater,NJ,SanofSyntholabeRecherche.Edition:E072006.
- Cooper TJ, Guazzi M, Al-Mohammad A, Amir O, Bengal T, Cleland JG, Dickstein K (2013) Sildenafil in Heart failure (SilHF). An investigator-initiated multinational randomized controlled clinical trial: rationale and design. Eur J Heart Fail 15:119–122
- Crowther M.A., Ginsberg J.S., Julian J., Denburg J., Hirsh J., Douketis J., Laskin C., Fortin P., Anderson D., Kearon C., et al. A Comparison of Two Intensities of Warfarin for the Prevention of Recurrent Thrombosis in Patients with the Antiphospholipid Antibody Syndrome. N. Engl. J. Med. 2003;349:1133–1138.
- Dale KM, White CM. Dronedarone: an amiodarone analog for the treatment of atrial fibrillation and atrial flutter. Ann Pharmacother. 2007; 41: 599–605.
- Devreese K.M.J., de Groot P.G., de Laat B., Erkan D., Favaloro E.J., Mackie I., Martinuzzo M., Ortel T.L., Pengo V., Rand J.H., et al. Guidance from the Scientific and Standardization Committee for lupus anticoagulant/antiphospholipid antibodies of the International Society on Thrombosis and Haemostasis: Update of the guidelines for lupus anticoagulant detection and interpretation. J. Thromb. Haemost. 2020;18:2828–2839.
- Dewey FE, Gusarova V, Dunbar RL, O'Dushlaine C, Schurmann C, Gottesman O, McCarthy S, Van Hout CV, Bruse S, Dansky HM, Leader JB, Murray MF, Ritchie MD, Kirchner HL, Habegger L, Lopez A, Penn J, Zhao A, Shao W, Stahl N, Murphy AJ, Hamon S, Bouzelmat A, Zhang R, Shumel B, Pordy R, Gipe D, Herman GA, Sheu WHH, Lee IT, Liang KW, Guo X, Rotter JI, Chen YI, Kraus WE, Shah SH, Damrauer S, Small A, Rader DJ, Wulff AB, Nordestgaard BG, Tybjærg-Hansen A, van den Hoek AM, Princen HMG, Ledbetter DH, Carey DJ, Overton JD, Reid JG, Sasiela WJ, Banerjee P, Shuldiner AR, Borecki IB, Teslovich TM, Yancopoulos GD, Mellis SJ, Gromada J, Baras A. Genetic and pharmacologic inactivation of ANGPTL3 and cardiovascular disease. N Engl J Med. 2017;377:211-21.
- Douketis JD, Berger PB, Dunn AS, et al. The perioperative management of antithrombotic therapy: American College of Chest Physicians Evidence-Based Clinical Practice Guidelines (8th Edition) Chest. 2008;133:299S–339S.
- Ehrlich JR, Biliczki P, Hohnloser SH, Nattel S. Atrial-selective approaches for the treatment of atrial fibrillation. J Am Coll Cardiol. 2008; 51: 787–792.CrossrefMedlineGoogle Scholar
- Evaluation of Major Cardiovascular Events in Patients With, or at High Risk for, Cardiovascular Disease Who Are Statin Intolerant Treated With Bempedoic Acid (ETC-1002) or Placebo (CLEAR Outcomes). ClinicalTrials.gov Identifier: NCT02993406.
- Ezekowitz M, Hohnloser SH, Lubinski A, Bandman O, Canafax D, Ellis DJ, Milner PG, Ziola M, Thibault B. PASCAL: a randomized double-blind, placebo-controlled study of budiodarone (ATI-2042) in patients with paroxysmal atrial fibrillation and pacemakers with atrial fibrillation data logging capabilities [abstract]. Presented at Heart Rhythm Society Annual Scientific Sessions, Boston, Mass, May 2009.Google Scholar
- Federal Dug Administration, Center for Drug Evaluation and Research. Minutes of the meeting of the Cardiovascular and Renal Advisory Committee, March 18, 2009.
- Fedida D, Orth PM, Chen JY, Lin S, Plouview B, Jung G, Ezrin AM, Beatch GN. The mechanism of atrial antiarrhythmic action of RSD1235. J Cardiovasc Electrophysiol. 2005; 16: 1227–1238

- Brandts J, Ray KK. Bempedoic acid, an inhibitor of ATP citrate lyase for the treatment of hypercholesterolemia: early indications and potential. Expert Opin Investig Drugs. 2020;29:763-70.
  Folsom AR, Peacock JM, Demerath E, Boerwinkle E. Variation in ANGPTL4 and risk of coronary heart disease: the Atherosclerosis Risk in Communities Study. Metabolism. 2008;57:1591-6.
- Food and Drug Administration, Center for Drug Evaluation and Research. Minutes of the meeting of the Cardio-Renal Advisory Committee, November 14, 2007. Accessed at http://www.fda.gov/ohrms/dockets/ac/07/briefing/2007-4327b1-02-fda-backgrounder.pdf.Google Scholar
- Gautier P, Gillemare E, Djandjighian L, Marion A, Plachenault J, Bernhart C, Herbert J, Nisato D. In vivo and in vitro characterization of the novel antiarrhythmic agent SSR149744C: electrophysiological, anti-adrenergic and anti-angiotensin II effects. J Cardiovasc Pharmacol. 2004; 44: 244–257.CrossrefMedlineGoogle Scholar
- Gelrud A, Digenio A, Alexander V, Williams K, Hsieh A, Gouni-Berthold I, Bruckert E, Stroes E, Geary R, Hughes S, Tsimikas S, Witztum J, Gaudet D. Treatment with Volanesorsen reduced triglycerides and pancreatitis in patients with FCS and sHTG vs Placebo; Results of Approach and Compass. J Clin Lipidol. 2018;12:537.
- González-López E, Gallego-Delgado M, Guzzo-Merello G, de Haro-Del Moral FJ, Cobo
- Marcos M, Robles C, Bornstein B, Salas C, Lara-Pezzi E, Alonso-Pulpon L, Garcia-Pavia P (2015) Wild-type transthyretin amyloidosis as a cause of heart failure with preserved ejection fraction. Eur Heart J 36:2585–2594
- Graham MJ, Lee RG, Bell TA 3rd, Fu W, Mullick AE, Alexander VJ, Singleton W, Viney N, Geary R, Su J, Baker BF, Burkey J, Crooke ST, Crooke RM. Antisense oligonucleotide inhibition of apolipoprotein C-III reduces plasma triglycerides in rodents, nonhuman primates, and humans. Circ Res. 2013;112:1479-90.
- Greinacher A., Langer F., Makris M., Pai M., Pavord S., Tran H., Warkentin T.E. Vaccine-induced immune thrombotic thrombocytopenia (VITT): Update on diagnosis and management considering different resources. J. Thromb. Haemost. 2021 doi: 10.1111/jth.15572.
- Greinacher A., Thiele T., Warkentin T.E., Weisser K., Kyrle P.A., Eichinger S. Thrombotic Thrombocytopenia after ChAdOx1 nCov-19 Vaccination. N. Engl. J. Med. 2021;384:2092–2101. doi: 10.1056/NEJMoa2104840. [PMC free article] [PubMed] [CrossRef] [Google Scholar]
- Gruel Y., Rupin A., Watier H., Vigier S., Bardos P., Leroy J. Anticardiolipin antibodies in heparin-associated thrombocytopenia. Thromb. Res. 1992;67:601–606. doi: 10.1016/0049-3848(92)90020-B. [PubMed] [CrossRef] [Google Scholar]
- Hohnloser SH, Crijns HJGM, van Eickels M, Gaudin C, Page RL, Torp-Pederson C, Connolly SJ, for the ATHENA Investigators. Effect of dronedarone on cardiovascular events in atrial fibrillation. N Engl J Med. 2009; 360: 668–678.CrossrefMedlineGoogle Scholar
- Horlocker TT, Wedel DJ, Rowlingson JC, et al. Regional anesthesia in the patient receiving antithrombotic or thrombolytic therapy: American Society of Regional Anesthesia and Pain Medicine Evidence-Based Guidelines (Third Edition) Reg Anesth Pain Med. 2010;35:64–101. doi: 10.1097/AAP.0b013e3181c15c70. [PubMed] [CrossRef] [Google Scholar]
- Kearon C, Hirsh J. Management of anticoagulation before and after elective surgery. N Engl J Med. 1997;336:1506–1511. doi: 10.1056/NEJM199705223362107. [PubMed] [CrossRef] [Google Scholar]
- King CS, Holley AB, Jackson JL, et al. Twice vs three times daily heparin dosing for thromboprophylaxis in the general medical population. A metaanalysis. Chest. 2007;131:507–516. doi: 10.1378/chest.06-1861. [PubMed] [CrossRef] [Google Scholar]
- Kober L, Torp-Pederson C, McMurray HJV, Getzsche O, Levy S, Crijns HJGM, Amlie J, Carlsen J, for the Dronedarone Study Group. Increased mortality after dronedarone therapy for severe heart failure. N Engl J Med. 2008; 358: 2678–2687.CrossrefMedlineGoogle Scholar
- Kowey PR, Aliot E, Cappucci A, Connolly SJ, Crijns H, Hohnloser SH, Kulakowski P, Roy D, Radzik D. Placebo-controlled double-blind dose-ranging study of the efficacy and safety of celivarone for the prevention of ventricular arrhythmia-triggered ICD interventions [abstract]. J Am Coll Cardiol. 2008; 51: A2.Google Scholar
- Kowey PR, Aliot EM, Cappucci A, Connolly SJ, Crijns HJ, Hohnloser SH, Kulakowski P, Roy D, Radzik D, Singh BN. Placebo-controlled, double-blind dose-ranging study of the efficacy and safety of SSR149744C in patients with recent atrial fibrillation/flutter [abstract]. Heart Rhythm. 2007; 5 (Suppl): S72.Google Scholar
- Kytömaa S, Hegde S, Claggett B, Udell JA, Rosamond W, Temte J, Nichol K, Wright JD, Solomon SD, Vardeny O (2019) Association of influenza-like illness activity with hospitalizations for heart failure: the atherosclerosis risk in communities study. JAMA Cardiol.
- Laufs U, Banach M, Mancini GBJ, Gaudet D, Bloedon LT, Sterling LR, Kelly S, Stroes ESG. Efficacy and safety of bempedoic acid in patients with hypercholesterolemia and statin intolerance. J Am Heart Assoc. 2019;8;e011662.
- Lim W, Dentali F, Eikelboom JW, Crowther MA. Meta analysis: low-molecular-weight heparinand bleeding in patients with severe renal insufficiency. Ann Intern Med. 2006;144:673–684. doi: 10.7326/0003-4819-144-9-200605020-00011.
- Linkins L.A., Warkentin T.E., Pai M., Shivakumar S., Manji R.A., Wells P.S., Wu C., Nazi I., Crowther M.A. Rivaroxaban for treatment of suspected or confirmed heparin-induced thrombocytopenia study. J. Thromb. Haemost. 2016;14:1206–1210.
- Mach F, Baigent C, Catapano AL, Koskinas KC, Casula M, Badimon L, Chapman MJ, De Backer GG, Delgado V, Ference BA, Graham IM, Halliday A, Landmesser U, Mihaylova B, Pedersen TR, Riccardi G, Richter DJ, Sabatine MS, Taskinen MR, Tokgozoglu L, Wiklund O; ESC Scientific Document Group. 2019 ESC/EAS Guidelines for the management of dyslipidaemias: lipid modification to reduce cardiovascular risk. Eur Heart J. 2020;41:111-88.
- Maurer MS, Schwartz JH, Gundapaneni B, Elliott PM, Merlini G, Waddington-Cruz M, Kristen AV, Grogan M, Witteles R, Damy T, Drachman BM, Shah SJ, Hanna M, Judge DP, Barsdorf AI, Huber P, Patterson TA, Riley S, Schumacher J, Stewart M, Sultan MB, Rapezzi C, ATTR-ACT Study Investigators (2018) Tafamidis treatment for patients with transthyretin amyloid cardiomyopathy. N Engl J Med 379:1007–1016
- McEvoy GK, editor. Protamine sulfate. In: AHFS drug information 2008. Bethesda: American Society of Health-System Pharmacists; 2008. p. 1595–7.
- McMurray JJ, Dunselman P, Wedel H, Cleland JG, Lindberg M, Hjalmarson A, Kjekshus J, Waagstein F, Apetrei E, Barrios V, Böhm M, Kamenský G, Komajda M, Mareev V, Wikstrand J, CORONA Study Group (2010) Coenzyme Q10, rosuvastatin, and clinical outcomes in heart failure: a pre-specified substudy of CORONA (controlled rosuvastatin multinational study in heart failure). J Am Coll Cardiol 56:1196–1204
- Modin D, Jørgensen ME, Gislason G, Jensen JS, Køber L, Claggett B, Hegde SM, Solomon SD, Torp-Pedersen C, Biering-Sørensen T (2019) Influenza vaccine in heart failure. Circulation. 139:575–586

- Morey TE, Seubert CN, Raatkainen MJP, Martynyuk AE, Druzgala P, Milner P, Gonzalez MD, Dennis DM. Structure-activity relationships and electrophysiological effects of short-acting amiodarone homologs in guinea pig isolated heart. J Pharmacol Exp Ther. 2000; 297: 260–266.
- Morisco C, Trimarco B, Condorelli M (1993) Effect of coenzyme Q10 therapy in patients with congestive heart failure: a long-term multicenter randomized study. Clin Investig 71(8 Suppl):S134–S136
- Musco S, Conway EL, Kowey PR. Drug therapy for atrial fibrillation.MedClinNAm.2008;92:12141.
- Nazy I., Sachs U.J., Arnold D.M., McKenzie S.E., Choi P., Althaus K., Ahlen M.T., Sharma R., Grace R.F., Bakchoul T. Recommendations for the clinical and laboratory diagnosis of VITT against COVID-19: Communication from the ISTH SSC Subcommittee on Platelet Immunology. J. Thromb. Haemost. 2021;19:1585–1588.
- Nilius H., Kaufmann J., Cuker A., Nagler M. Comparative effectiveness and safety of anticoagulants for the treatment of heparin-induced thrombocytopenia. Am. J. Hematol. 2021;96:805–815.
- Nutescu EA, Spinler SA, Wittkowsky A, Dager WE. Low-molecular-weight heparin in renal impairment and obesity: available evidence and clinical practice recommendations across medical and surgical settings. Ann Pharmacother. 2009;43:1064–1083.
- O'Gara PT, Kushner FG, Ascheim DD, et al. 2013 ACCF/AHA guideline for the management of ST-elevation myocardial infarction: a report of the American College of Cardiology Foundation/American Heart Association Task Force on Practice Guidelines. Circulation.
- Pavord S., Scully M., Hunt B.J., Lester W., Bagot C., Craven B., Rampotas A., Ambler G., Makris M. Clinical Features of Vaccine-Induced Immune Thrombocytopenia and Thrombosis. N. Engl. J. Med. 2021;385:1680–1689.
- Pemafibrate to Reduce Cardiovascular OutcoMes by Reducing TriglyceridesinpatiENtsWithdiabetes.ClinicalTrials.govIdentifier: NCT03071692.
  Platton S., Bartlett A., MacCallum P., Makris M., McDonald V.,
- Singh D., Scully M., Pavord S. Evaluation of laboratory assays for anti-platelet factor 4 antibodies after ChAdOx1 nCOV-19 vaccination. J. Thromb. Haemost. 2021;19:2007–2013.
- Raal FJ, Kallend D, Ray KK, Turner T, Koenig W, Wright RS, Wijngaard PLJ, Curcio D, Jaros MJ, Leiter LA, Kastelein JJP; ORION-9 Investigators. Inclisiran for the Treatment of Heterozygous Familial Hypercholesterolemia. N Engl J Med. 2020;382:1520-30.
- Raschke RA, Reilly BM, Guidry JR, et al. The weight-based heparin dosing nomogram compared with a "standard care" nomogram: a randomized controlled trial. Ann Intern Med. 1993;119:874–881
- Ray KK, Landmesser U, Leiter LA, Kallend D, Dufour R, Karakas M, Hall T, Troquay RP, Turner T, Visseren FL, Wijngaard P, Wright RS, Kastelein JJ. Inclisiran in patients at high cardiovascular risk with elevated LDL cholesterol. N Engl J Med. 2017;376:1430-40.
- Ruiz-Irastorza G., Hunt B.J., Khamashta M.A. A systematic review of secondary thromboprophylaxis in patients with antiphospholipid antibodies. Arthritis Care Res. 2007;57:1487–1495.
- Saour JN, Sieck JO, Mamo LAR, Gallus AS. Trial of different intensities of anticoagulation in patients with prosthetic heart valves. N Engl J Med. 1990;322:428–432.
- Savelieva I, Camm AJ. Anti-arrhythmic drug therapy for atrial fibrillation: current anti-arrhythmic drugs, investigational agents, and innovative approaches.Europace.2008;10:647665.
  Smith MS, Muir H, Hall R. Perioperative management of drug therapy, clinical considerations. Drugs. 1996;51:238–259. doi: 10.2165/00003495-199651020-00005. [PubMed] [CrossRef] [Google Scholar]
- Schulman S, Beth RJ, Kearon C, Levine MN. Hemorrhagic complications of anticoagulant and thrombolytic treatment: American College of Chest Physicians Evidence-BaseSingh BN, Connolly SJ, Crijns HJGM, Roy D, Kowey PR, Cappucci A, Radzik D, Aliot EM, Hohnloser SH, Investigators. Dronedarone for maintenance of sinus rhythm in atrial fibrillation or flutter. N Engl J Med. 2007; 357: 23–35. 11
- Tafreshi MJ, Rowles J. A review of the investigational antiarrhythmic agent dronedarone. J Cardiovasc Phamacol Ther. 2007; 12: 15–26.
- Touboul P, Brugada J, Cappucci A, Crijns HJGM, Edvardsso N, Hohnloser SH. Dronedarone for prevention of atrial fibrillation: a dose-ranging study. Eur Heart J. 2003; 24: 1481–1487.
- Tripodi A., de Laat B., Wahl D., Ageno W., Cosmi B., Crowther M. Monitoring patients with the lupus anticoagulant while treated with vitamin K antagonists: Communication from the SSC of the ISTH. J. Thromb. Haemost. 2016;14:2304–2307.
- Tschuppert Y, Buclin T, Rothuizen LE, Decosterd LA, Galleyrand J, Gaud C, Bioffaz J. Effect of dronedarone on renal function in healthy subjects. Br J Clin Pharmacol. 2007; 64: 785–791.MedlineGoogle Scholar
- Turpie AGG, Robinson JG, Doyle DJ, et al. Comparison of high-dose with low-dose subcutaneous heparin to prevent left ventricular mural thrombosis in patients with acute transmural anterior myocardial infarction. N Engl J Med. 1989;320:352–357.
- Wang X, Zhang Y, Tan H, Wang P, Zha X, Chong W, Zhou L, Fang F. Efficacy and safety of bempedoic acid for prevention of cardiovascular events and diabetes: a systematic review and meta-analysis. Cardiovasc Diabetol. 2020;19:128.
- Warkentin T.E., Pai M., Linkins L.-A. Direct oral anticoagulants for treatment of HIT: Update of Hamilton experience and literature review. Blood. 2017;130:1104–1113. doi: 10.1182/blood-2017-04-778993.
- Witztum JL, Gaudet D, Freedman SD, Alexander VJ, Digenio A, Williams KR, Yang Q, Hughes SG, Geary RS, Arca M, Stroes ESG, Bergeron J. Volanesorsen and Triglyceride Levels in Familial Chylomicronemia Syndrome. N Engl J Med. 2019; 381:531-542.

CHAPTER

Ocular images-based Artificial Intelligence In Diagnosis of Systemic Diseases Including Cardiovascular Ailments

Artificial intelligence (AI) is intelligence—perceiving, synthesizing, and inferring information—demonstrated by computers, as opposed to intelligence displayed by humans or by other animals. "Intelligence" encompasses the ability to learn and to reason, to generalize, and to infer meaning.Example tasks in which this is done include speech recognition, computer vision, translation between (natural) languages, as well as other mappings of inputs.

AI applications include advanced web search engines (e.g., Google Search), recommendation systems (used by YouTube, Amazon, and Netflix), understanding human speech (such as Siri and Alexa), self-driving cars (e.g., Waymo), generative or creative tools (ChatGPT and AI art), automated decision-making, and competing at the highest level in strategic game systems (such as chess and Go). This has changed the purchasing process, being the AI application functions a mediator between the consumer, product, and brand by providing personalized recommendations based on previous consumer purchasing decisions.

As machines become increasingly capable, tasks considered to require "intelligence" are often removed from the definition of AI, a phenomenon known as the AI effect. For instance, optical character recognition is frequently excluded from things considered to be AI, having become a routine technology Artificial intelligence was founded as an academic discipline in 1956, and in the years since it has experienced several waves of optimism, followed by disappointment and the loss of funding (known as an "AI winter"), followed by new approaches, success, and renewed funding. AI research has tried and discarded many different approaches, including simulating the brain, modeling human problem solving, formal logic, large databases of knowledge, and imitating animal behavior. In the first decades of the 21st century, highly mathematical and statistical machine learning has dominated the field, and this technique has proved highly successful, helping to solve many challenging problems throughout industry and academia. The various sub-fields of AI research are centered around particular goals and the use of particular tools. The traditional goals of AI research include reasoning, knowledge representation, planning, learning, natural language processing, perception, and the ability to move and manipulate objects.[a] General intelligence (the ability to solve an arbitrary problem) is among the field's long-term goals. To solve these problems, AI researchers have adapted and integrated a wide range of problem-solving techniques, including search and mathematical optimization, formal logic, artificial neural networks, and methods based on statistics, probability, and economics. AI also draws upon computer science, psychology, linguistics, philosophy, and many other fields.The field was founded on the assumption that human intelligence "can be so precisely described that a machine can be made to simulate it".[b] This raised philosophical arguments about the mind and the ethical consequences of creating artificial beings endowed with human-like intelligence; these issues have previously been explored by myth, fiction (science fiction), and philosophy since antiquity.Computer scientists and philosophers have since suggested that AI may become an existential risk to humanity if its rational capacities are not steered towards goals beneficial to humankind.[c] Economists have frequently highlighted the risks of redundancies from AI, and speculated about unemployment if there is no adequate social policy for full employment. The term artificial intelligence has also been criticized for overhyping AI's true technological capabilities

In Ayurvedic and TCM ,much stress had been layed in the examination of eyes for not only diagnosis of eye diseases but also many systemic ailments.

Chakshu- Eyes: (Changes in the eye condition are indicative of many health conditions. A big whitish slow moving eye is indicative of kapha, a sharp bright, moist pinkish eye indicative of pitta, and a small flickering, dry, dusky and pigmented eye is indicative of vata.
The shape of the eyes reveal the nature of the person's original constitution. Also on examination, the eyes reveal what is the nature of the ailment and the doshas responsible for it.

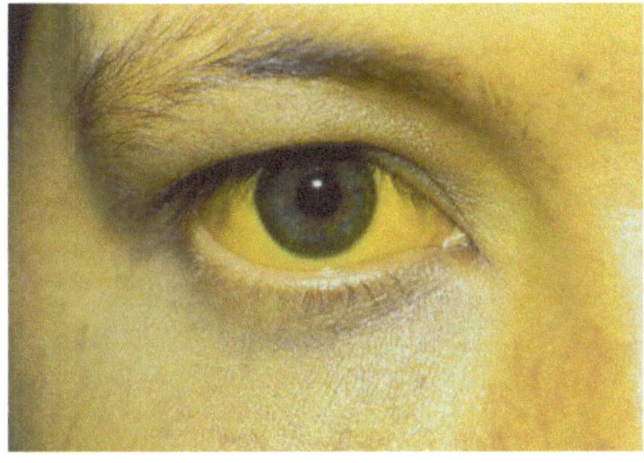

Fig 19.1 Showing face and eyes examination of a patient with jaundice in TCM in a patient with liver disease.

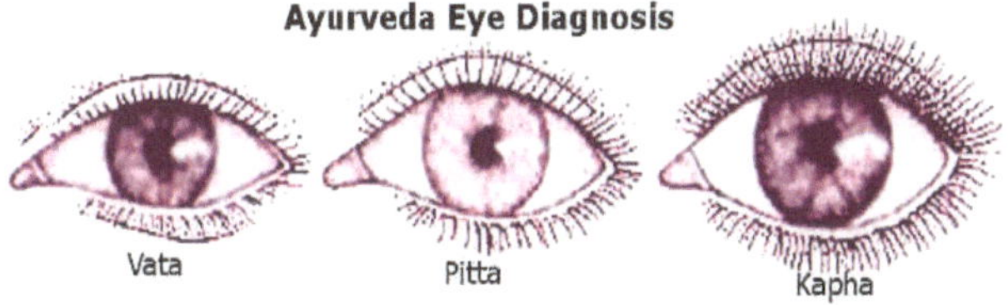

Fig 19.2: Changes in eyes in tridosha imbalance

Iriscopic Examination with TCM

- Iriscope is a diagnostic tool used to detect underlying signs of developing disease to recognize health problems at their earliest stages and to suggest ways to keep disease from developing.
- Safe, non-invasive and painless
- Analysis body constitutional strengths and weaknesses and nutritional deficiencies.
- Detect areas of injury, inflammation or degeneration and accumulation of toxins.
- Find emotional issues.
- Detect precancerous cell which may not be detected from western examination
- High percentage of accuracy in terms of diagnosis
- Right side reflects organs at right side such as Liver, Kidney etc and left side reflects organs at left side such as Heart, Spleen, Kidney etc.

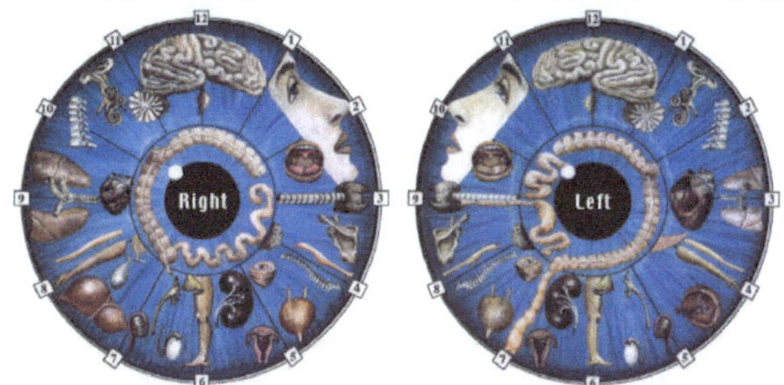

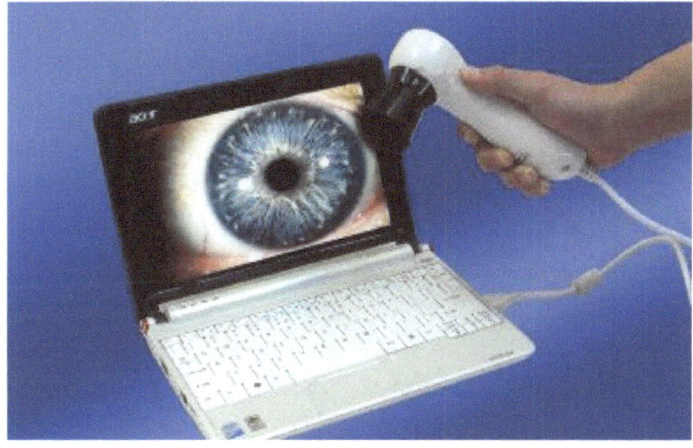

Fig.19.3 (Upper panel) shows diagnostic tool used for iris and (lower) localization of different bodly organs for detection of any developing disease .

artificial intelligence (AI), Ability of a machine to perform tasks thought to require human intelligence. Typical applications include game playing, language translation, expert systems, and robotics. Although pseudo-intelligent machinery dates back to antiquity, the first glimmerings of true intelligence awaited the development of digital computers in the 1940s. AI, or at least the semblance of intelligence, has developed in parallel with computer processing power, which appears to be the main limiting factor. Early AI projects, such as playing chess and solving mathematical problems, are now seen as trivial compared to visual pattern recognition, complex decision making, and the use of natural language

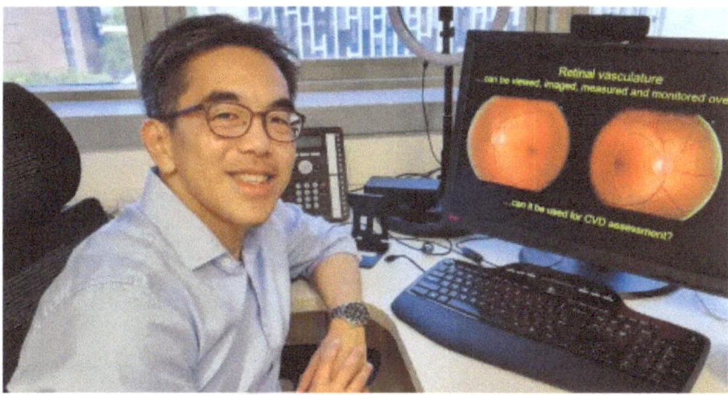

Fig.19.4 The application of AI to retinal image analysis may allow physicians, in milliseconds, to predict the risk for specific systemic diseases, according to Tien Yin Wong, MD, PhD

Artificial Intelligence (AI), which sprung from Alan Turing's paper in 1950, has revolutionized numerous real-world industries, such as translation, natural language processing, and image recognition after decades of development; and medicine is no exception. Machine learning (ML) and its important subset deep learning (DL) achieved prominent performance in multiple tasks of medical image processing: classification, object detection, tracking, and semantic segmentation.3 Powered by DL, AI is now used as a classifier and screening tool in some real-time in-vivo imaging processes, and also provides referral advice and reference diagnostics in image-centric specialties, such as ophthalmology,radiology, dermatology and cardiology. In ophthalmology, several AI-based diagnostic platforms based on retinal imaging such as IDx-DR and EyeArt AI Screening System for diabetic retinopathy (DR) have shown great application advantages in clinical practice. To date, the US Foodand Drug Administration (FDA) has approved more than 300 AI medical products, and ophthalmic disease screening applications are among the first to be approved. Given the rich information on pathological changes and accessibility of retinal images in primary care settings, retinal imaging-based AI models are widely used for detecting and predicting diseases such as type 2 diabetes mellitus (T2DM),4 cardiovascular diseases (CVD), hepatobiliary diseases,and chronic kidney disease (CKD)

Detection of Cardiocerebral Vascular Diseases and Risk Stratification

Detection of Retinal Microvascular Morphological Parameters for Stratification Certain visible changes in the retinal arterioles, such as vessel caliber , bi-furcation, or tortuosity , have been highly valuable for suggesting that altered arteriolar function may exist throughout the body

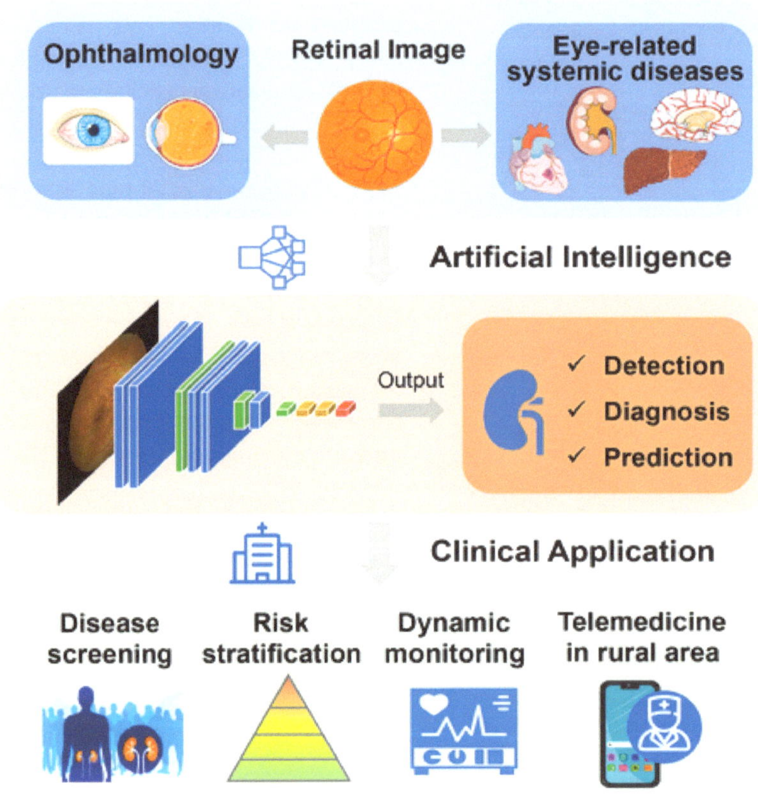

Fig.19.5 Graphical schematic illustration of retinal image-based artificial intelligence for the detection, diagnosis, and prediction of kidney diseases.

Deep learning models designed by Cheung et al. for the automatic measurement of retinal-vessel caliber in fundus photographs performed well. Their performance was comparable to expert graders in associations between measurements of retinal-vessel caliber, and cardiovascular disease (CVD) risk factors, including blood pressure, body-mass index, total cholesterol, and glycated-hemoglobin levels. This demonstrated that reduced retinal arteriolar caliber and increased retinal venular caliber were both independently associated with an increased risk of incident CVD events.

Zekavat et al. leveraged deep learning to quantify geometric microvasculature indices, and thereby characterized phenome-wide clinical associations and genomic risk factors. They reported that low retinal vascular fractal dimension and density were significantly associated with a higher risk of incident mortality, hypertension, and congestive heart failure. This novel framework emphasized how deep learning of images can quantify an interpretable phenotype that can then be integrated into clinical metadata, genetic data, and biomarker datasets to predict risk.

In another study, Duan et al. applied AI to assess morphological changes in retinal microvasculature and foveal avascular zone (FAZ) using optical coherence tomography angiography (OCTA), including three vascular parameters and four FAZ-related parameters. This investigation demonstrated that retinal microvascular and macular morphology exhibited damage patterns specific to different subtypes of ischemic stroke.

Prediction of Additional Risk Factors for Stratification

Given the anatomical and physiological similarity between cerebral and coronary circulation , non-invasive and accessible retinal abnormalities can directly reflect systemic vascular properties. Thus, in addition to demographic data including age and gender, coronary artery calcium (CAC) and carotid artery atherosclerosis are also frequently used to evaluate CVD risk index.

Poplin et al. proposed a deep-learning model to extract and quantify multiple cardiovascular risk factors from retinal images. The factors used by this model included age, gender, smoking status, HbA1c, and systolic blood pressure, all of which were considered essential for predicting incident CVD.

Retinal age has also been used as a proxy for predisposition to CVD. For example, Nusinovici et al. [19] evaluated the retina-based biological age (RetiAGE) based on a deep learning approach. They reported that RetiAGE, independently of phenotypic biomarkers (e.g., creatinine, glucose, C-reactiveprotein, etc.) and chronological age, indicated the potential presence of CVD. Moreover, retinal age prediction based on fundus images was also investigated by Zhu et al., who found that the retinal age gap (i.e., predicted retinal age minus chronological age) was significantly associated with arterial stiffness index, incident CVD events and stroke .

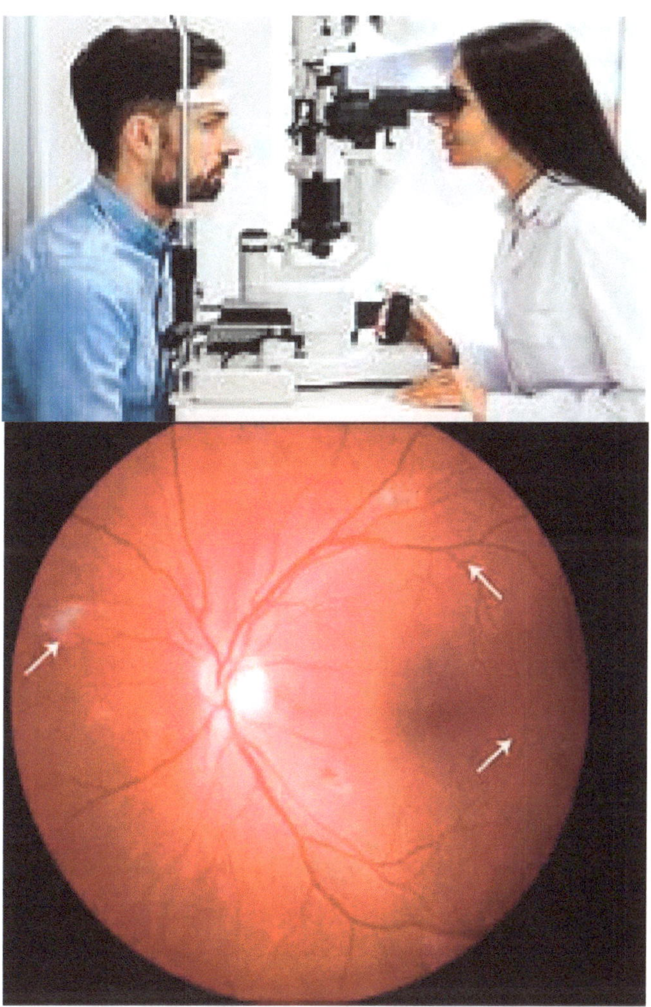

Fig.19.6 **Retinopathy Can Signal Coronary Heart Disease**

Retinal abnormalities usually have no symptoms in the early stages.It may not just be diabetics who have a higher risk of coronary heart disease (CHD) if they develop the eye condition retinopathy. Its reputation as a sign of systemic disease could extend to non-diabetics. "New studies have proven that retinopathy may occur parallel to small vessel disease in other organs such as the heart," says Jonathan Sears, MD, associate professor of ophthalmology at Cleveland Clinics Cole Eye Institute. "This means that a simple eye exam could potentially help assess a patients risk of CHD. Diabetes is a known risk factor, because this disease affects small vessels-but new clinical research has revealed a similar association in non-diabetics."

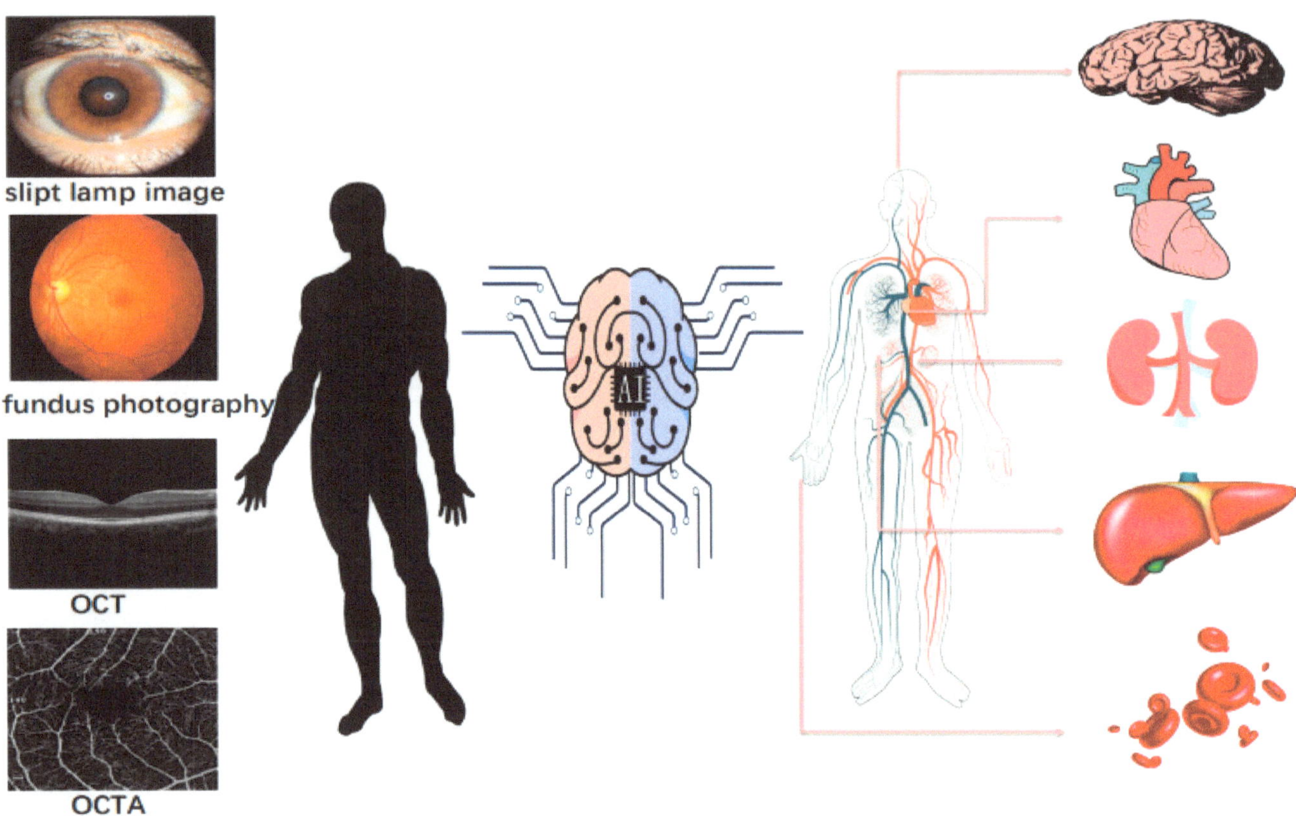

Fig.19.7 Overview of predictable systemic diseases capable of being assessed using primary ophthalmic imaging modalities and AI technology. These ocular images were derived from the authors' research database.

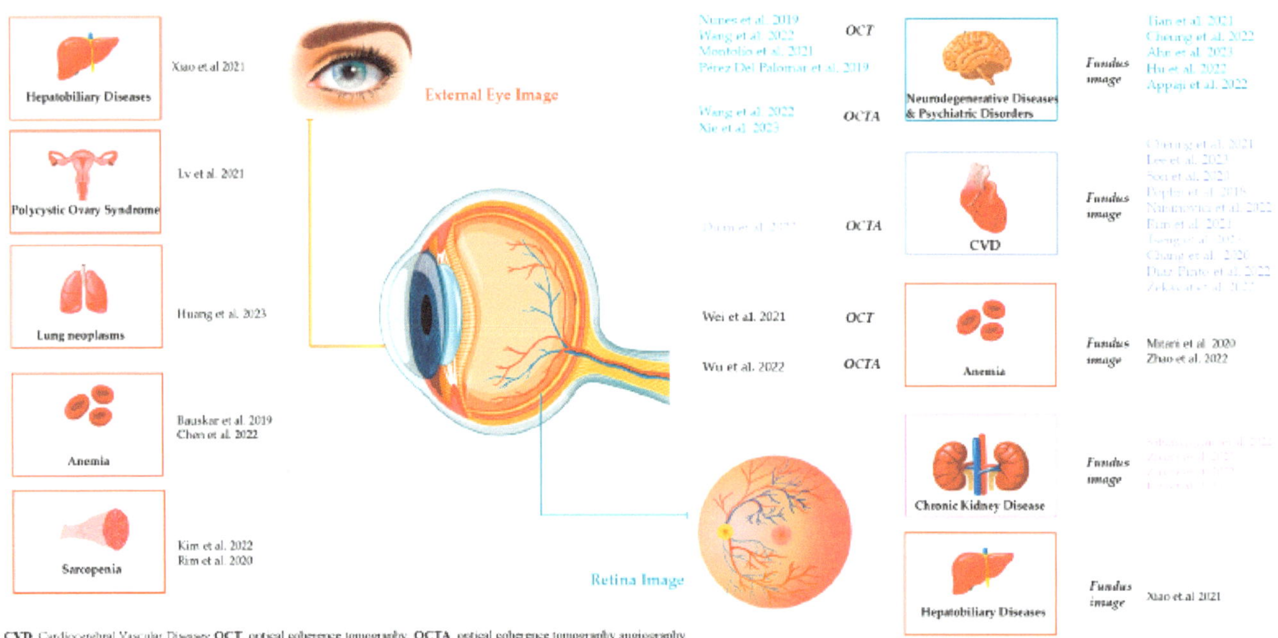

Fig.19.8 Classification of the included articles according to the image modalities used and the target systemic diseases

Many investigations have suggested that retinal image-based deep learning may be a beneficial alternative measure of CAC. For instance, a study conducted by Son et al. demonstrated a high accumulation of CAC. This accumulation was highly correlated with CVD and could be recognized by deep learning algorithms. In another study, Rim et al. developed a three-tier CVD risk stratification system based on Reti-CVD, which showed comparable effectiveness to traditional CT scan measurement in predicting future CVD risk. Furthermore, the authors validated the decent capabilities of Reti-CVD to serve as a risk enhancer tool to predict CVD events using UK biobank data

Using retinal fundus images, Chang et al. predicted atherosclerosis using a similar image analysis strategy. However, the low specificity (i.e., 0.404) suggested that the current algorithm was not suitable for the specific detection of atherosclerosis. Furthermore, they conducted a retrospective cohort analysis to prove that the deep-learning funduscopic atherosclerosis score (DL-FAS), as an independent predictor of CVD mortality, added predictive value over the standard Framingham risk score.

Prediction of Major Cardiocerebral Vascular Events

Previous studies have consistently suggested that major CVD events are predictable using AI algorithms. The aforementioned model by Poplin et al.] simultaneously predicted major adverse cardiac events (MACE) based on specific risk factors and obtained an area under the curve (AUC) value of 0.70 (0.65–0.74). Nevertheless, the retinal fundus algorithm did not have an additive effect on the predictive performance of SCORE risk calculation for MACE. In the hybrid system proposed by Diaz-Pinto et al. , retinal images and relevant clinical metadata were analyzed together to estimate cardiac indices—including left ventricular mass and left ventricular end-diastolic volume—and to predict incident myocardial infarction; this model showed an AUC of 0.80. In another study, a multimodal deep learning system was proposed by Lee et al. to predict current CVD and assess its performance against a clinical risk factors data-input model simultaneously. The authors found that the integrated network, which combined two networks using two different modalities and made full use of clinical metadata and fundus images, achieved the best performance, with an AUC of 0.872 in the external validation set. Given these results, many patients at high risk of future CVD events may benefit from available retinal image-based AI technology soon.

Detection of Chronic Kidney Disease and Renal Function

Homology in microvascular structure between the eye and the kidney suggests that incipient kidney diseases and renal function may be diagnosed using noninvasive ocular images

Sabanayagam et al. developed a deep learning algorithm to detect chronic kidney disease (CKD) from retinal images, and assessment of this model showed that it achieved both good performance and favorable generalization. Although slightly inferior to the combination model that incorporates clinical metadata of risk factors, it implied that accessible retinal photography can be used independently for CKD screening even without detailed medical history acquisition. In one interesting study, Zhang et al. further validated the potential value of an AI-derived image analysis system designed to predict the development of CKD in longitudinal cohorts. Risk stratification performance and the prognostic accuracy of the AI system were both positively assessed, and this model showed an AUC of 0.771 (0.677–0.840) for predicting the onset of CKD in four-year longitudinal data. To explore more predictive biomarkers, Zhang et al. conducted a prospective cohort study to assess the association between the retinal age gap (defined above) and incident kidney failure. Although a significant relationship was revealed, various confounding factors and selection bias were imputed for the limited generalizability of this model.

Additionally, deterioration of renal function reflects a propensity to advance to chronic kidney disease. Rim et al. attempted to use retinal photographs to predict the relative abundances of a series of systemic biomarkers, including creatinine, whose dynamic fluctuations are directly related to renal function. However, this analysis showed relatively poor predictive performance in the European external test. As a result, more comprehensive work is required to explore more precise predictive factors for incident CKD.

Application of retinal image-based AI models in diabetes

Currently, 425 million people are affected by diabetes mellitus worldwide.44 And at least one-third of patients with diabetes suffer from DR, leading to different stages of microaneurysms, exudates, hemorrhages, and eventually irreversible blindness. A DL algorithm developed by Gulshan et al.4 can check for signs of retinal photographs to help physicians screen more patients. A dataset of more than 128,000 images was created to train a deep neural network to detect DR, achieving 90.3% and 87.0% sensitivity

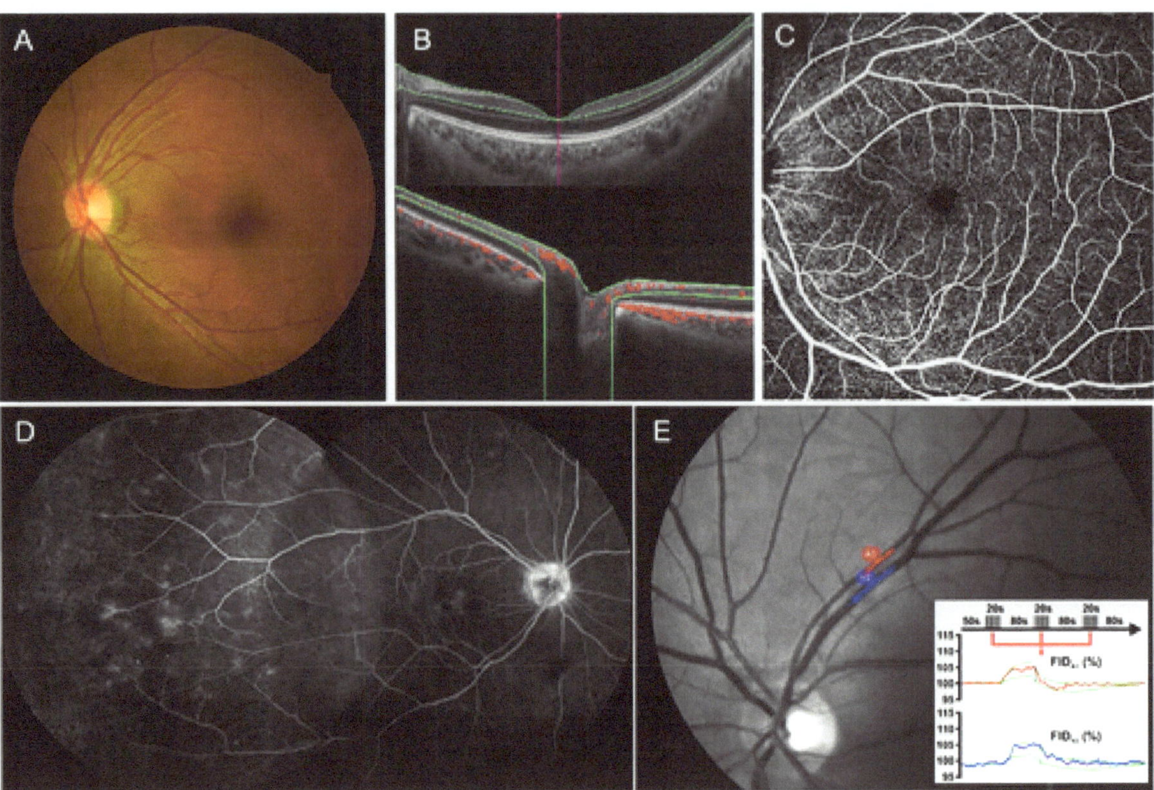

Fig.19.9 Retinal imaging modalities. (A) Color fundus photography; (B) Optical coherence tomography (OCT); (C) optical coherence tomography angiography (OCT-A); (D) Fluorescein angiography (FA); (E) dynamic retinal vessel analysis (DVA). Source: (D) Copyright 2021, Association for Research in Vision and Ophthalmology; (E) Copyright 2020, MDPI

and 98.1% and 98.5% specificity in 2 validation sets, performed with comparable accuracy as the ophthalmologists. Later numerous AI models detecting DR were developed and validated in multiethnic populations,45 multi-continent levels,46 and also in different levels of care.47 The system was put in a primary setting to help predict the DR development with an area under the curve (AUC) of 0.79 (95% confidence interval [CI]: 0.77–0.81) in the internal validation set and 0.70 in the external validation set. And the economic analysis has proved that the AI screening of DR combined with specialists can reach the lowest cost, which is US$62 per patient per year, compared to $66 for a fully automated model and $77 for the human assessment model

However, real-world studies have somehow shown that AI screening fell short in clinical practice, especially in remote rural areas with few medical resources. The project is being carried out in Thailand, where the same DL system has been installed in 11 clinics in the provinces of Pathum Thani and Chiang Mai.49 With inexperienced operators and unmet conditions, acquired images were somewhat different from the images required by the algorithm, and connect speed impeded the future applications of algorithms

TheEye/Kidney Connection: From Molecular To Clinical

The eye is a window for direct observation of many diseases, and the eye and kidney share similar development, structure, and pathogenic mechanisms. The alteration of ocular vascular structure and function is closely related to different kinds of kidney diseases, including diabetic nephropathy and hypertension nephropathy. Herein kidney diseases can be studied non-invasively by the in vivo visualization of the retinal microvasculature.

Shared physiological and molecular pathways of eye and kidney diseases

The link between kidney diseases and blindness was first reported by Richard Bright in 1836.60 Nowadays, scientists identify that both choroids of the eye and kidney develop from mesoderm around the fourth week, and they can be both affected by the same factors during this period. Basically, nephrons and choroids share some similar structures consisting of nerve fibers, stroma, and fenestrated microvessels, which are highly permeable to proteins and result in stroma edema. They both expressedrenin-angiotensin-aldosterone receptors,61 innervated by the autonomic nervous system, and regulated by systemic perfusion pressure

Epidemiologic and clinical association of eye and kidney diseases

Common risk factors of old age, smoking, diabetes mellitus, hyperlipidemia, and hypertension were reported shared

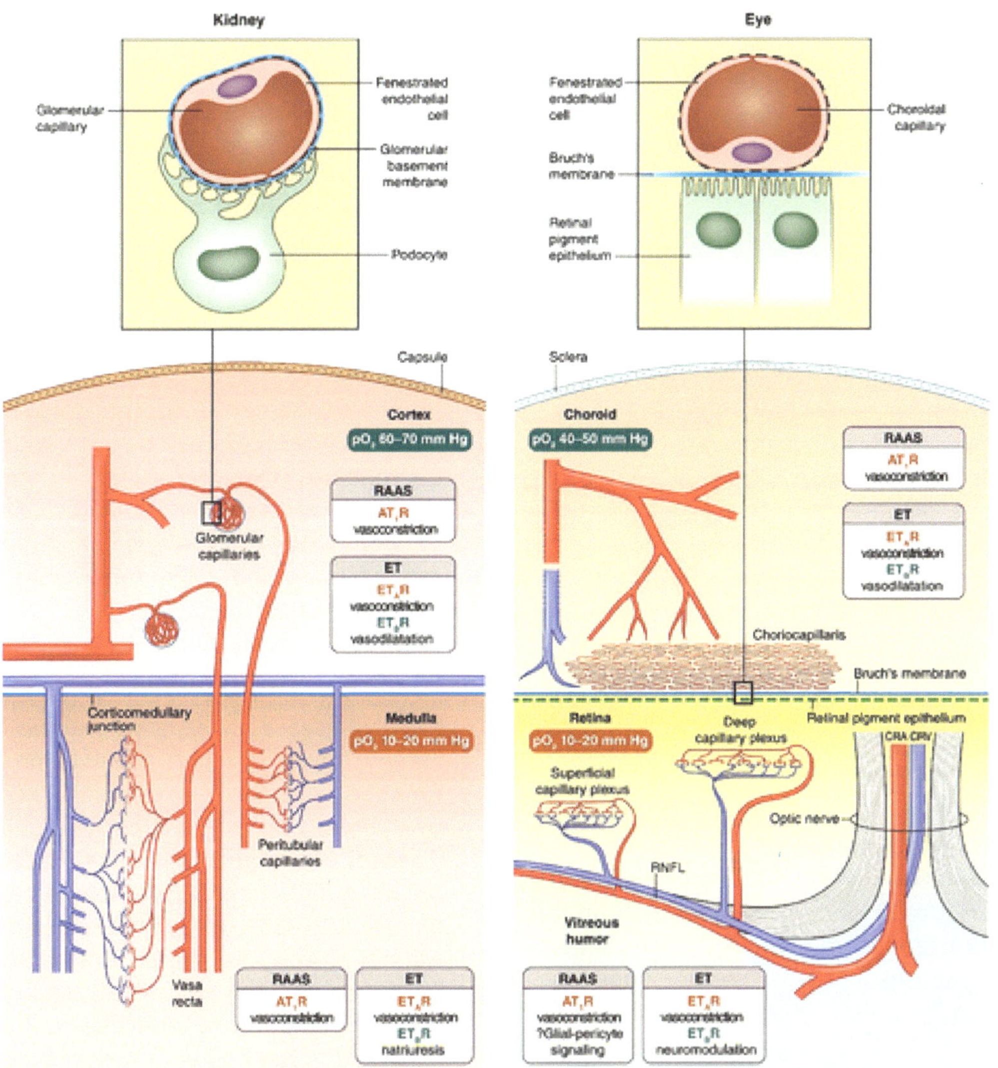

Fig. 19.10 The eye as a window to the kidney: common microcirculation organization and physiological regulation in kidney and eye. AT1R, angiotensin II type 1 receptor; CRA, central retinal artery; CRV, central retinal vein; ET, endothelin; ETAR, endothelin type A receptor; ETBR, endothelin type B receptor; pO2, partial pressure of oxygen; RAAS, renin-angiotensin-aldosterone system; RNFL, retinal nerve fiber layer. Source: Copyright 2020, Elsevier. Eye and kidney diseases have common embryonic, structural, pathogenic, and underlying molecular pathways. A variety of human congenital oculorenal syndromes have been described.63 Pax genes consist of a group of gene families that control development in encoding nuclear transcription factors, such as Waardenburg syndrome (Pax3), Aniridia (Pax6), Peter's anomaly (Pax6), and renal coloboma syndrome (Pax2).64 Bone morphogenetic protein-7 (BMP-7)41 is from another important growth factor-secreting family, the transforming growth factor-beta (TGF-beta) family. During embryogenesis of the mammalian kidney and eye, they would be both affected by the lack of BMP-7, exhibiting renal dysplasia and anophthalmia. Wilms' tumor suppressor (WT1)65 could also cause aniridia, cataract, corneal clouding, and nephroblastoma (Wilms' tumor) in children.

between CKD and ocular problems, either alone or in combination.66 Clinically, the comorbid eye diseases in patients with CKD and ESRD have some common manifestations.67, 68 Retinopathies and certain ocular fundus signs of cotton-wool spots and hemorrhages in superficial or deep capillaries of the retina were often found in CKD patients. Systemic or retinal edema is caused by hypoalbuminemia and retention of excess fluid accumulation in interstitial spaces or subretinal spaces.69 Renal anemia may cause retinal hypoxia, which leads to infarction of the nerve fiber layer and results in cotton wool spots. And the elevated blood cholesterol is associated with increased severity and extent of hard exudates Epidemiologic studies reveal a high prevalence of retinopathies in patients with CKD, independent of diabetes, hypertension, and other risk factors. A population-based cross-sectional study of 9670 Chinese participants in Beijing by Gao et al., found that retinopathy is more prevalent in patients with CKD (28.5% vs. 16.3%, $p < 0.001$). Also, the severity of retinopathy is associated with the level of kidney function loss (estimated glomerular filtration rate, eGFR) and predicts the future progression of CKD. In the Chronic Renal Insufficiency Cohort (CRIC) study70 of 1904 CKD patients in the United States found CKD patients with eGFR <30 ml/min/1.73m2 are associated with three times higher risk of retinopathies. A later serial study of 1583 CRIC participants showed that with the progression of retinopathy, the odds ratio (OR) for CKD progression was 2.24 (95% CI: 1.28–3.91) compared with participants with stable retinopathy, indicating a bidirectional link between the severity of kidney and eye diseases.Most kidney diseases and retinopathies start or worsen from vascular dysfunction and systemic diseases like diabetes mellitus and hypertension.72 The narrowing diameters of arterioles and widening of venules are thought to reflect the severity of both diseases. In the past two decades, studies have been focused on the qualitative measurement of retinal vessel calibers, including central retinal arteriolar equivalent (CRAE), central retinal venular equivalent (CRVE), arteriole-to-venule ratio (AVR), and the analysis of vessel network geometry, fractal dimension. Bao et al. aimed to examine the association between CRAE, CRVE, and AVR with CKD in rural China to provide the scientific basis for the early detection and diagnosis of CKD. After controlling for potential confounding factors, participants with the first quartile of AVR were shown to have a greater risk of albuminuria (OR = 1.261, 95% CI: 1.02–1.57) and CKD (OR = 1.240, 95% CI: 1.00–1.54) than the fourth quartile. It was investigated by Sabanayagam et al.75 if baseline retinal vessel diameters were related to future risk of impaired kidney function or vice versa, in prospective research involving numerous assessments of serum creatinine and retinal artery diameters (CRAE and CRVE). Retinopathy was also assessed whether it could predict future CVD events in participants of the CRIC study. Worsening early treatment DR study retinopathy scores were reported in 9.8% of individuals and were related to an elevated risk of incidence of any CVD (OR = 2.56, 95% CI: 1.25–5.22).A large scale of studies show that these retinal vascular indices are associated with CKD prevalence, but their abilities to predict CKD incidence or progression are equivocal..The measurement of consistent retinal vascular metrics may overlook the heterogeneity of different study populations and other information on fundus signs (e.g., microaneurysms, exudates, hemorrhages, and papilledema). And it also suggests that the sensitivity of conventional analysis of fundus photography cannot meet the need for precise identification of patients at risk.

Detecting And Diagnosing Kidney Diseases From Retinal Imaging

Kidney diseases, like glomerulonephritis and acute kidney injury, usually entail some decline in renal function, eventually developing CKD or kidney failure over time. CKD is the most common type of kidney disease. The high prevalence of CKD has become a major public health problem worldwide, affecting almost 10%–16% of the population in Asia, Europe, Australia, and the United States.With an increasing incidence of obesity and T2DM, combined with an aging population worldwide, a heavier burden is expected in the future decades, especially in low- and middle-income countries. Despite its severity, CKD is usually asymptomatic and progresses insidiously until the very late stage or ESRD, leading to complications like CVD and higher mortality. The idea of early detection is appealing because the inexpensive intervention can ameliorate renal function at an early stage and prevent continuous deterioration. The shortcomings of traditional analysis methods make a new comprehensive assessment approach urgently needed in kidney disease patients and a larger scale of population. The use of ML and DL combined withretinal imaging is a relatively prominent frontier in this research area

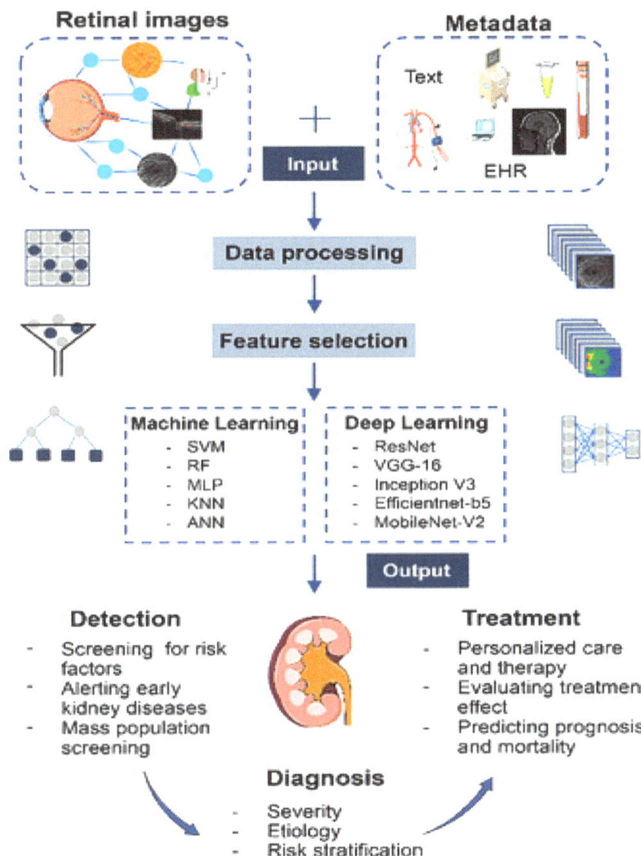

Fig.19.11 An illustration of the general workflow of retinal detection and prediction of kidney diseases. First, input data includes retinal information and metadata (text, electrical health record (EHR) and results from ultrasound or magnetic resonance imaging (MRI)), second: data processing (e.g., missing data imputation, image enhancement, etc.), third: feature selection, forth: model building with different machine learning (ML)/deep learning (DL) approaches, fifth: output classified into detection, diagnosis, and treatment of kidney diseases, and their applications in clinical practice and research. EHR, electrical health record; SVM, support vector machines; RF, random forest; MLP, multilayer perceptron; KNN, k-nearest neighbors; ANN, artificial neural network; RRT, renal replacement therapy.

Screening for risk factors of CKD

The increasing prevalence of kidney diseases worldwide is closely associated with risk factors, including smoking, obesity, hypertension, and metabolic syndromes like hyperlipidemia and diabetes.82 Retinal images were used to predict these important risk factors (age, gender, smoking, body mass index [BMI], etc.) in different studies. Kim et al. built a CNN model based on retinal fundus images to accurately predict age and sex. The R2 and MAE were 0.92 and 3.06 years for age prediction and sex was predicted with AUC>0.96 in test sets of normal, diabetes, and hypertensive participants, independent from the pathologic changes caused by systemic vascular diseases. Smokers and non-smokers were identified by a CNN model built by Vaghefi et al.83 using 165,104 retinal photographs, achieving 88.8% accuracy and 93.87% specificity in the contrast-enhanced model, while the skeletonized model was only 63.63% accuracy and 65.60% specificity. BMI, as well as other body composition factors like body muscle mass, weight, height, and percentage of body fat, were also predicted from retinal photographs, but the performance of current algorithms was generally poor with low R2 values (R2 = 0.13–0.17).

Other models were also developed to detect different factors related to kidney diseases, like dyslipidemia with elevated triglyceride (MAE = 0.49, R2 = 0.03), total cholesterol (MAE = 0.75, R2 = 0.03) and low-density lipoprotein cholesterol (LDL-c, MAE = 0.72, R2 = -0.03).80 The performance of the models was relatively poor in test sets and needed to be improved. Classification models of dyslipidemia81 identification show a better ability with an accuracy of 66.7% and an AUC of 0.703.

Diabetes and hypertension are common underlying conditions associated with CKD. In patients with diabetes, the prevalence of CKD is approximately 30% to 40%, and the numbers are rising with socioeconomic change and population aging. And hypertension accounts for 30% of all kidney diseases, only secondary to diabetes, leading to hypertensive nephropathy. The renal injury can be insidious and progressive, but the retinal signs can be the earliest findings to identify target organ damages, even before the presence of proteinuria and decrease of eGFR.

Alerting signs of early kidney diseases

CKD is often insidious, with patients remaining asymptomatic (stages G1 and G2) for long periods and consequential low awareness. When progressing to stage G3, a symptomatic stage with polyuria or fatigue caused by anemia, patients are at a significantly higher risk of complications and progression to ESRD. The assessment of kidney function chiefly depends on the level of GFR, and serum creatinine concentration is generally measured to calculate the value of eGFR by specific formula (for example, the CKD-EPI formula). CKD could also be alerted by abnormal laboratory blood tests of urea nitrogen, cystatin C, and proteinuria/ microalbuminuria from urine tests in routine health checks or population screening.Patients with increased blood urea nitrogen and creatinine were associated with the incidence of posterior subcapsular cataract84 (OR = 1.22, 95% CI: 1.03–1.54), late AMD85 (OR = 3.05, 95% CI: 1.51–1.61) and DR78 (OR = 3.20, 95% CI: 1.58–6.40). Vice versa, the change in retinal signs can indicate changes in kidney functions. The level of creatinine was predicted by Rim et al.86 with moderate performance (MAE = 0.11, R2 = 0.12) in the Korean dataset, however, it falls far short of robustness in multi-ethnic datasets (R2 = 0.06, 0.01 for Singapore Epidemiology of Eye Diseases and UK Biobank, respectively). Serum creatinine level may be affected by age, food intake, inflammation status, and drugs, the calculated eGFR was adopted as a more reliable indicator, whose decline could be observed at the early stage of kidney injury. Kang et al.87 attempted to predict early renal impairment, defined as eGFR < 90 ml/min/1.73m2, trained and tested with 25,706 fundus images from 6212 patients (Figure 4A). The AUC was 0.81 in the overall population, higher in subgroups of elevated serum hemoglobin A1c (HbA1c) level (0.81, 0.84, 0.85, and 0.87 for HbA1c level of ≤6.5%, >6.5%, >7.5%, and >10%, respectively), but observed poor specificity (60%) in diabetes patients. The performance of this model lacked external validation, and it should be noted that the concerned retinal-vessel features, and abnormal retina signs marked by saliency maps, like exudation and hemorrhage, may be due to pathological changes caused by other ophthalmic or systemic comorbidities. Proteinuria or microalbuminuria, which is defined as albumin/creatinine ratio (ACR) >17.0 for males or ACR>25.0 for females, is recommended as the preferred screening strategy for all patients with diabetes and hypertension. Lim et al.88 quantitatively measured fundus photographs by a semiautomated program to predict the presence of albuminuria, and the retinal vascular parameters were considered associated with renal function from regression models, showing better discriminative ability than the traditional risk factors model (AUC 0.80 vs. 0.77).

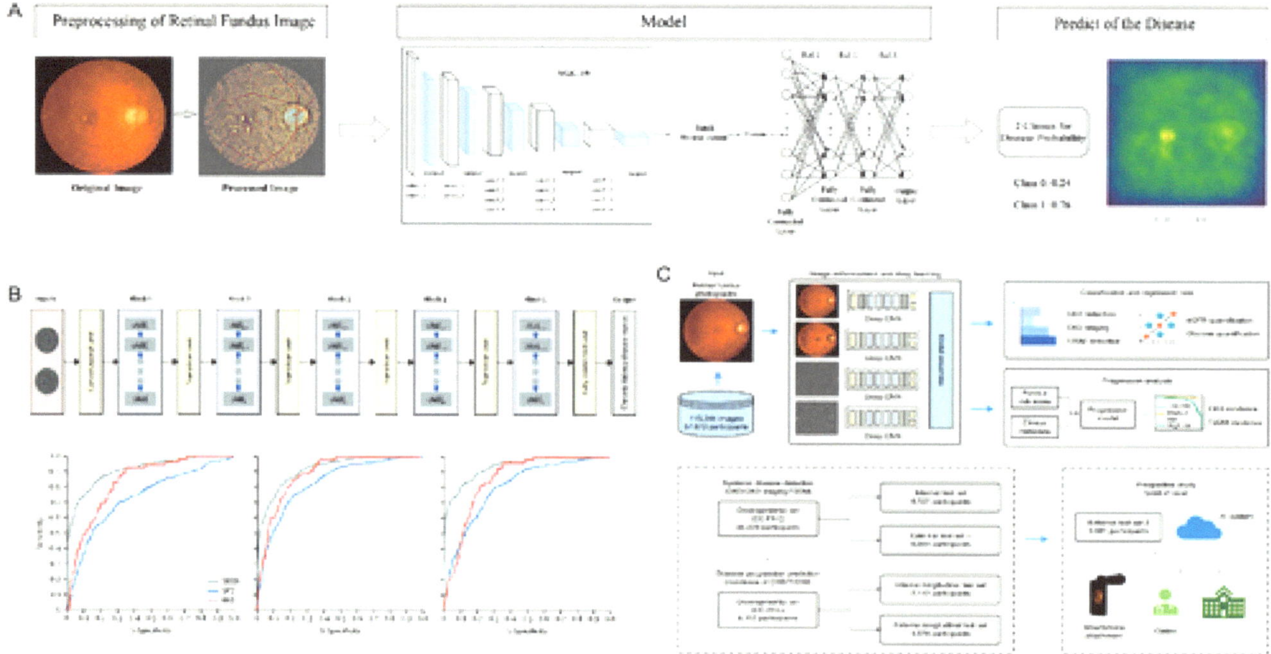

Fig.19.12 Retinal image-based AI models for screening and diagnosing kidney diseases: (A) schematic illustration of deep learning model detecting early renal function impairment; (B) Structure of deep learning models using retinal images to identify chronic kidney disease in community populations (upper panel) and the performance of image-only, risk factors and hybrid models (lower panel); (C) AI system for the diagnosis and incidence prediction of chronic kidney diseases using retinal fundus images. Source: (A) Copyright 2020, JMIR Publications; (B) Copyright 2020, Elsevier; (C) Copyright 2021, Springer Nature.

Diagnosing and grading CKD

For the early diagnosis of CKD in community and primary care clinics, two important studies have pointed out a new direction for renal disease screening mode based on retinal fundus images. In 2020, Sabanayagam et al.89 developed and validated a DL algorithm to detect CKDs in three population-based, multi-ethnic datasets (12,970 participants in total). In this study, multi-modal data were added into three models: a model of only fundus images, a model of CKD risk factors (age, sex, ethnicity, diabetes, and hypertension), and a hybrid model combining images and risk factors.They all showed similar good performance in the internal validation set (AUC = 0.911, 0.916, and 0.914, respectively) and moderate performance in the external validation cohort (AUC = 0.733–0.858). In subgroups of diabetes and hypertension patients, AUC was estimated similar to the whole population. Given that both the image-only model and the risk-factor model could predict CKD with high AUCs, and their combination only slightly improved the performance, fundus images alone could be employed as an auxiliary or opportunistic screening tool for CKDs in community populations, even without the collection of patient information. While the positive predictive value was high (54%) in the internal validation set, it was only 14% and 9% in external validation sets due to the high prevalence of CKD in the internal validation set. To improve the positive predictive value, the image-only model is recommended only to be applied to high-risk groups, such as diabetes and hypertension patients, however, this would limit its clinical utility in a larger population.Following this study, Zhang et al.16 built a DL model using ResNet-50 to identify CKD and early CKD patients only with fundus images or combined with clinical metadata (age, sex, height, weight, BMI, and BP). The models were trained and validated with 115,344 images from 57,672 patients. In the diagnosis model of CKD, the AUCs were 0.861 for the metadata model, and 0.918 for the model with only retinal images (Figure 4C). If the two models are combined, the accuracy rate will further increase (AUC = 0.930), providing better solutions for capturing features of CKDs. Then patient's eGFR, the key index of renal function and grading of CKD, was predicted using retinal fundus images with R2 of 0.327–0.507, and MAE of 11.1–13.4 ml/min/1.73m2, showing consistency with the measured eGFR (intraclass correlation coefficient [ICC] = 0.65, 95% CI: 0.63–0.66). For the grading of CKD, the thresholds of predicted eGFR were used to train regression models of differentiating advanced (stage G3) or severe+ CKD (stages G4 and G5) from early CKD (stages G1 and G2), which achieved good performance with AUCs of 0.853 and 0.825.Images captured by smartphone-based devices were introduced as an external test set to further evaluate the generalizability of the AI model and assess the feasibility of a massive population in a longitudinal cohort, achieving comparably good CKD detection performance (AUC = 0.897, 95% CI: 0.85–0.89, for image-only model) and non-inferior performance of eGFR prediction (ICC = 0.53, 95% CI: 0.50–0.55). The deployment of smartphone- and cloud-based AI diagnosis systems could build a bidirectional relationship between patients and clinics to improve the feasibility and broaden healthcare access by encouraging patients to self-monitor and allowing doctors to diagnose and follow up with patients remotely. However, current studies remain at the first stage of CKD diagnosis, only concerned about the qualitative value of eGFR, and did not include other important biomarkers for kidney function, like microalbuminuria or electrolytes. For CKD patients with different causes, such as glomerulonephritis or diabetic nephropathy, their treatment, and prognosis may vary. That's why the etiologic diagnosis (the so-called etiologic/GFR/albuminuria classification system) is emphasized. This helps to prioritize the diagnosis and treatment of the underlying disease to slow down the progression of CKD.

Individual management for common complications of CKD

The kidney is critical in maintaining volume, bone health, acid-base balance, electrolyte stability, and blood pressure. Decreased kidney function can lead to several serious complications such as anemia, hyperkalemia, mineral bone disease, hyperphosphatemia, hypertension, and CVDs. Renal anemia plays an important factor in affecting the quality of life and prognosis of the patients. Chen et al. applied retinal vessel images from OCT to directly and non-evasively observe the hemoglobin concentration in the retina for the first time. Later, Mitani et al.91 and Zhao et al. leverage retinal fundus images to predict hemoglobin concentration and detect the status of anemia accurately (MAE: 0.67, AUC: 0.87; MAE: 0.83, AUC: 0.93, respectively). For the predictions of electrolyte disorders, sodium was predicted with an R2 of 0.12 (95% CI: 0.10–0.13), while the performance was poor for potassium, calcium, and phosphorus (R2 = 0.07, 0.07, and 0.02, respectively).86 These studies indicate that retinal imaging has clinical potential to screen for and monitor renal anemia in patients with CKD, which could aid in deciding on treatment plans and improving patient outcomes.

Evaluating the treatment effect and predicting the complications of dialysis

When CKD patients progress to the end stage, their renal function fails to meet the basic need for body operation, and RRT is essentially needed, which consists of hemodialysis, peritoneal dialysis, and kidney transplant. The most common treatment for ESRD patients is hemodialysis, however, the occurrence of complications (intradialytic hypotension [IDH], adverse cardiovascular events, renal anemia, etc.) leads to dialysis failure and poor patient survival. To evaluate the treatment effect and prevent complications, many indicators were used to monitor and evaluate patients' fluid and metabolic status, which includes laboratory blood tests of creatine and bioimpedance for volume assessment. Retinal images and vessel measurements also represent novel and non-invasive methods to facilitate easy assessments of dialysis patients. It has been proved that the blood flow in the retina and choroid was significantly changed after a single session of hemodialysis93, 94 and the decrease in SBP was associated with the subfoveal choroidal thickness. Thus, Coppolino et al.96 performed OCT-A before the dialysis session and predict the risk of IDH within 30 days of follow-up. IDH was shown to be associated with baseline foveal vessel density of superficial and deep capillary plexus in logistic regression analysis but inversely associated with the choroid. These metrics predict the occurrence of IDH with AUCs of 0.674-0.783, with limited small and single-center data without external validation and robustness tests. But a significantly high proportion of patients reported experiencing IDH emphasizes the importance of prediction and prevention of complications with rapid and non-invasive retinal examinations.

In another cohort of hemodialysis patients, Werfel et al. adopted flicker-induced dynamic retinal vessel signals to assess the microvascular function and improve the predictions of individual cardiovascular risk. For patients with ESRD and other chronic diseases, these algorithms provide a new potential for future applications of these clinically relevant outcome-specific impairments of microvascular function and will fill the gap in predictive tools for CKDs.

Predicting the prognosis and mortality of CKD

Prediction of CKD prognosis or mortality at the onset and primary assessment could help physicians identify patients at risk of ESRD progression and deliver intensive care and timely interventions. Retinal arteriolar narrowing reflects CKD and other vascular processes and predicts renal disease progression or renal endpoints (50% renal function loss or start of RRT). The relative risk for renal endpoints of narrow arterioles was 3.7 (95% CI: 1.7-8.4) and the tertile of the narrowest arterioles was associated with more renal endpoints (log-rank $p < 0.001$).79 The incidence and severity of DR98, 99 also reveal that retinal vessel changes were associated with poor renal outcomes (hazard ratio (HR) = 1.69, 95% CI: 1.16–2.45).Zhang et al.16 implemented a DL-based AI model to predict the risk of progression to advanced (stage 3) and severe CKD (stages 4 and 5) based on a 6-year longitudinal cohort. Combined with clinical data, the model performed well with a C-index of 0.845 (95% CI: 0.789–0.910) on the internal test set and 0.719 (95% CI: 0.627–0.807) on the external test set. Applications also extend to healthy individuals, the Kaplan-Meier method was used to stratify participants into low, medium, and high-risk groups with high degrees of separation ($p < 0.001$). And the incidence of CKD or advanced CKD in high-risk groups was significantly different from medium-risk groups, while no differences were observed in low-risk groups of CKD ($p = 0.212$ and 0.689 in the internal and external longitudinal test sets, respectively). A DL model was developed by Zhang et al.100 to characterize retinal age from retinal images and the retinal age gap (difference between model-based retinal age and chronological age) was used to predict the risk of ESRD. Cox proportional hazards regression models showed a 10% increase in the risk of incident ESRD with each one-year increase in retinal age gap (HR = 1.10, 95% CI: 1.03–1.17). As the retinal images are highly amendable for early prediction and longitudinal evaluations, they could not only help estimate the progression of ESRD but also assist doctors to be a predictor of mortality,101 After multivariable adjustments, the retinal age gap was associated with a 2% increase in the risk of all-cause mortality (HR = 1.02, 95% CI: 1.00–1.03, $p = 0.020$) and a 3% increase in the risk of cause-specific mortality attributable to non-cardiovascular and non-cancer disease (HR = 1.03, 95% CI: 1.00–1.05, $p = 0.041$).

This research suggests that retinal images have the potential to be used as a screening tool for risk assessment and the delivery of personalized treatment

Conclusion

As AI is transforming almost every aspect of our lives, researchers felt an urgent need to incorporate AI in medicine, including ophthalmology and other diseases. Many studies proved the capability of retinal image-based AI models for predicting systemic diseases, such as diabetes, CVDs, and CKDs

Neurological diseases

The eye is referred to as the "window to the soul" in literature, and the retina is an anatomical extension of the central nervous system. In reaction to internal and external environmental stimuli, the eye has a physiological and pathological state that is similar to that of the brain and spinal cord. As a result, research into the link between the eye and the neurological system is becoming increasingly common. For example, patients with Parkinson's disease can also exhibit visual impairment. Their retinal ganglion cells (RGCs) are injured, and the retinal nerve fibers layer (RNFL) in the retina is thinning Similarly, alterations in the structure and function of the retina have been seen in people with Alzheimer's disease (AD). Aβ and pTau proteins were found in the retina of Alzheimer's disease patients, which were representative molecules of Alzheimer's disease pathogenesis. OCT has produced evidence for considerable thinning of the peripapillary NFL, macular volume loss, and nerve fiber density reduction in individuals with moderate to severe AD, indicating that thinning could develop early in disease progression Besides, among older adults, thinner RNFL thickness at baseline was associated with a greater decline in cognitive function scores at follow-up .

Given the retina's tight association with neurological illnesses, it's unsurprising that researchers have employed AI to investigate the eye's relationship with the neurological system.

Alzheimer's disease (AD)

The diagnosis of AD relies on clinical manifestations, imaging, and cognitive-psychological examinations, which may occur in the late stages of AD. As the aging process accelerates, early screening for AD is necessary. Cheung et al. retrospectively collected fundus images from AD patients and healthy individuals in 11 studies and different countries, to construct and validate a model for the diagnosis of AD . The AUCs of the external validation sets were from 0.73 to 0.91. They also found that the AI model was able to distinguish between beta amyloid-negative and positive patients, and had better performance in patients with ocular disease.Since retinal thickness correlates with AD , OCT images that present retinal thickness are a good source for constructing AI. The AI algorithm for texture acquisition from OCT images is well implemented for AD detection, with an AUC of 0.795 . In addition, the combination of multimodal imaging and clinical data may improve the efficacy of AI systems. Based on this, multimodal retinal images including OCT, OCT-A, Ultra-widefield scanning laser ophthalmoscopy, and the patients' data were combined to develop AI models to detect AD . Ganglion cell-inner plexiform layer thickness map in OCT and combined model made good results of AUC over 0.8.

Others Dysfunctions

For a subset of neurological diseases that are difficult and costly to diagnose, AI based on retinal images has provided a convenient tool of screening. An AI system to diagnose diabetic peripheral neuropathy based on retinal color images was developed , which could provide a chance to screen their peripheral neuropathy status when people with diabetes screened their eyes. In patients with diabetic retinopathy, the AUC reached over 0.85. Also, the retinal vascular trajectory was acquired with the help of an AI algorithm, which connected the retina with schizophrenia and bipolar disorder, and performed the accuracy of 0.86 and 0.73, respectively . Moreover, Lau et al. connected retinal images with MRI, and they detected white matter hyperintensities in healthy people, which was vital for the development of cerebral small vessel disease, and both of the sensitivity and specificity were over 0.9

Autoimmune diseases

Multiple sclerosis

The relationship between the eyes and the immune system is so close that there are many autoimmune diseases with ocular characteristics, such as Sjögren syndrome, inflammatory bowel disease, multiple sclerosis, and many others. The patients can present as dry eyes, uveitis, optic neuritis, etc. The studies of eyes and multiple sclerosis suggested that the thickness of the retina was thing with the development of multiple sclerosis, and measurement of retinal thickness with OCT could be a biomarker of multiple sclerosis. Based on this, among the ocular images, OCT images are currently the main image source for AI diagnosis of multiple sclerosis. Cavaliere et al. collected OCT images from multiple sclerosis and controls. They got different regions of the retina and choroid with OCT ETDRS scan and TNSIT scan modes and calculated the variables with the highest AUC (0.97) to create a diagnosis model using a support vector machine algorithm.Similarly, Martin et al. got OCT images from 48 early-stage multiple sclerosis patients and 48 healthy people They measured the thickness of each layer of retina and choroid, and tried to find regions with the greatest discriminant capacity that could be used as a classifier. The best classifier showed a great performance (sensitivity = specificity = 0.98). Their work showed that the papillomacular bundle may be the first layer affected in the early stage of multiple sclerosis, and the OCT images-based AI system could be a new direction for the early diagnosis of multiple sclerosis.

Hematological diseases

Anemia

Anemia is commonly defined as a low concentration of hemoglobin (Hb). Most of the anemia is easily corrected, while the key is to be detected. The "gold standard" of anemia is Hb concentration measured by venous blood samples. However, the invasive procedure is a risk of pollution for medical workers and painful for patients. Therefore, some non-invasive and painless methods of measuring Hb have been developed such as pulse oximetry, occlusion spectroscopy, photoplethysmography and reflectance spectroscopy Compared to the "gold standard", the stability and accuracy of these methods have yet to be proven.

During the physical examination, pallor of the skin mucosa such as lips and palpebral conjunctiva is often considered as an indication of anemia. Therefore, some researchers have attempted to estimate anemia status by AI through palpebral conjunctiva images. With the help of image processing programs, scientists extracted color information from segmented palpebral conjunctiva images. Early in 2007, Suner et al. took pictures of palpebral conjunctiva and got RGB values from them [43]. They developed an algorithm according to the manually delineated regions of the digital photos. This algorithm allowed for a crude calculation of the subjects' hemoglobin concentrations. However, the quality of the images was easily influenced by the environment. Algorithms and wearable devices were developed to overcome this challenge [44, 45]. However, despite the variety of methods, detecting Hb values seemed to be difficult for AI that relied on eye images. It might be easier to diagnose anemia rather than to detect Hb values for AI. On the other hand, the association between retina and anemia was discovered [46], and researchers tried to use AI based on retinal images to diagnose anemia. Mitani et al. proposed a hypothesis that anemia could be detected from retinal images using deep learning They collected data from UK Biobank, and developed deep learning systems based on fundus images and metadata to det Hb and anemia status. Also, the combined AI system made a good performance on diabetes patients (AUC = 0.89). Along with the wide application of OCT . technology in the field of ophthalmology, Wei et al. used retinal OCT images and deep learning to predict anemia for the first time [48]. Their work has led to a new level of efficacy in assessing anemia status, with a high accuracy of 98.65%.

Sleep disorders

Obstructive sleep apnea (OSA) and narcolepsy

These are two main types of sleep disorders. The former is characterized by recurrent apnea during sleep, and the latter is characterized by drowsiness when awake and disturbed sleep. The diagnosis of OSA depends on a sleep breathing test, while the "gold standard" for the diagnosis of narcolepsy is the multiple sleep latency test. Relatively difficult diagnostic criteria limit the diagnosis of sleep disorders. With the deeper research of sleep disorders, the sleep status of patients with sleep disorders was gradually being understood and it had been found that electroencephalogram (EEG) and pupil size can represent such alterations]. Based on this, Liu et al. developed a neural network method to detect OSA and narcolepsy according to EEG and pupil size The accuracy of the algorithm was above 90%

Hepatobiliary diseases

Previously, it appeared that ocular symptoms such as scleral yellowing due to jaundice and K-F rings due to hepatomegaly could only offer suggestive information for particular disorders. However, Xiao et al. innovated the use of ocular images in the detection of hepatobiliary diseases with AI . They collected clinical data and ocular images (fundus images and slit-lamp images) of patients with seven hepatobiliary diseases from multiple centers and built an AI detection system based on the ocular images. Their algorithm has achieved good results in diseases such as cirrhosis and liver cancer (both of AUCs were over 0.83). In comparison to the AI, it was difficult for the six ophthalmologists to determine whether the subjects had hepatobiliary disease based on the ocular images, let alone diagnose the specific type of diseases. When using the heat map to interpret AI concerns, the highlighted areas are the optic disc and blood vessels of the fundus images and the conjunctiva, sclera, and iris of the slit-lamp images. This may help to discover new mechanisms of hepatobiliary diseases

Systemic parameters

The previous studies demonstrated that we could observe the whole body non-invasively through the eye. The above discussion shows that ocular images can be used for diabetes, cardiovascular disease, anemia, and many other systemic diseases. In 2019, Banowati et al. detected cholesterol levels by iris images with the help of AI, whose accuracy was 97.45% . And in the same year, Vaghefi et al. were able to determine the smoking status of the subjects based on retinal images.However, as AI is still in the developmental stage, reflecting the the whole-body state through ocular images still requires careful and comprehensive research. Thus, Rim et al. did the largest study to date in a related field. Collecting more than 230,000 fundus photographs, as well as setting 47 systemic parameters (age, sex, body-mass index, blood pressure, and some laboratory measurements, such as creatinine) as outputs, they evaluated the diagnostic efficacy of the AI more comprehensively. And the impact of different races on AI was also compared. Despite the poor detection efficacy of AI systems in some biomarkers, especially in external validation sets, it demonstrated the relevance of the eye to the whole body from another perspective. In addition, considering parameters with poor predictive performance, Rim et al. suggested that retinal changes may better reflect chronic diseases such as cardiovascular disease and chronic kidney disease

Heighlights of ocular based Artificial studies in systemic studies

1. Current studies are mainly focused on diseases that are very closely associated with the eye, such as diabetes, cardiovascular disease, CKD and AD. Researchers haven't often used AI to examine the connection between other diseases and the eye because there hasn't been much study on intrinsic connections. And this relies on researchers to further explore the ocular features associated with systemic diseases. Most current studies have focused on the use of ocular images to diagnose systemic diseases, with a small number being predictions of future incidence or progression, while clustering tasks are rare. This is mainly due to the level of difficulty in obtaining data. Future researchers may focus more on the task of predicting disease progression and assisting physicians in developing treatment plans.

2. Ocular images-based AI has benefits in several aspects, including reducing screening costs, improving efficiency and coverage, and reducing the burden on physicians. In the future, ocular images-based AI may be more widely used in screening, as it is presently used clinically to detect retinal diseases . In places with limited medical resources, AI can perform routine screening by integrating software into fundus cameras. Fundus images can simultaneously detect retinal diseases, systemic diseases, and risk factors with the help of AI, which may help us to identify problems at an early or even pre-clinical stage of the disease.

3. In the future, many areas still require research. Firstly, apart from diagnosis, researchers can explore predicting the prognosis of diseases through eye imaging. This can help doctors in planning medical treatments. Secondly, most current researches use two-dimensional ocular images, and the acquisition of three-dimensional images from OCTA or other devices may be a new direction. Treating the entire eye as a single entity may help us uncover more differences in diseases. Thirdly, more innovative algorithms must be developed and incorporated to enhance disease detection performance.

4. Currently, the application of ocular images to detect systemic diseases confronts many challenges. First, a large number of images are needed in AI systems. Not only the construction of the model, but also testing the performance of the model requires an external validation set. In addition, the number of ocular images needed for each type of disease is currently unknown. However, for most departments, eye examinations are not routine. Therefore, to study the relationship between systemic diseases and the eyes, the acquirement of high-quality ocular images and a complete database of clinical information needs to be fully supported. This requires close collaboration between doctors in ophthalmology and other departments, as well as the assistance of AI engineers. To eliminate the interference of the number of images, the researchers must make images “better and more”.

5. There are a lot of “black boxes” in the field of AI. There is still a great deal unknown about the mechanisms of image recognition by artificial intelligence, especially by deep learning systems. Some scientists have attempted to debunk AI systems, but no better explanatory views have emerged yet. Therefore, although some studies have attempted to represent the regions of interest of AI in the form of heat maps, we cannot understand the principles by which the system establishes the association of ocular and systemic diseases. Machine learning algorithms apart from deep learning may have better interpretations and should be applied more often to obtain more highly interpretable eye features.

6. Some rare diseases are difficult to study with AI. Based on the need for AI systems to extract features, a large number of high-quality images are indispensable to build a diagnostic system. However, this is difficult to do for some rare diseases. In these areas, it is likely that manual diagnosis will still dominate in the future. Although there are algorithms to increase the number of images by image enhancement, this is still of limited help for diversity. Multicenter studies and interpretable machine learning algorithms may be the solutions.

7.Ophthalmic imaging devices vary widely and produce different types of images. For example, fundus images from different devices may differ in size, resolution, image format, and color. Using images from different devices to build AI models may reduce model performance. Conversely, if a model can perform well in different styles of image datasets, it indicates that the model has good robustness. Therefore, we need an algorithm or image standard to make different images easy for AI recognition.

8.There are many ethical and legal issues before AI can be used in the clinical setting. There is a risk of information leaking when using AI systems because they need a lot of patient data to build them. To make sure that patient information is not utilized in other ways, strict legal restrictions and information protection measures are required. Blockchain technology has been used in data transfer to ensure that patients' personal information was not misused.

Predicting Body Composition Factors From RFPBody composition factors predicted from RFP include body massindex (BMI), body muscle mass, height, weight, relative fat mass,and waist-hip ratio (WHR) . Performance of current algorithms in BMI prediction is generally poor withlow R2-values (R2: 0.13–0.17). Model generalizability across ethnically distinct datasets was poor as well. Rim et al. found that DL algorithms for prediction of height, body weight,BMI (and other non-body composition factors), trained on aSouth Korean dataset, showed limited generalizability in the UK Biobank dataset (majority White ethnicity) (R^2 ≤0.08).Proportional bias was observed, where predicted values in thelower range were overestimated and those in the higher rangewere underestimated. While BMI is a parameter of interest dueto its well-established associations with all-cause and cause-specific mortality,prediction of other plausible parametersof body composition have been described. The prediction of bodymuscle mass is noteworthy, as it is a potentially more reliablebiomarker than BMI for cardiometabolic risk and nutritionalstatus Rim et al. reported that body muscle masscould be predicted with an R^2 of 0.52 (95% CI: 0.51–0.53) i

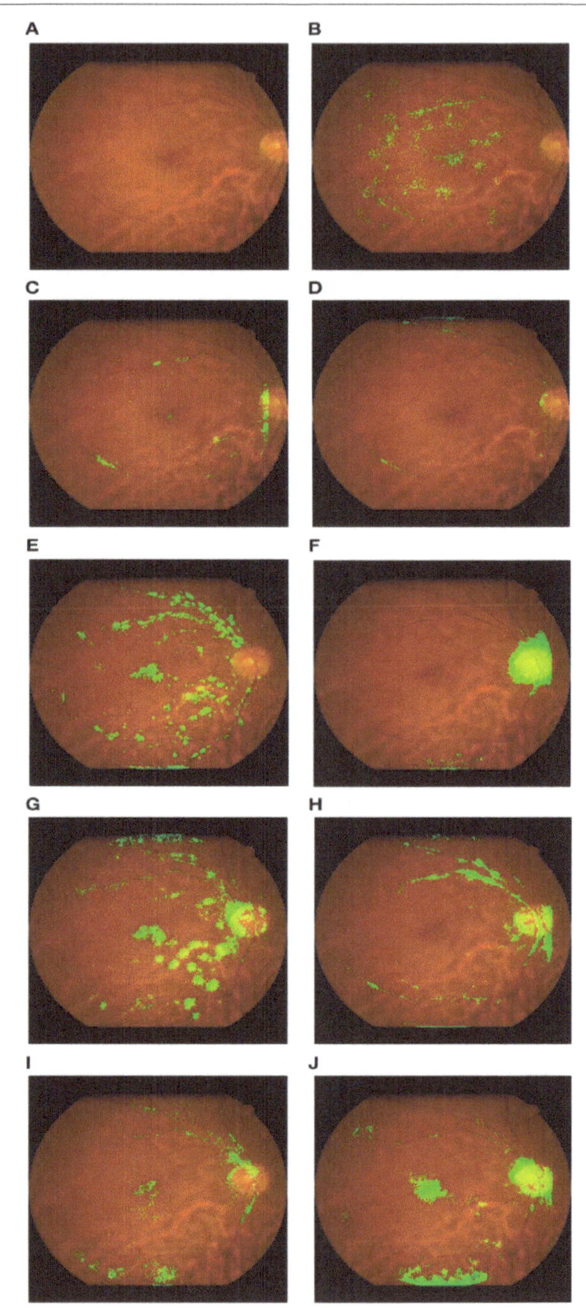

Fig 19.13 Example heatmaps overlaid on retinal fundus photographs highlighting areas of interest. These examples were derived from the authors' research database. (A) Original photograph with no overlay; (B) red blood cell count; (C) systolic blood pressure; (D) Weight; (E) age; (F) body mass index; (G) creatinine; (H) diastolic blood pressure; (I) hemoglobin; (J) height.

Bibliography and Acknowledgement

- Aldrich TK, Moosikasuwan M, Shah SD, Deshpande KS. Length-normalized pulse photoplethysmography: a noninvasive method to measure blood hemoglobin, Bronx, NY. Ann Biomed Eng. 2002;30(10):1291–1298.
- Appaji A, Nagendra B, Chako DM, Padmanabha A, Jacob A, Hiremath CV, et al. Examination of retinal vascular trajectory in schizophrenia and bipolar disorder. Psychiatry Clin Neurosci. 2019;73(12):738–744
- Banowati C, Novianty A, Setianingsih C. Cholesterol level detection based on iris recognition using convolutional neural network method. In: 2019 IEEE Conference on Sustainable Utilization and Development in Engineering and Technologies (CSUDET). Penang, Malaysia: IEEE; 2019. p. 116–21
- Barker SJ, Badal JJ. The measurement of dyshemoglobins and total hemoglobin by pulse oximetry. Curr Opin Anaesthesiol. 2008;21(6):805–810.
- Campbell JP, Kim SJ, Brown JM, Ostmo S, Chan RVP, Kalpathy-Cramer J, et al. Evaluation of a deep learning-derived quantitative retinopathy of prematurity severity scale. Ophthalmology. 2021;128(7):1070–1076. doi: 10.1016/j.ophtha.2020.10.025
- Cavaliere C, Vilades E, Alonso-Rodríguez M, Rodrigo M, Pablo L, Miguel J, et al. Computer-aided diagnosis of multiple sclerosis using a support vector machine and optical coherence tomography features. Sens. 2019;19(23):5323.
- Cervera DR, Smith L, Diaz-Santana L, Kumar M, Raman R, Sivaprasad S. Identifying peripheral neuropathy in colour fundus photographs based on deep learning. Diagnostics. 2021;11(11):1943.
- Chang J, Ko A, Park SM, Choi S, Kim K, Kim SM, et al. Association of cardiovascular mortality and deep learning-funduscopic atherosclerosis score derived from retinal fundus images. Am J Ophthalmol. 2020;217:121–130.
- Chen YM, Miaou SG. A Kalman filtering and nonlinear penalty regression approach for noninvasive anemia detection with palpebral conjunctiva images. J Healthc Eng. 2017;2017:9580385.
- Cheung CY, Ran AR, Wang S, Chan VTT, Sham K, Hilal S, et al. A deep learning model for detection of Alzheimer's disease based on retinal photographs: a retrospective, multicentre case-control study. Lancet Digit Health. 2022
- Cheung CY, Xu D, Cheng CY, Sabanayagam C, Tham YC, Yu M, et al. A deep-learning system for the assessment of cardiovascular disease risk via the measurement of retinal-vessel calibre. Nat Biomed Eng. 2021;5(6):498–508. doi: 10.1038/s41551-020-00626-4
- Dimauro G, Caivano D, Girardi F. A new method and a non-invasive device to estimate anemia based on digital images of the conjunctiva. Ieee Access. 2018;6:46968–46975.
- Frank Z, Timothy R, Robert W, James L, Jeanne S, Thomas R. Sleep-wake abnormalities in narcolepsy. Sleep. 1986;1:189–193
- Garcia-Martin E, Ortiz M, Boquete L, Sánchez-Morla EM, Barea R, Cavaliere C, et al. Early diagnosis of multiple sclerosis by OCT analysis using Cohen's d method and a neural network as classifier. Comput Biol Med. 2021;129:104165.
- Grzybowski A, editor. Artificial intelligence in ophthalmology. Cham: Springer; 2021
- Gu C, Wang Y, Jiang Y, Xu F, Wang S, Liu R, et al. Application of artificial intelligence system for screening multiple fundus diseases in Chinese primary healthcare settings: A real-world, multicentre and cross-sectional study of 4795 cases. Br J Ophthalmol. 2023 Mar 6
- Hannappe MA, Arnould L, Méloux A, Mouhat B, Bichat F, Zeller M, et al. Vascular density with optical coherence tomography angiography and systemic biomarkers in low and high cardiovascular risk patients. Sci Rep. 2020;10(1):16718. doi: 10.1038/s41598-020-73861-z.
- Hart NJ, Koronyo Y, Black KL, Koronyo-Hamaoui M. Ocular indicators of Alzheimer's: exploring disease in the retina. Acta Neuropathol. 2016;132(6):767–787
- He J, Baxter SL, Xu J, Xu J, Zhou X, Zhang K. The practical implementation of artificial intelligence technologies in medicine. Nat Med. 2019;25(1):30–36. doi: 10.1038/s41591-018-0307-0.
- Huang L, Zhang D, Ji J, Wang Y, Zhang R. Central retina changes in Parkinson's disease: a systematic review and meta-analysis. J Neurol. 2021;268(12):4646–4654.
- Kang EY, Hsieh YT, Li CH, Huang YJ, Kuo CF, Kang JH, et al. Deep learning-based detection of early renal function impairment using retinal fundus images: model development and validation. JMIR Med Inform. 2020;8(11):e23472
- Kim HM, Han JW, Park YJ, Bae JB, Woo SJ, Kim KW. Association between retinal layer thickness and cognitive decline in older adults. JAMA Ophthalmol. 2022
- Kim O, McMurdy J, Jay G, Lines C, Crawford G, Alber M. Combined reflectance spectroscopy and stochastic modeling approach for noninvasive hemoglobin determination via palpebral conjunctiva. Physiol Rep. 2014;2(1):e00192.
- Lau AY, Mok V, Lee J, Fan Y, Zeng J, Lam B, et al. Retinal image analytics detects white matter hyperintensities in healthy adults. Ann Clin Transl Neurol. 2019;6(1):98–105.
- Li F, Su Y, Lin F, Li Z, Song Y, Nie S, et al. A deep-learning system predicts glaucoma incidence and progression using retinal photographs. J Clin Invest. 2022;132(11):e157968.
- Liew G, Mitchell P, Wong TY, Iyengar SK, Wang JJ. CKD increases the risk of age-related macular degeneration. J Am Soc Nephrol. 2008;19(4):806–811
- Liu D, Pang Z, Lloyd SR. A neural network method for detection of obstructive sleep apnea and narcolepsy based on pupil size and EEG. IEEE Trans Neural Netw. 2008;19(2):308–318.
- Liu N, Liang G, Li L, Zhou H, Zhang L, Song X. An eyelid parameters auto-measuring method based on 3D scanning. Displays. 2021;1(69):102063.
- Margulies LJ. Ocular manifestations of cardiovascular and hematologic disorders. Curr Opin Ophthalmol. 1994;5(6):99–104
  Mitani A, Huang A, Venugopalan S, Corrado GS, Peng L, Webster DR, et al. Detection of anaemia from retinal fundus images via deeplearning. Nat Biomed Eng. 2020;4(1):18–27.
- Moraes G, Fu DJ, Wilson M, Khalid H, Wagner SK, Korot E, et al. Quantitative analysis of OCT for neovascular age-related macular degeneration using deep learning. Ophthalmology. 2021;128(5):693–705. doi: 10.1016/j.ophtha.2020.09.025
- Nunes A, Silva G, Duque C, Januario C, Santana I, Ambrosio AF, et al. Retinal texture biomarkers may help to discriminate between Alzheimer's, Parkinson's, and healthy controls. PLoS ONE. 2019;14(6):e0218826.
- O'Bryhim BE, Lin JB, Stavern GPV, Apte RS. OCT angiography findings in preclinical Alzheimer's disease: 3-year follow-up. Ophthalmology. 2021;128(10):1489–1491.
- Owen CG, Rudnicka AR, Welikala RA, Fraz MM, Barman SA, Luben R, et al. Retinal vasculometry associations with cardiometabolic risk factors in the european prospective investigation of cancer—norfolk study. Ophthalmology. 2019;126(1):96–106. doi: 10.1016/j.ophtha.2018.07.022.
- Pakzad-Vaezi K, Pepple KL. Tubulointerstitial nephritis and uveitis. Curr Opin Ophthalmol. 2017;28(6):629–635
  Pinto M, Barjas-Castro ML, Nascimento S, Falconi MNA, Zulli R, Castro V. The new noninvasive occlusion spectroscopy hemoglobin measurement method: a reliable and easy anemia screening test for blood donors. Transfusion. 2012;53:766.
- Poplin R, Varadarajan AV, Blumer K, Liu Y, McConnell MV,

Corrado GS, et al. Prediction of cardiovascular risk factors from retinal fundus photographs via deep learning. Nat Biomed Eng. 2018;2(3):158–164

- Rim TH, Lee CJ, Tham YC, Cheung N, Yu M, Lee G, et al. Deep-learning-based cardiovascular risk stratification using coronary artery calcium scores predicted from retinal photographs. Lancet Digital Health. 2021;3(5):e306–e316.
- Rim TH, Lee G, Kim Y, Tham YC, Lee CJ, Baik SJ, et al. Prediction of systemic biomarkers from retinal photographs: development and validation of deep-learning algorithms. Lancet Digit Health. 2020;2(10):e526–e536.
- Ruamviboonsuk P, Tiwari R, Sayres R, Nganthavee V, Hemarat K, Kongprayoon A, et al. Real-time diabetic retinopathy screening by deep learning in a multisite national screening programme: a prospective interventional cohort study. Lancet Digit Health Saarela V, Nuutinen M, Ala-Houhala M, Arikoski P, Ronnholm K, Jahnukainen T. Tubulointerstitial nephritis and uveitissyndrome in children: a prospective multicenter study. Ophthalmology. 2013;120(7):1476–1481.
- Sabanayagam C, Xu D, Ting DSW, Nusinovici S, Banu R, Hamzah H, et al. A deep learning algorithm to detect chronic kidney disease from retinal photographs in community-based populations. Lancet Digit Health. 2020;2(6):e295–302.
- Sarabi MS, Khansari MM, Zhang J, Kushner-Lenhoff S, Gahm JK, Qiao Y, et al. 3D retinal vessel density mapping with OCT-angiography. IEEE J Biomed Health Inform. 2020;24(12):3466–3479.
- Sayin N. Ocular complications of diabetes mellitus. World J Diabetes. 2015;6(1):92.
- Smoking on age and sex prediction from retinal fundus images. Sci Rep. 2020;10(1):4623.
- Son J, Shin JY, Chun EJ, Jung KH, Park KH, Park SJ. Predicting high coronary artery calcium score from retinal fundus images with deep learning algorithms. Transl Vision Sci Technol. 2020;9(2):28. doi: 10.1167/tvst.9.2.28
- Suner S, Crawford G, McMurdy J, Jay G. Non-invasive determination of hemoglobin by digital photography of palpebral conjunctiva. J Emerg Med. 2007;33(2):105–111.
- Tan TE, Anees A, Chen C, Li S, Xu X, Li Z, et al. Retinal photograph-based deep learning algorithms for myopia and a blockchain platform to facilitate artificial intelligence medical research: a retrospective multicohort study. Lancet Digit Health. 2021;3(5):e317–e329.
- Vaghefi E, Yang S, Hill S, Humphrey G, Walker N, Squirrell D. Detection of smoking status from retinal images; a convolutional neural network study. Sci Rep. 2019;9(1):7180.
- Wang H, Abbas KM, Abbasifard M, Abbasi-Kangevari M, Abbastabar H, Abd-Allah F, et al. Global age-sex-specific fertility, mortality, healthy life expectancy (HALE), and population estimates in 204 countries and territories, 1950–2019: a comprehensive demographic analysis for the global burden of disease study 2019. Lancet. 2020;396(10258):1160–1203.
- Wei H, Shen H, Li J, Zhao R, Chen Z. AneNet: a lightweight network for the real-time anemia screening from retinal vessel optical coherence tomography images. Opt Laser Technol. 2021;136:106773.
- Wisely CE, Wang D, Henao R, Grewal DS, Thompson AC, Robbins CB, et al. Convolutional neural network to identify symptomatic Alzheimer's disease using multimodal retinal imaging. Br J Ophthalmol. 2022;106(3):388–395.
- Wong CW, Wong TY, Cheng CY, Sabanayagam C. Kidney and eye diseases: common risk factors, etiological mechanisms, and pathways. Kidney Int. 2014;85(6):1290–1302.
- Wong TY, Coresh J, Klein R, Muntner P, Couper DJ, Sharrett AR, et al. Retinal microvascular abnormalities and renal dysfunction: the atherosclerosis risk in communities study. J Am Soc Nephrol. 2004;15(9):2469–2476.
- Xiao W, Huang X, Wang JH, Lin DR, Zhu Y, Chen C, et al. Screening and identifying hepatobiliary diseases through deep learning using ocular images: a prospective, multicentre study. Lancet Digit Health. 2021;3(2):e88–97.
- Yoss RE, Moyer NJ, Hollenhorst RW. Pupil size and spontaneous pupillary waves associated with alertness, drowsiness, and sleep. Neurology. 1970;20(6):545–554.
- Zhang B, Chou Y, Zhao X, Yang J, Chen Y. Early detection of microvascular impairments with optical coherence tomography angiography in diabetic patients without clinical retinopathy: a meta-analysis. Am J Ophthalmol. 2021;222:226–237.
- Zhang K, Liu X, Xu J, Yuan J, Cai W, Chen T, et al. Deep-learning models for the detection and incidence prediction of chronic kidney disease and type 2 diabetes from retinal fundus images. Nat Biomed Eng. 2021;5(6):533–545
- Zhang L, Wu Y, Hu M, Guo W. Automatic image analysis of episcleral hemangioma applied to the prognosis prediction of trabeculotomy in Sturge-Weber syndrome. Displays. 2022;1(71):102118.
- Zhang L, Yuan M, An Z, Zhao X, Wu H, Li H, et al. Prediction of hypertension, hyperglycemia and dyslipidemia from retinal fundus photographs via deep learning: a cross-sectional study of chronic diseases in central China. PLoS ONE. 2020;15(5):e0233166.

NEWER INNOVATIONS IN CARDIOLOGY -Brief Notes

CHAPTER

DIABETES UPDATE

Scientists Developed Low Cost Device For Monitoring Diabetes Through Sweat

A new, non-invasive option for controlling diabetes may be just around the corner. Scientists at the University of Texas at Dallas have developed a wearable that is capable of managing the condition just by monitoring a patient's sweat. The study was published in the journal Scientific Reports. Diabetes is a lifelong condition that causes a person's blood sugar level to become too high. Globally, it is estimated that over 380 million people suffer from the disease. People throughout the world are encouraged to learn about risks and warningsigns.

Scientists have been looking for a non-invasive way to monitor the levels of glucose in people with diabetes for a long time now. This is considered to be the holy grail of diabetes treatment. The current method involves pricking your fingers multiple times a day.The new wearable diagnostic biosensor can detect three interconnected compounds – cortisol, glucose and interleukin-6, for up to a week. The University of Texas at Dallas team showed that the measurents are accurate with just one to three microliters of the liquid, much less than the 25 to 50 previously believed necessary.

The Team wanted to make a product more useful than something disposable after a single use. Because the wearable measures and tracks multiple molecules over time, it also tells a story about a patients health. Further steps will include building in a small Bluetooth transceiver to send data to a smartphone, and developing an app There is no information when such a device would become available. Hopefully not too long. Prasad says, throughout the development process the Team used processes that could easily be scaled up to allow for mass production. Best of all, the cost of manufacturing will be as little as 10 to 15 cents – comparable to what it currently takes to make single-use glucose test strips.

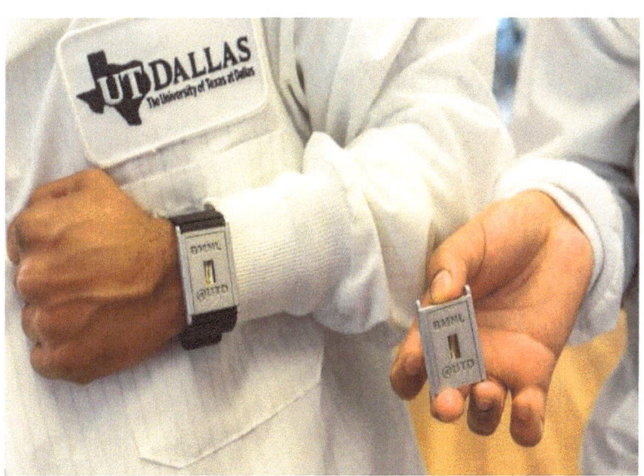

Fig. 20.1 Scientists at the University of Texas at Dallas have developed a wearable that is capable of managing the condition just by monitoring a patient's sweat

Gluco Track Gives You Freedom From Finger Pricking to Help You Manage Your Diabetes

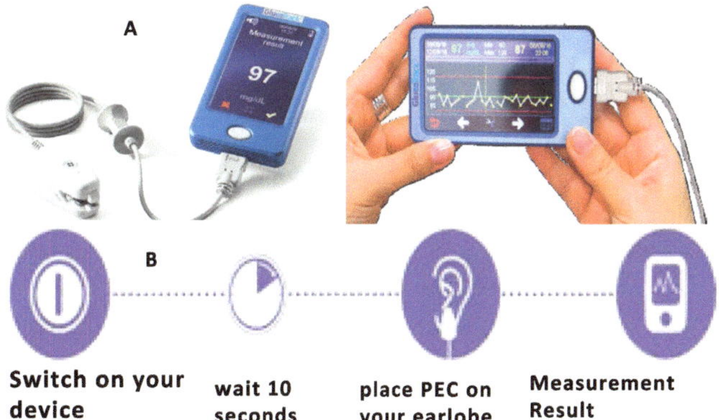

Fig.20.2 With Glucotrack, you can view your glucose profile by frequently measuring without using needles(A&B)

VALUE OF FFR IN CLINICAL PRACTICE

Key points

- FFR is a single highly reliable and reproducible invasive method to assess the ischemia producing potential of a lesion with accuracy of more than 90%.
- Currently a cutoff value of less than 0.8 is recommended for revascularization.
- Useful in assessment of intermediate coronary lesions in stable ischemic heart disease (left main disease, bifurcation disease, ostial disease, serial lesions, diffuse disease, old MI, collateralized vessels).
- In ACS patients it can be used for non-culprit lesions and after 7 days in the culprit lesions (not reliable in the culprit vessels in acute stage).
- While performing FFR important to equalize pressure sensor at the tip of the guide catheter after removing the introduced needle.
- Pressure sensor should be placed atleast 3 cm distal to thelesion. Although a number of resting indices (resting Pd/Pa, IFR etc) have been proposed, their diagnostic accuracy is around 80%. However if resting Pd/Pa is < 0.8 on maximal hyper-emia, the FFR will be < 0.8. If one is evaluating a single focal
- stenosis one can use the baseline criteria for revascularization.

Table 20.1. Vasodilators for testing Fractional Flow Reserve.

Epicardial vasodilators:
Nitroglycerin: 200–400 μg IC, administer 30 s before 1st measurement
Microvascular vasodilators:
Adenosine or ATP: ≥40 μg IC bolus in RCA, ≥ 80 μg IC bolus in LCA
Adenosine or ATP: 140 μg/kg/min IV (preferably through a central venous line)
Regadeonson (Rapiscan): 400 μg single bolus IC or peripheral IV
Papaverine: 10–12 mg in the RCA, 15–20 mg in the LCA

IC: intracoronary, IV: Intravenously, RCA: Right Coronary Artery, LCA: Left Coronary Artery, ATP: Adenosine triphosphate.

- Hyperemia is essential to achieve a steady state of minimal microvascular resistance to correctly interpret lesion physiology in all lesions (single or serial or diffuse disease).
- For hyperemia IV adenosine or Regadenoson is better than IC bolus for steady state and continuous pullback to assess serial lesions.
- Sometimes IV adenosine may not have adequate vaso-dilatory effect due to rapid peripheral metabolism. In such scenarios perform the response using incremental doses of IC adenosine bolus For multi-vessel evaluation, IV adenosine is preferred over Regadenoson because it has a longer lasting hemodynamic effect.
- Regadenoson has significantly larger blood pressure lowering effect than IV adenosine (caution in patients with border-line blood pressures).
- Slight variations in FFR values seen with respirations but use the lowest value in steady state.
- Pullback slowly along the entire length of the artery. Pullback to guide catheter to identify if there is any significant electronic drift.

COMPUTED FRACTIONAL FLOW RESERVE(FFR_{CT}) DERIVED FROM CORONARY CT ANGIOGRAPHY

Recent advances in image-based modeling and computational fluid dynamics permit the calculation of coronary artery pressure and flow from typically acquired coronary computed tomography (CT) scans. Computed fractional flow reserve is the ratio of mean coronary artery pressure divided by mean aortic pressure under conditions of simulated maximal coronary hyperemia, thus providing a non-invasive estimate of fractional flow reserve (FFRCT) at every point in the coronary tree. Prospective multicenter clinical trials have shown that computed FFRCT improves diagnostic accuracy and discrimination compared to CT stenosis alone for the diagnosis of hemodynamically significant coronary artery disease (CAD), when compared to invasive FFR as the reference gold standard. This promising new technology provides a combined anatomic and physiologic assessment of CAD in a single noninvasive test that can help select patients for invasive angiography and revascularization or best medical therapy. Further evaluation of the clinical effectiveness and economic implications of noninvasive FFRCT are now being explored.

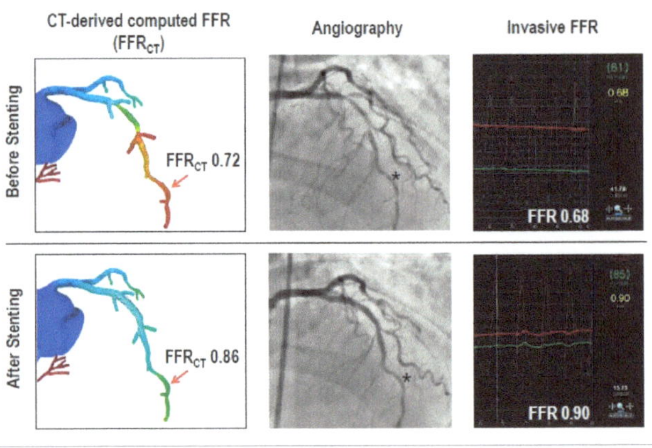

Fig.20.3 Invasive and Noninvasive Functional Assessment Before and After Revascularization (A) Noninvasive fractional flow reserve (FFR) from coronary computed tomographic angiography data (FFRCT) of the left anterior descending (LAD) coronary ar-tery was 0.72. Invasive coronary angiography and FFR confirmed the functionally significant LAD stenosis. (B) FFRCT demonstrated no ischemia in the LAD after virtual stenting, with a computed value of 0.86. Invasive FFR after stent implantation was 0.90.

VITAMIN D AND CARDIOVASCULAR DISEASE

Vitamin D is a fat soluble vitamin which also functions as a hormone. Now there is ample evidence that low levels of Vitamin D has been found to be associated with diabetes, systemic hypertension, metabolic syndrome, coronary heart disease (CHD), heart failure and vascular inflammation.

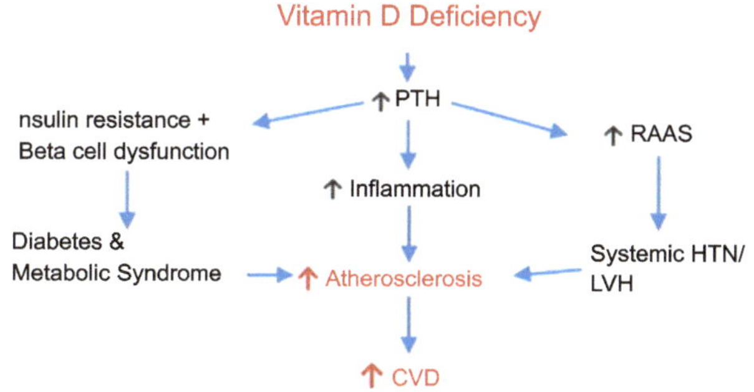

Fig. 20.4 The mechanisms of Vitamin D deficiency leading to atherosclerotic vascular disease. (PTH – parathyroid hormone, RAAS – renin angiotensin aldosterone system, HTN – hypertension, CVD – cardiovascular disease, LVH – left ventricular hypertrophy).

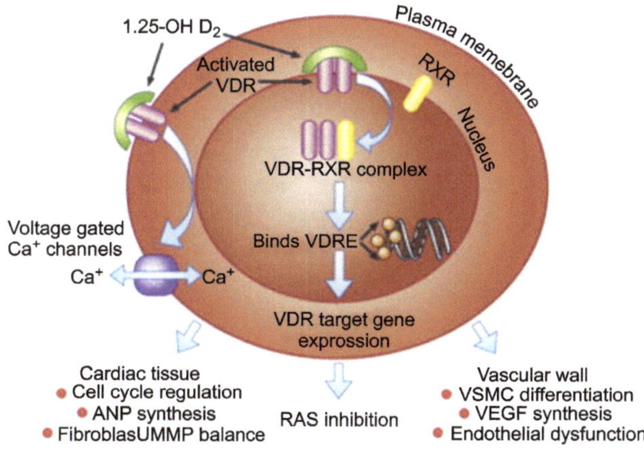

Fig. 20.5 Mechanisms by which vitamin D deficiency may confer cardiovascular risk. Potential effects of vitamin D metabolism on the cardiovascular system are divergent, but share common initial steps of nuclear and plasma membrane VDR activation. VDR, vitamin D receptor; 1, 25-OH D2, 1, 25-dihydroxyvitamin D; RXR, retinoid-X receptor; Ca+, calcium cation; ANP, atrial natriuretic peptide; MMP, matrix metalloproteinases; VDRE, vitamin D response elements (promoter region of target genes); RAS, renin–angiotensin system; VEGF, vascular endothelial growth factor; VSMC, vascular smooth muscle cells. (Published with permission from EHJ, Ibhar Al Mheid et al. Vitamin D and cardiovascular disease: is the evidence solid? Eur Heart J. 2013 Dec; 34(48): 3691–8).

The mechanism of Vitamin D deficiency leading to atherosclerotic vascular disease is complex. It involves raised parathormone levels leading to heightened RAAS (renin-angiotensin-aldosterone) activity, insulin resistance and inflammation. At the cellular level, vitamin D acts through the vitamin D receptor (VDR), which is found in virtually all tissues of the body including cardiovascular tissues like cardiomyocytes, endothelial, and vascular smooth muscle cells. Cardiovascular effects of vitamin D share the common initial steps of nuclear and plasma membrane VDR activation in the above cells.

There are few reports of association of CHD and vitamin D levels from India. An observational study of hospitalized patients with AMI from Bengaluru reported 83.5% prevalence of Vitamin D deficiency.6 The association between low vitamin D levels and cardiovascular risk factors have also been noted in previous studies from India.

THE ECG OF THE FUTURE

What is **Electrocardiography** (ECG), and why is it useful? ECG is the interpretation of the electrical activity of the heart over a period of time. It is used to measure the rate and regularity of heartbeats as well as the size and position of the chambers, the presence of any damage to the heart, and the effects of drugs or devices used to regulate the heart.

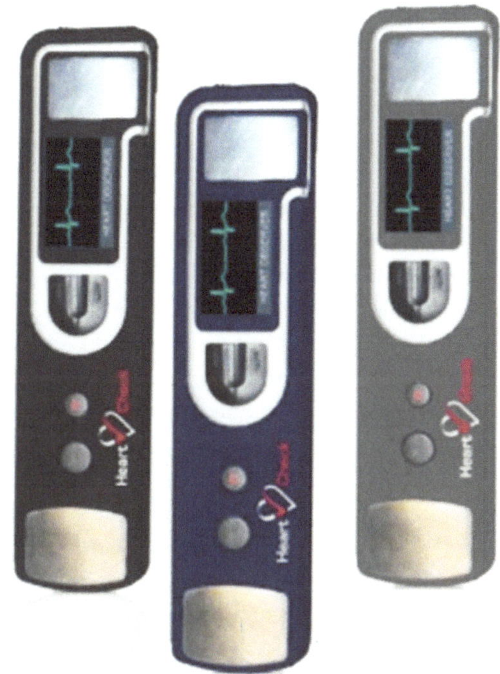

Fig. 20.6 Showing The HeartCheck Pen which would benefit any person interested in monitoring their health due to heart disease.

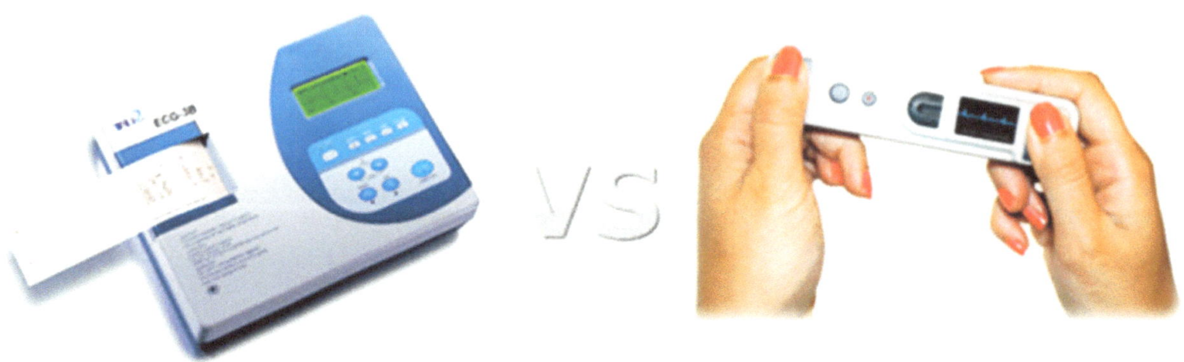

Fig. 20.7 showing comparing conventional (left) and pen type ECGs (right)

It sounds like having an ECG could be quite handy, right? Well yes, it would be, but who would want to spend thousands and have a large brick of a device lying around? Look at the size of that thing below, not me! How about something you can trust to deliver accurate results and slip into your shirt pocket? Now we are talking. CardioComm's new handheld **Heart Check TM Pen** does just that, it puts the benefits of an ECG in the palm of your hand. You may see hypochondriacs lining up for this device, but its use goes well beyond those who have health obsession on the mind.

The HeartCheck Pen would benefit any person interested in monitoring their health due to heart disease. It could also be used to determine potential heart disease by assessing abnormal heart rhythms and muscle defects. From athletes to seniors, a wide range of consumers could benefit from this device.

"We feel the HeartCheck Pen is a true remote monitoring device because it is compact, easy to use, and takes accurate heart readings in only 30 seconds. The Pen may be used from anywhere, including at home, the office, the gym or in remote areas which are often inaccessible to common ECG machines," said Etienne Grima, CardioComm Solutions' CEO.

The device makes sending and storing ECGs easy. Up to 20 ECGs can be stored on the device, and once you hit that mark you can download the ECGs to your computer and print them off, or save some trees and send them electronically to your doc or clinic. The data can also be downloaded to GEMSTM Home, where repeated recordings can be managed in a personal health data record.

"What makes this product unique," explained Grima, "is that after a consumer sends a selected heart rate recording to the C4 medical call-center over the internet using GEMSTM Home, the actual ECG recording will be reviewed and interpreted by an attending C4 physician. The ECG report will then be made available to the customer, again through GEM Home, where they may retrieve the ECG interpretation and use it in communicating with their own health care providers."

The HeartCheck Pen definitely has some interesting advantages over its big brother, but is it something you would use?.

NEW ANDROID ECG SYSTEM TO LET PATIENTS, ATHLETES KEEP A CLOSE EYE ON HEART

A new smartphone-based device that may replace Holter monitors and help athletes achieve endurance goals is under development at VTT Technical Research Centre of Finland. Some dangerous heart arrhythmias can be hard to detect since they often comes and go, and so can be missed at the doctor's office. Holter monitors have been used for decades to monitor the heart over extended periods of time, but they are bulky and inconvenient.

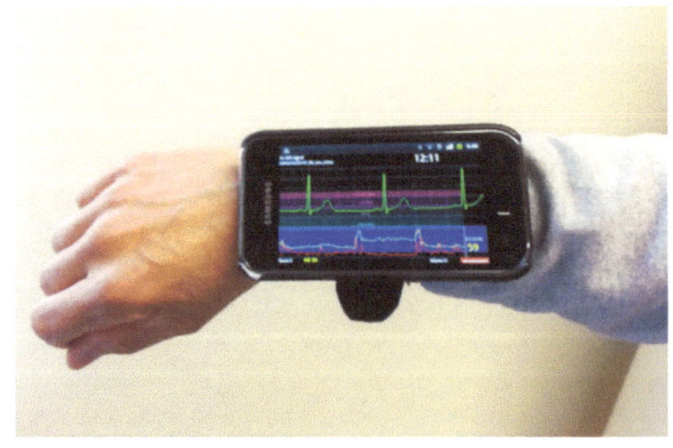

Fig. 20.8 showing New Android ECG System for monitoring heart rhythm on the wrist of a person

The new system straps on the chest of the user and sends ECG data over to an Android smartphone wirelessly over Bluetooth. A live chart can be examined and historical data can be passed to a cardiologist for review. Moreover, unlike the AliveCor and ECGCheck that are ECGs within an iPhone case, the form factor of the VTT device allows athletes to closely monitor their heartbeat during exercise, helping achieve goals while detecting **arrhythmia that top end athletes can be subject to**.

From VTT: The device measures ECG signals at a sufficiently high sampling rate, identifies individual heart beats and counts the interval between consecutive beats. The device is also equipped with an accelerometer. The signals are sent to a smart phone via Bluetooth. The application displays ECG, heart rate and its variability. The signal from the accelerometer can also be used as a step counter.

Beat2Phone is the first device and software application developed for Android phones that can be used to measure and save an ECG and to perform an extensive analysis of the data. The device also enables an advanced heart rate analysis, and GPS-based speed and distance measurements. Compared to wristband devices, smart phones represent the best available user interface technology.

SEEQ MOBILE CARDIAC TELEMETRY SYSTEM

Short-Term Heart Monitoring Up to 30 Days

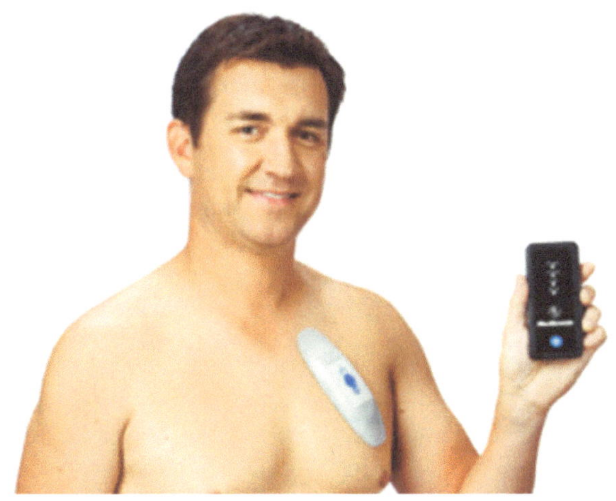

Fig. 20.9 The SEEQ™ Mobile Cardiac Telemetry System

It may help your doctor diagnose and treat irregular heartbeats related to:

- Unexplained fainting
- Heart palpitations
- Atrial fibrillation
- Unexplained stroke

The simplest solution

Unlike most external heart monitoring systems, SEEQ MCT features a discreet, patient-friendly design. You can easily apply the peel-and-stick wearable sensor yourself. It's like an adhesive bandage you wear on your chest. Once applied, the wearable sensor monitors your heart, records any irregular heart rhythms, and communicates through a cellular network to the Medtronic Monitoring Center via the Transmitter you carry with you.

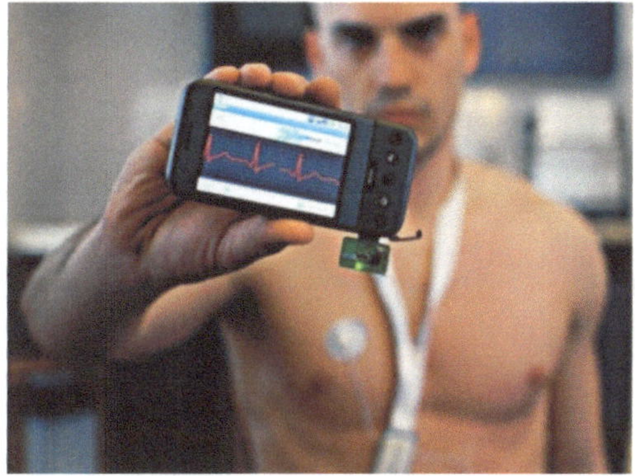

Fig. 20.10 ECG signals wirelessly transmitted to an Android mobile phone via a low-power interface.

MONITORING YOUR HEALTH WITH YOUR MOBILE PHONE ECG

The newly-developed low-power interface wirelessly transmits bio-signals retrieved by imec and Holst Centre's Human++ BAN sensor nodes to an Android mobile phone where the data are collected, stored, processed, and sent over the internet to make them available for authorized users such as a physician. The interface is based on a standard Secure Digital Input Output (SDIO) interface on Android mobile phones, enabling the integration of all the features available on Google's operating system (SMS, e-mail and data transmission over the internet, GPS to track user location). Moreover, the mobile phone's hardware is extended to operate with low-power communication protocols and low-power radios, enabling long-term medical telemonitoring. As the interface is based on the Linux kernel, the system is also easily portable on other Linux-based devices, such as PDA's or laptops. And, the system allows configuration of thresholds on the measured parameters and automatic sending of alerts such as SMS messages and e-mails based on these values.

CARDIODEFENDER SMARTPHONE-BASED ECG, A 21ST CENTURY HOLTER MONITOR

Everist Genomics, an Ann Arbor, Michigan company, is set to release its CardioDefender diagnostic system, a smartphone

ECG that can provide continuous readings throughout the day that can help detect arrhythmias that may be hard to spot in an office visit. The system uses a wrist watch-like device to collect data from electrodes and transmit it wirelessly via Bluetooth to a smartphone that can then share it with clinicians monitoring the patient. CardioDefender, that recently won both FDA approval and EU's CE Mark, can activate an alarm to rapidly notify a physician of any particularly unwelcome graph via an email, page, or other electronic means.

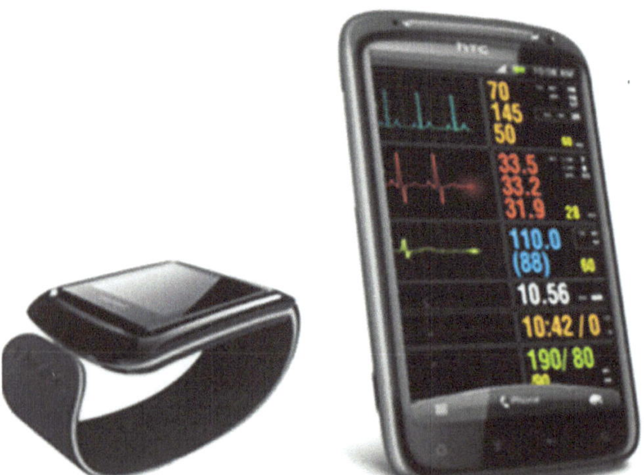

Fig 20.11 Showing CardioDefender Smartphone-based ECG, a 21st Century Holter Monitor "Real-time reporting of symptomatic and asymptomatic arrhythmias; CardioDefender has the ability to capture and report both symptomatic and asymptomatic ar-rhythmias

Fully mobile system; CardioDefender is the world's first ECG system which delivers hospital based quality ECG and arrhythmia analysis by integrating unique software, algorithms and data compression capabilities which enable a smartphone to perform as a mobile ECG.

Real time heart and rythm monitoring

Beat-by-beat analysis of heart rhythm (as opposed to sam-pling some heart beats or part of a heart beat). Long term monitoring capability; CardioDefender can perform up to 3 months of real-time, beat-by-beat quantitative patient monitoring and analysis. Quantitative analysis and reporting; CardioDefender is a fully automated, quantitative ECG monitoring and arrhythmia event reporting system. Comprehensive range of heart rhythm monitoring algo-rithms to enable automated detection and reporting of medically important arrhythmias to physicians and monitor-ing centers.Abnormal heart rhythms reported directly to physicians mobile phone or computer; innovative and patent protected software and data compression technology means Cardio Defender can -report real-time results to a physician's smartphone, tablets, laptop and desk top computer (in addition to a cardiac monitoring center).Access to full, detailed ECG data captured during the moni-toring period, including post heart monitoring data processing for additional measurements.Real-time reporting of symptomatic and asymptomatic arrhythmias; CardioDefender has the ability to capture and report both symptomatic and asymptomatic arrhythmias.

Echo and Heart Failure When Do People Need An Echo And When Do They Need Natriuretic Peptides?

Chronic heart failure (HF) represents a large societal burden of disease and has recently been characterized as an emerging epidemic.HF is associated with significant mortality and morbidity.Furthermore, healthcare expenditures are only expected to increase due to ageing of the population. As a result, strategies to prevent HF and improve the efficiency and quality of care are needed. HF is a clinical syndrome characterized by heterogeneities in both aetiology and phenotype, making management and intervention difficult. For example, it has become apparent that almost 50% of HF patients may have HF with preserved left ventricular (LV) ejection fraction (HFpEF), a disease that represents a diagnostic,prognostic and therapeutic challenge. Echocardiography provides a large amount of detailed information regarding cardiac structure and function in an easily accessible and cost-effective manner and is currently recommended in the diagnostic workup of patients in whom HF cannot be ruled out clinically. Additionally, biomarkers such as type B natriuretic peptides (BNP) and N-terminal prohormone BNP (NT-proBNP) may aid in the diagnosis of HF. This review summarizes the important features, strengths and limitations of echocardiography and BNP HF with respect to diagnosis, prognosis and risk prediction. Heart failure (HF) is a threat to public health. Heterogeneities in aetiology and phenotype complicate the diagnosis and management of HF. This is especially true when considering HF with preserved ejection fraction (HFpEF), which makes up 50% of HF cases. Natriuretic peptides may aid in establishing a working diagnosis in patients suspected of HF, but echocardiography remains the optimal choice for diagnosing HF. Echocardiography provides important prognostic information in both HF with reduced ejection fraction (HFrEF) and HFpEF. Traditionally, emphasis has been put on the left ventricular ejection fraction (LVEF). LVEF is useful for both diagnosis and prognosis in HFrEF.However, echocardiography offers more than this single parameter of systolic function, and for optimal risk assessment in HFrEF, an echocardiogram evaluating systolic, diastolic, left atrial and right ventricular function is beneficial.

In the assessment of echocardiographic modalities such as global longitudinal strain (GLS) by 2D speckle-tracking may be useful. LVEF offers little value in HFpEF and is neither helpful for diagnosis nor prognosis. Diastolic function quantified by E/e and systolic function determined by GLS offer prognostic insight in HFpEF. In HFpEF, other parameters of cardiac performance such as left atrial and right ventricular function evaluated by echocardiography also contribute with prognostic information. Hence, it is important to consider the entire echocardiogram and not focus solely on systolic function. Future research should focus on combining echocardiographic parameters into risk prediction models to adopt a more personalized approach to prognosis instead of identifying yet another echocardiographic biomarker. Natriuretic peptides are secreted in response to myocardial wall stress. HFpEF is characterized by a small LV cavity and thickened LV walls . Since the law of Laplace dictates that LV wall stress is inversely proportional with LV wall thickness and directly proportional to LV radius, HFpEF does not elevate LV wall stress in the same way as seen in HFrEF . Furthermore, it is known that values of natriuretic peptides are consistently lower in obese patients.Accordingly, it has been shown that obese HFpEF patients have lower levels of natriuretic peptides when compared to non-obese HFpEF patients.The mechanisms responsible for the lower levels of natriuretic peptides seen in obese HFpEF patients are currently unclear; however, it has been hypothesized that increased epicardial fat mass in obesity may subject the heart to an increased external pressure.This increased external pressure then attenuates some of the intraventricular pressure that is believed to stimulate natriuretic peptide release, leading to reduced natriuretic peptide release .

When considering that almost 50% of all HF patients display a preserved EF phenotype and that obesity is closely associated with HFpEF , caution must be taken when excluding a HF diagnosis on the basis of a BNP measurement of <35 pg/mL or a NT-proBNP <125 pg/mL as recommended in current guidelines The high prevalence of morbid obesity in HFpEF decreases the diagnostic value of natriuretic peptides, and it also complicates the estimation of jugular venous pressure and other diagnostic signs such as oedema. It should be noted that common cardiovascular medications such as angiotensin-converting enzyme inhibitors, angiotensin II receptor antagonists and diuretics may reduce circulating levels of BNP

VESSEL CLEANING MACHINE / WRIST REDUCING BLOOD PRESSURE

Product Description

Wrist reducing high blood pressure vessel cleaning machine.

Indications

High blood pressure, hyperviscosity, hyperlipidemia, hypertension, diabetes, cardiovascular and cerebrovascular diseases.

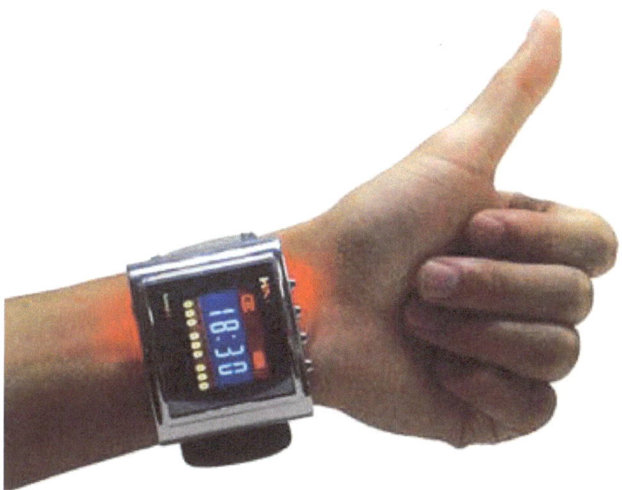

Fig. 20.12 showing Wrist Reducing High Blood Pressure Vessel Cleaning Machine

Advantage

1. Low level laser irradiation, non-invasive, no side effect, no cross infection, pure green physiotherapy.
2. Above 90% therapeutic effect with positive clinical trial report provided.
3. As household physiotherapy devices, small size, intelligent design, easy operation and convenient carrying.
4. Great marketing margin exists.
5. Certification and patents protection provided with the passing of CE, RoHs, ISO9001 and ISO13485.

Therapeutic Principle

HY30-D hypertention laser therapy watch is based on modern laser medicine and proven clinical practice. The device applies a low-level 650 nm wavelength laser. Our instrument utilizes explicit irradiation to change biological characteristics and remove fat layer/cholesterol from red blood cells, thereby improving the activity, deformability, and oxygen carrying capacity of cells to reduce the concentration of middle molecules in the bloodstream. This process improves hem rheological properties while lowering triglycerides and cholesterol for the effective treatment and prevention of heart and brain diseases.

Function and Performance

1. Improving blood viscosity through laser blood irradia-tion.
2. Improving blood oxygen carrying capacity through laser blood irradiation.
3. Reducing blood-fat and total cholesterol through laser blood irradiation.

4. Quickly and effectively correct the abnormity of lipid metabolism and maintain the equilibrium level of the lipid metabolism in the human body through laser blood irradiation.
5. Improving the partial blood circulation around the nasal cavities and the immunological competence of the nasal mucosa membranes through irradiation the nasal mucosa.
6. Therapeutic efficacy control on ischemic cardiac-cerebral vascular diseases.

Features

7. Good clinical therapeutic effect, laser irradiation to three parts or acupoints of human body at the same time can be reached.
8. A laser stabilizer specially added to perform with more stability.
9. Our semiconductor laser devices are used by high quality imported laser head which has the long life-span.
10. Products owned five patents protection.
11. Humanistic and scientific design to fit human physiological curve and ergonomics.
12. Medical use of high capacity lithium battery for the energy-saving.
13. Using high-class and durable metal enclosure which is conducive to heat diffusion for the power stable.
14. Time and power are adjustable, very smart memory system.
15. Two output modes: Pulse and Continues, which have manual and automatic switch available.
16. Pluggable laser wire, more convenience in use and easier maintenance.

Caution

1. Not suitable for the following groups: Cancer patient, pregnancy, patient with hemorrhagic diseases.
2. Children shall only use the instrument under the direction of their parents.
3. The elder patients and sensitive patients must accept the low-power and short-time treatment at the beginning, the rate of work could be increased as the body adjusts.

NEXT GENERATION OF VITAL AND BLOOD PRESSURE MEASUREMENT

- Wear your CARUNDA24 on your wrist, just like a watch and monitor your blood pressure around the clock.
- Measure your blood pressure easily and comfortably, without a cuff.
- Your blood pressure will be displayed (and stored) immediately.
- Your personal data can be transferred to external devices for further analysis.
- Continuous measurements – without a cuff – overcome a 100 year limitation of traditional methods of measuring blood pressure.
- Follow the exciting process of developing a brand new system on these pages.

Background

Today more than one billion people are suffering from high blood pressure (hypertension) and continuous surveillance should be available for these people. Over half of the population affected are not even aware of their disease according to the World Health Organisation. Monitoring vital functions is a must for these and other people suffering from other kind of serious diseases.

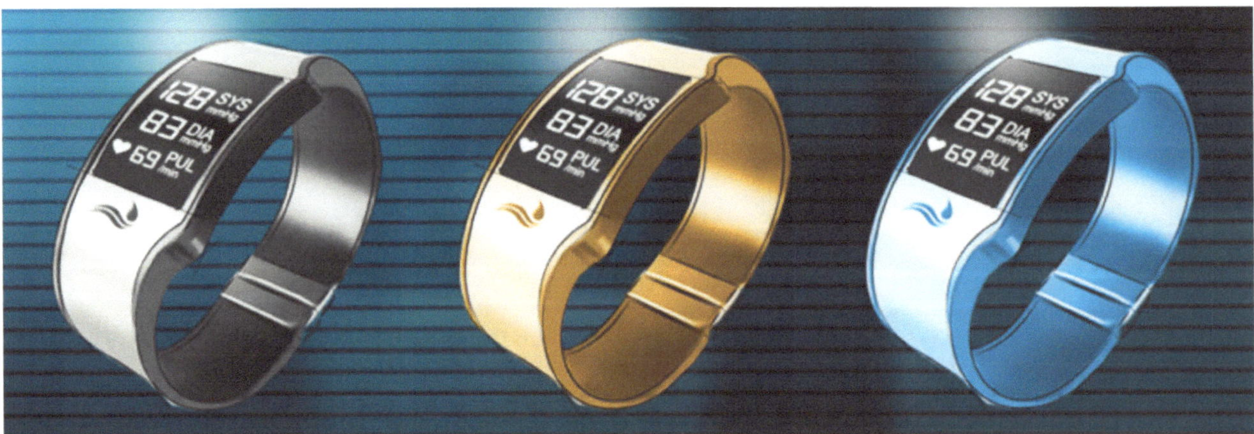

Fig 20.13 Showing next generation wrist watch type of vital and blood pressure measurement instrument

NON-INVASIVE GLUCOMETER FROM ORSENSE APPROVED IN EUROPE

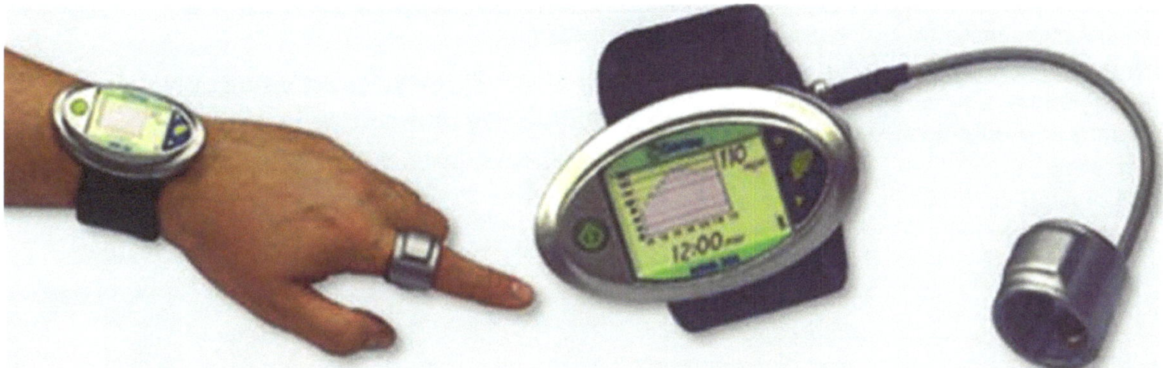

Fig. 20.14 OrSense Ltd., a Nes Ziona, Israel company, is reporting that its NBM-200G non-invasive continuous monitor of blood glucose for diabetics has been granted the CE Mark of approval in the EU. The bulky device is illustrated below, and the picture above shows expected appearance of the next generation device based on the company's proprietary technology. The NBM-200G is based on OrSense's proprietary breakthrough technology that allows non-invasive measurement of analytes including glucose, hemoglobin, and oxygen saturation with very high sensitivity. The NBM-200G is operated by placing a ring-shaped probe around the patient's finger, which applies a gentle pressure to the finger, similar to that applied during non-invasive blood-pressure measurement and temporarily occludes the blood flow. During the occlusion, optical elements in the sensor perform a sensitive measurement of the light transmitted through the finger. This method, called Occlusion Spectroscopy, provides a quick, accurate and painless measurement of the patient's blood glucose. The method was tested on over 400 subjects, exhibiting comparable accuracy to invasive solutions, while providing superior ease of use and safety. In addition, the NBM-200G enables the identification of glucose trends and the detection of hypo- and hyperglycemia events and may also optimally answer the growing need for tight glycemic control in acute care settings, thereby reducing morbidity and mortality.

24 HOURS SPO_2 AMBULATORY BLOOD PRESSURE MONITORING COLOR LCD SPO_2 ABPM BP MONITOR

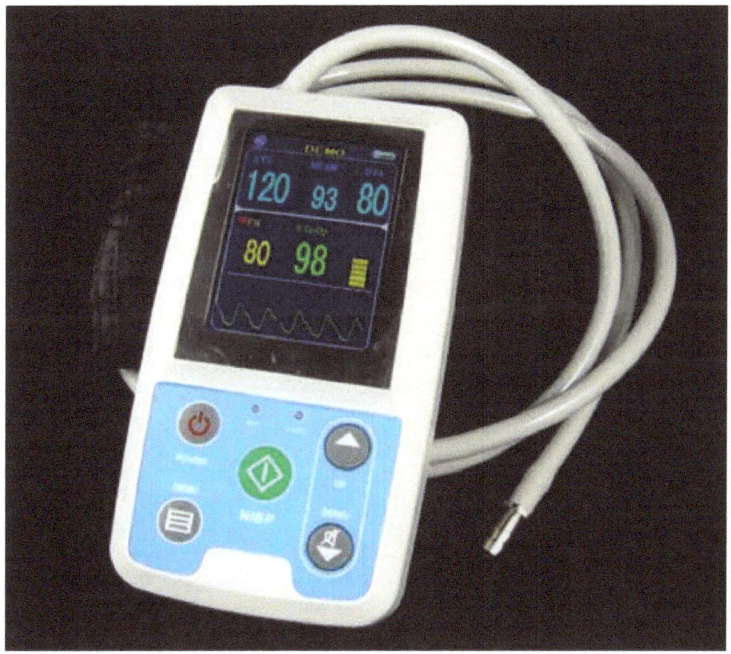

Fig. 20.15 Showing 24 hours SpO_2 ambulatory blood pressure monitoring Color LCD SpO_2 ABPM BP monitor.

Vital functions include breathing, body (core) temperature and the cardiovascular system, in particular arterial pulse (wave) and arterial blood pressure. Today there are a several systems which deliver a variety of data, but only very few in the field of blood pressure. The well-known and widely used heart-rate-monitors show only one aspect of the pulse and not the whole pulse-wave.

CARUNDA24 solves this problem. The continuous, non-invasive measurement of the pulse wave provides you and your physician or health-care professional not only with blood pressure (diastolic and systolic) but also critical information about the quality of your pulse including the number and regularity of your heart-beat and the rate of increase in blood pressure.

Whether you are affected by high blood pressure, or simply want to take preventive action, CARUNDA24 will help increase awareness and early recognition of potential adverse events, enabling you reduce their risk of related health problems.

What you can Expect

With CARUNDA24 we aim to offer a medically certified system that meets the highest technical and medical requirements and is suitable for use in hospitals, medical practices as well as at home. CARUNDA24 looks – and can be worn – just like an ordinary watch, measuring the pulse wave and therefore the blood pressure (continuously) on the surface of the wrist. Data is displayed and stored instantly and can be transferred wirelessly to external equipment for detailed analysis.

Measuring Blood pressure with CARUNDA24 is extremely simple – it can be measured for several hours; in fact all day long, if necessary...around the clock!

STBL aims to provide state of the art medical approved systems, that fullfil highest technological and medical standards. These systems should be able to be used in clinics, medical offices but also at home.

Risks and Challenges

Even after a successful "proof of concept", the road from clinical prototype to a commercially deliverable system is still full of challenges; which may be of a technical nature (as CARUNDA24 uses a new method which still has to be subjected to extensive testing) or in the validation process where unknown questions may arise.

At the start of 2014 the preperation of an extensive clinical proof of concept milestone was started which will lasted around nine months. With the preparation of a new generation of prototypes can be begun in the first quarter of 2015 the earliest. In this and all further steps unknown questions may arise whicht could lead to further delays.

Additional Applications

Due to the newly developed continuous measurement method and modern communication technologies CARUNDA24 systems could be used in the field of telemedicine, remote surveillance such as in nursing homes or intensive care units.

Three Scientist who got Nobel prize in Physiology or medicine in 2019

Three scientists have shared this year's Nobel prize in physiology or medicine for discovering how the body responds to changes in oxygen levels, one of the most essential processes for life.

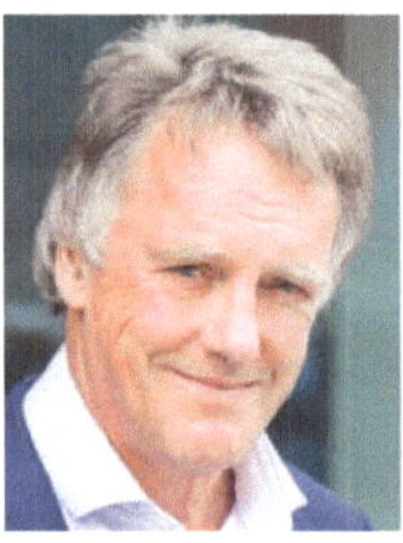
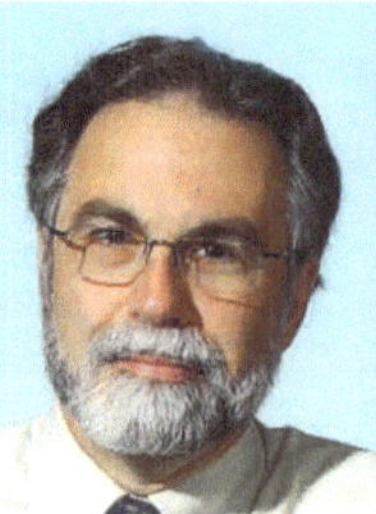
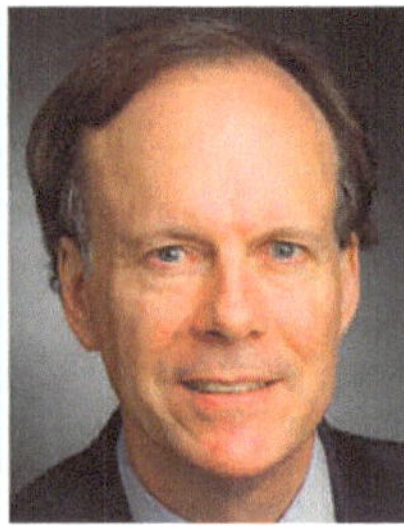

Fig.20.16 L-R: Sir Peter Ratcliffe, Gregg Semenza and William Kaelin. Their work has been hailed as having 'greatly expanded our knowledge of how physiological response makes life possible'. Photograph : EPA

William Kaelin Jr at the Dana-Farber Cancer Institute and Harvard University in Massachusetts, Sir Peter Ratcliffe at Oxford University and the Francis Crick Institute in London, and Gregg Semenza at Johns Hopkins University in Baltimore, Maryland, worked out how cells sense falling oxygen levels and respond by making new blood cells and vessels. Beyond describing a fundamental physiological process that enables animals to thrive in some of the highest-altitude regions on Earth, the mechanism has given researchers new routes to treatments for anaemia, cancer, heart disease and other conditions.

Ratcliffe was summoned from a lab meeting in Oxford to take the call from Stockholm. "I tried to make sure it wasn't some friend down the road having a laugh at my expense," he told the Guardian. "Then I accepted the news and had a think about how I was going to reorder my day."Ratcliffe had spent the weekend working on an EU synergy grant and had not imagined his morning taking such a turn. "When I got up this morning I didn't have any expectation or make any contingency plans for the announcement at all," he said. On finishing the call he returned to his meeting and, at the request of the Nobel committee, carried on without a word. At least one scientist had her suspicions, however, having noticed he had left a coffee in the room and returned with a tea. "She's a scientist, so trained to draw deductions from the things she observes," Ratcliffe said. "I'd decided I needed a little less agitation rather than more." The three laureates will share the 9m Swedish kronor (£740,000) prize equally, according to the Karolinska Institute in Stockholm. Asked what he intended to do with the windfall, Ratcliffe said : "I'll be discussing that with my wife in private. But it'll be something good." A party was on thecards, he said, but not immediately.

"I'm trying to stay sober because it's going to be a busy day." Kaelin said he was half-asleep when his phone went. "I was aware as a scientist that if you get a phone call at 5am with too many digits, it's sometimes very good news, and my heart started racing," he said. "It was all a bit surreal." The trio won the prestigious Lasker prize in 2016. In work that spanned more than two decades, the researchers teased apart different aspects of how cells in the body first sense and then respond to low oxygen levels. The crucial gas is used by tiny structures called mitochondria found in nearly all animal cells to convert food into useful energy. The scientists showed that when oxygen is in short supply, a protein complex that Semenza called hypoxia-inducible factor, or HIF, builds up in nearly all the cells in the body. The rise in HIF has a number of effects but most notably ramps up the activity of a gene used to produce erythropoietin (EPO), a hormone that in turn boosts the creation of oxygen-carrying red blood cells.Randall Johnson, a professor of molecular physiology and pathology at Cambridge University, said this year's Nobel laureates "have greatly expanded our knowledge of how physiological response makes life possible".He said the role of HIF was crucial from the earliest days of life. "If an embryo doesn't have the HIF gene it won't survive past very early embryogenesis. Even in the womb our bodies need this gene to do everything they do." The work has led to the development of a number of drugs such as roxadustat and daprodustat, which treat anaemia by fooling the body into thinking it is at high altitude, making it churn out more red blood cells. Roxadustat is on the market in China and is being assessed by European regulatorsSimilar drugs aim to help heart disease and lung cancer patients who struggle to get enough oxygen into their bloodstream. More experimental drugs based on the finding seek to prevent other cancers growing by blocking their ability to make new blood vessels

CLINICAL APPLICATION OF CENTRAL BLOOD PRESSURE

What is central blood pressure?

Central blood pressure is the pressure in the aorta, which is the large artery into which the heart pumps. The term '*central blood pressure*' usually refers to the pressure in the aorta near the heart.

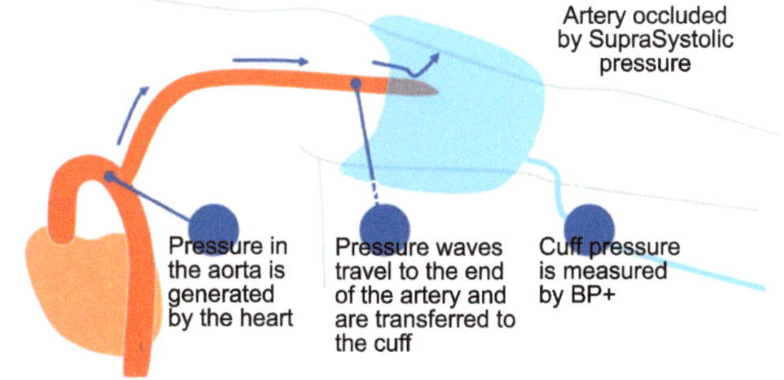

Fig. 20.17 Diagram explaining basic understanding of central blood pressure mechanism.

How is central blood pressure different from normal blood pressure?

Normally, blood pressure is measured in the upper arm, which is a 'peripheral' artery. Peripheral blood pressure is usually higher than central blood pressure due to the peripheral site being closer to locations from which echoes reverberate.

The degree to which the peripheral blood pressure is higher than central blood pressure depends partly on the stiffness of the arteries.

Why is central blood pressure important?

Central pressure has been shown to more strongly relate to vascular disease and outcome than traditional upper arm blood pressure. It also can distinguish between the effects of different hypertension medications when upper arm blood pressure and pulse wave velocity do not.

Central blood pressure is the pressure that the heart has to pump against to get blood to flow to the rest of the body. Higher central blood pressures mean that the heart must work harder to do its job. This can eventually lead to heart failure. Central blood pressure also determines the pressure in the blood vessels feeding the brain. If central pressure is too high, it may cause aneurysms and strokes.

How is central blood pressure measured?

Central blood pressure can be directly measured only using a pressure sensor or catheter inserted into the aorta (usually through an artery in the groin or wrist). This procedure is invasive and can lead to complications.

How does BP+ measure central blood pressure non-invasively?

BP+ calculates central blood pressure using a physics-based model of the arteries between the aorta and the cuff. This model relate how pressure waves travel between the aorta and the occluded artery under the suprasystolic cuff, as shown in the diagram that follows. More details are available in.

Central Aortic Systolic Pressure Monitoring Device

A-PULSE CASPal® is a simple device for the measurement of Central Aortic Systolic Pressure(CASP) in a simple clinic or home setting. It is a world-first portable CASP measurement device developed by HealthSTATS International. It is empowered by EVBP technology; a FDA listed and patented technology using modified applanation tonometry on the radial artery at the position of the wrist. It is completely non-invasive, painless and easy-to-operate. It is specially designed for home user for ease of use to obtain CASP.

A-PULSE CASPal® is a noninvasive blood pressure monitoring system which is designed to measure the Central

Aortic Systolic Pressure (CASP) and additional arterial pulse waveform related indices based on arterial tonometry at the radial artery of the wrist. The system consists of four main elements:

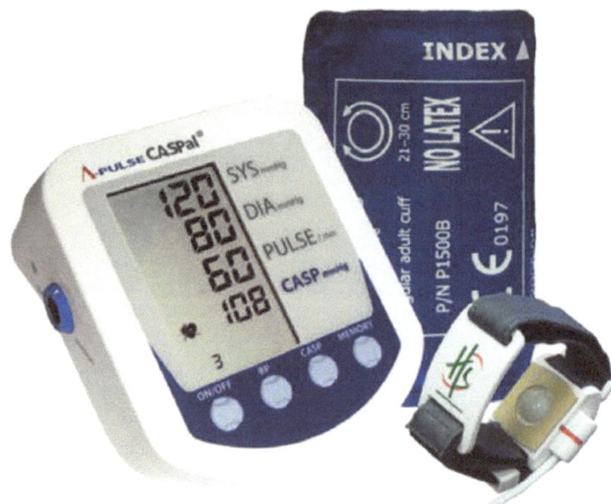

Fig 20.18 showing A-PULSE CASPal® is a simple device for the measurement of Central Aortic Systolic Pressure(CASP) in a simple clinic or home setting ,using modified applanation tonometry on the radial artery at the position of the wrist

- A-PULSE CASPal® monitor.
- Wrist sensor module based on the technology of the BPro® monitor device
- Built-in software algorithm for blood pressure measurement and calculation based on the A-PULSE CASP® software
- Integrated oscillometric blood pressure module for calibration.

What are the advantages of the BP+ approach to central pressure?

Central pressure is estimated non-invasively by using a mathematical relationship to a peripheral pressure. The degree to which this mathematical relationship matches any individual determines the accuracy of the central pressure estimate in that subject.

The BP+ technique has a number of advantages over empirical transfer function and statistical attempts at estimating central blood pressure.

Upper arm measurement means the distance between the sensor and the heart is much shorter than wrist or finger measurements, meaning less variability between the arterial geometry of individuals.

Cuff inflated to occlude the brachial artery means individual variations in downstream arteries can be ignored.

Physics-based model is applicable where statistical and empirical relationships are invalid. This is particularly true for stiff arteries.

Does BP+ require calibration to estimate central blood pressure?

No external calibration is necessary to estimate central blood pressure using BP+. Instead information already collected from the upper-arm blood pressure measurement is used.

Does BP+ assume central mean and diastolic pressures?

BP+ calculates central systolic, diastolic and mean pressures. Other technologies assume central diastolic and/or mean pressures are equal to peripheral blood pressures.

How accurate are BP+ central blood pressure estimates?

Central blood pressure estimates have been independently tested against an accepted non-invasive technique for central blood pressure estimation and indicates well within the requirements of American Association for the Advancement of Medical Instrumentation (AAMI) standard SP10. Details will be available in the Proceedings of Artery 2010.

Does the central pressure estimate require patient height, age, sex etc.?

The BP+ central pressure estimate is model-based, not statistics-based and does not require the use of any other patient measurements.

Does brachial artery, arm or cuff variation affect accuracy?

The suprasystolic waveform is calibrated from the peripheral blood pressure. Variations in the arm and cuff are therefore not significant.

The brachial artery isn't nearly as affected by cardiovascular disease as other major blood vessels and so does not influence the accuracy of the artery model in this way.

Is Augmentation Index related to Central Blood Pressure?

Both augmentation index and central blood pressure are known to increase with the age of the subject and be related to cardiovascular outcome. However, they are thought to measure different aspects of arterial stiffness.

Blood pressure plays a significant role in determining the arterial wall structure. Elevated blood pressure can lead to remodelling of the arterial structure, to compensate for changes in wall stress which would affect the augmentation index.

Are cholesterol and central blood pressure related?

Cholesterol is a blood chemical indicator, which may or may not relate to functional measures of cardiovascular health such as central blood pressure. Nevertheless, some research suggests that patients with hypercholesterolemia exhibit increased central pulse pressure compared with normocholesterolemic controls.

A POCKET SIZED ECHOCARDIOGRAPHY MACHINE?

Will Vscan ultrasound technology replace the Stethoscope?

Sometimes a never before seen idea is not necessary for frugal innovation. If a currently used product can be remade in such a way that it becomes more effective and valuable to society this is also an example of frugal innovation. GE has a great example of this type of innovation with their Vscan pocket sized ultrasound device.

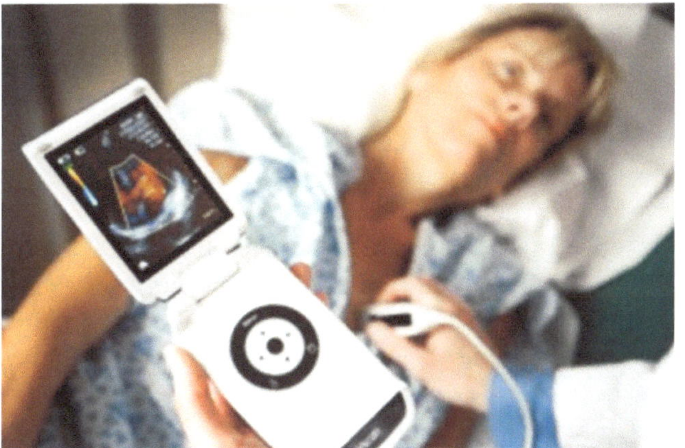

Fig. 20.19 showing patient being examined for his heart problem by a portable Vscan echocardiography.

The Vscan ultrasound device greatly increased the usability of ultrasound technology by making the device small enough that if can fit in a pocket. Traditional ultrasound equipment is much larger and often must be wheeled around on a large cart.

However the cost of Vscan is more impressive than it's size. Traditional ultrasound equipment can cost up to $150,000 but Vscan costs only $7,700. This makes the device not only portable but effective for use an many situations. MIT Technology Review compares Vscan with the traditional stethoscope. The stethoscope has become iconic in the medical world but it's primary use is only to listen to the heart. Now doctors have access to technology that lets them look at a patients heart in real time.

ELECTRONIC STETHOSCOPES: WHAT'S NEW FOR AUSCULTATION

Although there is nothing wrong with traditional stethoscopes, taking the time to learn the nuances of digital auscultation will improve your diagnostic capabilities

The stethoscope is perhaps the most iconic device associated with medical practice, and the most important part of the stethoscope will always be the part "between the ear tips." Because I last reviewed high-tech stethoscopes 5 years ago, I thought it appropriate to discuss the new technologies that can improve our ability to auscultate.

Murmurs are Common

The incidence of heart murmurs can be as high as 80 to 90% in children, yet the vast majority of auscultated murmurs in children are not associated with structural heart disease and therefore are considered merely "functional" or "innocent" murmurs. This creates a dilemma for the pediatrician who, upon hearing a previously undocumented murmur in a child, must decide whether the murmur merits further investigation.

Murmur Interpretation Software

Five years ago, murmur interpretation software was available from Zargis Medical, which had established a relationship with 3M Corporation (St Paul, Minnesota), manufacturer of the Littmann Model 3200 electronic stethoscope. The software, called Cardioscan, communicated via Bluetooth wireless connectivity to the stethoscope and prompted the user to record heart sounds from 4 positions on the patient's chest. The software would then analyze the recordings, report whether a murmur was present, and specify whether an echocardiogram was indicated.

An update and Review of Instrument-based Vision Screening

Unfortunately, Zargis Medical went out of business, and its excellent murmur analysis software became unavailable. However, a South African company, Diacoustic Medical Devices (Stellenbosch, South Africa) recently introduced its own SensiCardiac software to analyze murmurs. One study performed in Australia on a limited number of patients indicated that the SensiCardiac software has a sensitivity and specificity for detecting pathologic murmurs of 82% and 88%, respectively.7 This is much better than the performance of PCPs in identifying pathologic murmurs, but less than that of cardiologists.

The SensiCardiac software is used in conjunction with the Littmann Model 3200 stethoscope and is accessed via a subscription service that costs $25 per month for up to 20 tests; $49 per month for up to 100 tests; and $99 per month for unlimited testing. The software is growing in popularity in areas of the world where access to cardiologists is limited. Keep in mind that the majority of heart sounds and murmurs occur in the frequency range of 5 to 800 Hz. Because human ears are most sensitive to sounds in the 500-Hz to 4000-Hz frequency range, many murmurs ideally need to be amplified for them to be appreciated by examiners.8 Computers have

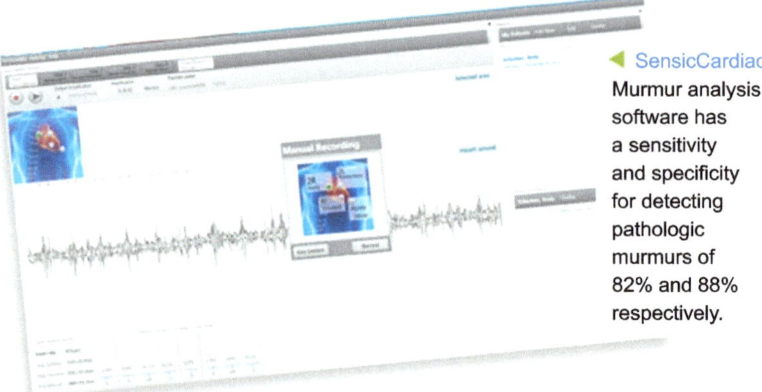

Fig. 20.20 Showing features of SensiCardiac stethoscope

no frequency limitations, and computer-assisted auscultation software such as SensiCardiac can improve the ability of physicians to diagnose pathologic murmurs.

Advantages of Digital Stethoscopes

As a reviewer of medical devices, over the years I have had the opportunity to use a variety of electronic stethoscopes. These stethoscopes convert the acoustic signal of auscultated sounds into digital signals that can be processed for optimal listening. While we refer to these devices as electronic stethoscopes, it is more appropriate to refer to them as digital stethoscopes.

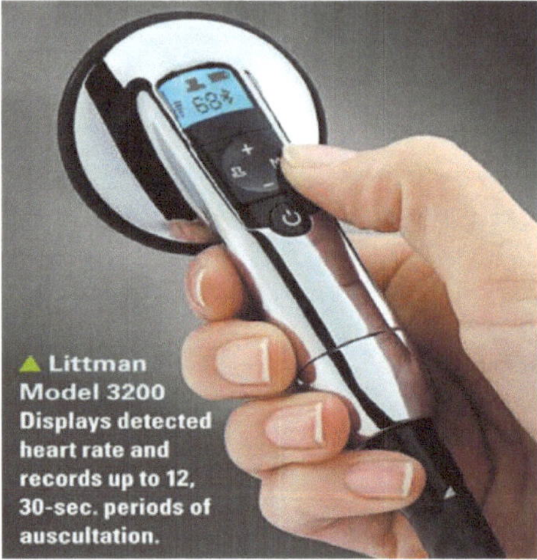

Fig. 20.21 Showing features of Littmann 3200 stethoscope.

I have been an avid user of the Littmann 3200stethoscope for many years and I will never go back to using a traditional stethoscope. Chief advantages of going electronic are the reduction or elimination of external sounds that interfere with optimal auscultation, as well as amplification of sounds across selected frequency ranges. Despite poor hearing, I can detect murmurs and lung sounds with my Littmann Model 3200 that colleagues using standard stethoscopes sometimes miss. The Littmann Model 3200 displays the detected heart rate and also enables me to record up to 12, 30-second periods of auscultation. Later, I can replay the recording for the parent merely by pushing a few buttons on the headpiece and placing the earpieces in the parent's ears. I find this extremely helpful in explaining a murmur or lung findings with parents and, as a consequence, they are more likely to understand and follow my recommendations.

While I have found the Littmann Model 3200 useful in detecting murmurs, its true utility, I think, lies in auscultation of lung sounds. Because it facilitates the auscultation of rales and rhonchi, I find I have substantially reduced the number of chest x-rays that I order. It does take time to learn the subtleties associated with auscultation with a digital stethoscope (distinguishing pathologic sounds from normal sounds), but given time and patience I am confident that most providers can become expert users of these devices.

LITTMANN MODELS 3200 AND 3100

In addition to the features discussed above, the Model 3200 is powered by a single AA battery and has a bell, diaphragm, and combined frequency mode. You can download the free StethAssist Heart and Lung Sound Visualization Software from the 3M website (bit.ly/StethAssist-software) to either a Mac or PC for storage and display. The recordings also can be sent to cardiologists for analysis via the Internet. The Littmann Model 3200 is quite affordable at about $400. If you want the acoustics of the 3200 but are not interested in its recording capability, combined frequency mode, and its ability to wirelessly connect to diagnostic software, you can purchase the Littman Model 3100 for about $60 less.

AN ICONOCLASTIC ELECTRONIC STETHOSCOPE

Thinklabs (Centennial, Colorado) is an interesting company headed by a very interesting entrepreneur. Clive Smith is both a musician and an electrical engineer with a graduate degree from the California Institute of Technology, Pasadena. After years of research and development, Thinklabs has developed a new digital stethoscope that utilizes an electromagnetic diaphragm with a conductive inner surface to provide outstanding acoustics for auscultation.

VISCOPE MD AND CARDIOSLEEVE

Two other electronic stethoscopes are worth your consideration. The ViScope MD from HD Medical Group (Santa Clara, California) is the first "visual" stethoscope that displays a simultaneous phonocardiogram on a high-resolution color screen.

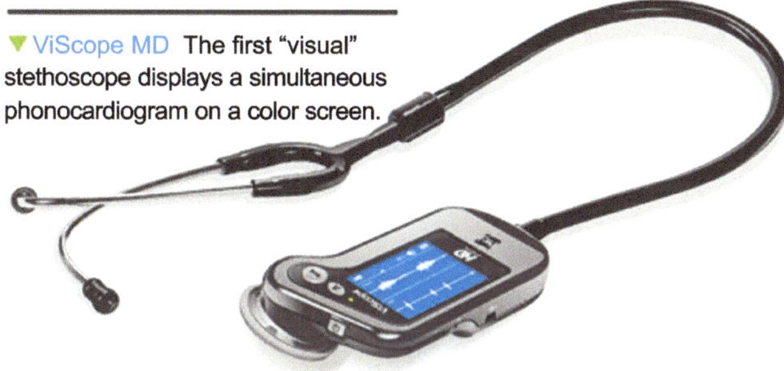

Fig. 20.22 Showing features of ViScope MD stethoscope.

With this device, you can essentially "see" what you hear. It can capture 4, 10-second recordings and transfer this data to a computer to document the sounds auscultated. Like the Littmann Model 3200, it features noise cancellation as well as sound amplification, and it has a bell, diaphragm, and combined frequency mode. The ViScope MD integrates an internal algorithm that indicates whether a murmur is present. It has a rechargeable battery and sells for $600.

Finally, in the next quarter of this year, physicians can look forward to a unique stethoscope accessory that not only provides improved auscultation and Bluetooth connectivity to mobile devices, but also adds 3-lead electrocardiogram capabilities as well. The device is called the **CardioSleeve** from Rijuven Corporation (Wexford, Pennsylvania) and it connects to most standard stethoscopes. The CardioSleeve communicates with a smartphone to display its results that can be uploaded to Rijuven servers for review and analysis. It is being promoted as a device that will improve our ability to detect pathologic murmurs as well as dysrhythmias, and it may be helpful in diagnosing long QT syndrome that is associated with sudden death in pediatric patients. The stethoscope accessory will be priced at $400, and a subscription to its online services will be reasonably priced. I look forward to trialing the device when it becomes available.

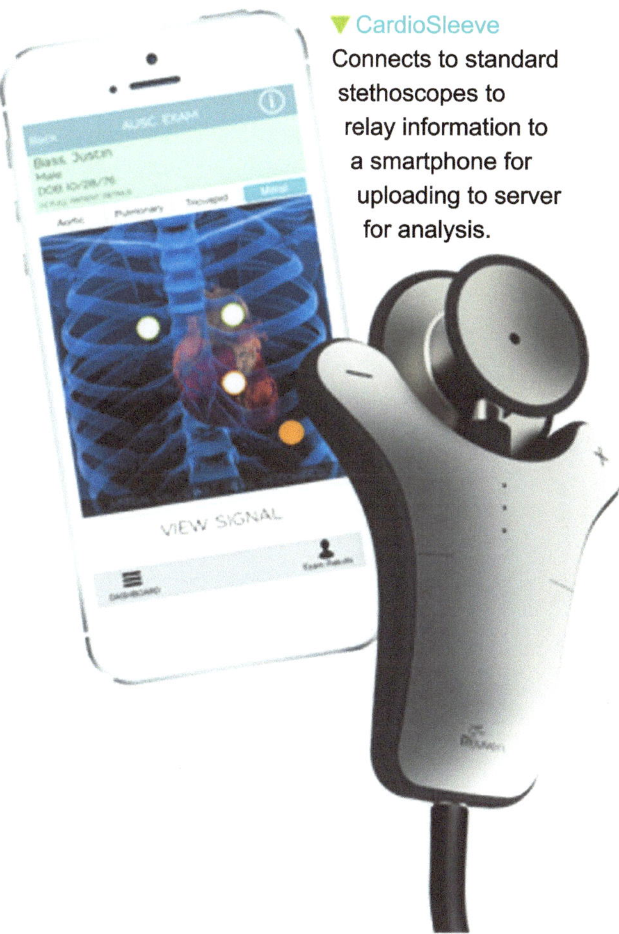

Fig. 20.23 Showing features of CardioSleeve stethoscope.

CARDIONICS AMPLIFIED FOR THE HARD OF HEARING AND HEARING IMPAIRED ELECTRONIC STETHOSCOPE FOR PHYSICIAN

Reviews

The Cardionics Electronic Stethoscope for the hard of hearing and hearing impaired is designed to be worn on the belt or lab coat. Delivers improved sound quality, making physical diagnosis faster and easier. Amplifies heart, breath and bowel sounds or Korotkoff sounds without amplifying outside noise. Can also be used in a stress test situation on a treadmill.

This product is compatible with Cardionics Extra Headphones.

Includes single adult diaphragm.

Output allows attachment to PDA, computer, tape recorder or external earphones.

Sound selector switch allows listening in proper frequency for heart or breath sounds.

Exceptional sound quality with 64 gain positions.

One-year warranty against manufacturer's defects.

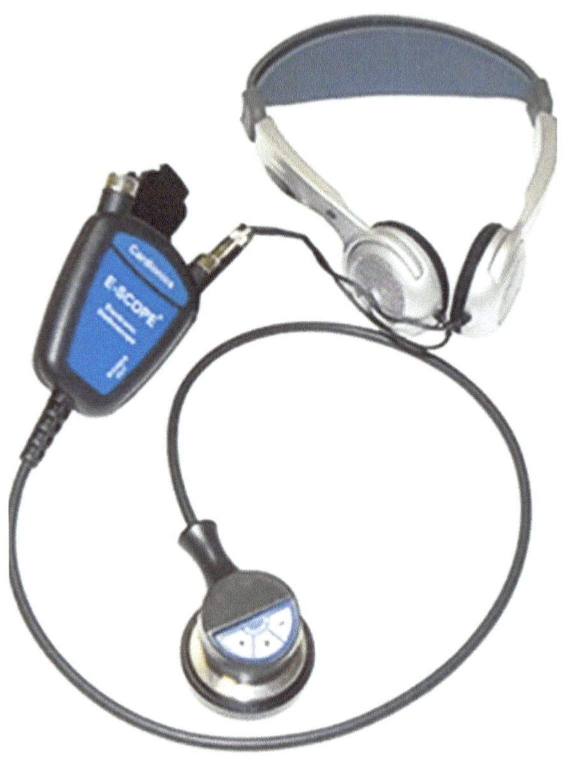

Fig. 20.24 Showing features of cardionics amplified for the hard of hearing and hearing impaired electronic stethoscope for physician.

CONTEMPORARY REVIEWS IN INTERVENTIONAL CARDIOLOGY

Bioabsorbable Coronary Stents

Percutaneous coronary intervention (PCI) with bioabsorbable stents has created interest because the need for mechanical support for the healing artery is temporary, and beyond the first few months there are potential disadvantages of a permanent metallic prosthesis. Stents improve immediate outcomes, including profoundly reducing acute vessel occlusion after PCI by scaffolding intimal tissue flaps that have separated from deeper layers and by optimizing vessel caliber. They limit restenosis by preventing negative remodeling. The intimal hyperplastic healing response to PCI that contributes to restenosis, especially after bare metal stenting, can be limited by coating stents with antiproliferative medications.

Potential advantages of having the stent disappear from the treated site include reduced or abolished late stent thrombosis, improved lesion imaging with computed tomography or magnetic resonance, facilitation of repeat treatments (surgical or percutaneous) to the same site, restoration of vasomotion, and freedom from side-branch obstruction by struts and from strut fracture-induced restenosis. Bioabsorbable stents have a potential pediatric role because they allow vessel growth and do not need eventual surgical removal. The progression of stenosis seen within stents 7 to 10 years after stenting has been attributed, at least in part, to inflammation around metallic struts, which might argue for an absorbable stent. Progression is also observed late after balloon angioplasty. Some patients say they prefer an effective temporary implant rather than a permanent prosthesis.

Although the concept of bioabsorbable stents has created interest for >20 years, there are challenges in making a stent that has sufficient radial strength for an appropriate duration, that does not have unduly thick struts, that can be a drug delivery vehicle, and where degradation does not generate an unacceptable inflammatory response. We will review the different bioabsorbable stents that have been studied clinically and discuss the duration of the need for mechanical support and the potential amelioration of late stent thrombosis risk.

Bioabsorbable Therapeutics Stent

The bioabsorbable therapeutics stent (Bioabsorbable Therapeutics Inc, Menlo Park, Calif), a fully bioabsorbable sirolimus-eluting stent that also releases salicylic acid, has a polymer backbone that gives the stent the physical structure and a polymer coating that contains and controls the release of the antiproliferative.

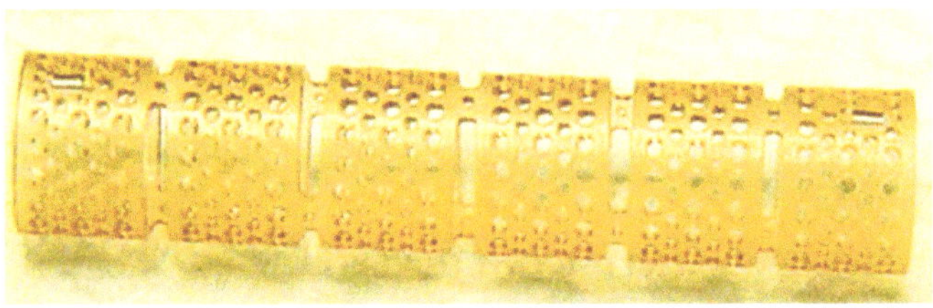

Fig. 20.25 The bioabsorbable therapeutics stent has absorbable backbone and coating polymers constructed from repeating salicylate molecules joined by linker molecules. The coating contains and controls the release of sirolimus. The stent has a high stent to artery ratio of 65%. It has a strut thickness of 200 μm and crossing profile of 2.0 mm. It is balloon expandable and radiolucent.

The structure of the coating polymer is repeating salicylate molecules linked by adipic acid molecules. The stent backbone polymer structure is also repeating salicylate molecules but joined by different linker molecules. During absorption, the bonds between salicylic acid and linker molecules are hydrolyzed releasing the anti-inflammatory drug, salicylic acid. This anti-inflammatory agent is expected to counter the inflammation associated with PCI17 and with polymer degradation.6Sirolimus is dissolved in the coating polymer that is applied to the abluminal surface of the stent backbone releasing the antiproliferative drug at a rate and dose similar to that of Cypher stents. Absorption of the stent, expected to be complete within 6 to 12 months, is by surface erosion.

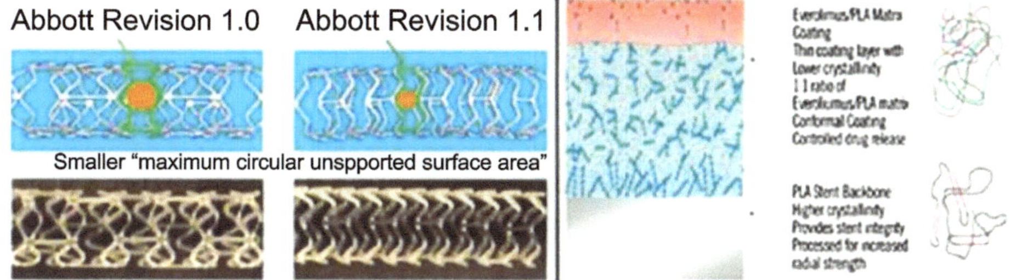

Fig. 20.26 Left panel: the changes in scaffold design between revision 1.0 and revision 1.1 o.

In the first-in-man Whisper trial, a stent with strut thickness of 200 μm and a crossing profile of 2.0 mm with a stent-to-artery coverage of 65% was implanted in 8 patients. Because of higher-than-expected intimal hyperplasia, a subsequent design iteration will have thinner struts, a higher dose of sirolimus, and a lower percent wall coverage.

How Long Do Coronary Arteries Need the Mechanical Support of a Stent?

Stents, essential components of contemporary PCI, scaffold intimal flaps that have separated from deeper layers, prevent early constrictive remodeling, and deliver antiproliferative drug to limit excessive healing. After this, a permanent implant is unnecessary and has potential disadvantages. After balloon angioplasty, preclinical and human studies have shown that restenosis is caused mainly by early constrictive remodeling (vessel shrinkage) and to a lesser extent by an hyperplastic healing response. Not all patients experience constrictive remodeling and some indeed have positive remodeling. Prevention of constrictive remodeling is the major reason stents limit restenosis. Over time, during the absorption process, an absorbable stent gradually loses its radial strength and ability to resist constrictive remodeling forces long before it is fully absorbed. What is not clear is how long the artery needs the support of a stent. the Abbott Absorb bio-vascular scaffolds (BVS). Revision 1.1 has a higher radial strength as a consequence of reduced ‘maximum circular unsupported surface area’. Right panel: shows the material structure of the scaffolds, which is unchanged between the two revisions. (Images adapted and reprinted from Onuma Y et al with permission from Europa Digital & Publishing15; BVS 1.0 and BVS 1.1 images reprinted with permission from data on file at Abbott Vascular). Access the article online to view this figure in colour.

In a clinical study using serial angiography and IVUS after angioplasty and directional coronary atherectomy, there was some early positive remodeling up to 1 month and then between 1 and 6 months there was luminal reduction due mainly to negative remodeling (reduction in external elastic lamina). Most angiographic restenosis after balloon angioplasty occurs between 1 and 3 months and is rare thereafter. Absorption of a magnesium alloy stent in humans was rapid and mechanical support lasting days or weeks was too short to prevent constrictive remodeling and restenosis. These data taken together suggest that a mechanically intact stent is needed to counter negative remodeling and limit restenosis for somewhere between 1 and 3 months. Stents are required to limit the constrictive remodeling in the first 6 months after balloon angioplasty. Because most patients have luminal enlargement between 6 months and 5 years after balloon angioplasty, a stent is not needed beyond 6 months. If, as has been postulated but not proven, the late luminal enlargement after balloon angioplasty is due to adaptive positive arterial remodeling, a circumferentially rigid stent may be disadvantageous in that it may obstruct this normal component of vessel healing.

In the Absorb trial, the polylactide BVS stent struts resisted the constrictive remodeling forces sufficiently, such that by 6 months on IVUS there was no vessel shrinkage (no change in external elastic lamina) although the stent itself had reduced in cross-sectional area by 11 to 12%.9 Between 6 months and 2 years, IVUS showed no change in vessel area (external elastic lamina), but the lumen increased in size and the stent was no longer identifiable by 2 years.The BVS stent clearly did its job of preventing negative remodeling; however, the duration for which radial support was provided is unclear.

Will Bioabsorbable Stents Eliminate the Risk of Late Thrombosis at the PCI Site?

DES are a major breakthrough in interventional cardiology because they more than halve the need for repeat intervention compared with BMS.Although a small increase in thrombosis is offset by a reduced risk of complications associated with repeat revascularization. late (6 month to 1 year) or very late (beyond 1 year) thrombosis is the feared complication of stenting that may result in myocardial infarction and death. Although late-stent thrombosis occurs with both BMS and DES, that after DES occurs later and as primary thrombosis, whereas that after BMS can be secondary to repeat intervention for restenosis. A worst case scenario is that the problem of late-stent thrombosis after first-generation DES implantation may be ongoing indefinitely as a registry of >8000 patients reported that it occurred at a constant rate of 0.6% per annum without diminution by 4 years. Indefinite continuation of dual antiplatelet therapy is not a practical solution because of expense and because a quarter of late-stent thromboses occurred in patients receiving dual antiplatelet therapy. In addition, dual antiplatelet therapy may be discontinued because of troublesome minor bleeding or to reduce the risk of bleeding during surgery.

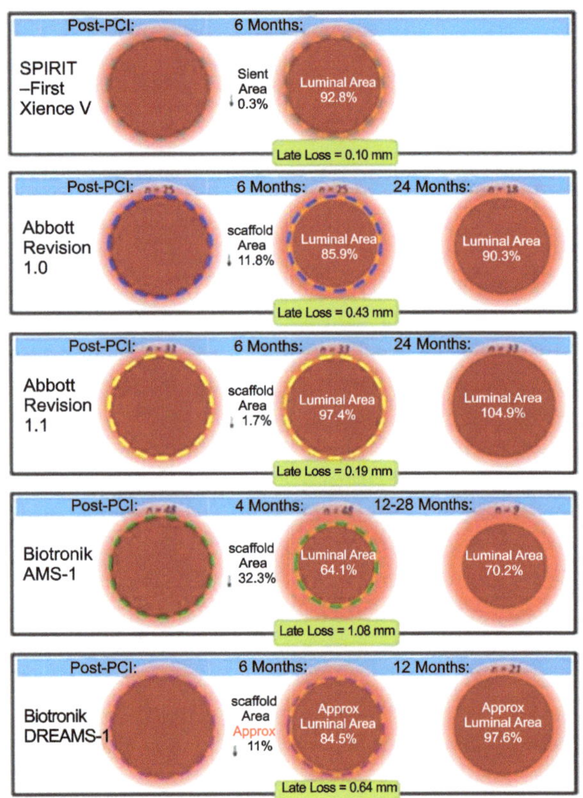

Fig. 20.27 Comparison of bioabsorbable stent/scaffold and Xience V DES luminal area at follow-up (adapted from Garg and Serruys, Serruys Pres. TCT 2008 and 2011.

An ideal DES would have no risk of late thrombosis and a fully bioabsorbable drug-eluting stent may fulfill this hope. Primary thrombosis at the treated site almost never occurred late after balloon angioplasty and has been described as the bane of stenting from the very beginning. Although multiple factors predispose to late thrombosis, it is reasonable to hope that it will be rare if a stent is completely absorbed because there would be no permanent metallic or polymeric foreign body exposed to blood even if endothelialization were functionally abnormal, delayed, or incomplete. If stent struts disappear, there can be no late stent malapposition. If the stent struts and coating are completely absorbed and the drug gone, there may be none of the ongoing chronic inflammation known to predispose to thrombosis. The endothelial regrowth after first-generation Taxus or Cypher stenting may be delayed but, in addition, may be functionally abnormal. Preliminary reports from some patients 2 years after BVS stent implantation raise the possibility of return of a functionally normal endothelium at the stented site because there was vasodilatation or absence of vasoconstriction downstream after acetylcholine administration. These observations will need to be confirmed in a larger trial. When the bioabsorbable coating of a metallic DES has been absorbed, all that remains is a BMS, and so the risk of late thrombosis may be limited to that of a BMS. However, even BMS have an ongoing risk of thrombosis that may be improved if there were no permanent foreign body in the vessel wall. An additional reason that a fully bioabsorbable DES may have a low risk of late thrombosis, perhaps lower than even late after balloon angioplasty, is that the

Summary

An ideal stent should furnish best acute outcomes after PCI by sealing intimal flaps and optimizing lumen size. It should control restenosis by limiting negative remodeling and by controlling excessive healing by delivery of an antiproliferative drug. Beyond 6 months, a permanent implant has no useful function and has possible disadvantages including the potential for late thrombosis. The concept of a stent that does its job and disappears has appeal A number of different materials ranging from magnesium to a variety of polymers have been used to construct stents of different designs. Some of these are being tested in clinical trials. The best outcomes to date have been with the BVS everolimus-eluting PLLA stent where in the Absorb trial, cohort A at 2 years, the stent was safe in the small number of patients with simple lesions Indeed, there is a suggestion of luminal enlargement between 6 months and 2 years, return of vasomotion, and endothelial function. These findings need to be confirmed in larger trials in more complex lesions. A hope is that a healed, normally functioning vessel free of foreign body and restenosis will be free of the risk of late thrombosis. Time will tell if this dream will come true.

TRANSCATHETER AORTIC VALVE REPLACEMENT (TAVR) OR TVI

Transcatheter aortic valve replacement (TAVR) is a procedure for select patients with severe symptomatic aortic stenosis (narrowing of the aortic valve opening) who are not candidates for traditional open chest surgery or are high-risk operable candidates. TAVR is performed on a beating heart and does not require cardio-pulmonary bypass. The TAVR valve is made of bovine (cow) pericardium and is supported with a metal stent. There are currently three approaches:

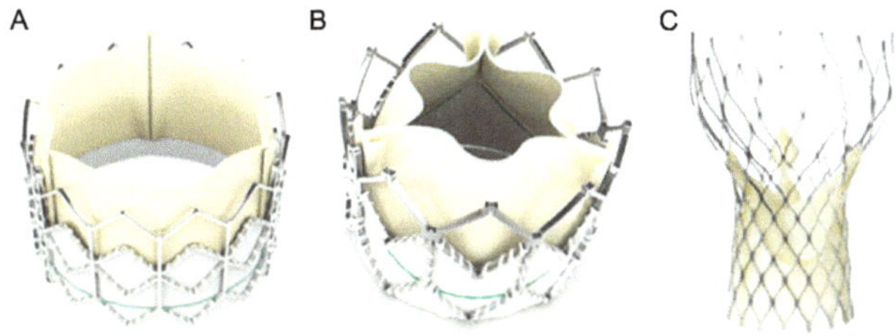

Fig. 20.28 Current Widely Available Transcatheter Valves (A) The Edwards SAPIEN THV balloon-expandable valve (Edwards Lifesciences, Irvine, California) incorporates a stainless steel frame, bovine pericardial leaflets,x and a fabric sealing cuff. (B) The SAPIEN XT THV (Edwards Lifesciences) utilizes a cobalt chromium alloy frame and is compatible with lower profile delivery catheters. (C) The Medtronic CoreValve (Medtronic, Minneapolis, Minnesota) incorporates a self-expandable frame, porcine pericardial leaflets, and a pericardial seal.

Transfemoral Approach

A catheter is placed in the femoral artery (in the groin) similar to angioplasty, and guided into the chambers of the heart. A compressed tissue heart valve is placed on the balloon catheter and is positioned directly inside the diseased aortic valve. Once in position, the balloon is inflated to secure the valve in place. This procedure is performed with general anesthesia in a hybrid suite (which has both catheterization and surgical capabilities). A team of iterventional cardiologists and imaging specialists, heart surgeons and cardiac anesthesiologists work together, utilizing fluoroscopy and echocardiography to guide the valve to the site of the patient's diseased heart valve.Cleveland Clinic was one of three early pioneering centers in the USA and one of more than 20 centers involved in the randomized PARTNER trials (Placement of Aortic Transcatheter Valve) of TAVR. The one-year results of the PARTNER-B trial were released in September 2010. The inoperable patients involved in the PARTNER-B trial had severe symptomatic aortic stenosis and were not candidates for surgery. The patients were randomly selected to receive either TAVR or standard medical care. Among the inoperable patients who had TAVR, the procedure reduced their absolute risk of dying within a year by 20% (the risk of mortality at one year went from 50 to 30%).

The transfemoral approach is now approved by the FDA for patients who have severe, symptomatic aortic stenosis who are ineligible for open surgical replacement, based on the PARTNER-B trial results. It is not approved for patients who are eligible for traditional aortic valve surgery, patients with bicuspid aortic valves, endocarditis, or cannot tolerate anticoagulation/antiplatelet therapy.

Investigational Transfemoral Approach

TAVR via femoral artery is now being tested for moderately high risk and high risk operable patients as well as inoperable patients in a new research trial PARTNER-II.

Transapical Approach

The transfemoral approach requires the use of catheters large enough to place the transcatheter aortic valve replacement through. Patients with peripheral artery disease may not have arteries large enough to support the transfemoral approach. In this case, patients can be evaluated to participate in a research study (PARTNER-II) which uses the alternative transapical approach.

During the transapical procedure, the surgeon makes a 4 inch incision between the ribs. A compressed tissue heart valve is placed on the balloon catheter, inserted through the ribs into the apex of the left ventricle and positioned directly inside the diseased aortic valve. Once in position, the balloon is inflated to secure the valve in place. This procedure is performed under general anesthesia, in a hybrid operating room. A team of imaging and interventional cardiologists and heart surgeons

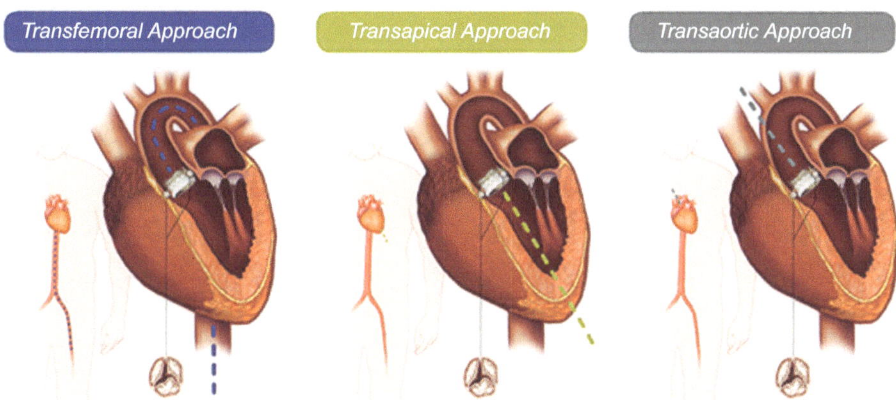

Fig. 20.29 Diagrams showing different routes of aortic valve implantation

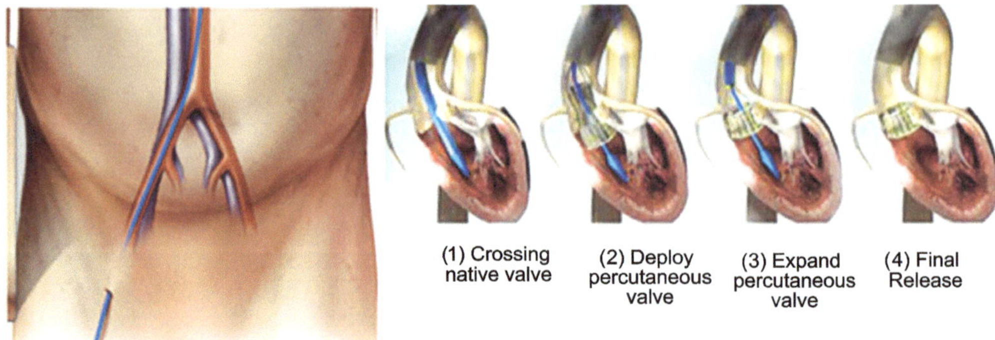

Fig. 20.30 Diagram illustrating different steps in transfemoral implantation of aortic valve

work together, utilizing fluoroscopy and echocardiography to guide the valve to the site of the patient's diseased heart valve.

Investigational Transaortic Approach

During the transaortic procedure, the surgeon makes a J shaped incision at the top of the sternum in between the manubrium and the sternum. A compressed tissue heart valve is placed on the balloon catheter, inserted into the aorta and positioned directly inside the diseased aortic valve. Once in position, the balloon is inflated to secure the valve in place.

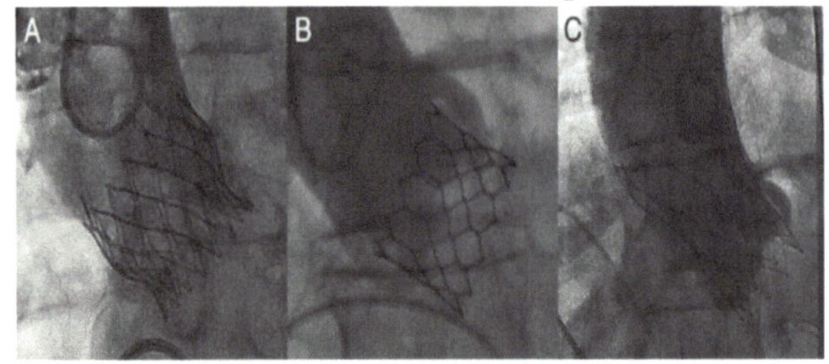

Fig. 20.31 Fluoroscopic Images of Some Newer Valves Undergoing Early Evaluation in Patients The CENTERA valve (A) is self-expandable and utilizes an electronic motorized release and retrieval system, while the S3 valve (B) incorporates an improved sealing system and utilizes a 14-F expandable sheath (Edwards Lifesciences, Irvine, California). (C) The Portico valve (St. Jude Medical Inc., St. Paul, Minnesota) is self-expandable, retrievable, and repositionable.

What You Should Know About TAVR

TAVR is performed in high-risk and inoperable patients with aortic stenosis. All patients are careful evaluate to see if they are candidates for traditional surgical aortic valve replacement and then TAVR can be considered for treatment. The goal is to provide the best treatment for each individual patient.

Cleveland Clinic was involved in TAVR research since 2006 and has evaluated around 2000 patients and performed more than 220 procedures

Transfemoral TAVR was recently approved by the FDA for inoperable patients.

There are ongoing research trials for TAVR for high-risk operable, moderate risk operable and inoperable patients. The positive results seen in the PARTNER trial were related to procedures performed at valve centers where there is a team approach between interventional cardiologists and surgeons.

The one year survival results for PARTNER-A, the high-risk patient population were similar in those who received surgery vs. those who received TAVR.

There are still risks associated with TAVR as there is with surgical AVR. These should be taken into consideration in decision making.

Total Endoscopic Aortic Valve Replacement (TEAVR

Surgical aortic valve replacement (SAVR) is continually evolving with minimal access procedures becoming more widespread thanks to the latest turning point: sutureless technology. Beyond the advantages linked to the elimination of sutures and knots (some of those devices carrying a Nitinol frame offer the possibility of being compressed, enabling their passage through a thoracoscopic trocar.

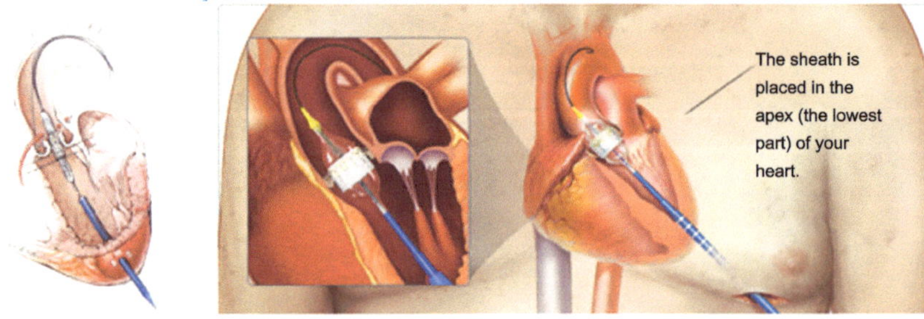

Fig.20.32 Diagram illustrating transapical approach in implantation of aortic valve.

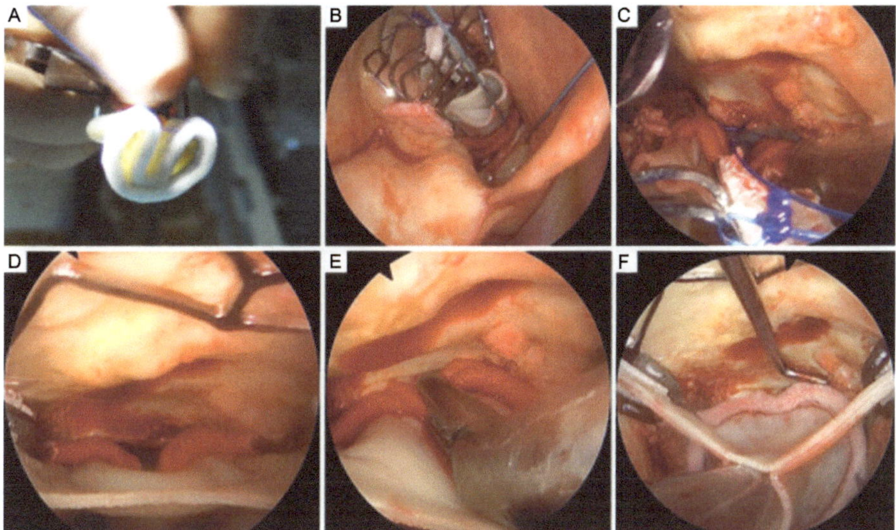

Fig. 20.33 Deployment of the 3f Enable valve through endoscopic technique. (A) The 3f Enable valve is kept compresssed by a prolene stitch before introduction in the trocar; (B) positionning of the non-coronary portion of the bioprosthesis; (C) positionning of the right portion of the bioprosthesis; (D) initial deployment of the folded leaflet after cutting the prolene stitch; (E) final deployment of the right portion of the bioprostehsis cuff; (F) final control of the sitting of the 3f Enable valve (including hook control around the valve).

Total endoscopic aortic valve replacement (TEAVR) aims to further reduce surgical wall chest trauma by avoiding sternal fractures or costal spreading. Clinical advantages have already been shown during atrial septal defect (ASD) closure surgery (8), thus favoring total endoscopic approach over ministernotomy and minithoracotomy.

WATCHMAN AND LARIAT PROCEDURES IN PREVENTION OF ATRIAL FIBRILLATION STROKE

The Watchman and Lariet procedures are among the newest procedures available to prevent A-fib related stroke.The most serious risk from atrial fibrillation is thromboembolic stroke. The left atrial appendage (LAA) is a pouch-like extension of the left atrium about the size of your thumb with a narrow opening into the left atrium. With atrial fibrillation, blood can pool and form clots in this appendage. If a blood clot breaks loose it may travel through the blood vessels and eventually plug a smaller vessel in the brain or heart. Doctors often prescribe the blood thinning medications such as Coumadin to prevent blood clots, however, it can often cause serious side effects. Today, the doctors at PHCVI can offer many patients an alternative such as the Watchman Device and Lariat procedure to prevent blood clots associated with atrial fibrillation.

What is the Watchman Device?

The Watchman Device is a small, fabric-covered device permanently placed in the opening of the left atrial appendage to prevent harmful-sized blood clots from exiting and entering the bloodstream. It is made of materials that are well-tolerated by most patients, and intended for those with non-valvular atrial fib, who require treatment for potential blood clotting and can tolerate Coumadin.

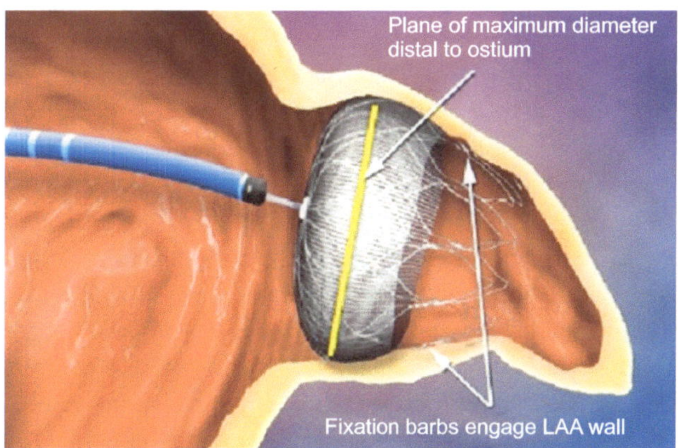

Fig. 20.34 showing watchman device for occlusion of left atrial appendage in the prevention stroke in atrial fibrillation.

The Procedure: Watchman LAA closure is performed under local or general anesthesia in the cathaterization lab. The heart is reached through a hole made in the femoral vein in the upper thigh and the device is delivered to the LAA through a catheter under X-ray and ultrasound guidance. The procedure takes about an hour and requires an overnight hospital stay. It takes at least 45 days for the heart tissue to heal. It will be important to continue taking Coumadin (your doctor will prescribe a lower dosage) and a daily aspirin. Your physician may also prescribe an antibiotic to prevent infection after surgery.

What is the Lariat Procedure?: This permanent, one-time procedure has been found to be highly successful and poses fewer risks and less discomfort to patients than surgery. Performed under general anesthesia, the Lariat procedure uses two catheters carrying the Lariat Suture Delivery Device. One of these catheters is inserted under the patient's rib cage; the other is sent to the heart's left atrial appendage (LAA). Once the catheters are in place, the device places and then tightens a loop stitch around the base of the left atrial appendage, sealing it off from the rest of the heart, blocking stroke-causing blood clots from traveling to the brain.

Benefits of the Lariat Procedure

- The Lariat procedure is a minimally invasive procedure that:
- Can reduce the risk of stroke by 85 to 90 percent
- Is suitable for patients who cannot undergo surgery
- Minimizes discomfort and promotes faster healing and quicker recovery.

BIO-HYBRID KIDNEY POWERED BY HEART IN THE OFFING

Washington, Feb 16 (PTI) Scientists are developing a first-of-its kind implantable artificial kidney with microchip filters and living cells that will be powered by the patient's own heart. "We are creating a bio-hybrid device that can mimic a kidney to remove enough waste products, salt and water to keep a patient off dialysis," said William H Fissell IV, from Vanderbilt University Medical Centre in US. The goal is to make it small enough, roughly the size of a soda can, to be implanted inside the body, Fissell said. The key to the device is a microchip, researchers said. "It uses the same processes that were developed by the microelectronics industry for computers," said Fissell. The chips are affordable, precise and make ideal filters. Researchers are designing each pore in the filter one by one based on what they want that pore to do. Each device will hold roughly fifteen microchips layered on top of each other. However, the microchips have another essential role beyond filtering, researchers said. "They're also the scaffold in which living kidney cells will rest," said Fissell. N Researchers use live kidney cells that will grow on and around the microchip filters. The goal is for these cells to mimic the natural actions of the kidney. "We can use kidney cells that fortunately for us grow well in the lab dish, and grow them into a bioreactor of living cells that will be the only 'Santa Claus' membrane in the world - the only membrane that will know which chemicals have been naughty and which have been nice," said Fissell." Then they can reabsorb the nutrients your body needs and discard the wastes your body desperately wants to get rid of," said Fissell. Since this bio-hybrid device sits out of reach from the body's immune response, it is protected from rejection. "The issue is not one of immune compliance, of matching, like it is with an organ transplant," said Fissell. The device operates naturally with a patient's blood flow." We must transform that unsteady pulsating blood flow in the arteries and move it through an artificial device without clotting or damage," he said. Researchers are using fluid dynamics to see if there are certain regions in the device that might cause clotting. They use computer models to refine the shape of the channels for the smoothest blood flow. Then they rapidly prototype the new design using 3D printing and test it to make the blood flow as smoothly as possible

DELHI BASED DUO BUILD WORLD'S CHEAPEST AND SMALLEST VENTILATOR THAT FITS IN POCKET

Good news for patients who are advised to stay on aventilator. They can now breathe comfortably by using this mini ventilator. The world's cheapest and smallest ventilator, developed by AIIMS in collaboration with a private company, can easily fit into your pocket, according to PTI. This invention is the is the brainchild of Dr Deepak Agrawal, professor in the department of neurosurgery at AIIMS, who joined with Diwakar Vaish, a robotics researcher at A-SET Robotics to make the device. Diwakar Vaish (25) said, "It is almost 450 times smaller than the conventional ventilators and can be moved around easily," as per Hindustan Times.

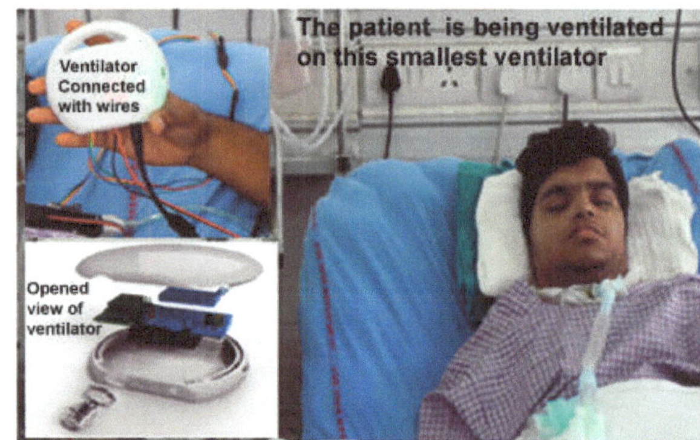

Fig 20.35 The world's cheapest and smallest ventilator, developed by AIIMS in collaboration with a private company, can easily fit into your pocket.

There are lot of patients in AIIMS and in hospitals across India who are required to be on ventilator for a prolonged period and are unable to arrange them because of the exorbitant costs and the technical expertise required to operate them. "We have 10 to 15 such patients in the neurosurgery department itself who are on ventilator for the lasttwo years or more," said Dr Agrawal. This ventilator is easyto use and soon will be available in the market for a priceat less than `15,000. "We are using the ventilator on some patients as pilot," he added. Currently, a basic ventilators is priced above 2.5 lakhs in the market, as per PTI. our whole lives."

The ventilator can be controlled with an Android app and it uses an artificial intelligence algorithm to adjust air supply for normal breathing of the patient, as per HT. Vaish said, "There is no requirement for oxygen cylinders, which cost between ` 3,000 and ` 4,000 a day." "It works by pushing the atmospheric air into the lungs of the patients who cannot breathe on their own. The disposable ventilators currently in use also push in air, but they do it at a fixed frequency that does not necessarily match the patient's breathing pattern, which may cause low oxygen saturation. This device synchronises ventilator air support with the normal breathing pattern," Dr Agrawal was quoted as saying by HT.

CURRENT INNOVATIONS IN PACEMAKER THERAPY

In recent years, more and more pacemakers have been implanted, with the result that not only cardiological specialists are increasingly being confronted by such patients. In view of the multiplicity of the implanted systems, every general practitioner should have a basic knowledge of their various functions. Functional pacemaker disorders may result in an acute emergency that requires immediate attention. Current Innovations in Pacemaker Therapy would be discussed under the following headings such as:

1. Leadless pacemaker therapy.
2. Left ventricular resynchronization therapy with Leadlesspacemaker.
3. Leadless pacing: current status and future perspectives.
4. Advances in Implantable Cardioverter Defibrillator(ICD) Technology.
5. Battery Life, MRI-safe ICDs, Reducing Shocks andReducing Implanted Hardware.

A *pacemaker* is a device that sends small electricalimpulses to the heart muscle to maintain a suitable heart.

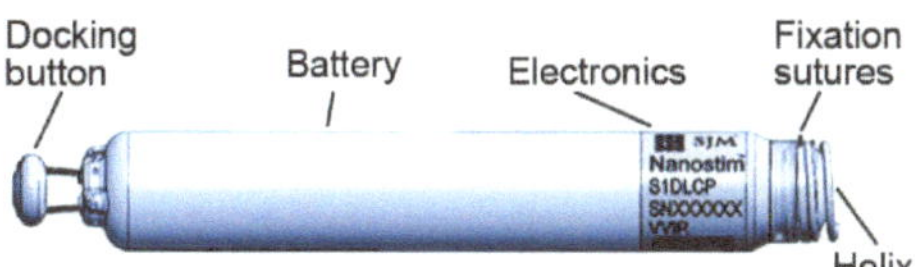

Fig 20.37 The St. Jude Medical Nanostim™ leadless pacemaker(reproduced with permission from St. Jude Medical Inc.). The various components of the pacemaker have been shown in this figure. rate or to stimulate the lower chambers of the heart (ventricles).

What is Leadless Pacemaker ?

Pacemakers are used to treat patients with brady-arrythmias, slow heart rhythms that may occur as a result of disease in the heart's conduction system (such as the SA node, AV node or His-Purkinje network). A leadless pacemaker is small self-contained device that is inserted in the right ventricle of the heart.

What are the Benefits of a Leadless Pacemaker?

- It does not require connecting leads (wires) or agenerator, or a creation of a surgical pocket on the chest. These are the most common causes of traditional pacemaker complications over the long-term, and may affect up to 1 in 10 patients.
- When the leadless device is in place, there is no lumpunder the skin on the chest or leads anchored to themuscle bed. Sometimes these cause minor discom-

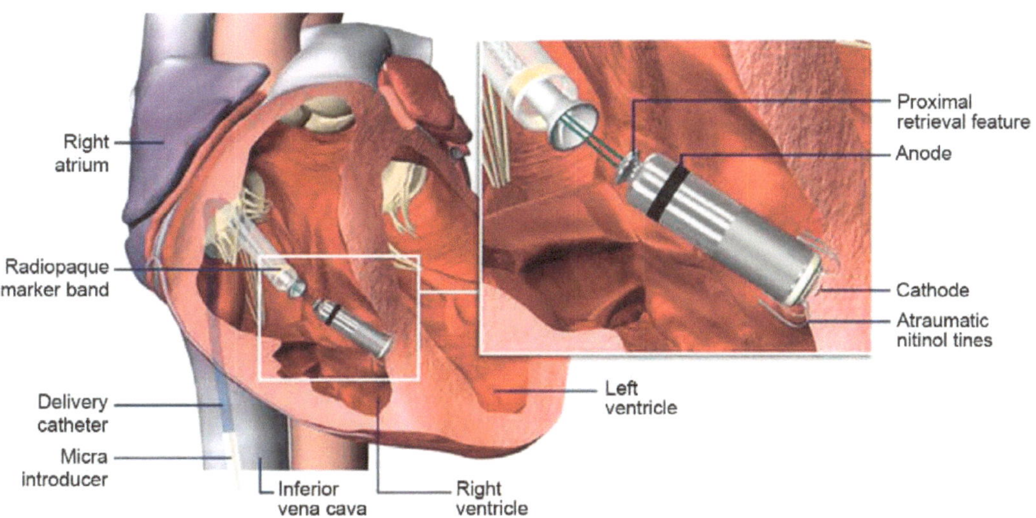

Fig 20.36 Illustration demonstrates the route,site and morphological features of leadless pacemaker.

fort for patients who live with traditional pacemakers. The incisional access for a traditional pacemaker and each generator replacement leaves a scar that is a cosmetic concern for some patients.

- The procedure uses a catheter to place the device. The procedure typically takes less time than a traditional pacemaker implant procedure.
- Because there are no wires or generator, you do not need to limit upper body activity after the implant.

Who is a Candidate for a Leadless Pacemaker?

Not everyone is a candidate for a leadless pacemaker. Currently, the device is available only for patients with certain medical conditions and a slow heart rate (brady-cardia) who need single-chamber pacing only. Like all pacemakers, leadless pacemakers require approval by the Food and Drug Administration (FDA) and sometimes there are additional restrictions upon availability for an indi-vidual patient. Your doctor can tell you if you are a candi-date for a leadless pacemaker after a review of your medical history, heart rhythm, and the results of medical tests. You may need an echocardiogram (ultrasound of the heart) or other noninvasive tests.

Contraindications in Leadless Pacemakers

These devices are contraindicated in individuals who require:

- Dual-chamber pacing or who have demonstrable pacemaker syndrome.
- Current devices are not MRI compatible.
- Leadless pacemakers are contra indicated in patients with implantable cardioverter-defibrillators, as high-voltage-shocks could damage the pacemaker, and the effect of the pacemaker on shock effectiveness is unknown.
- Leadless devices should be avoided in individuals with-elevated right ventricular pressures because of high ertheoretical risk of embolization.
- The presence of mechanical tricuspid valves or inferior vena cava filters also precludes the use of leadless pacemakers.

How is the Leadless Pacemaker Implanted?

After puncture of the right femoral artery, a 12F vascularintroducer was inserted in conjunction with an arterial closure device (ProStar XL or Perclose Proglide 6F, Abbot Vascular Inc.). A 12F deflectable sheath (WiCS-LV) was introduced into the LV via a transaortic approach using a180 cm soft-tip guide wire (0.032? or 0.035?) and a dilator. Intravenous heparin was administered to attain and maintain an activation clotting time level in the range of 200–250. The dilator/wire was exchanged for a catheter with the electrode at the distal tip and equipped with a detachable connection to the electrode. This connection retains the electrode on the catheter prior to deployment and also provides a direct electrical contact to the cathode of the electrode for electrogram monitoring and pacing. With the electrode retained within the tip of the sheath, the sheath was steered under fluoroscopic guidance to a targeted LV implant site. Radiopaque contrast was administered through the catheter and used to discernsheath contact with the LV. Tissue viability was confirmed using the electrogram and by pacing threshold. The procedure takes about 30 minutes to complete, although this can vary patient-to-patient based on individual anatomical consideration.

What Happens after the Procedure?

You will need to lie flat and keep the leg straight for two to six hours after the procedure. This prevents bleeding from the access site. Do not try to sit or stand. A sterile dressing will be placed on your groin area to protect it from infection. You will spend the night in the hospital and will be able to go home after your device check and a chest X-ray.

What are the Risks of a Leadless Pacemaker Implant?

Every procedure has complications associated with it. The most common possible problems after a leadless pacemaker implant involve the incision site, such as swelling and bleeding. These are not typically life threatening but may lead to a longer hospital stay or slower recovery.

More serious but rare complications include the device moving out of place (dislodgement) or internal bleeding, such as pericardial effusion or tamponade.

Follow-up: Follow up after a leadless pacemaker is similar to a traditional schedule with non-invasive checks.

First-in-man implantation of leadless ultrasound-based-cardiac stimulation pacing system: novel endocardial left ventricular resynchronization therapy in heart failure patients *Transthoracic echocardiography imaging* was performed to view the distal end of the sheath and to insure proper alignment. By advancing the catheter the electrode's anchorbarbs were attached to the LVendo wall. Contrast injections through the catheter in two fluoroscopic views confirmed insertion of the anchor barbs, the electrode was released, and detachment was confirmed by changes in the electrogram signal. The sheath was withdrawn, the artery was secured with the closure device, and heparin was stopped to reduce the ACT level to below 180 s prior to the implantation of the transmitter.

A 3 cm incision in a left lateral or in an abdominal position and a 6 cm incision over the previously identified ICS were made to create the subcutaneous pockets for the battery and transmitter. Tunnelling between the two incisions passed the interconnect cable from the transmitter to connect the battery, then both were inserted in their pockets.

Programming the transmitter was performed to enable sensing the RV pacing signal and to trigger acoustic transmissions to the electrode in the LV. After observation of bi-ventricular pacing on 12-lead ECG, the transmitter and battery were sutured in place.

The importance of specific-site pacing is increasingly recognized in cardiac resynchronization therapy (CRT). Using current pacing technology, site selection is still largely limited by coronary vein anatomy, whereas left ventricular(LV) endocardial pacing using current lead technology is risky and challenging. To overcome limitations and complications with current LV pacing, the feasibility of anew technology enabling LV endocardial stimulation without the use of a lead is being evaluated in patients.

Methods and Results

Patients presented in this report are part of the Wireless-Stimulation Endocardially for CRT Trial (WiSE-CRT) study investigating the safety and performance of the WiCS®-LV system, an implantable cardiac pacing system capable of leadless pacing based on converting ultrasound energy to electrical energy. Three patients are presented: (i) a patient with an existing implantable defibrillator, (ii) a patient with a CRT system whose LV lead does not capture, and (iii) a CRT patient classified as a non-responder. All three patients were successfully treated. Acute electrical pacing thresholds ranged from 0.7 to 1.0 V at 0.5 ms; all patients retained captured at 6 months. Functional New York Heart Association class significantly changed (Pre: III in two patients, and IV in one patient; Post: I in one patient, II in one patient, and II–III in one patient), and LV ejection fraction increased from 23.7 ± 3.4 to 39 ± 6.2% ($P < 0.017$).

Leadless pacing: current status and future perspectives

Despite all the enthusiasm generated by these novel and remarkable devices, it has to be stressed that the peri-procedural risks associated with implantation require attention. For two out of the three systems, clinical trials have either been terminated or put temporarily on hold because of severe complications, including death. Cardiac perforation and tamponade seem to be issues that need to be addressed. Device design, especially as regards the fixation mechanism, should be carefully evaluated and if necessary adapted. A safe implantation technique that is applicable to a broad clinical setting is desirable. This will also require proper education and training of implantingphysicians. Evaluation of these devices in clinical studies and registries will be necessary to judge the benefit-to-risk profile, especially in the long-term.Future steps that may be taken are the development of leadless multichamber devices that communicate with each other. Such new devices would make leadless pacing suitable for a much larger population. Boston Scientific is currently developing a leadless pacemaker system, which may in the future be complementary to their subcutaneous ICD (*e.g.*, for delivering antitachycardia or anti-bradycardia pacing, or for enhancing arrhythmia diagnosis). Research is currently underway for harvesting kinetic energy from cardiac motion to fuel pacemaker function (similarly to automatic watches). Intracardiac pacemakers may one day profit from such technology, thereby dispensing with the need for device replacement. Intravascular defibrillators are another next step, and initial results of an investigational device have recently been published.

Advances in Implantable Cardioverter Defibrillator (ICD) Technology

There have been several recent advancements in implantable cardioverter defibrillator (ICD) technology to extend battery life, improvements in patient monitoring to avoid needless shocks, the introduction of quadripolar lead devices to improve device programming and to improve therapy effectiveness, and development of magnetic resonance imaging (MRI)-safe ICDs. ICDs are implanted in patients who are at high risk for sudden cardiac arrest (SCA) due to sustained ventricular tachycardia or fibrillation.

These devices also are used to improve the heart's pumping-ability in heart failure patients. ICDs are incorporated intocardiac resynchronization therapy defibrillator (CRT-D)devices, which resynchronize the contractions of both ventricles and have defibrillation capabilities. Several newerICDs offer pacing functions, and many vendors offer wireless remote monitoring/ interrogation of the device data with bedside sending units so patients do not need tocome in for regular office visits.

Quadripolar Leads Expand Therapy Options

One of the biggest innovations has been the introduction of quadripolar lead devices. The leads use four electrodesto allow more programming options for pacing and overcoming issues with lead placement. This can help optimize CRT-D therapy and decrease the number of patients who do not respond. Up to 10 percent of heart failure patients' left ventricular (LV) lead placements are not successful because of anatomical challenges, phrenic nerve stimulation (PNS) or poor electrical measurement. Use of a quadripolar LV lead instead of a bipolar option during CRT can decrease complications at six months, according to preliminary results presented at the 2014 European Society of Cardiology (ESC) Congress. The MORE-CRT

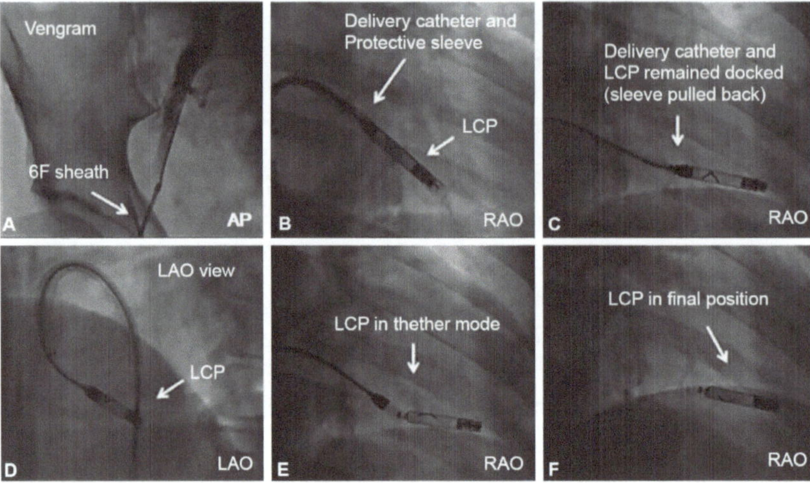

Fig. 20.38 (a) Leadless cardiac pacemaker implantation steps. (A) A venogram may optionally be performed;(B)The LCP is positioned into the RV by deflecting the catheter and placed ~0.5–1 cm from the RV apex; (C andD)Protective cover is pulled back to expose the flexible part of the catheter; (E) The pacemaker is undocked fromthe delivery catheter while a tethered connection is maintained. In case the position is suboptimal, the LCP canbe re-engaged, unscrewed, and repositioned. (F) The LCP is released by rotating the release knob of the catheter.

trial demonstrated the safety and efficiency of the quadripolar lead technology in providing more options to manage CRT patients. The MORE-CRT study included 1,068 heart failure patients scheduled for CRT from 63 centers in 13 countries. The study includes more than 1,000CRT patients with either a bipolar lead or a quadripolar lead. The study showed that at six months, compared to controls, patients with quadripolar leads were significantly more likely to be free from a composite endpoint of bothintra- and post-operative LV lead-related complications(85.97 percent versus 76.86 percent, P=0.0001) — a relative risk reduction (RRR) of 40.8 percent. The driver of this benefit was mainly intra-operative complications, which were reduced by more than 50 percent in the quadripolar group (5.98 percent vs. 13.73 percent, P<0.0001, RRR 56.4percent). Additional data released in 2014 show use of quadripolar LV leads was associated with significantly reduced hospitalizations specific to heart failure and LV lead surgical revision.

Presented at Heart Rhythm 2014. The Hospitalization Rates and Associated Cost Analysis of Quadripolar versus Bipolar CRT-D: a comparative analysis of a single-center prospective Italian registry presentation, demonstrated quadripolar leads reduced the number of hospitalizations by 53 percent when compared to the non-quadripolar group. This hospitalization rate reduction translated into a statistically significant 62 percent reduction in overall costs for both healthcare systems and patients. St. Jude Medical was the first to gain U.S. Food and Drug Administration (FDA) approval for a quadripolar pacing lead in January 2012, on its Unify Quadra CRT-D, which uses the Quartet left ventricular quadripolar pacing lead.

SUBCUTANEOUS ICD TECHNOLOGY

The FDA granted market clearance in October 2012 for Boston Scientifics' S-ICD system, the world's first commercially available subcutaneous ICD (S-ICD). The S-ICD sits entirely just below the skin without the needfor implantable leads to be placed inside the heart. This leaves the heart and blood vessels untouched, offering patients an alternative to transvenous ICDs, which require leads to be placed in the heart itself.

External Defibrillator Offers Bridge

Therapy for patients at risk for SCA who are being evaluated for a permanent ICD, Zoll offers the LifeVest wearable exter-

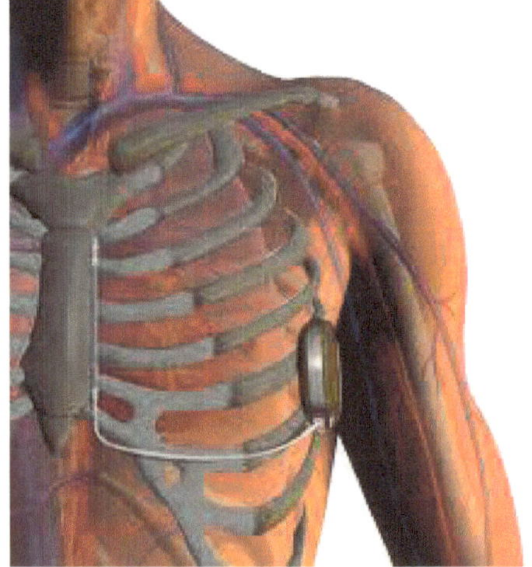

Fig.20.39 (b) Subcutaneous ICD (S-ICD). The S-ICD sits entirely just below the skin without the need for implantable leads to be placed inside the heart.

nal defibrillator as a temporary solution. The LifeVest allows a physician time to assess a patient's long-term arrhythmic risk and make appropriate plans. The LifeVest is light-weight and easy to wear under a patient's clothing, allowing them to return to their daily activities while having the peace of mind that they are protected from SCA. The LifeVest continuously monitors the patient's heart and, if a life-threatening heart rhythm is detected, the device delivers a treatment shock to restore normal heart rhythm. This device continuously monitors the patient's heart with dry, non-adhesive sensing electrodes to detect life-threatening abnormal heart rhythms. If a life-threatening heart rhythm is detected, the device alerts bystanders and delivers a treatment shock to restore normal heart rhythm. The entire event, from detecting a life-threatening arrhythmia to automatically delivering a treatment shock, usually occurs in less than a minute.

The LifeVest is used for a range of patient conditions or situations, including following a heart attack and before or after bypass surgery or stent placement, as well as for those with cardiomyopathy or congestive heart failure that places them at particular risk. Zoll said the LifeVest has been prescribed to more than 100,000 patients. Zoll intregrates this device with the LifeVest Network online patient data management system. It allows clinicians to monitor patient data online, downloaded from a patient's LifeVest. It gives the clinician options to customize events that generate an alert, or to be notified for a number of events, such as detected arrhythmias, treatments, patient-recorded electrocardiograms (ECGs) and patient use.

MRI-safe ICDs

It is estimated that about 60 percent of ICD patients will need an MRI within 10 years of receiving a device. Until the availability of MR-conditional ICD systems, patients with devices have been contraindicated from receiving MRI scans because of potential interactions between the MRI and device function. There are several MRI-compatible ICDs now available in Europe and two undergoing FDA investigational device exemption (IDE) pivotal trials in the United States The ProMRI trial is evaluating Biotronik's DX ICD system, which gained CE mark in Europe in 2011, becoming the first MRI-compatible ICD on the market. In May 2014, Medtronic announced the first U.S. trial implant of its Evera MRI SureScan ICD system. Medtronic gained European CE mark approval for the device in April 2014.

Reducing Shocks

Patients' quality of life and faith in their ICDs can be significantly decreased if their ICD shocks the patient needlessly. Some vendors now include technology to help reduce inappropriate shocks. St. Jude Medical's Assura ICD and CRT portfolio features Secure Sense RV Lead Noise Discrimination, an algorithm that expands St. Jude's ShockGuard technology and offers advanced sensing options designed to reduce the incidence of inappropriate shocks. The algorithm provides advanced alerts as well as more proactively lowering the risk of lead-related complications through its ability to automatically withhold tachycardia therapy in the presence of lead noise (over-sensing of electrical signals). The technology differentiates lead noise from true ventricular tachycardia (VT) or ventricular fibrillation (VF) episodes that require life-saving therapy.In addition, ShockGuard technology features specific programming that distinguishes between rhythms that require defibrillation therapy and those that do not, such as benign arrhythmias. DecisionTx programming offers advanced sensing technology designed to avoid sensing unwanted signals (T-waves) and more anti-tachycardia pacing options, which can convert many fast ventricular arrhythmias painlessly and avoid the need for high-voltage shocks. Medtronic's Evera MRI includes SmartShock 2.0, a shock reduction algorithm that enables the device to better differentiate between dangerous and harmless heart rhythms. Medtronic said studies estimate about 20 percent of patients with implantable defibrillators might experience inappropriate shocks in response to a benign arrhythmia or electrical noise sensed by the device. Lead failure is another source of inappropriate shocks. In late 2013, Medtronic gained FDA clearance for its Lead Integrity Alert (LIA) software for use with non-Medtronic leads. LIA can report performance issues on Durata and Riata (St. Jude Medical) and Endotak (Boston Scientific) defibrillator leads when connected to a Medtronic device.

Reducing Implanted Hardware

Biotronik's Ilesto family of ICD/CRT-D devices includes the Ilesto DX.The platform allows for a 15 percent size reduction and 29percent fewer components with no compromise in longevity orclinical features. It is the first defibrillator system equipped to providefull atrial diagnostic information with just one specialized defibrillatorlead. The DX system offers an alternative with more monitoringcapability than a single-chamber device, and without additional leadsrequired for dual-chamber devices.

VACCINE TO LOWER CHOLESTEROL

A vaccine that could reduce LDL cholesterol and atherosclerosis is currently being tested in human trials.Daily statin use to lower cholesterol may soon be a thing of the past. A new study reveals how a vaccine successfully lowered "bad" cholesterol in mice and reduced atherosclerosis, which is a narrowing of the arteries caused by a buildup of plaque.The vaccine is called AT04A and has already entered a human clinical trial, which is expected to deliver results by the end of this year.If the vaccine is found to be safe and effective in humans, researchers say that it would offer a long-term therapeutic strategy for high cholesterol; rather than taking statins every day, patients could simply have an initial injection, followed by an annual booster.

CARDIOVASCULAR COMPLICATIO IN COVID-19 PATIENTS

The prevalence of hypertension and other cardiovascular disease has been reported as 15% to 32.6% and 2.5% to 15%, respectively. Patients with underlying cardiovascular disease are more prone to develop cardiac injury, be severely ill,or require intensive care. Cardiac injury, which is indicated by elevated cardiac troponin I (cTnI), also has been confirmed in COVID-19 patients. The incidence of cardiac injury has ranged from 7.2% to 27.8%, and its incidence in intensive care unit patients and deaths has been reported as 22.2% and 77%, respectively. Patients with elevated cTnI levels have shown a higher rate of cardiovascular disease, and cTnI was significantly increased in severely ill or deceased COVID-19 patients compared with patients with milder symptoms. A higher cTnI level also was associated with greater complications and mortality. Elevated N-terminal pro-brain natiuretic peptide (NT-proBNP) level also has been demonstrated, and patients with elevated cTnI levels were more likely to have elevated levels of NT-proBNP. All these findings suggested the relationship between cardiac injury, cardiac dysfunction, and poor outcome. Monitoring cTnI longitudinally during hospitalization may help predict the progression of the disease.Left ventricular dysfunction, persistent hypotension, acute myopericarditis, myocarditis, arrhythmia, and heart failure also have been reported in COVID-19 patients. Interstitial mononuclear inflammatory infiltration in heart tissue also provides evidence of myocarditis in COVID-19 patients. However, in a recent report of case series from critically ill patients in the Seattle, WA, region, no cardiac dysfunction was detected on echocardiograms. Both echocardiography and cardiac magnetic resonance imaging have been used widely in the evaluation of cardiac structural and functional changes, and the upcoming reports about their role in the diagnosis and prognostication of patientswith COVID-19 are awaitedAt present, the exact pathophysiological mechanisms of myocardial injury are not fully understood. Patient characteristics, the severity of infection, and host reaction all participate in the development of cardiac complications.Direct damage by the virus, systemic inflammatory responses, instability of coronary plaque, and hypoxia have been proposed as possible mechanisms

Instability of coronary atherosclerotic plaques, increased coagulation activation46 and platelet-aggregating activity, and hypoxemia due to abnormal ventilation/perfusion lead to decreased myocardial oxygen supply and myocardial ischemia. Activation of the sympathetic nervous system leads to increased heart rate and peripheral resistance, which will further compromise coronary perfusion.

Transient disturbance of endothelial function and vascular tone, volume overload due to impaired sodium and water metabolism,51 and cardiac arrhythmia8 may contribute to decreased left ventricular function or worsening of heart failure Direct pathogen invasion in severe pneumonia patients has been confirmed. In patients with severe pneumococcal disease, Streptococcus pneumoniae was detected in the myocardium, leading to cardiac injury and local proinflammatory responses.30 In addition SARS-CoV has been detected in 35% of patients with SARS, which suggests the possibility of direct damage to cardiomyocytes by the virus

COVID-19 is rapidly spreading globally. At present, very little is known about this virus. Before vaccination is available, there is no effective therapy at present. As new clinical evidence emerges, the diagnosis and treatment may change. Clinical trials are necessary to determine the risk factors of cardiac complications, the mechanisms of cardiac injury, and possible treatments to improve the outcome of patients with COVID-19.

NOBEL PRIZE IN MEDICINE IS AWARDED TO 3 AMERICANS FOR WORK ON CIRCADIAN RHYTHM

Jeffrey C. Hall, Michael Rosbash and Michael W. Young are the joint winners of the 2017 Nobel Prize in physiology or medicine, winning for their discoveries about how internal clocks and biological rhythms govern human life. The three Americans won "for their discoveries of molecular mechanisms controlling the circadian rhythm," the Nobel Foundation says. From the Nobel Assembly at Karolinska Institutet, which announced the prize early Monday morning: "Using fruit flies as a model organism, this year's Nobel laureates isolated a gene that controls the normal daily biological rhythm. They showed that this gene encodes a protein that accumulates in the cell during the night, and is then degraded during the day. Subsequently, they identified additional protein components of this machinery, exposing the mechanism governing the self-sustaining clockwork inside the cell. We now recognize that biological clocks function by the same principles in cells of other multicellular organisms, including humans. "With exquisite precision, our inner clock adapts our physiology to the dramatically different phases of the day. The clock regulates critical functions such as behavior, hormone levels, sleep, body temperature and metabolism." Hall, 72, was born in New York and has worked at institutions from the University of Wash-ington to the California Institute of Technology. For decades, he was on the faculty at Brandeis University in Waltham, west of Boston; more recently, he has been associated with the University of Maine.Rosbash, 73, was born in Kansas City, Mo., and studied at the Massachusetts Institute of Technology and at the University of Edinburgh in Scotland. Since 1974, he has been on faculty at Brandeis University in Waltham, Mass.

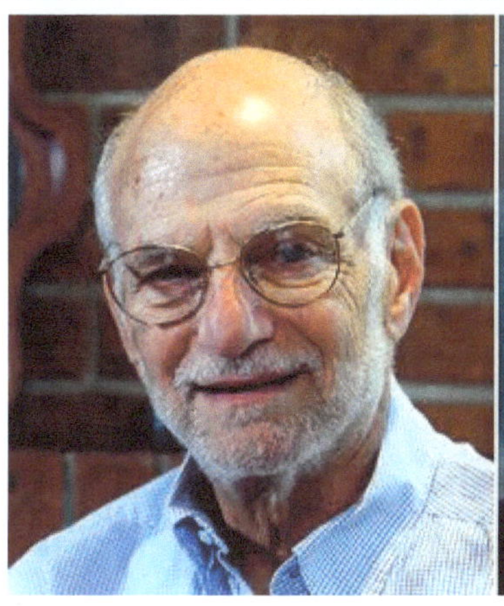
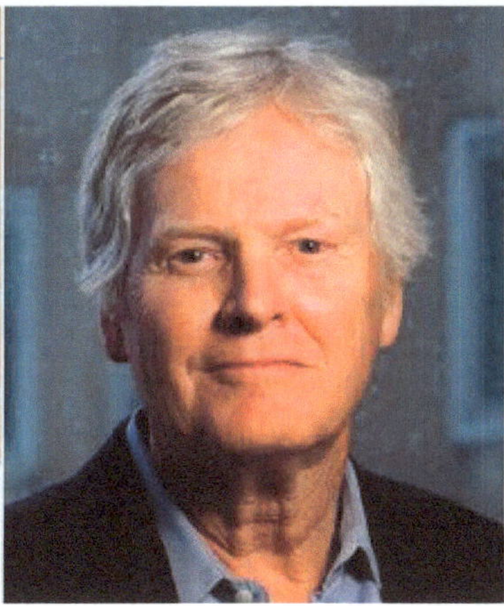
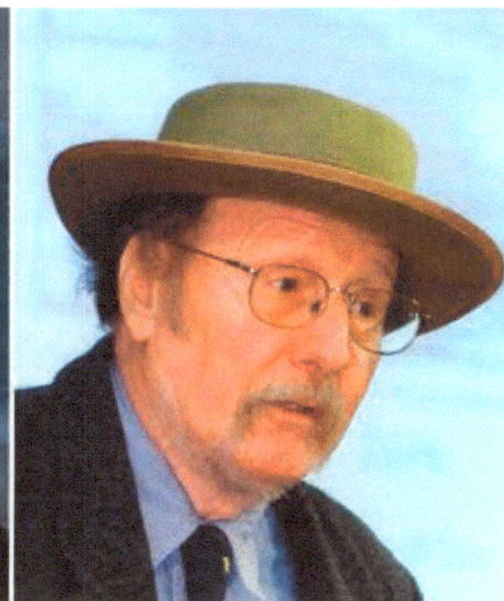

Fig 20.40 Nobel prize is awarded to 3 Americans for work on Circadian Rhythm. Jeffrey C. Hall, Michael Rosbash and Michael W. Young (From left ---Right)

Young, 68, was born in Miami, Fla., and earned his doctoral degree at the University of Texas in Austin. He then worked as a postdoctoral fellow at Stanford University in Palo Alto before joining the faculty at the Rockefeller University in 1978.

SCIENTISTS CREATED A PIG-HUMAN HYBRID EMBRYO FOR HUMAN ORGAN TRANSPLANTATION

Scientists at the Salk Institute in California have created a part-human, part-pig embryo. Bioethicist Arthur Caplan told us about the ethical concerns involved in mixing human and animal DNA.An experiment reported on Thursday in Cell, a peer-reviewed scientific journal, announced a purported break through in bioengineering: the successful creation of an embryo with both human and pig DNA (and to be clear, the artwork above is just a photo of a sculpture). The results, "raise the possibility of xeno-generating transplantable human tissues and organs towards addressing the world-wide shortage of organ donors," according to the paper. But while the embryo was only allowed to develop for a few days, the genesis of this early-stage creature revives an uncomfortable debate about whether animal-human hybrids are, well, horrifying monsters waiting to happen.In November 2015, shortly after the National Institutes of Health(NIH) put a hold on its own experiments that combined human and animal cells, the federal government hosted a meeting of the minds to discuss that very question. More specifically, the NIH feared "the specter of an intelli-gent mouse stuck in a laboratory somewhere screaming 'I want to get out," NIH ethicist David Resnik, told Technology Review magazine.

NIH may have been acting out of an abundance of caution, but there are still potentially icky dilemmas to work out. We still don't know how these early-stage bundles of fetal cells translate into human parts on or inside a pig. Some areas for human cells, like the stomach, are less troubling than if they materialized in, say, the brain. To find out we're on the verge of a horror movie scenario, I talked to medical ethicist Arthur Caplan of New York University's Langone Medical Center. He told me more oversight for scientists like Wu might be a good idea, but not for the reason I thought he would. He also said we're kinda-sorta, already animal-human hybrids.Transplant breakthrough as scientists implant human stem cells into pigs genetically modified to accept them

- New line of pigs do not reject transplants .Scientists at the Salk Institute in California have created a part-human, part-pig embryo.
- Will allow for future research on stem cell therapies
- Pigs are much closer to humans than many other test-animalsScientists have successfully transplanted human stem cells into pigs that were genetically modified not to reject them. The cells were able to thrive, raising hopes of potential stem cells treatments for debilitating diseases. The breakthrough could also aid in developing treatments for patients suffering from severe immune deficiency.

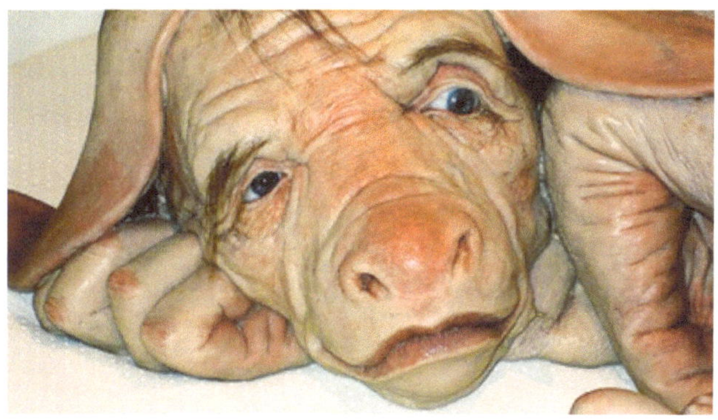

Fig. 20.41 Scientists at the Salk Institute in California have created a part-human, part-pig embryo.

HEART CELLS TRANSFORMED INTO 'BIOLOGICAL PACEMAKER'

'New Biological PacemakerIn healthy people, a small region of the heart, called the sinoatrial node, fires the electrical impulses that determine heart rate. If this region is not working properly, people can develop heart rhythm problems, and have symptoms such as fatigue, fainting or even cardiac arrest. Such patients may have electronic pacemakers put in to monitor the heart rhythm, which sends electrical pulses to keep the heart beating normally.In the study, the researchers used pigs with a condition called complete heart block, in which the heart beats very slowly. The researchers injected a gene called TBX18 into a small area of the heart muscle. This gene converted this area of heart muscle cells into sinoatrial node cells."In essence, we create a new sinoatrial node in a part of the heart that ordinarily spreads the impulse, but does not originate it," study researcher Dr. Eduardo Marbán, director of the Cedars-Sinai Heart Institute, said in news conference about the findings. "The newly created node then takes over as a functional pacemaker, bypassing the need for implanted electronics and hardware."Within a few days, the pigs that received the TBX18 gene had faster heartbeats than pigs that did not receive the gene. In addition, the hearts of pigs with the biological pacemaker were able to speed up during exercise, and slow down during rest much better than the hearts of pigs without the biological pacemaker. The pigs with the TBX18 gene were also more physically active than the pigs without the gene, according to the study.The treatment was designed to be temporary, and the researchers tested it for only two weeks. Toward the end of the study, the treatment was slightly less effective, likely because, over time, the pigs' bodies started to reject cells with the injected virus. The researchers are now testing how long the treatment lasts.IIT Guwahati Team Develops Silk Patch to Repair Damaged Heart TissueBy Prasad Ravindranath posted on August 12, 2017 The heart cells grew and proliferated filling the membrane 7–10 days after it was seeded with cells," say Biman Mandal and Shreya Mehrotra.Unlike current scaffolds, the 3D patch has high cell density, a foremost requirement for heart tissue.Scientists at the Indian Institute of Technology (IIT) Guwahati have fabricated a 3D cardiac tissue patch using silk protein membranes seeded with heart muscle cells. The patch can potentially be used for regenerating damaged heart tissue. "The 3D patch that we fabricated can be implanted at the site of damage to help the he2art regain normal function. It can also be used for sealing holes in the heart," says Prof. Biman Mandal from the Department of Biosciences and Bioengineering, IIT Guwahati, who led the research.Cardiac tissue gets permanently damaged when oxygen supply is reduced or cut off during heart attack. The damaged portion gets scarred and does not contract and relax leading to a change in the shape of the heart over time and reduced pumping capacity. While grafts currently available fail to mimic the structure and the function of the native heart tissue as well as maintain high cell numbers, the patch developed by the IIT Guwahati researchers scores over them on many counts. The results were published in the Journal of Materials Chemistry .The team led by Prof. Mandal tested both mulberry (Bombyx mori) and non-mulberry (Antheraea assama) silk to fabricate the membrane.

Non-invasive Cardiac Radiation for Ablation of Ventricular Tachycardia

Recent advances have enabled noninvasive mapping of cardiac arrhythmias with electrocardiographic imaging and noninvasive delivery of precise ablative radiation with stereotactic body radiation therapy (SBRT). We combined these techniques to perform catheter-free, electrophysio-logy-guided, noninvasive cardiac radioablation for ventricular tachycardia.Invesgators targeted arrhythmogenic scar regions by combining anatomi-

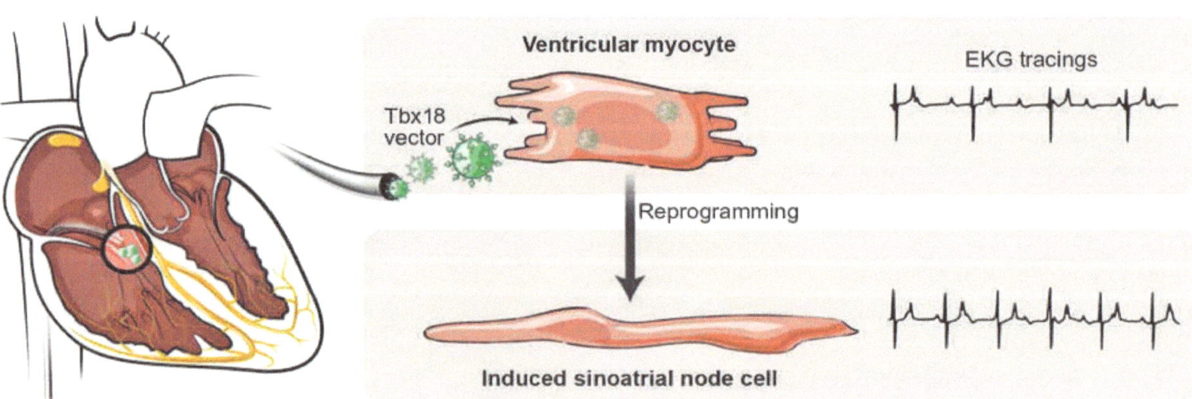

Fig.20.42 Tbx18 adenovirus reprograms heart muscle cells into sinoatrial node cells. Reprogrammed cells then generate electrical impulses to restore normal heart rate. Image from Science 345(6194):268–269.

cal imaging with noninvasive electro-cardiographic imaging during ventricular tachycardia that was induced by means of an implantable cardioverter–defibrillator (ICD). SBRT simulation, planning, and treat-ments were performed with the use of standard techniques. Patients were treated with a single fraction of 25 Gy while awake. Efficacy was assessed by counting episodes of ventricular tachycardia, as recorded by ICDs. Safety was assessed by means of serial cardiac and thoracic imaging. Results obtained from April through November 2015, five patients with high-risk, refractory ventricular tachycardia underwent treatment. The mean noninvasive ablation time was 14 minutes (range, 11 to 18). During the 3 months before treatment, the patients had a combined history of 6577 episodes of ventricular tachycardia. During a 6 week postablation "blanking period" (when arrhythmias may occur owing to postablation inflammation), there were 680 episodes of ventricular tachycardia. After the 6-week blanking period, there were 4 episodes of ventricular tachy-cardia over the next 46 patient-months, for a reduction from baseline of 99.9%. A reduction in episodes of ventricular tachycardia occurred in all five patients. The mean left ventricular ejection fraction did not decrease with treat-ment. At 3 months, adjacent lung showed opacities consistent with mild inflammatory changes, which had resolved by 1 year.It is therefore inferred that patients with refractory ventricular tachycardia, non-invasive treatment with electrophysiology-guided cardiac radioablation markedly reduced the burden of ventricular tachycardia (Funded by Barnes–Jewish Hospital Foundation and others).

Telomeres and Telomerase in Cardio-Vascular Diseases

Cardiovascular Risk Factors

The amount of telomere lost during each cell division variesamong people. Previous evidence indicated that increasedoxidative stress and chronic inflammation are associated with a higher telomere loss and accelerated telomereshortening. Several common risk factors for CVD such as smoking, diabetes mellitus, hypercholesterolemia, hypertension,obesity, physical inactivity, alcohol consumptionand psychosocial problems have been associated with short TL. However, the mechanism underlying the associationof telomere shortening with these risk factors remains hypothetical. Most studies have reported that telomere shortening is associated with these risk factors through increased tissue inflammation and oxidative stress. For example, animal studies demonstrated that hyperglycemiaattenuates nitric oxide production in endothelial cells, promotes inflammation and oxidative stress, and accelerates LTL shortening and vascular atherosclerotic processes. In additional, we found disrupted circadian rhythm results in loss of rhythmic telomerase activities with shortened TL and premature aging in mice. Similar observations also showed in the emergency physicians working in rotating shifts.

BCG VACCINE IN TYPE 1 DIABETES MELLITUS

BCG Vaccine could restore proper immune recsponse in type 1 diabe-tes Faustman's team was the first to document type 1 diabetes reversal in mice and in a subsequent phase I trial demonstrated successful human clinical results who had received the BCG vaccination. Long-term data from the study is expected to be published later this year. Now a five-year, 150-person, phase II trial is enrolling to assess whether repeat BCG vaccination can improve or even reverse advanced type 1 diabetes in adults. Earlier this year Belgian biotech company, Imcyse, announced they will begin human trials across Europe of a separate type 1diabetes vaccine, with results expected in 2 018

L -WAVE IN ECHO DOPPLER STUDY

An L wave in pulse wave Doppler and M mode echocardiography represents continued pulmo-nary vein mid diastolic flow through the left atrium in to LV across mitral valve after early rapid filling. Presence of an L wave in these patients associated with higher E/E is indicative of advance diastolic dysfunction. This has been attributed to combination of elevated filling pressure, delayed myocardial relaxation, and slow heart rate.Triphasic mitral inflow in patients with LV systolic dysfunction has been associated with clinical heart failure, where as in patients with left ventricular hypertrophy and normal LV ejection fraction it was associated with elevated LV filling pressures and high risk of hospitaliza-tion for heart failure.Therefore although uncommon, finding of L and Lwave is an important marker of severe diastolic dysfunction and management should be directed accordingly

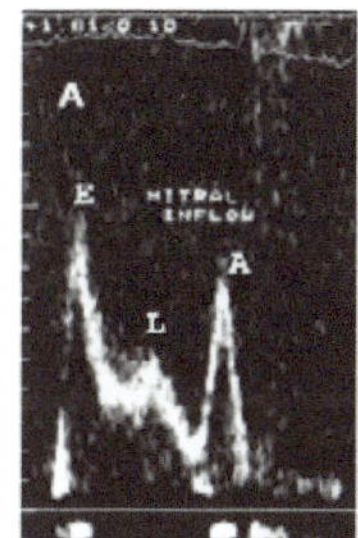

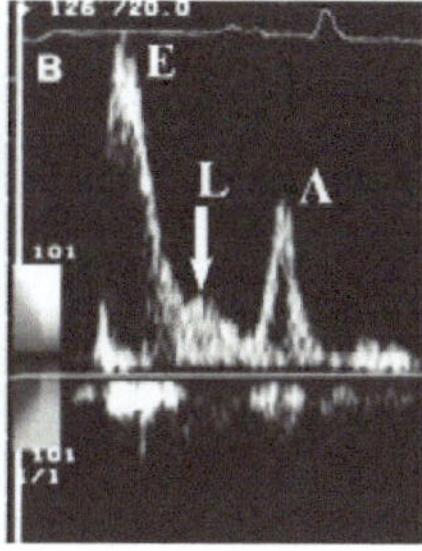

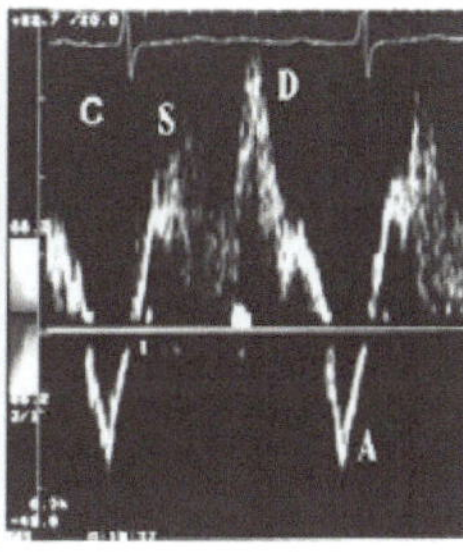

Fig 20.43 L-wave is seen on mitral Doppler inflow in patient with longstanding hypertension and moderate mitral regurgitation B Mitral Doppler inflow and C Pulmonary vein flow in an elderly hypertensive patient with left ventricular hypertyrophy .The mitral inflow E/A ratio >1 and blunted systolic/diastolic S/D pulmonary vein flow ratios along with prominent pulmonary vein ,atrial wave (A) are consistent with pseudonormaliztion .An L-Wave though not as prominent as in (A&B) is also noted in (C) With permission from: Kerut EK, McIlwain EF, Plotnick GD: Handbook of Echo-Doppler Interpretation, 2nd Ed. Elmsford, New York, Blackwell Publishing, Inc., 2004, p. 71.)

Health Care Automated Teller Machine (ATM)

Health ATM is a one-stop digital touch-point integrated machine designed to diagnose all the chronic disease, delivering primary care and diagnostics. ATM for healthcare, is built-in with the latest diagnostic equipment for the diagnosis of basic vitals, cardiology, neurology, pulmonary testing, gynecology, clinical diagnostic and life-saving equipment and emergency facilities. Like an Automated Teller Machine (ATM) in a bank, Health ATM is a touch-screen kiosk hardware, designed for managing health-related information which allows individuals to access their personal health information through any Internet connected web browser.

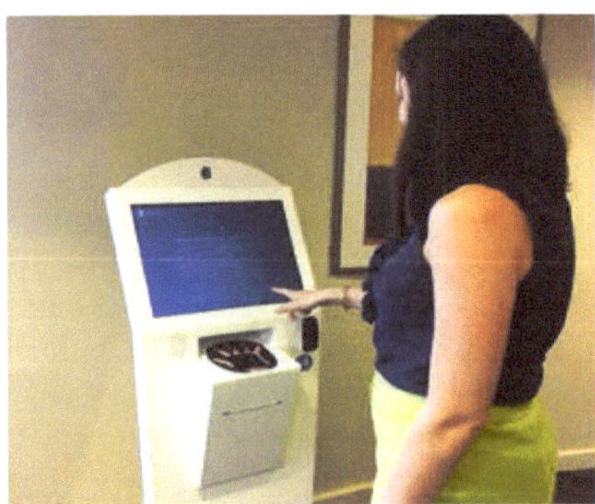

Fig.20.44 A young lady is facing automated medical ATMs machine for their health screening.

It is a combination of FDA and CE approved Medical diagnostic devices combined with HIPAA compliant software backend. It allows patients to be more empowered, allows them to actively participate in managing their health needs with access to world class medical facilities. HealthATM, resolves the problems of primary health services in rural and remote areas. It's modern, sophisticated, simplified, accurate & automated healthcare kiosk. The multifaceted kiosk helps in easy diagnosis of the medical problem for people in remote locations, where hospitals are not within reach. It also provides a central platform for the patients to interact with the specialist of the fields through Telemedicine (video conferencing).

Smart Health Kiosk connects:- For the remote peripheral site: Health ATM with integrated medical devices for real time audio video consultation & real time diagnostics allows to connects to specialist doctor

For the Doctor: Web & Mobile application to consult with the patient, view his health reports, integrated chat feature for follow up

For the Patient: Fosters health self- management via web & Mobile application to book an appointment, view his health reports, check basic health checkup on kiosk, book prescribed lab-test on kiosk, generate waiting token on kiosk, and consult in-house doctor etc. **Smart Health Kiosk monitors** vital signs for the following

- Blood pressure
- Blood glucose
- Lipid Profile
- Blood Oxygen Saturation
- HD video conferencing for doctor consultation
- Temperature
- Instant report

Ocular images-based artificial intelligence on systemic diseases

With the progress of AI and medical big data, ocular images have already been used in the detection of endocrine, cardiovascular, neurological, renal, hematological, and many other diseases. These studies have further deepened our understanding of the eye as a reflection of the whole body.

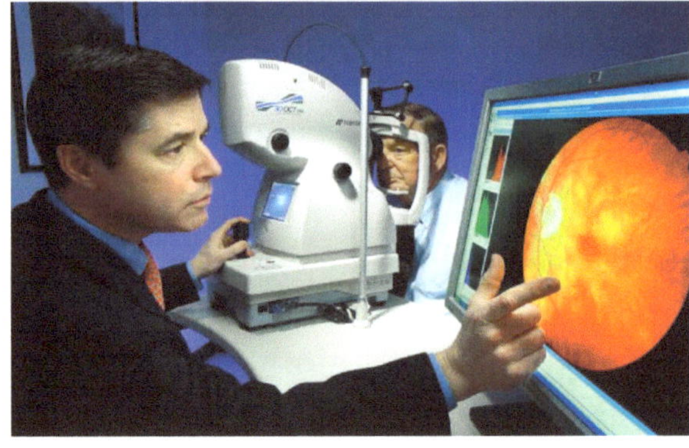

Fig.20.45 Doctor is studying retinoscopic image based on AI in a patient with cardiovascular disorder.

Artificial intelligence (AI) is a subfield of computer science in which computer algorithms are trained to perform tasks associated with human intelligence . AI research encompasses a wide range of topics, including machine learning, deep learning, natural language processing, decision support systems, robotics, and many others. AI can learn from previous experiences, make sound decisions, and respond quickly. Because of this trait, AI is frequently employed in recommendation algorithms, search engines, autonomous driving, health care, and other industries, and has made significant progress.The eye has unique anatomical structure—its transparent refractive interstitium, that permits light to pass through the pupil to the retina, allowing the eye to serve as a window to examine the state of the blood vessels and nerves.

Systemic diseases, such as hypertension and diabetes, can manifest as distinct ocular presentations. The optical transparency of ocular structures enables non-invasive observation of changes in vasculature and nerves, a unique diagnostic capacity not available through alternative examination modalities. Therefore, the reflection of whole-body status based on ocular features has always been hot. With the advancement of AI techniques, images are commonly used in studies to diagnose ocular diseases such as diabetic retinopathy , age-related macular degeneration , retinopathy of prematurity glaucoma and others. Furthermore, the use of ocular images has been expanded beyond the study of ocular disorders and has aided in the discovery of various previously unknown connections with systemic diseases. AI can uncover a wealth of information that doctors previously couldn't see with their naked eyes, widening the breadth of disease diagnosis. In recent years, there are many studies connecting ocular features with systemic diseases and risks, such as diabetes, cardiovascular disease, Alzheimer's disease, kidney disease, and so on. However, advances about ocular images-based AI on systemic diseases have yet to be summarized in detail. This review aims to highlight the recent progress in various systemic diseases.

Umblical Cord In The Management Of Various Diseases .

For over four years Cells4 Life has offered the additional option of storing umbilical cord tissue stem cells alongside those found in the cord blood. But what is so special about these cells and why is it important to preserve them? The benefits of storing umbilical cord tissue stem cells Cord tissue is one of the richest sources of mesenchymal stem cells available. These are the cells that are thought to have the most potential in the field of regenerative medicine. Cord tissue is currently being investigated for use in the treatment of the following conditions:

- Alzheimer's disease
- Aplastic anaemia
- Cardiomyopathy
- Cartilage repair
- Cerebral Palsy
- Connective tissue diseases
- Diabetes (type 2)
- Erectile Dysfunction
- Liver failure
- Multiple Sclerosis
- Myocardial infarction
- Osteoarthritis
- Ovarian failure
- Parkinson's disease
- Psoriasis
- Retinitis pigmentosa
- Rheumatoid arthritis
- Sepsis
- Spinal cord injury
- Stroke
- Traumatic optic neuropathy
- Ulcerative colitis
- And many more...

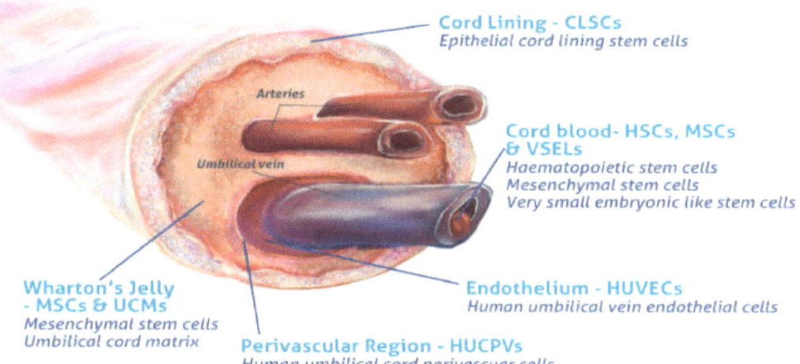

Fig.20.46 *Illustration showing various types of stem cells found in cord tissue*

Israeli researchers have successfully established a new approach for pacing the heart

This novel biologic strategy employs light-sensitive genes that can be injected into the heart and then activated by flashes of blue light. More than 3 million people worldwide have had electronic pacemakers implanted. The most common indication for a pacemaker is the treatment of a slow heart beat which can put patients at risk for fainting, heart failure, and even death. Pacemakers work by sending electrical signals to the heart to regulate the heart beat. Pacemakers can also be used for cardiac resynchronization therapy (CRT), an approach aiming to synchronize the contraction of the heart's two ventricles in order to improve heart function, symptom status and decrease mortality in some patients who suffer from heart failure. The new optogenetic approach for cardiac pacing and resynchronization was developed by Prof. Lior Gepstein and Dr. Udi Nussinovitch of the Technion-Israel Institute of Technology's Rappaport Faculty of Medicine, and Rambam Medical Center.

Transplant breakthrough as scientists implant human stem cells into pigs genetically modified to accept them

- New line of pigs do not reject transplants
- Will allow for future research on stem cell therapies
- Pigs are much closer to humans than many other test animals

Scientists have successfully transplanted human stem cells into pigs that were genetically modified not to reject them. The cells were able to thrive, raising hopes of potential stem cells treatments for debilitating diseases. The breakthrough could also aid in developing treatments for patients suffering from severe immune deficiency.

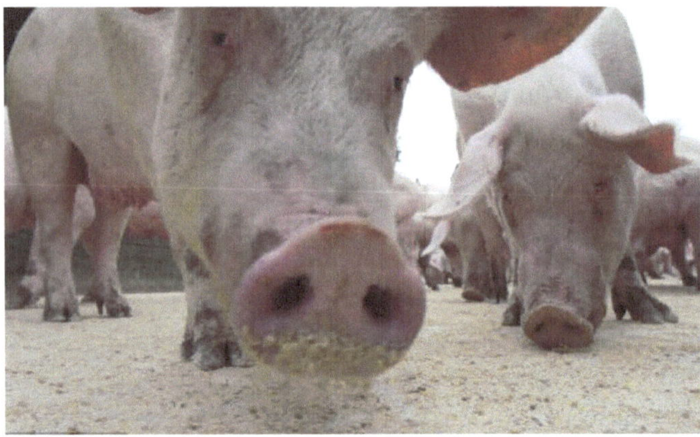

Fig.20.47 : Scientists have successfully transplanted human stem cells into pigs that were genetically modified not to reject them in am major breakthrough for stem cells treatments

What is the Technique

The team of researchers implanted human pluripotent stem cells in a special line of pigs developed by Randall Prather, an MU Curators Professor of reproductive physiology. Prather created the pigs with immune systems that allow the pigs to accept all transplants or grafts without rejection. Once the scientists implanted the cells, the pigs did not reject the stem cells and the cells thrived.

One of the biggest challenges for medical researchers studying the effectiveness of stem cell therapies is that transplants or grafts of cells are often rejected by the hosts. This rejection can render experiments useless, makingresearch into potentially life-saving treatments a long and difficult process. 'The rejection of transplants and grafts by host bodies is a huge hurdle for medical researchers,' said Michael Roberts at the University of Missouri. 'By establishing that these pigs will support transplants without the fear of rejection, we can move stem cell therapy research forward at a quicker pace. 'Hopefully this means that we are one step closer to therapies and treatments for a number of debilitating human diseases.' The team of researchers implanted human pluripotent stem cells in a special line of pigs developed by Randall Prather, an MU Curators Professor of reproductive physiology. Prather created the pigs with immune systems that allow the pigs to accept all transplants or grafts without rejection. Researchers created the pigs with immune systems that allow the pigs to accept all transplants or grafts without rejection. Once the scientists implanted the cells, the pigs did not reject the stem cells and the cells thrived. Prather says achieving this success with pigs is notable because pigs are much closer to humans than many other test animals. 'Many medical researchers prefer conducting studies with pigs because they are more anatomically similar to humans than other animals, such as mice and rats,' Prather said. 'Physically, pigs are much closer to the size and scale of humans than other animals, and they respond to health threats similarly. 'This means that research in pigs is more likely to have results similar to those in humans for many different tests and treatments.'

Telomeres and Telomerase in Cardiovascular Diseases

Implications for Cardiovascular Diseases Measurement of Telomere Length

Peripheral leukocyte DNA has been most commonly used in epidemiological studies to measure TL because a blood sample can be easily obtained. A consistent synchrony exists between LTL and somatic cells, including vascular cells, within people. The two methods most commonly used in clinical studies are Southern blotting and quantitative polymerase chain reaction (qPCR). Southern blotting has an advantage of measuring the absolute LTL, including the proportion of very short telomeres. Cells with very short TL are closely associated with cellular senescence, regardless of mean TL, because only one critically short telomere can force a cell to enter senescence. However, Southern blotting requires numerous DNA samples (2–3 µg per assay) and is time-consuming and expensive. Thus, qPCR is used in most epidemiological studies. The fundamental difference in laboratory methods among individual studies might contribute to controversial results. Recently, a study compared these laboratory methods performed in two independent laboratories to measure the same samples. Both the q-PCR and Southern blotting provided highly reproducible and correlated results. The overview of TL and associated cardiovascular diseases.

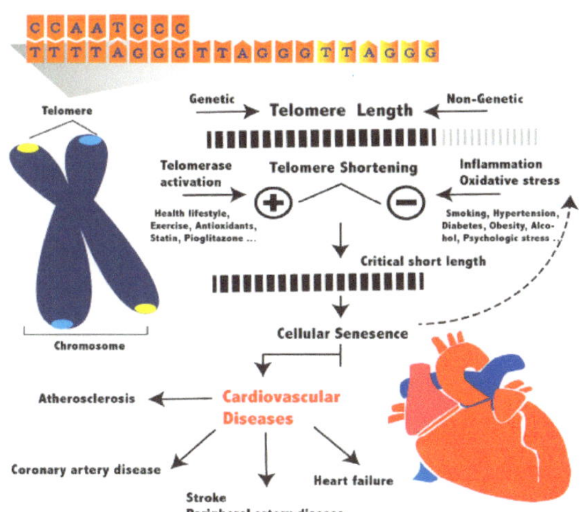

Fig.20.48: Schematic overview of telomere length and cardiovascular diseases. Individual variations of telomere length are affected by genetic and non-genetic factors. Critically short telomeres lead to cellular senescence and dysfunction, which contribute to atherogenesis and reduce repair and regenerative capacity in cardiovascular system. Disease promoting factors, such as smoking and hypertension, accelerate telomere shortening through inflammation or increased oxidant stress. However, disease protective factors, such as exercise and statin use, can activate telomerase activity and maintain telomere length.

Cardiovascular Risk Factors

The amount of telomere lost during each cell division varies among people. Previous evidence indicated that increased oxidative stress and chronic inflammation are associated with a higher telomere loss and accelerated telomere shortening. Several common risk factors for CVD such as smoking, diabetes mellitus, hypercholesterolemia, hypertension, obesity, physical inactivity, alcohol consumption and psychosocial problems have been associated with short TL. However, the mechanism underlying the association of telomere shortening with these risk factors remains hypothetical. Most studies have reported that telomere shortening is associated with these risk factors through increased tissue inflammation and oxidative stress. For example, animal studies demonstrated that hyperglycemia attenuates nitric oxide production in endothelial cell, promotes inflammation and oxidative stress, and accelerates LTL shortening and vascular atherosclerotic processes. In additional, we found disrupted circadian rhythm results in loss of rhythmic telomerase activities with shortened TL
and premature aging in mice. Similar observations also showed in the emergency physicians working in rotating shifts. However, some dietary and lifestyle factors such as marine omega-3 fatty acid , antioxidants , vitamin intake, physical activity, and healthy lifestyle were reported to decrease rates of LTL shortening. These factors might contribute to reduced reactive oxygen species, inhibitinflammation, increase endothelial nitric oxide synthase (eNOS) activity, and increased telomerase activity. In an experimental study, voluntary wheel running in mice for three weeks upregulated the activity of telomerase, increased the expression of TRF2, and reduced the expression of vascular apoptosis regulators. However, these exercise-induced changes were absent in both TERT-/- and endothelial nitric oxide synthase (eNOS)-/- mice, indicating the beneficial effects are medicated by TERT and Enos. A human study also reported that comprehensive lifestyle changes significantly increased telomerase activity and consequently telomere maintenance capacity in human immune system cells

Consequently, telomere shortening is a reflection of cellular aging and a marker of the health status of the aging population. Absolute TL at birth is determined by genetic materials from both parents. During aging, the mean TL declines with cell replication and turnover. The process of telomere shortening is accelerated by exposure to disease-promoting factors such as smoking, obesity, and psychosocial stress. Furthermore, telomerase activation has been considered a possible target for reversing the telomere shortening.

Coronary Artery Diseases

Several studies in diverse populations have reported an association of shorter telomeres in circulating leukocytes with CAD. The precise mechanisms connecting short telomeres and CAD are yet to be established. Current evidence from epidemiologic and experimental studies supports the role of telomeres in CAD development. First, cardiovascular risk factors such as smoking, hypertension, insulin resistance, and hyperlipidemia, are associated with short LTL. Second, the progression of atherosclerotic plaques in vasculature have been shown to be associated with short TL and cell senescence in vascular cells such as endothelial and vascular smooth muscle cells. Furthermore, short mean LTL represents a greater degree of telomere attrition and senescence in immune cells. Low grade systemic inflammation, which is thought to be mediated by immunosenescence, has been shown to be associated with numerous age-related conditions, including atherosclerosis and cardiovascular diseases.However, many studies are cross-sectional design and because most cardiovascular risk factors also affect LTL, the causal or consequential relationship between shorter TL and CAD remains controversial. Recently, some prospective longitudinal studies may support the hypothesis that telomere shortening causes CAD, rather than telomere shortening is a consequence of CAD. In a large prospective WOSCOPS study, compared with people in the highest tertiles of LTL, those in the lowest tertiles of LTL had a 44% increased risk of coronary artery events in a mean follow-up period of 5.5 years after adjustment for risk factors for CAD. In addition, a recent meta-analysis of prospective studies reported that the estimated relative risk of the shortest versus the longest third of LTL was 1.4 (95% confidence interval : 1.15–1.70). LTL was measured in these prospective trials before the diagnosis of a CVD, thus avoiding the concern of the confounding of reverse causality. Furthermore, reports about the association of genetic variants affecting TL with the risk of CAD also provide evidence for the causal association. The genotypes are randomly determined during conception and thus their associations could be not susceptible to bias and confounding. A meta-analysis of 14 GWASs including up to 22,233 patients with CAD and 64,762 controls revealed that seven SNPs have been identified for the variation in mean LTL. For example, a mean TL decrease of 117 base pairs per TERC telomere-shortening allele accounts for approximately 10% drop in functional telomere reserves in a typical middle-aged adult, and thus increases susceptibility to telomere dysfunction and replicative senescence. The effect of inter-individual variations in LTL is also illustrated in this meta-analysis, which found that the allele associated with shorter LTL increases the risk of CAD; one SD decrease in LTL was estimated to increase the CAD risk by 21%.

LTL in patients with CAD has prognostic value. A prospective cohort study of 780 patients conducted for a follow-up period of 4.4 years reported an association of decreased LTL with all-cause mortality, with an adjusted hazard ratio of 1.8 in the lowest TL quartile compared with the highest TL quartile. Moreover, LTL has been observed to be shorter in patients with premature acute MI (aged <50 years) than in healthy, age-matched controls. According analysis in previous studies, patients with MI have TL that the allele associated with shorter LTL increases the risk of CAD; one SD decrease in LTL was estimated to increase the CAD risk by 21%.

LTL in patients with CAD has prognostic value. A prospective cohort study of 780 patients conducted for a follow-up period of 4.4 years reported an association of decreased LTL with all-cause mortality, with an adjusted hazard ratio of 1.8 in the lowest TL quartile compared with the highest TL quartile. Moreover, LTL has been observed to be shorter in patients with premature acute MI (aged <50 years) than in healthy, age-matched controls. According analysis in previous studies, patients with MI have TL that is equivalent to that in controls older than 8–12 years. This might partially explain some young patients with MI without traditional cardiovascular risk factors. Biological aging can reflect the effects of cumulative oxidative stress and inflammatory burden on the aging vasculature. Compared with chronological aging, biological aging may provide superior risk stratification for CVDs. Accurate risk assessment is essential to provide appropriate therapeutic interventions and to further reduce the occurrence of morbid cardiovascular events. New network analysis systems, including genetic traits, imaging characters, and biological risk factors, should be developed for determining the risk of atherosclerosis. We thick LTL could be a sensitive score in the risk prediction system, and additional clinical trials are required to validate the observation and hypothesis.

In the coronary intervention field, researchers observed shorter LTL and increased proinflammatory activity in high-risk unstable plaque (calcified thin capped fibroatheroma) on virtual histology intravascular ultrasound in patients with acute coronary syndrome also. Furthermore, delayed re-endothelialization after drug-eluting stent (DES) implantation with uncovered stent struts can increase the risk of stent thrombosis. A small clinical trial reported an inverse association of LTL with the percentage of uncovered stent struts, as assessed through optical coherence tomography. Shorter LTL may indicate functional exhaustion and impaired proliferative capacity of EPCs, which are responsible for re-endothelialization after a vascular injury. Additional large-scale prospective studies should be conducted to investigate the clinical application of

LTL as a predictive marker for stent thrombosis and target vessel outcomes after DES implantation.

Heart Failure

In a clinical study of 803 patients, LTL was decreased by approximately 40% in patients with HF, and TL in the patients with HF was related to the disease severity.A study investigating the association of a lower left ventricular ejection fraction with decreased TL reported an association of one SD decrease in TL with a 5% lower ejection fraction. Moreover, LTL was significantly associated with cardiovascular outcomes in patients with ischemic HF. HF with a normal ejection fraction was not well recognized until the two previous decades. Approximately half of patients hospitalized for HF have a normal ejection fraction, and outcomes in these patients are equivalent to those in patients with a lower ejection fraction. Aging leads to an increase in the deposition of extracellular matrix components, principally collagen, with an increase in the ratio of type I to type III collagen and a decrease in the elastin content, contributing to impaired ventricular relaxation. Furthermore, blunted beta-adrenergic responsiveness, excitation–contraction coupling, and altered calcium-handling proteins contribute to diastolic dysfunction. Studies have reported that the left ventricular relaxation function deteriorates with normal aging and is positively associated with LTL. Older people with shorter LTL have a significantly lower E/A ratio

BCG vaccine could restore proper immune response in type 1 diabetes

Faustman's team was the first to document type 1 diabetes reversal in mice and in a subsequent phase I trial demonstrated successful human clinical results who had received the BCG vaccination. Long-term data from the study is expected to be published later this year. Now a five-year, 150-person, phase II trial is enrolling to assess whether repeat BCG vaccination can improve or even reverse advanced type 1 diabetes in adults. Earlier this year Belgian biotech company, Imcyse, announced they will begin human trials across Europe of a separate type 1 diabetes vaccine, with results expected in 2018. Data presented at American Diabetes Association meeting describes a potential new mechanism by which the BCG vaccine may restore the proper immune response to the insulin-secreting islet cells of the pancreas. Presented by Denise Faustman, MD, PhD, director of the Massachusetts General Hospital Immunobiology Laboratory and principal investigator of the trial, the findings suggest that BCG may induce a permanent increase in expression of genes that restore the beneficial regulatory T cells (Tregs) that prevent the immune system from attacking the body's own tissue.

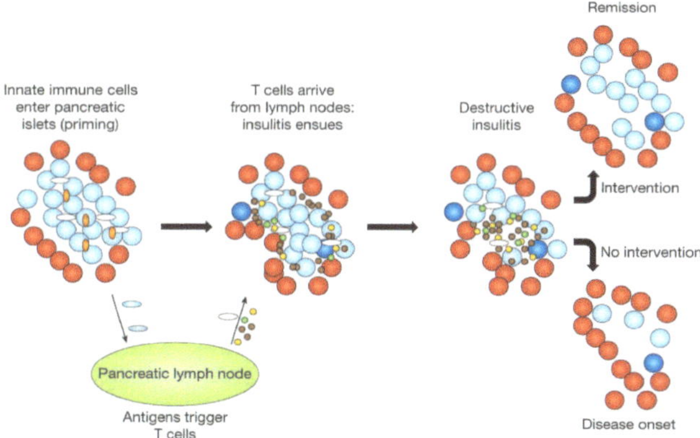

Fig.20.49: BCG vaccine is being tried for reversal type 1 diabetes mellitus Immunologic history of type 1 diabetes. Potential Mechanism for BCG Vaccine Reversal of Type 1 Diabetes

"Many groups are looking at the ability of BCG vaccination to reverse autoimmunity," says Faustman, who is an associate professor of Medicine at Harvard Medical School. "We and other global efforts have known for some time that restoring beneficial Treg cells might halt the abnormal self-reactivity in type 1 diabetes and other autoimmune diseases, but therapies to restore this immune balance have not achieved long-lasting results. The discovery that BCG restores Tregs through epigenetics – a process that modulates whether or not genes are expressed – is exciting. This now provides a better idea of how BCG vaccination appears to work by powerfully modulating Treg induction and resetting the immune system to halt the underlying cause of the disease."Best known for its role in tuberculosis prevention, the BCG vaccine is based on a harmless strain of bacteria related the one that causes tuberculosis. A generic drug with over 100 years of clinical use and safety data, BCG is currently approved by the FDA for vaccination against tuberculosis and for the treatment of bladder cancer. Multiple international studies are currently investigatingthe potential of repeat BCG vaccinations to prevent and reverse autoimmune diseases including type 1 diabetes and multiple sclerosis.

"BCG is interesting because it brings into play so many areas of immunology that we as a community have been looking at for decades, including Tregs and the hygiene hypothesis," says Faustman. "Repeat BCG vaccination appears to permanently turn on signature Treg genes, and the vaccine's beneficial effect on host immune response recapitulates decades of human co-evolution with myocbacteria, a relationship that has been lost with modern eating and living habits. It is incredible that a safe and inexpensive vaccine may be the key to stopping these terrible diseases." Faustman's research team was the first group to document reversal of advanced type 1 diabetes in mice and subsequently completed a successful phase I human clinical trial of BCG vaccination. The 5-year, 150-person, phase II trial is investigating whether repeat BCG vaccination can clinically improve type 1 diabetes in adults with existing disease and is almost fully enrolled. Long-term follow-up data from the phase I trial will be published later this year. The phase II trial is entirely funded by private philanthropy from individuals and family foundations

IIT Guwahati team develops silk patch to repair damaged heart tissue

By Prasad Ravindranathposted Onaugust 12, 2017 The heart cells grew and proliferated filling the membrane 7-10 days after it was seeded with cells," say Biman Mandal (left) and Shreya Mehrotra. Unlike current scaffolds, the 3D patch has high cell density, a foremost requirement for heart tissue. Scientists at the Indian Institute of Technology (IIT) Guwahati have fabricated a 3D cardiac tissue patch using silk protein membranes seeded with heart muscle cells. The patch can potentially be used for regenerating damaged heart tissue. "The 3D patch that we fabricated can be implanted at the site of damage to help the heart regain normal function. It can also be used for sealing holes in the heart," says Prof. Biman Mandal from the Department of Biosciences and Bioengineering, IIT Guwahati, who led ther research.

Cardiac tissue gets permanently damaged when oxygen supply is reduced or cut off during heart attack. The damaged portion gets scarred and does not contract and relax leading to a change in the shape of the heart over time and reduced pumping capacity. While grafts currently available fail to mimic the structure and the function of the native heart tissue as well as maintain high cell numbers, the patch developed by the IIT Guwahati researchers scores over them on many counts. The results were published in the Journal of Materials Chemistry .The team led by Prof. Mandal tested both mulberry (Bombyx mori) and non-mulberry (Antheraea assama) silk to fabricate the membrane.

Making a 3D patch

The single membranes with proliferating cells were then stacked one over the other to form a 3D patch. "In 5-6 days, the cells present on top of the membrane bound to the membrane above it leading to the layers sticking to each other," Prof. Mandal says. "Stacking the membranes to form a 3D patch overcomes the drawbacks of current scaffolds used for cardiac tissue engineering in terms of creating a high cell dense anisotropic patch, a foremost requirement for this tissue," he stresses. The silk in the patch supports the cells till the newly formed cardiac tissue integrates with the native heart tissue and degrades once the integration takes place. "This method is better than the conventional direct delivery of cardiac cells to repair the damaged portion of the heart as the cells get washed out from the injected site," says Ms. Mehrotra. Animals studies will be carried out in collaboration with AIIMS.

Role of Nano-Robotics in Medicine

Advancement in technology has really manipulated the world around us on an ever decreasing scale. These robots play a key role in the field of biomedicine particularly used for the removal of kidney stone, treatment of cancer & elimination of defected part in the DNA structure etc.

A nanorobot is an extremely small robot that is designed to perform specific tasks at the nanoscale dimension of few nanometers i.e. 1 nm = 10-9 meter. In healthcare IT industry, this technology brings a great boom & helps in protecting & maintaining the human body against viruses or bacteria. Researchers in robotics industry will use the pollution-free process to build cheapest & inexpensive nanorobots.

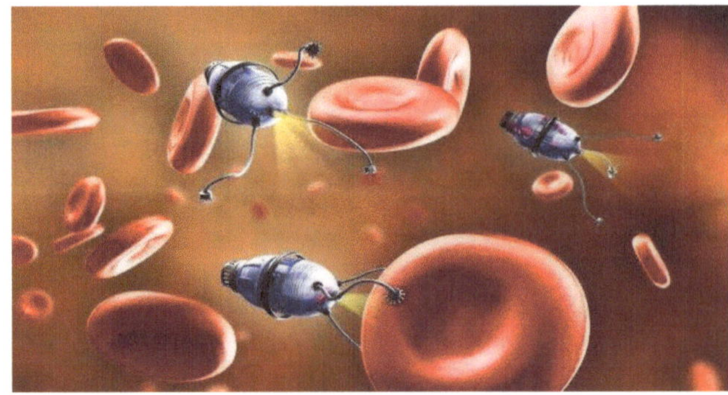

Fig.20.50 showing nonorobits working inside the blood circulation system

To replace worn out units, nanorobots might also produce a replica of themselves known as self-replication. Other common names of Nanorobots are Nanomites, Nanobots, Nanites etc ranging from 0.01 to 0.1 micrometres.

How Nanorobots Work?

Suppose you visit a doctor for a common disease treatment, instead of giving treatment he/she sends you to a special team who implants small robots in your bloodstream. These robots will recognise the cause of your illness and provide a dose of medication directly to an infected area. It feels awesome when you got to know quickly about the cause of your problem. These robots are known as Nanorobots which greatly transforms the future of healthcare& eventually cure everything from cancer to haemophilia. As per research theories, nanorobots will possess at least two-way communication. Through sound waves, these robots will receive power or even reprogramming instructions from an external source and will respond to acoustic signals. A special network of stationery nanorobots will be positioned throughout the body which will keep the track of each active nanorobot passes & then report the results. Physicians or doctors could not only monitor a patient progress but can also change the instructions of the nanorobots in vivo to progress to another stage of healing. After treating, these nanorobots would be flush out of the body immediately.

Nanorobots in cancer treatment

Cancer is a big disease which would be untreatable if not diagnose early. At the time of cancer treatment, the patient had to undergo long chemotherapies which will adversely affect other human cells. This traditional radiation treatment of chemotherapy kills not only the cancer cells but also the healthy human cells which lead to hair loss, depression, nausea & fatigue. The other alternative of this painful chemotherapies is nanorobots. Doctors would offer the patient an injection of a special type of nanorobot that would check & destroy the cancer cells without touching the healthy ones. This great enhancement would raise the standard of healthcare at great extent.

Applications of Nanorobots in Medical Field

Nanorobots in the medical field can perform a wide range of tasks in monitoring, diagnosis & treating diseases. Inside the human body, these robots deliver specific drugs or medicine into the specific targets & sites. Let's have a look at nanorobots applications in the medical field.

Treatment & Diagnosis of Diabetes: To maintain the human metabolism, glucose molecules are carried through the bloodstream. To determine the need for injecting insulin inside the body, glucose monitoring nanorobots uses the chemosensor.

Dentistry: For dental treatment, the nanorobots used are dentifrobots which induce desensitise tooth, oral analgesia, straighten irregular set of teeth. Deliver the drug: Nanorobots used for drug delivery is Pharmacytes which will transport the drug to the targeted point. The dosage of the drug will be loaded into the payload of the pharmacyte.

Surgery: Surgical nanorobots can act as a semi-autonomous onsite surgeon will perform various functions such as diagnosing, detection of pathology, correcting lesions by nanomanipulation etc

Cancer Detection & treatment: Nanorobots are made up of a mixture of protein & a polymer known as transferrin which is capable of detecting tumour cells. These robots kill the cancer cells without damaging the healthy cells which will lead to hair loss, nausea etc

Gene Therapy: Genetic disease can be treated by nanorobots by comparing the molecular structure of both proteins & DNA found in the cell

Nattokinase: A Promising Alternative in Prevention and Treatment of Cardiovascular Disease

Cardiovascular diseases (CVDs) are the most prevalent cause of deaths worldwide. In 2015, the number of CVD-related deaths represented 31% of all deaths globally To date, there are limited approaches available for the control and/or management of CVD-related mortality. Natto, a cheese-like food made of soybeans fermented with Bacillus subtilis, has been consumed as a traditional food in Asian countries for more than 2000 years. Natto consumption is believed to be a significant contributor to the longevity of the Japanese population. Recent studies demonstrated that a high natto intake was associated with decreased risk of total CVD mortality and, in particular, a decreased risk of mortality from ischaemic heart diseases. Before the 1980s,very little was known about the mechanism by which natto consumption led to overall cardiovascular health. In 1987, Sumi et al discovered that natto contained a potent fibrinolytic enzyme called nattokinase (NK). Since then, a considerable amount of NK research has been performed on NK in Japan, Korea, China, and the

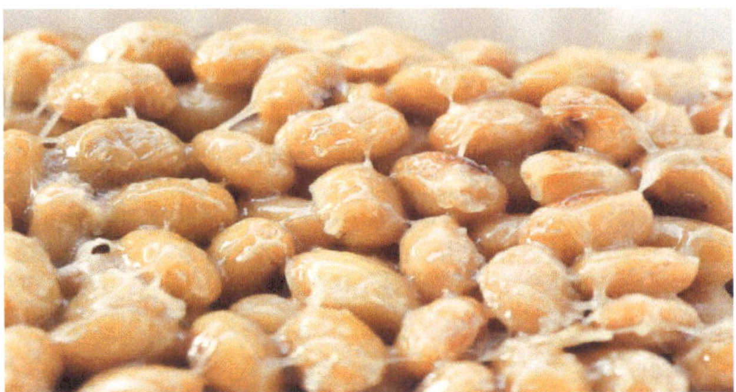

Fig.20.51: showing features of fermented Natto beans (Soya beans)

United States, and these studies confirmed that NK, an alkaline protease of 275 amino acid residues with a molecular weight of approximately 28 kDa, is the most active ingredient of natto and is responsible for many favourable effects on cardiovascular health. First, NK has potent fibrinolytic/fibrinolytic enzyme called nattokinase (NK). Since then, a considerable amount of NK research has been performed on NK in Japan, Korea, China, and the United States, and these studies confirmed that NK, an alkaline protease of 275 amino acid residues with a molecular weight of approximately 28 kDa, is the most active ingredient of natto and is responsible for many favourable effects on cardiovascular health. First, NK has potent fibrinolytic antithrombotic activity. In addition, in both animal and human studies, NK also has an antihypertensive, anti-atherosclerotic, lipid-lowering antiplatelet/anticoagulant, and neuroprotective actions. All these pharmacologic actions of NK have relevance to the prevention and treatment of CVD. Indeed, NK supplementation has shown to enhance markers of fibrinolysis and anticoagulation and to decrease blood pressure (BP) and atherosclerosis in human subjects

The most unique feature of NK is that, as a single compound, it possesses multiple CVD preventative and alleviating pharmacologic effects (namely, antithrombotic, antihypertensive, anticoagulant, anti-atherosclerotic, and neuroprotective effects). There are no other drugs or drug candidates with multiple pharmacologic properties similar to NK. In addition, NK is a natural product that can be administered orally, has a proven safety profile, is economical to use, and provides distinct advantages over other pharmaceutical products. It therefore has the potential to be developed as a new-generation drug for the prevention, treatment, and long-term care of CVD.The present review aims to concisely summarise the key pharmacologic effects and mechanisms of action of NK with a focus on their relevance to, and potential for, the prevention and treatment of CVD. The advantages of NK as an agent for the management of CVD will be outlined. Some remaining issues surrounding NK as a drug candidate for CVD will be criticallyreviewed and analysed.

Pharmacologic Actions of NK

The pharmacologic effects and mechanisms of action of NK will be reviewed and summarised under the followingsubheadingsfibrinolytic/antithrombotic effects, anti-atherosclerotic and lipid-lowering effects, antihypertensive effects, antiplatelet /anticoagulant effects,and neuroprotectiveactions Potent fibrinolytic/antithrombotic effects of NK Although natto has been consumed in Asia for thousands of years, the fibrinolytic property of NK was only discovered in 1987. Since this initial discovery, multiple laboratory and human studies have consistently reported the potent antithrombolytic action of NK

A considerable amount of work has been performed to evaluate the thrombolytic effects of NK in vitro and in animal models. Using a rat model, Fujita et al examined the effect of NK on chemically induced thrombi in the common carotid artery (CCA) and found NK to be 4 times more potent than plasmin in thrombus dissolution. At a concentration of 2836 FU, NK lysed 88% of thrombi within 6 hours, and NK exhibited significant prophylactic antithrombotic effects in vivo. The efficacy of NK against thrombosis was confirmed in a carrageenan-induced tail thrombosis model. The survival rate of mice with pulmonary thrombosis was increased by NK and the formation of thrombosis in mice was remarkably inhibited by NK, demonstrating significant antithrombotic effects. In addition, in a model of rat experimental pulmonary thrombosis, oral administration of NK led to a decrease in thrombus count and plasma euglobulin lysis time (ELT), as well as an increase in tissue plasminogen activator (tPA), indicating that NK is capable of activating plasma fibrinolysis in vivo. Omura et al further found that a purified protein layer, NKCP, which mainly consisted of NK, had both fibrinolytic and antithrombotic effects, which they described as being similar to that of heparin. In rats, Natto treatment shortened ELT and significantly prolonged partial thromboplastin time compared with a nontreated rat group.

APPENDIX

Associated Contributors To This Manuscript

Alan C. Kwan , Amir Pourmorteza, Dan Stutman, David A. Bluemke, João A. C. LimaNext-Generation Hardware Advances in CT: Cardiac Applications Nov17 2020https:

Alyssa M. Flores,Falen Demsas,Nicholas J. Leeper and Elsie Gyang Ross Leveraging Machine Learning and Artificial Intelligence to Improve Peripheral Artery Disease Detection, Treatment, and Outcomes Jun2021Circulation Research. 2021;128:1833–1850

Amarinder Bindra Shelley :-A New Drugs for the Treatment of Heart Failure. Hallhttps://doi.org/10.15420/usc.2017:17:1

Ananya Mandal. Reviewed by Kate Anderton, B.Sc. (Editor) Scientists create a functioning 3D printed heart Apr 15 2019 Andreas A. Giannopoulos, Dimitris Mitsouras, Shi-Joon Yoo, Peter P. Liu, Yiannis S. Chatzizisis & Frank J. Rybicki Applications of 3D printing in cardiovascular diseases Nature Reviews Cardiology volume 13, pages701–718 (2016)

Andrew Lin, BMedSci,Márton Kolossváry, Manish Motwani, , Ivana Išgum, Pál Maurovich-Horvat Piotr J. Slomka, and Damini Dey, Artificial Intelligence in Cardiovascular Imaging for Risk Stratification in Coronary Artery Disease Radiol Cardiothorac Imagin2021 Feb 25;3(1):e200512. doi: 10.1148/ryct.2021200512.

Bayoumy K, Gaber M, Elshafeey A, Mhaimeed O, Dineen EH, Marvel FA, et al. Smart wearable devices in cardiovascular care: where we are and how to move forward. Nat Rev Cardiol. (2021)

Calvin H. Yeh, Kerstin Hogg and Jeffrey I. Weitz Arteriosclerosis, Thrombosis, and Vascular Biology Vascular Biology Vol. 35, No. 5

Chun-Li Wang1,2*, Kuo-Chun Hung Recent Advances in Echocardiography Received 1 March 2017; accepted 23 March 2017

Darren Turner, B.A.,1 Angela C. Rieger, M.S., M.D.,1 Wayne Balkan, Ph.D.,1,2 and Joshua M. Hare, M.D.1,2,*Clinical-based Cell Therapies for Heart Disease—Current and Future State Rambam Maimonides Med J. 2020 Apr; 11(2): e0015.

Gremmel T, Yanachkov IB, Yanachkova MI, Wright GE, Wider J, Undyala VV, Michelson AD, Frelinger AL, Przyklenk K. Synergistic inhibition of both P2Y1 and P2Y12 adenosine diphosphate receptors as novel approach to rapidly attenuate platelet-mediated thrombosis.Arterioscler Thromb Vasc Biol. 2016; 36:501–509.

Gremmel T, Michelson AD, Frelinger AL, Bhatt DL. Novel aspects of antiplatelet therapy in cardiovascular disease.Res Pract Thromb Haemost. 2018; 2:439–449.

David Sanders, MD, Leo Ungar, MD, Michael A. Eskander, MD and Arnold H. Seto, MD, MPAAmbulatory ECG monitoring in the age of smartphones Cleveland Clinic Journal of Medicine July 2019, 86 (7) 483-493;

Ethan Grooby, Chiranjibi Sitaula, T'ng Chang Kwok, Don Sharkey, Faezeh Marzbanrad & Atul Malhotra Artificial intelligence-driven wearable technologies for neonatal cardiorespiratory monitoring: Part 1 wearable technology Pediatric Research volume 93, pages413–425 (2023)

Hannah JoyArtificial Intelligence Helps Predict Heart Attack and Stroke The Medindia Medical Review Team on February 14, 2020 at 4:22 PM

Hannah Tredway Nikhil Pasumarti, Matthew A. Crystal Kanwal M. Farooqi 3D printing applications for percutaneous structural interventions in congenital heart disease Department of Pediatrics, New York Presbyterian/Columbia University Irving Medical Center, New York, NY 10032, USA. Division of Pediatric Cardiology, Department of Pediatrics, New York Presbyterian/Columbia University Irving Medical Center, New York, NY 10032, USA.

Jacek Kwiecinski, Evangelos Tzolos, Mohammed N. Meah, Sebastien Cadet, Philip D. Adamson, Kajetan Grodecki, Nikhil V. Joshi, Alastair J. Moss, Michelle C. Williams, Edwin J.R. van Beek, Daniel S. Berman, David E. Newby, Damini Dey, Marc R. Dweck and Piotr J. Slomka Machine Learning with 18F-Sodium Fluoride PET and Quantitative Plaque Analysis on CT Angiography for the Future Risk of Myocardial InfarctionJournal of Nuclear Medicine January 2022, 63 (1) 158-165

James J. Glazier, MD1 and Amir Kaki, MD1-The Impella Device: Historical Background, Clinical Applications and Future DirectionsInt J Angiol. 2019 Jun; 28(2): 118–123

Johannes Bonatti, George Vetrovec, Celia Riga, Oussama Wazni & Petr Stadler;- Robotic technology in cardiovascular medicine Nature Reviews Cardiology volume 11, pages266–275 (2014)

Karim Bayoumy, Mohammed Gaber, Abdallah Elshafeey, Omar Mhaimeed, Elizabeth H. Dineen, Francoise A. Marvel, Seth S. Martin, Evan D. Muse,

Mintu P. Turakhia, Khaldoun G. Tarakji & Mohamed B. ElshazlySmart wearable devices in cardiovascular care: where we are and how to move forward Nature Reviews Cardiology volume 18, pages581–599 (2021)

Malini Madhavan , Siva K Mulpuru , Christopher J McLeod , Yong-Mei Cha , Paul A Friedman Advances and Future Directions in Cardiac Pacemakers J Am Coll Cardiol 2017 Jan 17;69(2):211-235.

Nature Biotechnology First pig-to-human heart. Publisher: Springer NatureFeb 15, 2022

Nitesh Gautam , Prachi Saluja , Abdallah Malkawi Mark G Rabbat , Mouaz H Al-Mallah , Gianluca Pontone , Yiye Zhang ,Benjamin C Lee Subhi J Al'Aref Current and Future Applications of Artificial Intelligence in Coronary Artery Disease.Healthcare (Basel) 2022 Jan 26;10(2):232.

O'Donoghue ML, Bhatt DL, Wiviott SD, Goodman SG, Fitzgerald DJ, Angiolillo DJ, Goto S, Montalescot G, Zeymer U, Aylward PE, Guetta V, Dudek D, Ziecina R, Contant CF, Flather MD; LANCELOT-ACS Investigators. Safety and tolerability of atopaxar in the treatment of patients with acute coronary syndromes: the lessons from antagonizing the cellular effects of Thrombin–Acute Coronary Syndromes Trial.Circulation. 2011; 123:1843–1853.

Peter Manning and Pirooz Eghtesady :- 3D Printing in Complex Congenital Heart Disease: Across a Spectrum of Age, Pathology, and Imaging Techniques .J Am Coll Cardiol Img. 2017 Aug, 10 (8) 953–956

R. C. Joshi, J. S. Khan, V. K. Pathak and M. K. Dutta, "AI-CardioCare: Artificial Intelligence Based Device for Cardiac Health Monitoring," in IEEE Transactions on Human-Machine Systems, vol. 52, no. 6, pp. 1292-1302, Dec. 2022,

ShafkatAnwarGautamK.SinghJacob MillerMonica SharmaPeterManningJosephJ.BilladelloPirooz Eghtesady and Pamela K. Woodard . 3D Printing is a Transformative Technology in Congenital Heart Disease J Am Coll Cardiol Basic Trans Science. 2018 Apr, 3 (2) 294–312

Steven G. Chrysant & George S. Chrysant. New and emerging cardiovascular and antihypertensive drugs https://doi.org/10.1080/14740338.2020.1810232

Ungerer M, Li Z, Baumgartner C, et al. The GPVI – Fc fusion protein revacept reduces thrombus formation and improves vascular dysfunction in atherosclerosis without any impact on bleeding times.PLoS One. 2013; 8:e71193.

Ungerer M, Rosport K, Bültmann A, Piechatzek R, Uhland K, Schlieper P, Gawaz M, Münch G. Novel antiplatelet drug revacept (Dimeric Glycoprotein VI-Fc) specifically and efficiently inhibited collagen-induced platelet aggregation without affecting general hemostasis in humans.Circulation. 2011; 123:1891–1899.

Vardas P, Cowie M, Dagres N, Asvestas D, Tzeis S, Vardas EP, et al. The electrocardiogram endeavour: From the Holter single-lead recordings to multilead wearable devices supported by computational machine learning algorithms. Europace. (2020) 22:19–23.

Vaduganathan M, Bhatt DL. Simultaneous platelet P2Y12 and P2Y1 ADP receptor blockade: are two better than one?Arterioscler Thromb Vasc Biol. 2016; 36:427–428.

Vaduganathan M, Qamar A, Badreldin HA, Faxon DP, Bhatt DL. Cangrelor use in cardiogenic shock.JACC Cardiovasc Interv. 2017; 10:1712–1714. doi: 10.1016/j.jcin.2017.07.009

Venkat D Nagarajan, Su-Lin Lee, Jan-Lukas Robertus, Christoph A Nienaber, Natalia A Trayanova, Sabine Ernst Artificial intelligence in the diagnosis and management of arrhythmias European Heart Journal, Volume 42, Issue 38, 7 October 2021, Pages 3904–3916,

Yanyan Ma, Peng Ding, Lanlan Li, Yang Liu, Ping Jin, Jiayou Tang & Jian Yang Three-dimensional printing for heart diseases: clinical application reviewBio-Design and Manufacturing volume 4, pages 675–687 (2021

Yang W, Wang Y, Lai A, et al. Discovery of 4-aryl-7-hydroxyindoline-based P2Y1 antagonists as novel antiplatelet agents.J Med Chem. 2014; 57:6150–6164. doi: 10.1021/jm5006226CrossrefMedlineGoogle Scholar

Wong PC, Watson C, Crain EJ. The P2Y1 receptor antagonist MRS2500 prevents carotid artery thrombosis in cynomolgus monkeys.J Thromb Thrombolysis. 2016; 41:514–521.

Xu XR, Carrim N, Neves MA, McKeown T, Stratton TW, Coelho RM, Lei X, Chen P, Xu J, Dai X, Li BX, Ni H. Platelets and platelet adhesion molecules: novel mechanisms of thrombosis and anti-thrombotic therapies.Thromb J. 2016; 14(suppl 1):29. doi: 10.1186/s12959-016-0100-6

INDEX

A

B

C

D

E

F

G

H

P

R

S

T

V

W

Recently Published Books By The Author

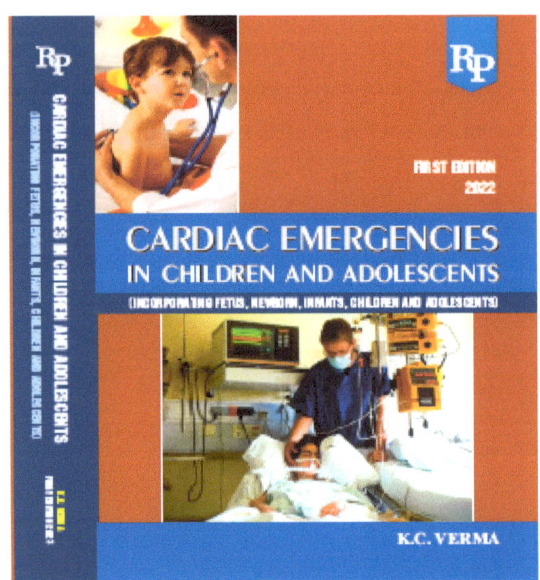

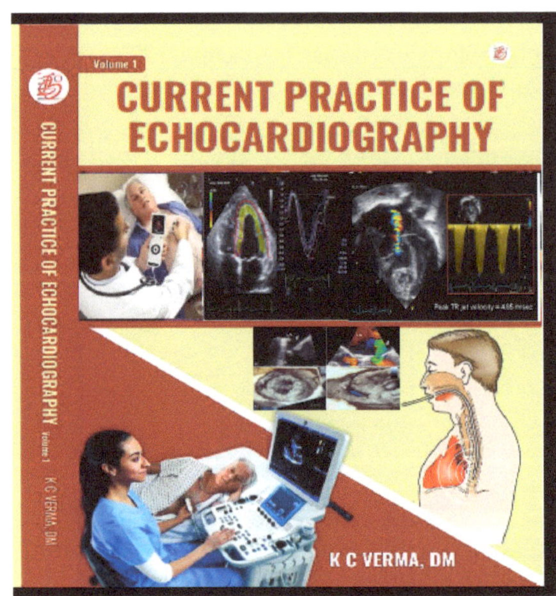

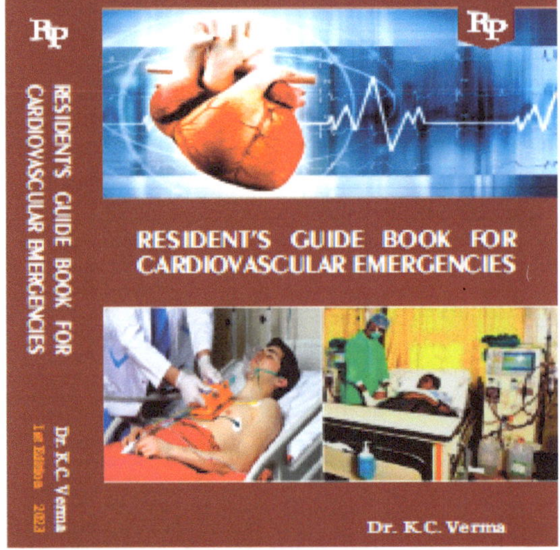

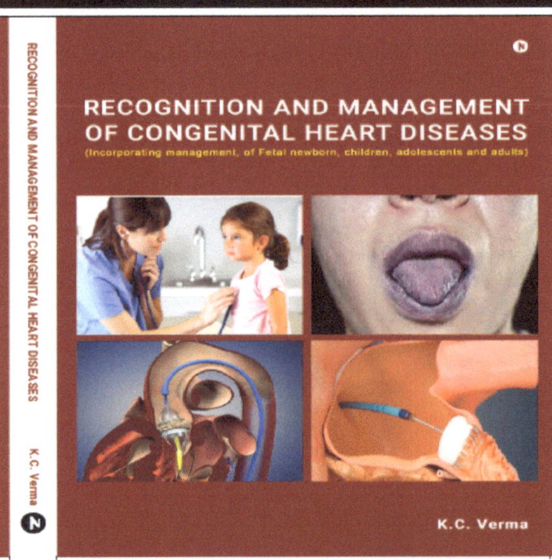

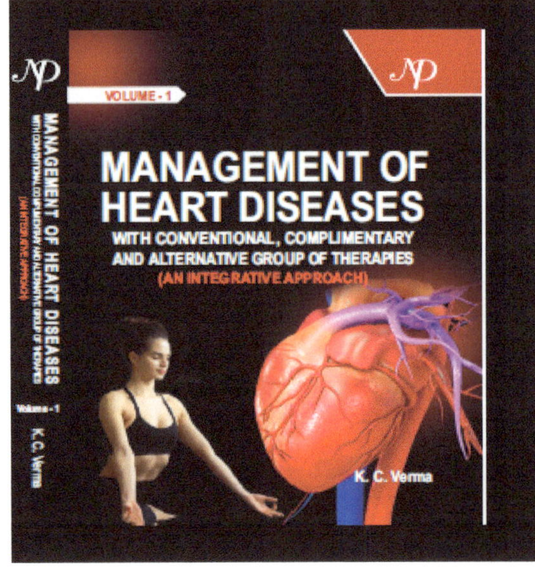

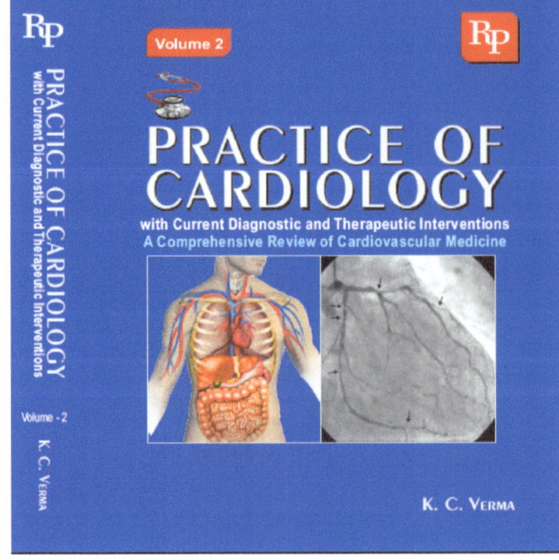

www.ingramcontent.com/pod-product-compliance
Ingram Content Group UK Ltd.
Pitfield, Milton Keynes, MK11 3LW, UK
UKHW060039010826
14090UKWH00041B/251

* 9 7 9 8 8 9 0 6 6 9 8 0 3 *